Student Resources

Online Student Resources are **included** with this textbook.
Visit **http://nursing.pearsonhighered.com** for the following assets and activities:

- Learning Outcomes
- Chapter Review Questions
- Case Studies

- Activities
- Additional content updates
- Weblinks

- Links to additional nursing resources

Additional resources available. For more information and purchasing options visit nursing.pearsonhighered.com

Pearson's Nurse's Drug Guide

- Published annually to be your current, comprehensive, and clinically relevant source for drug information

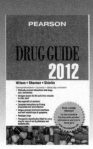

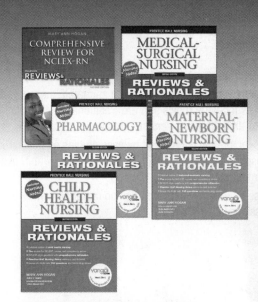

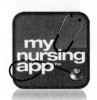

- Your complete mobile solution!

Real Nursing Skills

- Video demonstrations of over 200 clinical nursing skills
- Each skill includes Purpose, Preparation, Procedure, Post-Procedure, Expected and Unexpected Outcomes, Documentation and References and Resources

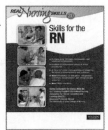

- Concentrated review of core content
- Thousands of practice questions with comprehensive rationales

PEARSON

ALWAYS LEARNING

Instructor Resources—Redefined!

PEARSON NURSING CLASS PREPARATION RESOURCES

New and Unique!

- Use this preparation tool to find animations, videos, images, and other media resources that cross the nursing curriculum! Organized by topic and fully searchable by resource type and key word, this easy-to-use platform allows you to:
  - Search through the media library of assets
  - Upload your own resources
  - Export to PowerPoint or HTML pages

Use this tool to find and review other unique instructor resources:

Pearson Nursing Lecture Series

- Highly visual, fully narrated and animated, these short lectures focus on topics that are traditionally difficult to teach and difficult for students to grasp
- All lectures accompanied by case studies and classroom response questions for greater interactivity within even the largest classroom
- Use as lecture tools, remediation material, homework assignments and more!

MYTEST AND ONLINE TESTING

- Test questions even **more accessible** now with both pencil and paper (MyTest) and online delivery options (Online Testing)
- **NCLEX-style** questions

BOOK-SPECIFIC RESOURCES
Also available to instructors:

- Comprehensive **PowerPoint** lecture note presentation
- **Online course management systems** complete with instructor tools and student activities

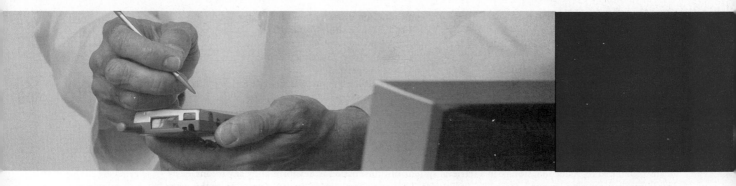

Handbook of Informatics for Nurses & Healthcare Professionals

Fifth Edition

Toni Hebda, RN, MNEd, PhD, MSIS
Professor of Nursing Programs
Chatham University, Pittsburgh, PA

Patricia Czar, RN
Information Systems Consultant
Pittsburgh, PA

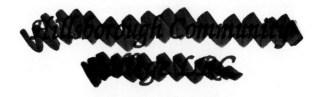

PEARSON

Boston   Columbus   Indianapolis   New York   San Francisco   Upper Saddle River
Amsterdam   Cape Town   Dubai   London   Madrid   Milan   Munich   Paris   Montréal   Toronto
Delhi   Mexico City   São Paulo   Sydney   Hong Kong   Seoul   Singapore   Taipei   Tokyo

Publisher: Julie Levin Alexander
Publisher's Assistant: Regina Bruno
Senior Acquisitions Editor: Kelly Trakalo
Assistant Editor: Lauren Sweeney
Director of Marketing: David Gesell
Marketing Manager: Phoenix Harvey
Marketing Specialist: Michael Sirinides
Marketing Assistant: Crystal Gonzalez

Production Project Manager: Debbie Ryan
Production Editor: Yagnesh Yani
Art Director: Jayne Conte
Cover Desinger: Suzanne Behnke
Cover Image: Fotolia
Composition: PreMediaGlobal
Printer/Binder: Edwards Brothers Malloy
Cover Printer: Lehigh-Phoenix Color/Hagerstown

Many of the designations by manufacturers and seller to distinguish their products are claimed as trademarks. Where those designations appear in this book, and the publisher was aware of a trademark claim, the designations have been printed in initial caps or all caps.

Library of Congress Cataloging-in Publication Data

Hebda, Toni.
 Handbook of informatics for nurses & healthcare professionals / Toni Hebda, Patricia Czar.—5th ed.
  p. ; cm.
 Handbook of informatics for nurses & healthcare professionals
 Includes bibliographical references and index.
 ISBN-13: 978-0-13-257495-2 (alk. paper)
 ISBN-10: 0-13-257495-0 (alk. paper)
 I. Czar, Patricia.   II. Title.   III. Title: Handbook of informatics for nurses & healthcare professionals.
[DNLM: 1. Nursing Informatics.   2. Allied Health Personnel.   WY 26.5]
 LC Classification not assigned
 610.730285—dc23

                                                              2011045850

10 9 8 7

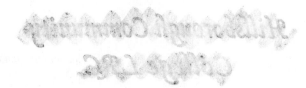

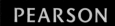

ISBN 10: 0-13-257495-0
ISBN 13: 978-0-13-257495-2

Contents

Preface

The idea for this book first came from the realization that there were few comprehensive sources available that provided practical information about computer applications and information systems in healthcare. From its inception, this book was seen as a guide for nurses and other healthcare professionals who needed to learn how to adapt and use computer applications in the workplace. Over time, it has also come to serve as a text for students in the healthcare professions who need to develop informatics competencies, whether that might be at a basic or more advanced level such as that required of informatics nurse specialists, clinical nurse leaders, or doctoral students, or healthcare professionals.

The fifth edition contains updates and revisions to reflect rapid changes in healthcare information technology. Some chapters have been reorganized, and eight new chapters have been added. The authors endeavor to provide an understanding of the concepts, skills, and tasks that are needed for healthcare professionals today and to achieve the national information technology goals set forth first by President Bush in 2004 and later by President Obama as a means to help transform the healthcare delivery system. This edition brings in the expertise of several contributors. Both the primary authors and the contributors share an avid interest and involvement in HIT and informatics, as well as experience in the field, involvement in informatics groups, and a history of presenting at both national and international levels.

NEW TO THIS EDITION

- Eight new chapters!

   Chapter 5: Professional Use of Electronic Resources
   Chapter 9: Improving the Usability of Health Informatics Applications
   Chapter 15: The Role of Standardized Terminology and Language in informatics
   Chapter 16: Personal Health Records
   Chapter 17: Health Information Exchanges
   Chapter 18: Health Policy and Health Information Technology
   Chapter 24: Consumer Education and Informatics
   Chapter 26: Public Health Informatics

- Extensive HIPAA and legislative updates.
- **New information** on the integrated use of smart technology in Chapter 6
- **Updated information** on the relationship between HIT and reform initiatives, support for the Magnet Hospital journey, patient-centered medical homes, and accountable care organizations (Chapter 1)
- **New information** on the American Recovery and Reinvestment Act of 2009 and Meaningful Use
- **New information** on Web 2.0 technologies
- **New content** on virtual training (Chapter 11)
- **New appendix** on robotic applications

ORGANIZATION

The book is divided into three sections: General Computer Information, Healthcare Information Systems, and Specialty Applications. The major themes of privacy, confidentiality, and information security are woven throughout the book. Likewise, project management is a concept introduced in the strategic planning chapter and carried through other chapters.

Section I: General Computer Information

This introductory section reviews information common to all information systems. It assumes no prior knowledge or experience with computers.

- **Chapter 1:** Introduces informatics as an area of specialty, addresses major issues in healthcare that are driving the adoption of information technology, and talks about nurses as knowledge workers and the TIGER initiative as a means to transform the profession by establishing informatics competencies for all nurses and by promoting active involvement in the advancement of information technology.
- **Chapter 2:** Reviews basic information and terminology related to computer hardware and software. It is geared toward persons with a limited knowledge in this area.
- **Chapter 3:** Emphasizes the significance of good data integrity and management. It also addresses the burgeoning area of data mining, its applications within the healthcare delivery system, and the role of the nurse with knowledge discovery in databases.
- **Chapter 4:** Addresses basic concepts and applications of the Internet and World Wide Web inclusive of basic search strategies and criteria for evaluating the quality of online information.
- **Chapter 5:** Discusses professional use of electronic resources.

Section II: Healthcare Information Systems

This section covers information and issues related to computers and information systems in healthcare. It bridges the gap between the theory and practice of nursing informatics. Chapters 7 through 22 discuss all aspects of selecting, implementing, and operating information systems. Chapters 7 through 10 discuss the processes of overall and system strategic planning, system selection, improving the usability of health informatics applications, and implementation.

- **Chapter 6:** Covers basic information on healthcare information systems, including computerized provider order enter (sometimes referred to as computerized physician or provider order entry), decision support and expert systems, and pharmacy systems. Smart technology, as well as physician practice management systems, long-term and homecare systems are included.
- **Chapter 7:** Discusses the need to integrate information technology into the strategic plan of the organization and introduces project management, which appears as a thread in subsequent chapters.
- **Chapter 8:** Provides practical advice on the selection of an information system.
- **Chapter 9:** Addresses the concepts of human factors, ergonomics, human–computer interaction, and usability, all of which play a vital role in the adoption and use of technology.
- **Chapter 10:** Covers information system implementation and routine maintenance.
- **Chapter 11:** Explores information systems training from plans to evaluation of acquired competencies and matters in between.
- **Chapter 12:** Discusses information security and confidentiality; it includes practical information on ways to protect information housed in information systems and on mobile devices.
- **Chapter 13:** Addresses issues that impact the exchange of data from one information system to another as well as its significance for healthcare professionals.
- **Chapter 14:** Discusses the development of the electronic record, Meaningful Use incentives to encourage adoption of technology, and benefits associated with the EHR and Meaningful Use.
- **Chapter 15:** New chapter devoted to the role of standardized terminology and language in informatics.
- **Chapter 16:** Content on the personal health record that was previously incorporated into the EHR chapter now has its own chapter, so that examples, issues, and developments in this area can be addressed more fully.

- **Chapter 17:** This chapter identifies exchange health information as a key step in the process of developing a birth-to-death electronic record for every individual. Exchange models, obstacles, and the current status of HIE are included in the discussion.
- **Chapter 18:** New chapter on health policy and HIT in recognition of the fact that this important area received scant attention in prior editions.
- **Chapter 19:** Addresses the following legislation in terms of its impact on healthcare and nursing informatics: Electronic Signatures in Global and National Commerce Act (ESIGN) of 2000, Health Insurance Portability and Accountability Act (HIPAA) of 1996, Medicare Improvements for Patients and Providers Act of 2008, and the American Recovery and Reinvestment Act of 2009 (ARRA).
- **Chapter 20:** Provides insight into the complexity of regulatory and reimbursement issues.
- **Chapter 21:** Covers accreditation issues for information system design and use.
- **Chapter 22:** Discusses the relationship between strategic planning for the organization and the significance of maintaining uninterrupted operations for patient care as well as legal requirements to maintain and restore information. Much of this chapter is geared for the professional working in information services or preparing to work in this area.

Section III: Specialty Applications

This section covers specialty applications of computers and informatics.

- **Chapter 23:** Details ways that computers can support education of healthcare professionals. It includes a section on the use of mobile devices.
- **Chapter 24:** A new chapter devoted to consumer education and informatics.
- **Chapter 25:** Discusses the applications and issues associated with telehealth with a special section on telenursing.
- **Chapter 26:** A new chapter on public health informatics.
- **Chapter 27:** Looks at ways that informatics supports evidence-based practice, translational research, and comparative effectiveness research and application to practice.

Five appendices are included on the Online Student Resources at http://nursing.pearson highered.com. Appendices A and B provide detailed information on getting up and running on the Internet and using the Internet for career purposes. Appendix C is on robotic applications. Appendix D provides suggested responses to end-of-chapter case studies. The fifth and final appendix provides a guide to Web 2.0 applications.

HOW TO USE THIS BOOK

This book may be used in the following different ways:

- It may be read from cover to cover for a comprehensive view of nursing informatics.
- Specific chapters may be read according to reader interest or need.
- It may serve as a reference for nurses and other clinicians involved in system design, selection and implementation, and ongoing maintenance.
- It may be useful for the educator or researcher who wants to make better use of information technology.
- It can serve as a review for the American Nurses Association's Informatics Credentialing examination.

Each chapter contains pedagogical aids that help the readers learn and apply the information discussed.

Learning Objectives—Learning Objectives are listed at the beginning of each chapter to let the readers know what they can expect to learn from their study of it.

Future Directions—As the last section in each chapter, Future Directions forecasts how the topic covered in the chapter might evolve in the upcoming years.

Case Study Exercises—Case studies at the end of each chapter discuss common, real-life applications, which review and reinforce the concepts presented in the chapter.

Summary—To assist in the review of the chapter, the Summary at the end of each chapter highlights the key concepts and information from the chapter.

References—Resources used in the chapter are listed at the end.

Online Student Resources—At the end of each chapter, you are encouraged to access the online student resources at http://nursing.pearsonhighered.com for application exercises that enhance the learning experience, build on knowledge gained from the textbook, and foster critical thinking.

Glossary—The glossary at the end of the book serves to familiarize readers with the vocabulary used in this book and in healthcare informatics. We recognize that healthcare professionals have varying degrees of computer and informatics knowledge. This book does not assume that the reader has prior knowledge of computers. All computer terms are defined in the chapter, in the glossary at the end of the book, and on the Online Student Resources Web site.

About the Authors

Toni Hebda, RN, MNEd, PhD, MSIS, is a professor with the Chamberlain College of Nursing. MSN Online Program. She has held several academic and clinical positions over the years and worked as a system analyst. Her interest in informatics provided a focus for her dissertation and subsequently led her to help establish a regional nursing informatics support group and obtain a graduate degree in information science. She is a reviewer for the *Online Journal of Nursing Informatics.* She is a member of informatics groups and has presented in the field.

    Patricia Czar, RN, is an information systems consultant. She has been active in informatics for more than 25 years, serving as manager of clinical systems at a major medical center where she was responsible for planning, design, implementation, and ongoing support for all of the clinical information systems. Patricia has been an active member of several informatics groups and has presented nationally and internationally. She has also served as a mentor for many nursing and health informatics students.

Acknowledgments

We acknowledge our gratitude first and foremost to our families for their support as we wrote and revised this book. We are grateful and excited to have work from our contributors in this edition. We are grateful to our coworkers and professional colleagues who provided encouragement and support throughout the process of conceiving and writing this book. We appreciate the many helpful comments offered by our reviewers. Finally, we thank Kelly Trakalo, Senior Acquisitions Editor, and Lauren Sweeney Moraes, Assistant Editor, the staff at Pearson Health Science, and all of the persons who worked on the production of this edition for their encouragement, suggestions, and support.

When we first started to write together, we knew each other only on a professional basis. As we worked on this book, we found that our different professional backgrounds, experiences, and personalities complemented each other well and added to the quality of the final product. The best part of this project, however, has been the friendship that we have developed as we worked together and the new acquaintances that we have made as we worked with our contributors.

Thank You

This edition brings in work from additional contributors for a robust coverage of topics throughout the book. We thank them for their time and expertise. We would also like to thank all of the reviewers who carefully looked at the entire manuscript. You have helped shaped this book to become a more useful text for everyone.

Contributors

Jane Brokel, PhD, RN
Chapter 17: Health Information Exchanges
Assistant Professor, College of Nursing University of Iowa, Iowa City, IA

Terri L. Calderone, EdD, RN
Chapter 11: Information Systems Training
Chapter 25: Telehealth
Assistant Professor, Department of Nursing and Allied Health Professions, Indiana University of Pennsylvania, Indiana, PA

Pam Charney, PhD, RD
Chapter 24: Consumer Education and Informatics
Affiliate Associate Professor Pharmacy, University of Washington, Seattle, WA

Vicky Elfrink Cordi, PhD, RN-BC
Chapter 24: Consumer Education and Informatics
Clinical Associate Professor, Emeritus College of Nursing, The Ohio State University Columbus, Ohio and Senior Associate, iTeleHealth, Inc., Cocoa Beach, FL

Patricia Czar, RN
Chapter 1: Informatics in Healthcare Professions
Chapter 6: Healthcare Information Systems
Chapter 13: System Integration and Interoperability
Chapter 14: The Electronic Health Record
Chapter 21: Accreditation Issues for Information System Design and Use
Appendix B: Career Resources on the Internet
Appendix C: Robotic Applications in Healthcare
Appendix D: Case Study Exercises—Suggested Responses
Information systems consultant, Pittsburgh PA

Janice Unruh Davidson, PhD, RN-BC, FNP-BC, NEA-BC, CNE, FAANP
Chapter 3: Ensuring Quality of Information
DNP Program Professor, Chamberlain College of Nursing, Downing Grove, IL

Sue Evans, RN, MSN, CMSRN
Chapter 10: System Implementation and Maintenance
Clinician–Medical Unit/Admission Team, University of Pittsburgh Medical Center, Pittsburgh, PA

John Gosney, MA
Mobile Technology in Chapter 23: Mobile Applications for Healthcare Education
Faculty Liaison, Learning Technologies Lecturer in American Studies Indiana University-Purdue University, Indianapolis, IN

Wanda Govan-Jenkins, MS, MBA, DNP, RN
Chapter 20: Regulatory and Reimbursement Issues
Program Coordinator for EHR Implementation, Office of the National Coordinator for Health Information Technology, Washington, D.C.

Toni Hebda, RN, MNEd, PhD, MSIS
Chapter 1: Informatics in Healthcare Professions
Chapter 6: Healthcare Information Systems
Chapter 13: System Integration and Interoperability

Chapter 14: The Electronic Health Record
Chapter 18: Health Policy and Health Information Technology
Chapter 21: Accreditation Issues for Information System Design and Use
Chapter 26: Public Health Informatics
Appendix B: Career Resources on the Internet
Appendix C: Robotic Applications in Healthcare
Appendix D: Case Study Exercises—Suggested Responses
Professor, Chamberlain College of Nursing Online MSN Program

Katherine Holzmacher, MS, RN-BC, NP, CPHIT, CPEHR
Chapter 8: Selecting a Healthcare Information System
Director of Clinical/Nursing Informatics, Stony Brook University Medical Center, Stony Brook, NY

Kathleen Hunter, PhD, RN-BC
Chapter 5: Professional Use of Electronic Resources
Chapter 19: Legislation
Associate Professor, Chamberlain College of Nursing Online MSN Program

Karen Koziol, RNC, MS
Chapter 23: Integrating Technology, Informatics, and the Internet Into Nursing Education
Information Coordinator Mercy College—Dobbs Ferry Campus Dobbs Ferry, NY
Clinical Coordinator Dominican College Orangeburg, NY

Darlene Lovasik, RN
Smart Technology in Chapter 6: Smart Technology
University of Pittsburgh Medical Center, Pittsburgh, PA

Cynthia Lundberg, RN, BSN
Chapter 15: The Role of Standardized Terminology and Language in Informatics
Clinical Informatics Educator, SNOMED Terminology Solutions, A Division of the College of American Pathologists Lake Cook Road, Deerfield, IL

Christine Malmgreen, RN-BC MA, MS
Chapter 23: Integrating Technology, Informatics, and the Internet Into Nursing Education
Adjunct Professor, Mercy College—Dobbs Ferry Campus Dobbs Ferry, NY

Susan Matney, MSN, RN-C, FAAN
Chapter 15: The Role of Standardized Terminology and Language in Informatics
Medical Informaticist HDD Team 3M Health Information Systems Adjunct Faculty, College of Nursing at University of Utah, Salt Lake City, UT

Marcia McCaw, RN, BSN
Smart Technology in Chapter 6 Healthcare Information Systems
University of Pittsburgh Medical Center, Pittsburgh, PA.

Keith McInnes, ScD, MSc
Chapter 16: Personal Health Records
Center for Health Quality Outcomes and Economic Research, Bedford VA Medical Center, Department of Health Policy and Management, Boston University School of Public Health

Nicholas Molley, MBA, MIDS
Chapter 2: Hardware, Software, and the Roles of Support Personnel
Ursuline College Pepper Pike OH; Senior Consultant, IBM Corporation

Toni Morrison, RN
Smart Technology in Chapter 6 Healthcare Information Systems
Intermediate Product Manager, SmartRoom LLC/UPMC International & Commercial Services, Pittsburgh, PA

Lauren Panton, MA
Chapter 4: The Internet and the World Wide Web: An Overview
Appendix E: Guide to Web 2.0 Applications
Manager, Instructional Technology and Media, Chatham University, Pittsburgh, PA

Dr. Carol Patton, Dr. PH, FNP-BC, RN, CRNP, CNE
Chapter 26: Public Health Informatics
Chapter 27: Evidence-Based Practice and Research
Associate Clinical Professor, Drexel University School of Nursing Philadelphia, PA

Dr. Wichian Premchaiswadi, BEng, MSC, MEng, DEng
Chapter 12: Information Security and Confidentiality
Associate Professor, Dean, Graduate School of Information Technology and Assistant President, Siam University, Bangkok, Thailand

Carol Curio Scholle, RN, MSN
Smart Technology in Chapter 6 Healthcare Information Systems
Clinical Director, Transplant, Dialysis and Inpatient Surgical Services, University of Pittsburgh Medical Center, Pittsburgh, PA

Nancy Staggers, PhD, RN, FAAN
Chapter 9: Improving the Usability of Health Informatics Applications
Professor, Informatics School of Nursing University of Maryland Baltimore, MD

Barbara Treusch, RN, BSN, MS, MBA
Chapter 11: Information Systems Training
System Analyst, eRecord IView Team, University of Pittsburgh Medical Center, Pittsburgh PA

William G. Weppner, MD, MPH
Chapter 16: Personal Health Records
Department of Medicine, University of Washington Seattle, WA and Boise Veterans Administration Medical Center Boise, ID

Dr. James G. Williams, BS, MS, PhD
Chapter 12: Information Security and Confidentiality
Chapter 22: Continuity Planning and Management (Disaster Recovery)
Professor Emeritus and Past Chair of the Department of Information Science and Telecommunications, University of Pittsburgh, Pittsburgh, PA

Marisa Wilson, DNSc., MHSc., RN-BC
Chapter 7: Strategic Planning for Information Technology Projects
Assistant Professor, University of Maryland School of Nursing, Baltimore, MD

Susan S. Woods, MD, MPH
Chapter 16: Personal Health Records
Department of Medical Informatics and Clinical Epidemiology, Oregon Health and Science University; Portland VA Medical Center

Cynthia K. Zidek, PhD, RN
Chapter 25: Telehealth
Assistant Professor, Department of Nursing and Allied Health Professions, Indiana University of Pennsylvania, Indiana, PA

Reviewers

Carol Kilmon, PhD, RN
The University of Texas, Tyler, TX

Charlotte Seckman, PhD, RN-BC
University of Maryland, Baltimore, MD

Cynthia W. Kelly, PhD, RN
Xavier University, Cincinnati, OH

Dawn Zwick, RN, MSN, APRN-BC
Kent State University, North Canton, OH

Eli Collins-Brown, EdD
Methodist College of Nursing, Peoria, IL

Elizabeth Wright, MSN, RN
Indiana Wesleyan University, Marion, IN

John E. Jemison, MS
Southwestern AG University, Waxahachie, TX

Leanne M. Waterman, MS, RN, CNS, FNP
Onondaga Community College, Syracuse, NY

Marisa L. Wilson, DNSc, MHSc, RN-BC
University of Maryland, Baltimore, MD

Mary K. Pabst, PhD, RN
Elmhurst College, Elmhurst, IL

Mary T. Boylston, RN, MSN, EdD
Eastern University, St. Davids, PA

Rhonda Reed, MSN, RN, CRRN
Indiana State University, Terre Haute, IN

Richard Jeffery Lyons, RN, BSN, MS
University of Indianapolis, Indianapolis, IN

Rosie Williams, RN, MSN
Alcorn State University, Natchez, MS

Susan H. Lynch, MSN, RN, CNE
University of North Carolina, Charlotte, NC

Tresa Kaur Dusaj, PhD(c), RN-BC
Monmouth University, West Long Branch, NJ

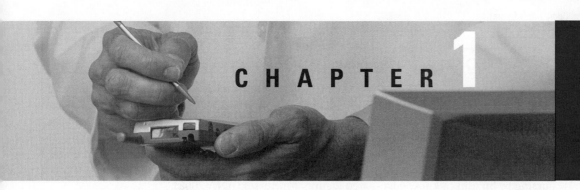

CHAPTER 1

Informatics in the Healthcare Professions

After completing this chapter, you should be able to:

1. Define the terms *data, information, knowledge,* and *wisdom.*

2. Describe the role of the nurse as knowledge worker.

3. Discuss the significance of good information and knowledge management for healthcare delivery, healthcare disciplines, and healthcare consumers.

4. Distinguish between *medical informatics, nursing informatics,* and *consumer informatics.*

5. Differentiate between *computer* and *information literacy.*

6. Discuss the Technology Informatics Guiding Education Reform Initiative and contrast the different informatics competencies needed for nurses entering into practice, experienced nurses, and informatics nurses and nurse specialists.

7. Discuss the relationship between major issues in healthcare and the deployment of information technology.

8. Identify characteristics that define nursing informatics as a specialty area of practice.

9. Provide specific examples of how nursing informatics impacts the healthcare consumer as well as professional practice, administration, education, and research.

10. Forecast the roles that nursing informatics and health information technology will play in the healthcare delivery system 5 years from now.

11. Compare the types of educational opportunities available in nursing informatics.

DATA, INFORMATION, KNOWLEDGE, AND WISDOM

During the course of any day, nurses handle large amounts of data and information and apply knowledge. This is true for all nurses, whether they provide direct care or serve as administrators, educators, or researchers or in some other capacity. Informatics provides tools to help process, manage, and analyze data and information collected for the purposes of documenting and improving patient care, as well as to support knowledge that adds to the scientific foundation for nursing; provides value to nursing knowledge and work; and improves the public image for nursing by building a knowledge-based identity for nurses (ANA 2008).

Data are a collection of numbers, characters, or facts that are gathered according to some perceived need for analysis and possibly action at a later point in time (Anderson 1992). Examples of data include a client's vital signs. Other examples of data are the length of hospital stay for each client; the client's race, marital status, or employment status; and next of kin. Sometimes these types of data may be given a numeric or alphabetic code, as shown in Table 1–1.

A single piece of datum has little meaning. However, a collection of data can be examined for patterns and structure that can be interpreted (Saba & McCormick 1996; Warman 1993). **Information** is data that have been interpreted. For example, individual temperature readings are data. When they are plotted onto a graph, changes in the client's temperature over time and comparison with normal values become evident, thus turning into information. Table 1–2 provides examples of data and information. Although it is possible to determine whether individual values (data) fall within the normal range, the collection of several values over time creates a pattern, which in this case demonstrates the presence of a low-grade fever (information).

Data and information are collected when nurses record the following activities:

- Initial client history and allergies
- Initial and ongoing physical assessment
- Vital signs such as blood pressure and temperature
- Response to treatment
- Client response and comprehension of educational activities

Knowledge is a more complex concept. **Knowledge** is the synthesis of information derived from several sources to produce a single concept or idea. It is based on a logical process of analysis and provides order to thoughts and ideas and decreases uncertainty (Ayer 1966; Engelhardt 1980). It is dynamic and derives meaning from its context (Steyn 2004). Validation of information provides knowledge that can be used again. Historically, nursing has acquired knowledge through tradition, authority, borrowed theory, trial and error, personal experience, role modeling, reasoning, and research. Current demands for safer, cost-effective, quality care require evidence of the best practices supported by research. Computers and information technology (IT)

TABLE 1–1	Example of Coded Data: Employment Status Codes	
Code	**Status**	**Explanation**
1	Employed full time	Individual states that he or she is employed full time
2	Employed part time	Individual states that he or she is employed part time
3	Not employed	Individual states that he or she is not employed full time or part time
4	Self-employed	Self-explanatory
5	Retired	Self-explanatory
6	On active military duty	Self-explanatory
7	Unknown	Individual's employment status is unknown

TABLE 1–2	Examples of Data and Information		
Time	Temperature (°C)	Pulse	Respirations
7 AM	37.8	88	24
12 noon	38.9	96	24
4 PM	38	84	22
8 PM	37.2	83	20

The values in this table represent data: a client's vital signs over the course of a day. Each individual value is limited in meaning. The pattern of the values represents information, which is more useful to healthcare.

provide tools that aid data collection and the analysis associated with research to support the overall work of nurses. **Information technology** is a general term used to refer to the management and processing of information with the assistance of computers.

An example of knowledge can be seen in the determination of the most effective nursing interventions for the prevention of skin breakdown. If a research study produces data related to the prevention of skin breakdown achieved through specific interventions, these data can be collected and analyzed. The trends or patterns depicted by the data provide information regarding which treatment is more effective than others in preventing skin breakdown. The validation of this information through repeated studies provides knowledge that nurses can use to prevent skin breakdown in their clients.

Wisdom occurs when knowledge is used appropriately to manage and solve problems (Ackoff 1989; ANA 2008). It results from understanding and requires human effort. The trip from data to wisdom is neither automatic nor smooth (Murray 2000). Wisdom comes from cumulative experiences, as the result of learning skills and ways of thinking that can be viewed as predecessors to wisdom, and via the creation of conditions that help participants to use their accumulated knowledge effectively (Gluck & Baltes 2006). It represents the human part of the equation in the move along the continuum from data to information to knowledge to wisdom.

Large-scale use of data, information, and knowledge requires that they be accessible. Traditionally, client data and information have been handwritten in an unstructured format on paper and placed in multiple versions of the patient record at hospitals, clinics, physician offices, and long-term and home health agencies. This process makes the location, abstraction, and comparison of information slow and difficult, limiting the creation of knowledge. Increasing demands for improvements in healthcare delivery call for the use of IT as a means to automate and share information for quality measurement and improvement, research, and education. Technology exists to move from paper-based to computer-based records. It is essential that nurses collaborate with technical personnel to plan what information to include, the source of the information, and how it will be used. Nurses must be active participants in the design of automated documentation to ensure that information is recorded appropriately and in a format that can be accessed and useful to all healthcare providers. Nurses also have a responsibility to safeguard the security and privacy of client information via education, policy, and technical means.

Harsanyi, Lehmkuhl, Hott, Myers, and McGeehan (1994) argued that understanding current and evolving technology for the management and processing of nursing information helps the nursing profession assume a leadership position in health reform. That argument remains true now. If nurses understand the power of informatics, they can play an active role in evaluating and improving the quality of care, cost containment, and other consumer benefits. For example, nurses who are able to understand and use an information system (IS) that analyzes trends in client outcomes and cost can initiate appropriate changes in care. Nurses empowered by IT may also design computer applications that enhance client education, such as individualized discharge instructions, medication instructions and information, and information about diagnostic procedures. In these and other ways, nurses can integrate IT into nursing practice and administration as a means to manage client care, document observations, and monitor client outcomes for ongoing improvement of quality.

Nurses also handle information in the roles of educator and researcher. For example, educators must track information about students' classroom and clinical performance. Computers facilitate this process and allow educators to compare individuals with group norms. Nursing education must also prepare students to handle data. This is accomplished in several steps: teaching basic computer and information literacy, using nursing information systems, realizing the significance of automated data collection for quality assurance purposes, and recognizing the benefits of using computers to manage clinical data for research.

Researchers use computers to expedite the collection and analysis of data. One possible project, for example, uses data obtained from nursing documentation systems to study the relationship between frequent turning and positioning and the client's skin integrity. Nursing information systems are rich in data to support this type of research, and the growing prevalence of information systems increases research opportunities. As a result, nurses can expand the scientific base of their profession.

THE NURSE AS KNOWLEDGE WORKER

Healthcare professionals need to know more today to perform their daily jobs than at any previous point in history. Healthcare delivery systems are knowledge-intensive settings with nurses as the largest group of knowledge workers within those systems. Advancements in knowledge, skills, interventions, and drugs are growing at an exponential rate. This makes it impossible for any one individual to keep up with all the knowledge needed to practice nursing or any of the other healthcare disciplines without making use of available resources and continuing education. Unfortunately there is a failure on the part of the present healthcare delivery system to consistently translate new knowledge into practice and apply new technologies safely, appropriately, and expediently (IOM 2007). Several years typically elapse before new knowledge and advancements make it into the clinical setting. At the same time, the acuity level of clients continues to rise, changing the actual work that healthcare workers do and how they do it. One constant in this scenario is the ongoing need for knowledge and evidence. IT can bridge the gap as healthcare delivery continues its evolution from a task-based to a knowledge-based industry. Nurses need to be adept at using patient-centered IT tools to access information to expand their knowledge in a just-in-time, evidence-based fashion. There must be a shift from critical thinking to critical synthesis. In short, nurses must optimize their value as intellectual capital (Haase-Herrick & Herrin 2007; Simpson 2007). Work must also be done to develop workload measurements for knowledge workers. Pesut (2006) noted that a change has occurred in the nursing process and how nurses represent clinical thinking. The development of standardized nursing languages, electronic record systems, and sophisticated analyses all serve to facilitate this transformation to knowledge work.

The nurse assumes several roles during the course of client care (Snyder-Halpern, Corcoran-Perry, & Narayan 2001). Each role requires a different level of decision making and a different type of decision support. These roles include:

- *Data gatherer.* In this role the nurse collects clinical data such as vital signs.
- *Information user.* The nurse interprets and structures clinical data, such as a client's report of experienced pain, into information that can then be used to aid clinical decision making and patient monitoring over time. Quality assurance and infection control activities exemplify other ways in which nurses use information to detect patterns.
- *Knowledge user.* This role is seen when individual patient data are compared with existing nursing knowledge.

- *Knowledge builder.* Nurses display this role when they aggregate clinical data and show patterns across patients that serve to create new knowledge or can be interpreted within the context of existing nursing knowledge.

IT can support the nurse in each of these roles. Computerized assessment and documentation forms facilitate data collection by including prompts to help nurses to remember questions that they should ask and facts that they should record. These same tools strengthen the quality of clinical databases. The data gatherer role is also facilitated when input from monitoring devices is fed directly into clinical documentation systems. The information user role is supported when computer capability quickly discerns patterns that help translate data into information. This saves time and labor for the nurse and provides useful information in a timely fashion. Applications to support the knowledge user in clinical settings at the point of care are becoming more prevalent. These might include clinical practice guidelines, expert systems to support decision making, or research that supports evidence-based care and/or online drug databases. Although clinical information systems have the capability to aggregate data, this capability is not available at the bedside in all facilities. Knowledge builders examine aggregate data for relationships among variables and interventions. According to Davenport, Thomas, and Cantrell (2002), managers of knowledge workers have the responsibility to optimize the work process through improvements in the design of the workplace as well as the application of technology. The unfortunate reality is that resource allocation for health information technology (HIT) has lagged behind other industries, and the current healthcare environment has yet to fully realize its potential. IT can streamline paperwork, transform data into information and knowledge, and eliminate redundancy. A common factor found in a recent survey of the 100 top U.S. hospitals was the use of technology, EHRs, and health information exchange (Thomson Reuters 2011a, 2011b).

As healthcare delivery systems continue to evolve, additional changes in the ways that nurses and other healthcare professionals work are expected. The next expected metamorphosis is from knowledge worker to self-directed innovator. The innovator uses a holistic view, works across settings, and is enabled by access to information. This information is derived from multiple sources and formats but ideally may be accessed from a single platform (Hulford, Gough, & Krieger 2007).

THE SIGNIFICANCE OF GOOD INFORMATION AND KNOWLEDGE MANAGEMENT

Good information management ensures access to the right information at the right time to the people who need it. Vast amounts of information are produced daily. This information may or may not be readily available when it is needed. Its volume exceeds the processing capacity of any single human being. Part of good information management ensures that care providers have the resources that they need to provide safe, efficient, quality care. Some examples of these resources include clinical guidelines, standards of practice, policy and procedure manuals, research findings, drug databases, and information on community resources. IT can help to ensure access to the most recent versions of these types of resources via tools such as intranets, electronic communities, or blogs (Watson 2007). This solution eliminates the uncertainties of whether reference books are available in all clinical areas of any given facility and whether all areas have the most recent version. Good information management also eliminates redundant data collection. Redundant data collection wastes time and irritates clients (HIMSS 2002).

Although the terms *information management* and *knowledge management* are sometimes used interchangeably, **knowledge management** refers to the creation of systems that enable organizations to tap into the knowledge, experiences, and creativity of their staff to improve their performance (Davidson & Voss 2002). It is a structured process for the generation, storage, distribution, and application of both tacit knowledge (personal experience) and explicit knowledge (evidence) in organizations (Sandars & Heller 2006).

THE DEFINITION AND EVOLUTION OF INFORMATICS

Informatics is the science and art of turning data into information. The term can be traced to a Russian document published in 1968 (Bemmel & Musen 1997). It is an adaptation of the French term *informatique,* which refers to "the computer milieu" (Saba 2001). Broadly, informatics has been defined as "the study of the application of computer and statistical techniques to the management of information" (Academic Medical Publishing & CancerWEB 1997). The term has been applied to various disciplines. **Medical informatics** refers to the application of informatics to all of the healthcare disciplines as well as to the practice of medicine. Some sources distinguish medical informatics from health informatics in the following manner. Medical informatics focuses primarily upon information technologies that involve patient care and medical decision making while health informatics refers to the use of educational technology for healthcare clients or the general public. Informatics has subsequently emerged as an area of specialization within the various healthcare disciplines and is one of the fastest growing career fields in healthcare. Overlap occurs among medical, dental, and nursing informatics primarily in the areas of information retrieval, ethics, patient care, decision support, human-computer interactions, information systems, imaging, computer security, and computerized health records (Guenther & Caruth 2006). Table 1–3 displays some informatics terms and definitions; many are similar, but not all can be used interchangeably.

    Nursing informatics may be broadly defined as the use of information and computer technology to support all aspects of nursing practice, including direct delivery of care, administration, education, and research. The definition of nursing informatics is evolving as advances occur in nursing practice and technology; there have been many different definitions throughout the years as the discipline has evolved. According to the American Nurses Association (ANA) (2001) and Staggers and Thompson (2002), these may be broken down into the following categories: (1) definitions with an IT focus, (2) conceptually oriented definitions, and (3) definitions that focus on roles. Early definitions emphasized the role of technology. This may be seen

---

TABLE 1–3   Some Important Definitions in Informatics

Informatics. The science and art of turning data into information.

Medical informatics. May be used to refer to the application of information science and technology to acquire, process, organize, interpret, store, use, and communicate medical data in all of its forms in medical education, practice and research, patient care, and health management; the term may also refer more broadly to the application of informatics to all of the healthcare disciplines as well as the practice of medicine.

Health informatics. The application of computer and information science in all basic and applied biomedical sciences to facilitate the acquisition, processing, interpretation, optimal use, and communication of health-related data. The focus is the patient and the process of care, and the goal is to enhance the quality and efficiency of care provided.

Bioinformatics. The application of computer and IT to the management of biological information including the development of databases and algorithms to facilitate research.

Consumer health informatics. Study of patient use of online information and communication to improve health outcomes and decisions.

Dental informatics. Computer and information sciences to improve dental practice, research, education, and management.

Clinical health informatics. Multidisciplinary field that focuses on the enhancement of clinical information management at the point of healthcare through improvement of information processes, implementation of clinical information systems, and the use and evaluation of CDS tools as a means to improve the effectiveness, quality, and value of the services rendered.

Public health informatics. Application of information and computer science and technology to public health practice, research, and learning.

in the statement by Scholes and Barber (1980) that nursing informatics is the "application of computer technology to all fields of nursing." Ball and Hannah (1984) later used a definition of medical informatics to define nursing informatics as the "collected informational technologies which concern themselves with the client care decision-making process performed by healthcare practitioners" (p. 3). In 1985 Hannah added the role of the nurse within nursing informatics to the definition that she and Ball developed. It retained its technical focus. The emphasis on technology remained evident in several later definitions as well.

Critics note that many definitions emphasize technology and downplay the role of the informatics nurse (IN) in processing information that can be done without the aid of a computer. Staggers and Thompson (2002) also note that when clients are mentioned, it is usually in the role of passive recipients of care rather than as active participants in the care process.

The conceptually driven definitions started to appear in the mid-1980s as models and relationships were added to definitions (ANA 2001; Staggers & Thompson 2002). Schwirian (1986) used Hannah's 1985 definition but added a model that depicted users, information, goals, and computer hardware and software connected by bidirectional arrows. Schwirian called for a solid foundation of nursing informatics knowledge built on research that was model driven and proactive rather than problem driven. Graves and Corcoran (1989, p. 227) built on Hannah's definition to include "a combination of computer science, information science and nursing science designed to assist in the management and processing of nursing data, information and knowledge to support the practice of nursing and the delivery of nursing care." This definition addressed the purpose of technology and provided a link between information and knowledge. It built on an earlier model developed by Graves and Corcoran. In 1996, Turley introduced his model, which shows nursing informatics using theory from cognitive science, computer science, and information science on a base of nursing science with information present at the point that all areas overlap.

Role-oriented definitions began to appear at the same time that nursing informatics gained acceptance as an area of specialty practice. In 1992 the ANA's Council on Computer Applications in Nursing incorporated the role of the informatics nurse specialist (INS) into a definition derived from work by Graves and Corcoran. According to this definition, the purpose of nursing informatics was "to analyze information requirements; design, implement and evaluate information systems and data structures that support nursing; and identify and apply computer technologies for nursing." The ANA revised its definition again in 1994 to "legitimize the specialty and to guide efforts to create a certification examination" (ANA 2001, p. 16). The 1994 definition follows:

> Nursing informatics is the specialty that integrates nursing science, computer science, and information science in identifying, collecting, processing, and managing data and information to support nursing practice, administration, education, research, and expansion of nursing knowledge. Nursing informatics supports the practice of all nursing specialties in all sites and settings whether at the basic or advanced level. The practice includes the development of applications, tools, processes, and structures that assist nurses with the management of data in taking care of patients or in supporting their practice of nursing. (p. 3)

The ANA revised its definition of nursing informatics again in 2001, noting the need to address the core elements of "nurse, patient, health environment, decision making and nursing data, information knowledge, information structures, and information technology" (p. 17). The ANA prepared its definition for North America. This definition attempted to recognize the more active role of the patient in his or her own care and to more clearly articulate the role of the IN in the healthcare environment. This definition follows:

> Nursing informatics is a specialty that integrates nursing science, computer science, and information science to manage and communicate data, information, and knowledge in nursing practice. Nursing informatics facilitates the integration of data, information, and knowledge to support

patients, nurses, and other providers in their decision making in all roles and settings. This support is accomplished through the use of information structures, information processes, and information technology. (ANA 2001, p. 17)

Groups and individuals in other parts of the world also continued their work on definitions. The Nursing Informatics Special Interest Group of the International Medical Informatics Association (IMIA) (2003) amended its definition of *nursing informatics* in 1998 to read that nursing informatics "is the integration of nursing, its information, and information management with information processing and communication technology, to support the health of people worldwide." At approximately the same time, a National Steering Committee in Canada solicited feedback via the National Nursing Informatics Project (Hebert 1999) from nursing organizations, educational institutions, and employers to arrive at the following definition for Canada.

> Nursing Informatics (NI) is the application of computer science and information science to nursing. NI promotes the generation, management and processing of relevant data in order to use information and develop knowledge that supports nursing in all practice domains. (p. 5)

Despite national differences, there was a consensus on the need for a definition to shape the specialty, obtain funding for studies, design educational programs, and help other disciplines define informatics practice within their own areas and to set expectations for employers (Hebert 1999; Staggers & Thompson 2002). There was also agreement that the goal of nursing informatics was to ensure that data collected and housed within automated record systems would be available as information that can be used by healthcare professionals at the bedside as well as by those in administrative and research positions (Newbold 2002).

In subsequent years the practice of nursing informatics has continued to evolve, leading to a review and revision of both the definition and scope of practice statements by the ANA (2008). This recent definition incorporates the concept of wisdom to read as follows:

> Nursing informatics is a specialty that integrates nursing science, computer science, and information science to manage and communicate data, information, knowledge and wisdom into nursing practice. Nursing informatics facilitates the integration of data, information, knowledge and wisdom to support patients, nurses, and other providers in their decision making in all roles and settings. This support is accomplished through the use of information structures, information processes, and information technology. (ANA 2008, p. 1)

MEDICAL INFORMATICS, NURSING INFORMATICS, AND CONSUMER INFORMATICS

Medical informatics is generally used as a broad term to include all the disciplines in the field with specific health-related areas beneath it, including nursing informatics and consumer informatics. Consumer informatics is driven by several factors including technological advances, an increasingly Internet-savvy population, a need for increased accountability in the selection of healthcare services, an acceptance of online and telephone transactions in lieu of face-to-face interactions, concerns for safety, the advent of health savings accounts, and a change in the revenue model that calls for individuals to assume greater responsibility for payment for services (Singh, Hummel, & Walton 2005).

COMPUTER AND INFORMATION LITERACY

The terms *computer literacy* and *information literacy* are not synonymous. **Computer literacy** is a popular term used to refer to a familiarity with the use of personal computers, including the use of software tools such as word processing, spreadsheets, databases, presentation graphics, and e-mail. The majority of students admitted to nursing schools now enter with some level of computer literacy.

Information literacy has a broader meaning. Information literacy is defined as the ability to recognize when information is needed as well as the skills to find, evaluate, and use needed information effectively (Association of College and Research Libraries [ACRL] 2002). Information literacy is particularly important in today's environment of rapid technological change and knowledge growth, with information available from many sources and in different formats, including text, graphics, and audio. Information literacy is important to all disciplines because it forms the basis for ongoing learning. In its related definition of information and communication literacy, the Educational Testing Service (2007) focuses on the ability to use digital technology, communication tools, and networks as tools to problem solve and communicate, and to maintain a fundamental understanding of ethical and legal issues. In healthcare the definition of information literacy must also include an awareness of the conceptual differences between various classifications and standardized languages, critical thinking skills, the ability to use the tools offered by technology to solve information problems, as well as an understanding of the ethical and legal issues surrounding the access and use of information (Kisilowska 2006; Skiba 2005).

The significance of information literacy for nursing is that it represents an important step in promoting evidence-based nursing practice because the information-literate nurse can weigh the quality and significance of research findings for application (DiCecco 2005). Despite the recognition of information literacy as a bridge to evidence-based practice, the connection is not automatic. Problems include a lack of awareness of the importance of evidence-based practice, inconsistent role modeling by registered nurses (RNs), a lack of comfort in using database searches, and a lack of exposure to evidence-based clinical practice (Courey, Benson-Soros, Deemer, & Zeller 2006; Pravikoff, Tanner, & Pierce 2005).

In a survey of U.S. nurses to determine perceptions of access to tools to obtain evidence and assess skill levels with these tools, Pravikoff et al. (2005) found that the majority of respondents recognized the need for information to support practice, but the most frequently consulted resources included peers and general searches of the Internet. There was limited use of established bibliographic databases or crucial evaluation of research findings for application in practice. The majority of the respondents had never conducted a database search and claimed that they had never received instruction in the use of electronic resources. While the researchers noted that the majority of participants had graduated prior to the mid-1980s, these findings raise questions about the true levels of information literacy among practicing nurses and have led many nursing leaders to call for an evaluation of nursing curricula for the incorporation of information literacy and evidence-based practice. In another study of undergraduate nursing programs, McNeil et al. (2005) found that approximately one-half of undergraduate nursing programs were teaching information literacy skills and required students to enter with proficiency in word processing and e-mail. However, the inclusion of content on data standards and unified language systems was less obvious. Another study that relied upon self-reports by baccalaureate students found a significant improvement in skills over an 8-year period ending in 2005 but concluded that nursing education may not be providing entry-level nurses with all the skills needed in today's technology-rich environment, noting low reported levels of experience with databases, spreadsheets, and statistical packages (McDowell & Ma 2007).

This situation has ramifications for both nursing education and current practice. Ornes and Gassert (2007) found nursing faculty to be the greatest block to incorporating technology into curricula. Faculty need to examine their own knowledge and skills in information literacy, attitudes, the incorporation of information literacy throughout the curriculum, and assessment measures for information literacy. An important part of this evaluation includes consideration of how these foundation level skills are used and whether students and graduates progress to the critical review of research and its application into practice (Booth 2006; Skiba 2005). Institutions also need to put mechanisms into place to help develop information literacy among staff and to encourage evidence-based practice (McBride 2006).

INFORMATICS COMPETENCIES FOR HEALTHCARE PROVIDERS

For many years there was little agreement on the skills required for informatics competencies and the level of competencies required for each level of practice. This situation made it difficult for educators and employers to ensure that all nurses possessed appropriate skills. Arnold (1996) noted the need for familiarity with presentation graphics, data analysis, and decision support for administrators and educators. In 1998 the American Association of Colleges of Nursing (AACN) identified information management as a skill needed by baccalaureate nursing graduates. More specifically, the AACN wanted graduates to be able to use existing and evolving methods of discovering, retrieving, and using information in their practice. This requirement was partially addressed through the requirement for courses in basic computer skills as a gateway to information literacy and information management skills. Hobbs' (2002) review of previous studies of informatics competencies found conceptual, methodology, and measurement problems that made it difficult to make generalizations across the research, although there was agreement that nurses should have skills in basic word processing and the ability to use databases, spreadsheets, document care, and e-mail. Yee (2002) found that employers wanted graduates to have these skills as well as Internet search skills and the ability to use statistical software, clinical information systems, and scheduling systems. Heller, Oros, and Durney-Crowley (2003) observed a need for nurses to be adept at accessing patient information in electronic records and the use of telehealth applications. Garde, Harrison, and Hovenga (2005) called for the development of a comprehensive health informatics education framework for nurses as well as other health professionals. An increasing number of nursing leaders have called for greater attention to the development of informatics competencies, including information literacy, as a necessary stepping stone to evidence-based practice (Barton 2005; Desjardins, Cook, Jenkins, & Bakken 2005; Dreher & Miller 2006; Skiba 2005). McDowell and Ma (2007) emphasized the need for competence in e-mail, Web and database searches, spreadsheets, and statistical analysis for use in quality improvement activities, the creation and monitoring of budgets, and a better understanding of research findings. The very manner of how health information is accessed has changed as a result of the Internet and the migration toward electronic records. The federal mandate for an electronic medical record for all Americans by 2014 makes informatics competencies necessary for all healthcare professionals (Ornes & Gassert 2007). The tools and technology that nurses need to perform their work efficiently are changing in such a way that informatics competencies play a greater role.

Key Initiatives and Organizations

Several landmark reports from the Institute of Medicine (IOM) called for technology as a tool to help create a safer, more efficient healthcare delivery system along with workforce preparation that would enable healthcare professionals to use that technology to realize purported benefits. These IOM reports included *To Err is Human: Building a Safer Health System* (1999), *Crossing the Quality Chasm: A New Health System for the 21st Century* (2001), and *Keeping Patients Safe: Transforming the Work Environment of Nurses* (2004). The American Hospital Association (AHA, 2002) and the Robert Wood Johnson Foundation (Bleich, Connolly, Davis, Hewlett, & Hill 2006) espoused support for the increased use of technology to both create a better healthcare delivery system and improve the preparation of professionals to work in a high-technology healthcare delivery system.

Several parties—including individual researchers; academics; employers; and various professional organizations such as the ANA, the American Medical Informatics Association (AMIA), the Nursing Informatics Working Group of the Healthcare Information Management System Society (HIMSS), the National League for Nursing (NLN) Task Group on Informatics Competencies, the Healthcare Leadership Alliance, and the Alliance for Nursing Informatics—have turned their attention to the issue of informatics competencies. Informatics competencies are deemed essential as a means to facilitate the delivery of safer, more efficient care, to add to the knowledge base for the profession, and to transition toward evidence-based practice (Smedley 2005). The *Scope and Standards of Nursing Informatics Practice* (ANA 2008) included an updated matrix of competencies that expanded earlier work by Staggers, Gassert, and Curran (2001). The ANA document categorized competencies into one of three areas—computer literacy, information literacy, and professional development/leadership—considering the knowledge and skills needed at each level of practice.

The Technology Informatics Guiding Education Reform Initiative The Technology Informatics Guiding Education Reform (TIGER) Initiative emerged from a national gathering of leaders from nursing administration, practice, education, informatics, technology, and government, as well as other key stakeholders, who realized that nursing must transform itself as a profession to realize the benefits that electronic patient records can provide (HIMSS Nursing Task Force 2007; Sensmeier 2007; TIGER 2007). Its purpose was to create a vision for the future of nursing to provide a safer, higher-quality patient care through the use of IT. It requires informatics competencies for every nurse and active involvement in advancing HIT. The group identified leadership, education, technology-enabled processes that facilitate teamwork and relationships throughout the care continuum, systems that support education and practice, and a supportive culture and policies as key factors to attain this vision. It received federal funds and grants from the Robert Wood Johnson Foundation. The TIGER Initiative (n.d.) called for the redesign of nursing education to keep up with rapid changes in technology, active participation by nurses in the design of informatics tools, and increased visibility by nurses in the national health IT agenda. It organized teams to work toward the common goals; obtained additional funding; developed work plans and outcomes for each team; and identified informatics competencies for all levels of nursing personnel, including nursing assistants.

The QSEN Project This Robert Wood Johnson funded project seeks to prepare future nurses with the knowledge, skills, and attitudes (KSAs) needed to continuously improve the quality and safety of the healthcare delivery system (QSEN 2011). Five of the six competencies defined in phase I of the project were recommended by the IOM for all healthcare professionals. These six competencies include:

- Patient-centered care
- Teamwork and collaboration
- Evidence-based practice
- Quality improvement
- Safety
- Informatics

The QSEN Web site (http://www.qsen.org/) provides links to KSAs identified as needed for both prelicensure and graduate students as well as strategies for development.

The American Association of Colleges of Nursing AACN is the organization that provides a voice for baccalaureate and higher-degree nursing education programs in the United States, providing curriculum elements and a framework for baccalaureate and higher-degree nursing programs (AACN 2011a). AACN has established informatics as a curriculum element for baccalaureate, master's level, and doctoral programs, albeit expectations differ by level of education. Baccalaureate programs are expected to provide the skills needed to manage information and apply patient care technology (AACN 2008). MSN graduates are expected to:

- Use patient care technologies to deliver and enhance care
- Use communication technologies to integrate and coordinate care

- Analyze data to improve patient outcomes
- Manage information for evidence-based care and patient education
- Use and facilitate electronic health records (EHRs) to improve patient care (AACN 2011b, p. 5)

Advanced practice graduates should be able to answer questions that arise in practice, use new knowledge to analyze the outcomes of interventions and initiate change, use technology inclusive of information systems for the purpose of storage and retrieval of data, and query databases for the purpose of using available research in practice (AACN 1996). DNP graduates should be active participants in the design, selection, and use of IT for the purpose of supporting patient care and healthcare systems (AACN 2006).

The National League for Nursing The NLN position paper, *Preparing the Next Generation of Nurses to Practice in a Technology-rich Environment: An Informatics Agenda*, called for nursing education and the NLN itself to take steps to ensure that every nursing graduate demonstrate computer and information literacy as well as up-to-date skills in informatics (NLN 2007, 2008). The intent of the position paper was to reform nursing education to support quality measures to produce a graduate capable of working in a technologically rich healthcare delivery system.

International Council of Nurses Professional Organizations This federation of national nurses associations from more than 130 countries works to ensure quality nursing care for all through programs in three critical areas—practice, regulation, and social welfare (International Council of Nurses 2010). The International Classification for Nursing Practice (ICNP), a common code language for data, falls under the professional practice arena. The ICNP is extremely important for meaningful exchange of electronic data in a format that retains its meaning across settings and countries.

Competency Levels

The *Scope and Standards of Nursing Informatics Practice* (ANA 2008) delineated nursing informatics competency levels for different levels of practitioners.

Entry-Level Core Competencies The beginning nurse focuses primarily on developing and using skills that rely upon the ability to retrieve and enter data in an electronic format that is relevant to patient care, the analysis and interpretation of information as part of planning care, the use of informatics applications designed for nursing practice, and the implementation of policies relevant to information. The *Scope and Standards of Nursing Informatics Practice* (ANA 2008) calls for the following competencies for the beginning nurse:

- Basic computer literacy, including the ability to use basic desktop applications and electronic communication
- The ability to use IT to support clinical and administrative processes, which presumes information literacy to support evidence-based practice
- The ability to access data and perform documentation via computerized patient records
- The ability to support patient safety initiatives via the use of IT
- Recognition of the role of informatics in nursing

The Experienced Nurse The experienced nurse builds upon the competencies required for entry-level practitioners using basic computer skills to information regarding the patient. This practitioner has the expertise to serve as a content expert in system design, to see relationships among data elements, to execute judgments based on observed data patterns, to safeguard access to quality of information, and to participate in efforts to improve information management and communication. The ANA (2008) has identified competencies to include the following:

- Proficiency in his or her area of specialization and the use of IT and computers to support that area of practice including quality improvement and other related activities (ANA 2008)
- Knowledge representation methodologies for evidence-based practice
- The ability to use information systems and work with informatics specialists to enact system improvements
- Proficiency in using evidence-based databases
- The promotion of innovative applications of technology in healthcare

The Informatics Nurse This individual has advanced preparation in information management and possesses the following skills (ANA 2008):

- Proficiency with informatics applications to support all areas of nursing practice including quality improvement activities, research, project management, system design, development, analysis, implementation, support, maintenance, and evaluation
- Fiscal management
- Integration of multidisciplinary language/standards of practice
- Skills in critical thinking, data management and processing, decision making, and system development, and computer skills
- Identification and provision of data for decision making

The Informatics Nurse Specialist The INS possesses a sophisticated level of understanding and skills in information management and computer technology, demonstrating most of the competencies seen at the previous three levels. The INS is the innovator who sees the broad vision of what is possible and how it may be attained. The *Scope and Standards of Nursing Informatics Practice* (ANA 2008) calls for educational preparation for the INS that enables him or her to conduct informatics research and generate informatics theory. This preparation and expertise makes the INS well suited to work in a variety of areas and functional roles including project management and administration.

HEALTHCARE REFORM

Healthcare reform has re-emerged as a policy imperative in recent years. In 2004 President George W. Bush created the position of the national health information technology coordinator and called for the establishment of an EHR for every American by 2014 (Miller & West 2009). However, it was not until President Obama signed the American Recovery and Reinvestment Act (ARRA) and the Health Information Technology for Economic and Clinical Health (HITECH) Act into law in 2009 that the Department of Health and Human Services (HHS) was given authority to establish programs to improve healthcare quality, safety, and efficiency through the use of HIT and that funds were provided to support widespread adoption of HIT (McDermott Will & Emery 2009; Walker 2010). One aspect of ARRA necessitated that healthcare providers comply with mandated reporting requirements that were structured to provide information deemed critical to improve the overall quality of care. Compliance with reporting requirements were tied to the adoption and use of EHR systems certified as capable of collecting and sharing the specified data. Financial incentives were designated for providers that met mandatory reporting requirements.

Focus areas in reform efforts included hospital-physician integration, improved care management, the adoption and widespread use of information systems, and changes in service distribution and payer relationships. These changes require new competencies as well as excellent planning and analysis, which in turn make information systems, and a workforce skilled in their use, even more critical (Kim, Majka, & Sussman 2011).

THE PUSH FOR PATIENT SAFETY

Patient safety is a priority for health systems, professionals, and consumers around the world. In 2004 the World Health Organization (Joint Commission International Center for Patient Safety 2007; WHO 2007) launched the World Alliance for Patient Safety in response to a World Health Assembly Resolution urging the WHO and member states to consider the problem of patient safety. The Alliance addressed 10 major action issues, which included a focus on new technologies as a means to improve patient safety. In 2005 WHO designated the Joint Commission and Joint Commission International as the WHO Collaborating Centre on Patient Safety Solutions. The Collaborating Centre established an international network of experts and organizations with expertise in patient safety to identify, evaluate, adapt, and disseminate patient safety solutions across the globe. WHO defines patient safety solutions as "any system design or intervention that has demonstrated the ability to prevent or mitigate patient harm stemming from the processes of healthcare." The Centre plans to identify problems and present evidence-based solutions along with supporting documentation. In 2007 the International Steering Committee of the Centre approved solutions for the following:

- Look-alike, sound-alike medication names
- Patient identification
- Communication during patient handover
- Correct procedure and body site
- Electrolyte solution concentration control
- Medication accuracy
- Catheter and tubing misconnections
- Needle reuse and injection device safety
- Hand hygiene

The Centre then began work on the second round of patient safety solutions. The latter group of patient safety issues include follow-up on critical test results, falls, hospital-acquired central-line infections, pressure ulcers, care of the rapidly deteriorating patient, patient and family involvement in care, provider apology and disclosure, and medications with names that look or sound similar. The Centre coordinates the High 5s Project, which is developing standard operating procedures to address widespread patient safety problems across the globe (WHO 2011).

The Institute for Healthcare Improvement (IHI) (2011) is another group dedicated to the improvement of global healthcare. IHI (2007) challenged U.S. hospitals to join in a campaign to save 100,000 lives during an 18-month period that commenced in 2005. The 3,100 participating hospitals managed to save an estimated 122,000 lives during that period through the implementation of specific evidence-based and life-saving protocols that included:

- Special Rapid Response Teams that were called at the first sign of patient decline
- Evidence-based care for acute myocardial infarction
- Medication reconciliation as a means to prevent adverse drug events (ADEs)
- Steps to prevent central-line infections
- Prophylactic use of perioperative antibiotics to prevent surgical site infections
- Preventive measures against the development of ventilator-associated pneumonia

In 2006, IHI kicked off the 5 Million Lives Campaign, with the goal of sparing 5 million lives from medical harm during a 2-year period based upon estimates that nearly 15 million instances of medical harm occur in the United States each year. Four thousand U.S. hospitals participated in the adoption of 12 interventions designed to save lives and reduce injuries. Earlier standards were retained, and the following new standards were added:

- Reduce the incidence of surgical complications
- Reduce methicillin-resistant *Staphylococcus aureus* (MRSA) infection
- Prevent pressure ulcers
- Prevent harm from high-alert medications starting with anticoagulants, sedatives, narcotics, and insulin
- Decrease readmissions for the treatment of congestive heart failure
- Obtain cooperation from hospital boards of directors to accelerate organizational progress toward safe care

These and many other concurrent efforts are the outgrowth of the landmark reports published by the IOM, *To Err Is Human: Building a Safer Health System* and *Crossing the Quality Chasm: A New Health System for the 21st Century*, which served to heighten awareness of safety issues in the healthcare delivery system. The IOM is a division of the National Academy of Sciences, which was created by the U.S. government to advise in scientific and technical matters. Its Committee on the Quality of Health Care in America was formed in 1998 with the charge to develop a strategy that would substantially improve the quality of healthcare over a 10-year period. According to the IOM (1999), at least 44,000 to 98,000 deaths per year in U.S. hospitals are due to medication errors. The IOM included recommendations for the use of IT to prevent adverse drug interactions, inappropriate doses, potential side effects, and other types of mistakes.

The Joint Commission, formally known as the Joint Commission for Accreditation of Healthcare Organizations (2007), is an independent, nonprofit organization dedicated to improving the safety and quality of healthcare. The Joint Commission provides accreditation of healthcare organizations and related services to ensure that safety and quality standards are met. National Patient Safety Goals are identified annually to address problem areas. Accredited facilities must demonstrate compliance. Medication reconciliation became an accreditation requirement because it was noted that medication errors often occurred when patients were transferred from unit to unit and from one level of care to another and at the time of discharge (Rogers et al. 2006; Thompson 2005). Medication reconciliation entails obtaining a list of all preadmission meds, which is then used as a basis for comparison when medications are ordered, and at the time of admission, transfer, and discharge, to note discrepancies.

Many other organizations and groups also have an interest in patient safety. A partial list includes:

- American Nurses Association (ANA)
- American Medical Association
- Healthcare Information and Management System Society
- Agency for Healthcare Research and Quality (AHRQ)
- American Hospital Association (AHA
- Centers for Medicare & Medicaid Services
- Leapfrog Group
- National Advisory Council on Nurse Education and Practice (NACNEP)
- Council on Graduate Medical Education
- National Committee for Quality Assurance
- National Patient Safety Agency (United Kingdom)
- National Patient Safety Foundation
- Patient Safety Institute
- Patient Safety Task Force of the U.S. Department of Health and Human Services

- Institute for Healthcare Improvement
- Institute for Safe Medication Practice
- Centers for Disease Control
- U.S. Food and Drug Administration (FDA)
- Partnership for Patient Safety

Interest in patient safety spawned legislation. The Patient Safety and Quality Improvement Act of 2005 sought to improve patient safety by encouraging voluntary and confidential reporting of events that adversely affect patients. It created patient safety organizations to collect, aggregate, and analyze confidential information reported by healthcare providers. The bulk of other federal legislative efforts focus on incentives to the adoption of IT as a means to promote efficiency and improve safety. The Patient Safety Act represents an important move in the correct direction where information is shared about adverse events for learning purposes for the benefit of all. Approximately one-half of the states have passed their own medical error reporting laws, with a few establishing patient safety centers. Pennsylvania's Medical Care Availability and Reduction of Error (MCARE) Act requires the submission of reports of both adverse events and near misses (Rabinowitz et al. 2006). The National Reporting and Learning System in England and Wales coordinates the national reporting of patient safety incidents and determines solutions (Cousins & Baker 2004). This type of reporting allows institutions to compare their error rates with the statewide rate and produces safety alerts that help organizations to act proactively (Simpson 2005). Prior to this time institutions neither shared this type of data nor was there widespread learning from incidents and failures.

The IOM reports heightened public awareness of the threat of medical errors. Burroughs et al. (2007) found that inpatients defined medical errors more broadly to include falls, communication problems, and responsiveness. Many of the problems that threaten patient safety result from failed process or communication particularly when patients are transferred or shifts change. For this reason some experts call for a review of practices used by other fields, including the aviation industry and military, for guidance in creating a safer environment (Bauer 2006; Doucette 2006; Hohenhaus, Powell, & Hohenhaus 2006). The Federal Aviation Authority requires the development and use of practices designed to improve the recognition and utilization of all available resources to achieve safe operations. These practices include cross-monitoring and situational awareness in a cooperative, nonpunitive environment to create a culture of safety. Cross-monitoring is a process for double-checking high-risk work and verification of inaccurate or ambiguous information. This process may be manual or built into information systems. Situational awareness is awareness of what's going on. Unfortunately awareness may be decreased with poor communication, group think/mindset, and task overload/underload. Situation, background, assessment, recommendations (SBAR) represents an adaptation of aviation procedures by the U.S. Navy for the express purpose of improved communication of critical information. SBAR has since been used with success in healthcare. Its reliance upon redundancy establishes an expected pattern of communication, making deviations from the pattern and errors obvious. Situation and background are used to communicate objective information, whereas assessment and recommendation allow the sharing of opinion and requests. Variations of the technique to standardize report information have also been successful (Shendell-Falik, Feinson, & Mohr 2007). Prompts can be built into information systems to facilitate this process and improve care (Sidlow & Katz-Sidlow 2006). Some examples of information that nurses identify as important to care but are sometimes not communicated include attending physician, code and allergy status, reason for admission, identification of anticipated status changes, and daily plan of care inclusive of discharge plans.

The creation of a culture of safety requires a nonpunitive environment in which errors, near misses, and potential problems can be reported without fear of reprisal. Nurses are committed to patient safety initiatives because they are involved in care at all levels (Manno, Hogan, Heberlein, Nyakiti, & Mee 2006).

The Joint Commission announced plans to provide a data management system to accredited hospitals in 2007 to help identify and prioritize areas for improvement using current data, past survey findings, complaints, and reports of sentinel events. Resulting information could be used to drive quality and safety improvement efforts through comparative performance information, benchmark reports, and quality risk profiles. Aggregate data could be used to identify trends or common areas for improvement. States also launched efforts to improve patient safety. The Minnesota Alliance for Patient Safety was established as a collaborative effort to encourage statewide sharing of key safety information through electronic databases (Apoid, Daniels, & Sanneborn 2006).

Patient Identification

Errors in the patient identification process threaten patient safety. For this reason, the Joint Commission required organizations to investigate and plan for technology that could assist with the process of positive patient identification when it designated improving the accuracy of patient identification as a potential National Patient Safety Goal for 2008. There have also been national initiatives to reduce identification errors for procedures and during medication administration, laboratory testing, bedside glucose checks and blood transfusion, and the administration of intravenous (IV) fluids (Wickham et al. 2006). Barcodes and radio frequency identification (RFID) are the dominant technologies for this area. For example, the results of a recent Agency for Healthcare Research and Quality (AHRQ 2010) study demonstrated that barcode technology when used in conjunction with an electronic medication administration record substantially reduced errors.

Barcodes have been used in sales and various businesses for many years. Sometimes known as UPC codes, they can be found on most products including medications and IV fluids. Barcodes come in simple linear format or two-dimensional forms. Linear codes can include a medical record number, while two-dimensional forms can include more information such as name, age, provider, and gender. Barcode technology is inexpensive. Barcode technology does require line-of-sight scanning, which requires awakening or repositioning the patient. It may not read well on objects that have been bent, wrinkled, wet, or torn.

RFID tags are used in merchandise tags. RFID technology is durable, can contain more information, does not require direct visualization, and may be reprogrammable (VanVactor 2008). It is available in passive and active forms. The passive form contains a chip and antenna, is generally small, and may be flat. It broadcasts data when stimulated by radio frequency energy. Active RFID uses batteries and transmitters to constantly provide location information, making it ideal for tracking equipment, patient, and even staff. RFID tends to be more expensive, although research developments may soon make it more cost effective. Consequently there is no single technology solution for ensuring patient identification although RFID has been shown to be effective (Yang, Huang, & Huang 2009).

Information Technology Safeguards

Hospitals and healthcare providers have been slow to adopt IT that is commonly found in the business sector. IT advocates claim that it can support the work of healthcare professionals and benefit consumers by improving efficiency, quality, and safety. The desire to reduce or eliminate medication errors focuses attention on computerized physician (or provider/prescriber) order entry (CPOE), barcode medication administration (BCMA), and e-prescribing. When properly used, technologies such as automated drug dispensing systems, smart IV pumps, electronic medical records, computerized documentation at the beside, barcoding, and CPOE reduce adverse events through the introduction of additional checks and balances to existing systems (Manno et al. 2006). There are also IT applications for evidence-based medical error reporting, risk management, clinical alerts, electronic medication administration, and clinical decision support (CDS) that provide information that allows clinicians to be proactive. Evidence-based error identification and reporting applications collect data from external sources such as extant databases and applications to determine where errors occur to help focus resources (Simpson 2005).

Computerized Physician (or Provider/Prescriber) Order Entry

Computerized Physician (or Provider/Prescriber) Order Entry (CPOE) is the process by which the physician or another healthcare provider, such as a nurse practitioner, physician's assistant, or physical or occupational therapist, directly enters orders for client care into a hospital information system. Its benefits include a reduction in transcription errors; a decrease in elapsed time from order to implementation; standardization and more completeness of orders; fewer medication errors; and the ability to incorporate CDS, alerts for critical lab values, and prompts when certain tests are due. Information is drawn from separate systems such as the hospital, pharmacy, and laboratory systems with drug databases to warn prescribers of potential problems with dosages, potential drug interactions, allergies, and contraindications such as pregnancy or other health conditions (Alliance for Health Reform 2006; Simpson 2005).

Despite its purported benefits it is essential to recognize that CPOE is a tool, not a guarantee, of safety. There have been a few reports that CPOE has contributed to errors, particularly since not all CPOE are created equal. Several factors need to be considered when factoring actual CPOE efficiencies. These include ease of use, integration with clinical information systems, and design and training. Basic CPOE includes entry of orders with simple checking for allergies and drug interactions. At the intermediate level CPOE allows some flexibility in displaying results. Advanced clinical order management (ACOM) is a subset of CPOE. ACOM incorporates guided ordering or mentored ordering with formulary management. At its most advanced level ACOM makes use of artificial intelligence and collective knowledge from national standards of care, order sets, alerts, and best practices in workflow efficiencies (McCoy 2006).

Until recently widespread adoption of CPOE by U.S. physicians was slow. This was due to several factors including the perception that CPOE required additional time with few benefits for the provider, physician dislike of clerical or repetitive tasks, resentment over "cookbook" order sets by physicians who believe that they already provide high-quality care and do not need to have their decisions made for them, and a lack of a national policy (Aarts & Koppel 2009). Systems also need to be responsive to the user or risk not being used (Khajouei & Jaspers 2008; Rahimi, Timpka, Vimarlund, Uppugunduri, & Svensson 2009). The HITECH Act of 2009 has since provided financial incentives for the adoption of EHRs with corresponding Meaningful Use criteria proposed by the Centers for Medicare & Medicaid Services that mandate CPOE use (Devine et al. 2010).

E-Prescribing

E-prescribing refers to the electronic transmission of drug prescriptions from a hospital-based inpatient ordering system (CPOE) or handheld device (Gooch 2006). It may be done from a location at, or near, the patient. Associated advantages include fewer errors, improved communication, greater efficiency, improved compliance with recommended treatment guidelines, lower costs, and less time to fill prescriptions. Errors are reduced because problems with illegible handwriting are eliminated, and the system incorporates lists of patient allergies and other medications. Information may also be available that suggests the best drug for a particular problem, dosing recommendations, drug interactions, contraindications, off-label uses, allowable formulary drugs for a particular individual, and insurance co-payments. Like CPOE, e-prescribing has also been identified as a Meaningful Use criterion for adoption by eligible providers seeking to qualify for financial incentives available through Meaningful Use (CMS n.d.).

Barcode and RFID Medication Administration

The FDA issued a rule in 2004 requiring bar codes on most prescription and some over-the-counter medications as a means to decrease medication errors. Barcode scanning technology for medication administration automates the storage, dispensing, returning, restocking, and crediting of barcoded medications, improving safety by ensuring that the right medication is dispensed to the right patient particularly when used with barcoded patient ID bands. It is frequently referred to as BCMA.

Several varieties of barcode software and multiple barcode formats exist. Matching organizational needs to the appropriate hardware and software requires interdisciplinary collaboration between clinical, IS, financial, and supply management teams. According to the FDA (2004), barcode implementation will reduce medication errors by 50%. Barcode technology is also available for IV infusion pumps for integration into the medication administration system, point-of-care glucose meters, and blood products. RFID technology can be used in lieu of barcode technology for medication administration purposes. It offers several advantages but comes with a higher cost and is not widely used at present.

Decision-Support Software

Decision-support software (DSS) is a type of computer application that analyzes data and presents them in a fashion that facilitates decision making. It can incorporate lab values, standards of care, and other patient-specific information. It also contains alerts that help to promote safety. The underlying premise of DSS is that the amount of knowledge today exceeds the retention abilities of any one person. DSS is a tool that extends human capabilities. It may be an integral part of CPOE and e-prescribing programs. It can be found in other settings as well. An example that is relevant to nurses is when DSS guides the triage nurse through a series of observations, questions, and interventions when a patient presents with a specific complaint. There are also tools related to drugs and clinical pathways. The value of DSS is contingent upon both the quality of the individual tools and the willingness of users to use them. The selection of a tool has the potential to directly and indirectly impact patient care and outcomes (Middleton 2009). Clinical decision support has also been identified as a Meaningful Use criterion for adoption by eligible providers seeking to qualify for financial incentives available through Meaningful Use (CMS n.d.).

Smart Technology

The term **smart technology** has been used to refer to technology that is integrated, saves time and physical burdens, and improves patient outcomes (American Academy of Nursing 2010). The American Academy of Nursing Workforce Commission was established in 2000 to develop strategies for dealing with the nursing shortage. The Commission focused upon identifying changes that would allow nursing to improve patient outcomes, developing and deploying a model to analyze workflow processes, and finding ways to use technology and recommending design principles for technology that would complement the way that nurses work. This work was done in conjunction with 25 participating hospitals and healthcare delivery sites. The results from this effort have implications that extend beyond supporting the work that nurses do as safety and enhanced efficiencies may be other outcomes (Bolton, Gassert, & Cipriano 2008). Cumulative benefits may be seen as individual technologies are integrated. One example of these benefits may be seen when smart infusion pumps are used in conjunction with CPOE.

OTHER MAJOR ISSUES IN HEALTHCARE WITH INFORMATICS IMPLICATIONS

The Nursing Shortage

There are numerous projections of a severe global nursing shortage. The nursing shortage has the attention of the public and healthcare providers because numerous studies have shown a relationship between the number of patients assigned to a nurse and clinical outcome. This shortage comes at a time when the overall population is aging, placing greater demands on the healthcare system. Unfilled positions force hospitals to close units and curtail services. The ramifications of the shortage extend beyond vacant positions. There is also an issue of lost knowledge as nurses retire or opt to leave the profession, which can seriously impact an organization's performance (Hatcher et al. 2006; Trossman 2006a).

The causes of the nursing shortage are numerous. They include dissatisfaction, a decreased interest in the field, and decreased enrollment. The situation necessitates redesign of care delivery models and the way that nurses are educated. There must be an increased emphasis upon the development of problem-solving and analytical skills in an increasingly complex, rapidly changing environment where there is an exponential growth of knowledge that exceeds any individual's ability to keep up-to-date (Donley 2005). Technology cannot solve problems that result from staffing shortages, but it can help prevent errors by giving busy nurses a system of double checks. As already noted the American Academy of Nursing Workforce Commission conducted an investigation on ways that technology might address the nursing shortage.

Work Flow Changes

The way that nurses and other healthcare providers work is changing for many reasons. There is a shift away from tasks to knowledge work and the demand for best practices. This change in clinical thinking is likely to continue its evolution. It is enabled through nursing informatics, standardized nursing knowledge and language systems, electronic records, and more sophisticated data analysis techniques. Hospitalized patients are more acutely ill. More treatment is rendered in outpatient settings. Rising costs demand greater efficiencies, forcing individual nurses and administrators to look for innovative, better methods to utilize all resources.

Information Technology as a Means to Retain Aging Nurses

The Robert Wood Johnson Foundation report *Wisdom at Work* examines retention of the older nurse to retirement age and beyond as a means to deal with the "nursing shortage," noting that aging baby boomers represent the largest untapped labor market and the value of the accumulated wisdom found within this group (Hatcher 2006). It emphasizes the need to use well-designed technology to enable the work of the nurse, not complicate it. This is in concert with the ANA view that technology has a crucial role in healthcare with the potential to benefit nurses and patients if it is well used (Trossman 2006b). Technology-enhanced environments make it easier to direct care. Electronic records eliminate the need for a centralized nurses' station; automated alerts facilitate safety and remind staff when medications and treatments are due and when tasks need to be done. Smart technology tracks devices, eliminating wasted steps and time. Cell phone communication serves to decrease steps, quickly relay call light messages, and provide a means to record or listen to shift report.

Hart (2007) notes the need to plan for an aging workforce. From a technology perspective this includes improved ergonomics in both high-tech equipment and low-tech applications that allow older workers to effect patient transfers safely without risk of injury to either the patient or themselves.

Additional modifications include better product design for the older nurse such as the use of white letters on a dark background; efforts to reduce glare, lowering monitor placement to accommodate for bifocal wearers; and better lighting. All nurses, including older nurses, need to be active participants in technology design and testing.

Evidence-Based Practice

Nursing leaders have long emphasized the need to establish a set of knowledge that is uniquely nursing. Evidence provides the means necessary to provide consistent, quality care. Current practice leaves little time or opportunity to conduct literature searches, evaluate research, and make clinical decisions based upon research. Even fewer nurses have actually conducted research. The current work environment does not support these efforts. The widespread adoption of electronic patient records, CPOE, and other point-of-care technologies that support nursing workflow is expected to help remove barriers to information and evidence-based practice (Simpson 2006).

Genomics

The delivery of quality care increasingly calls for an understanding of the genetic contribution to diseases and human response to illness and interventions. For this reason an interdependent group of nurse leaders drafted *Essential Nursing Competencies and Curricula Guidelines for Genetics and Genomics* in 2005 to establish the minimum requirements to prepare nurses to deliver competent genetic- and genomic-focused care (ANA 2006). Information literacy and informatics skills are essential to the attainment of these competencies, which call for all RNs to:

- Demonstrate knowledge of the relationship of genetics and genomics to health, prevention, screening, and monitoring
- Identify clients who may benefit from genetic information and services and provide appropriate, accurate information
- Make referrals as needed
- Provide appropriate services
- Evaluate the effectiveness of current technology and interventions

The Magnet Hospital Journey

Magnet designation is one of the healthcare industry's most celebrated indicators of quality patient care. Magnet recognition was developed by the American Nurses Credential Center (ANCC) as a measure to recognize organizations that provide the very best nursing care. Magnet facilities use technology to promote, support, and improve patient and staff safety; integrate research and evidence-based practice into clinical processes; and support communication among the disciplines. Healthcare information technology provides a means to reduce errors and improve efficiency, patient safety, and knowledge. It facilitates the incorporation of evidence-based guidelines into documentation and helps to compensate for the nursing shortage while improving care (ANCC 2011). The IN plays a key role to obtaining and maintaining magnet hospital status. For this reason ANCC has worked with the TIGER Initiative to align their forces and integrate IT into practice.

Consumer-Driven Healthcare

As consumers become more sophisticated and knowledgeable about medical and information technologies they hold providers to higher standards (Consumer Influence 2006). They are not content to wait for care but increasingly expect to have a voice in determining what services are delivered and how. This has been particularly clear with the Veterans Health Administration where customer desires and needs have driven changes (Wertenberger, Yerardi, Drake, & Parlier

2006). It has implications for investment in technology as well so that providers can maintain a competitive edge. Another expectation is 24-hour availability of health information via interactive services that allow consumers to schedule appointments, e-mail their physicians, look up benefit information, and learn about their conditions. Marketing and delivery of promised services is extremely important in this situation. Consumers expect quality and often have already reviewed information about the quality of services provided. The personal health record is one example of a consumer-centric innovation, which, by definition is subject to the review and control of consumers who view, and sometimes supply information for the record, and dictate what other entities may view their record.

Online Report Cards

The concept of healthcare quality report cards has existed for several years. These documents contain evaluated care data of individual physicians, facilities, health plans, and other care providers, serving as a tool to help healthcare consumers by allowing them to compare the quality and other characteristics of providers and health plans. The AHRQ (n.d.) supports the Healthcare Report Card Compendium Web page, a searchable directory of over 200 sources of comparative information.

Remote Clinical Monitoring

An aging population, a shortage of healthcare professionals, and a move to keep the ill and elderly in their homes as long as possible—all while trying to contain costs—has led to a spate of programs that use technology to remind people to check their blood sugar or blood pressure, take their medications, and otherwise monitor them in their own homes. Measures range from monitoring glucose levels, weight, general well-being, and cardiac rhythms, to checking pace maker function, to determining whether the refrigerator was opened. This type of monitoring helps individuals to better manage their own health, minimize travel, and forestall moving to a facility for care (Nugent, Wallace, Kernohan, McCreight, Mulvenna, & Martin 2007).

Patient-Centered Medical Homes and Accountable Care Organizations

The patient-centered medical homes (PCMH) is a model of primary care intended to improve coordination of care, provide better access to care, and improve patient satisfaction. According to the AHRQ the PCMH is defined by the following attributes:

- Patient-centered
- Comprehensive
- Coordinated care
- Accessible
- Subject to continuous improvement through a systems-based approach to quality and safety (AHRQ 2011)

The PCMH had been advocated as one tool needed to achieve healthcare reform (Wang 2009). More recently the Department of Health and Human Services (HHS) released new rules intended to help providers better coordinate care for Medicare patients through accountable care organizations (ACOs). ACOs are the result of the Affordable Care Act, which provides financial incentives for providers to work across settings to coordinate care. Substantial savings are expected in Medicare spending as a result. Much like the medical home, patients and providers are seen as partners in this model (Healthcare.gov 2011).

Disease Management

Successful disease management requires two-way communication between providers and consumers, with active participation and involvement in treatment decisions. Consumers may not have the skills to accomplish these tasks or have difficulty understanding healthcare information and instructions due to language and culture differences and difficulty navigating the healthcare system (Nath 2007). Health literacy is needed. Health literacy connotes that an individual possesses the problem-solving and decision-making skills needed to comprehend and use new information and to navigate the healthcare system. Nurses need to be sensitive to the health literacy levels of their clients particularly as it impacts their outcomes, and assist them to develop a greater understanding of their health issues.

Research

The move to evidence-based practice as a means to meet demands for quality and cost-effective care now lies within the grasp of virtually every healthcare professional with the implementation of the electronic record. Electronic records and the systems that house them make it easier and faster to collect information. Data stripped of individual patient identifiers can then be downloaded into other applications for the identification of patterns and further analysis. Much of this process can be performed automatically so that the time frame from data collection to interpretation is shortened and findings can be disseminated and applied more quickly. The recent adoption of Meaningful Use requirements and subsequent collection of data will also foster comparative effectiveness research (CER). Comparative effectiveness research provides evidence on the efficacy, benefits, and harms of treatment options so as to better inform healthcare decisions. The ARRA of 2009 allocated monies for CER (HHS.gov/Recovery 2011).

Payment for Performance

In years past healthcare institutions, nurses, and consumers were affected by managed care. This system imposed limits upon what providers could charge, and payers provided a set reimbursement by diagnosis. Downsizing, acquisitions, and mergers occurred in an attempt to increase efficiency along with automation and cross-training of personnel. One legacy of this era was that fewer people were left to do the work. Another result was that remaining providers had the ability to extend their reach by offering a more comprehensive set of services and encouraging consumers to stay within their healthcare network. These types of alliances foster the sharing of information as merged entities gravitate to computer systems that can exchange information and as administrators turn to IT as a means to maximize efficiencies. While the emphasis remains on the bottom line the healthcare delivery system is moving toward a model where providers are paid for performance (Donley 2005). An IOM report (2006) noted problems with the healthcare delivery system, including incentives for a high volume of services rather than quality services and better outcomes. This same report calls for better coordination of care among providers and across episodes of illness and identifies design principles for payment for performance and its implementation. An earlier report provides a set of starter measures. The IOM notes that public reporting of outcomes would motivate improved provider behavior and provide consumers with information that they could use to make treatment decisions.

Patient Privacy

Emerging trends in healthcare delivery bring benefits as well as new threats to privacy and private health information. A growing number of Americans favor the use of electronic records as a means to improve the quality of care and lower costs (Gaylin, Moiduddin, Mohamoud, Lundeen, & Kelly 2011). Most feel that the benefits of electronic records outweigh risks to privacy, but concerns over privacy remain one of the biggest obstacles related to health information exchange. A 2011 survey of 1000 U.S. adults found that 49% thought that electronic access to health data would have a negative impact on the privacy of their personal health information (CDW Healthcare 2011). Rath (2011) noted that quality patient care includes the protection of patients' private health information. This protection is mandated through the Health Insurance Portability and Accountability Act. Individual healthcare organizations employ a variety of safeguards to protect the privacy of health information. Despite these measures data security is a real issue in healthcare, with many hospitals reporting a lack in confidence in their ability to prevent data security breaches ("EHR Coming" 2011). Several well-publicized breaches have occurred in recent years leading to fines, litigation, damaged reputations, credit issues, and identity theft concerns (Dodge 2010; Pike 2008). Some of the greatest risks have come from off-line data such as stolen or lost storage media or computers (Kegley 2010), although increased access to patient healthcare information from points both inside and outside of healthcare facilities and from mobile devices such as personal digital assistants (PDAs), laptops, and smartphones also raise the potential risk of unauthorized access to private health information (Holt 2011). The Growing use of e-mail and Web 2.0 applications for health education, reminders, and other patient-provider communication further increases this risk.

NURSING INFORMATICS AS A SPECIALTY AREA OF PRACTICE

Nursing informatics was first recognized as a specialty by the ANA in 1992. INs are knowledgeable about patient care and technology; for that reason, they provide a valuable communication link between healthcare and technology professionals (Abbott 2002). INs work in hospitals and other healthcare settings, in educational facilities, in research, as consultants, with medical device and software vendors or Web content providers, and in government agencies focusing on disease management.

The *Scope and Standards of Nursing Informatics Practice* (ANA 2001) noted that nursing informatics displays 5 of the 12 defining characteristics that must be present for a nursing specialty. These attributes were derived from earlier work by Styles (1989) and later modified by Panniers and Gassert (1996) and include the following:

- *A differentiated practice.* Nursing informatics differs from other specialties within nursing because it focuses on data, information, and knowledge; the structure and use are the same; and efforts to guarantee that nursing information is represented in efforts to automate health information. It shares an interest in the client, the environment, health, and nurses in other areas of specialty practice.
- *Defined research priorities.* Target areas for research were identified and published in the early 1990s. These centered primarily on the development of a standard language for use within nursing, which would allow nurses from different regions of a country or the world to establish that they were describing the same phenomenon and to conduct studies that could be replicated. In more recent years, survey results identified additional areas deemed critical for research, although the development of a standard nursing language remains crucial. The development of databases for clinical information is another priority area.
- *Representation by one or more organization(s).* This criterion is met because nursing informatics interests are represented by work groups within the AMIA and the IMIA, in a number of regional groups within the United States, and in national groups abroad. Table 1–4 displays some of these groups.
- *Formal educational programs.* Early leaders in nursing informatics obtained their expertise through experience as well as classes in related areas such as computer science and information science. Grant monies from the Division of Nursing of the Health Resources and Services Administration (National Advisory Council on Nurse Education and Practice 1997) were used to establish the first two graduate programs in nursing informatics at the University of Maryland in 1988 and at the University of Utah in 1990.

TABLE 1–4   A Partial Listing of Nursing Informatics Organizations and Groups National
American Medical Informatics Association (AMIA): Nursing Informatics Working Group
Canadian Nursing Informatics Association
Canadian Organisation for Advancement of Computers in Health (COACH)
Health Informatics New Zealand (HINZ): Nursing Informatics Working Group
National League for Nursing (NLN): Nursing Education Research, Technology, and Information Management Advisory Council (NERTIMAC)
American Medical Informatics Association (AMIA): Nursing Informatics Working Group Informatics Special Interest Group
Health Information and Management Systems Society (HIMSS): Nursing Informatics Community
Nursing Specialist Group (NSG) (http://www.bcs.org/category/10013) ANIA-CARING
Regional
Boston Area Nursing Informatics Consortium (BANIC)—Greater Boston Area
Central Savannah River Area Clinical Informatics Network (CSRA—CIN)
Delaware Valley Nursing Computer Network (DVNCN)
Informatics Nurses from Ohio (INFO)
Midwest Nursing Research Section—NI Research Section (MNRS)
North Carolina State Nurses Association Council on NI (CONI)
Nursing Information Systems Council of New England (NISCNE)
Ontario Nursing Informatics Group (ONIG)
International
Health Informatics Society of Australia (HISA)
Nursing Informatics Australia (NIA)
IMIA Nursing Informatics Special Interest Group

There are now several graduate programs as well as certificate programs and doctoral education in this area. Some nurses still elect to enter programs in healthcare informatics and medical informatics as a means to pursue their interests.

- *A credentialing process.* The American Nurses Credentialing Center (ANCC 2001) used the foundation provided by the ANA in its 1994 definition of nursing informatics and scope and standards of practice.

Applicants for the credentialing examination are required to meet the following criteria:

a. A baccalaureate or higher degree in nursing or a baccalaureate in a relevant field
b. A current, active license as a professional nurse in the United States or a legally recognized equivalent in another country
c. The equivalent of 2 years of full-time professional practice as a nurse
d. Thirty contact hours of continuing education applicable to nursing informatics within the past 3 years
e. A minimum of 2,000 hours of practice in informatics nursing in the past 3 years, or a minimum of 12 semester hours of graduate credits in nursing informatics courses with at least 1,000 hours of practice in informatics nursing within the previous 3 years, or completion of a graduate program in nursing informatics that includes at least 200 hours of faculty supervised clinical practicum

The certification examination covers content on the theory; information management principles and database management; human factors; and the analysis, design, implementation, evaluation, support, and marketing of information systems as well as trends and issues (ANCC 2007).

Nursing informatics is a specialty practice within a broader field that shares commonalities with other informatics areas (ANA 2007). It is interdisciplinary in nature. It is important to nursing because it represents the nursing perspective, identifies a practice base for nurses, produces unique knowledge, and provides needed standardized nursing language. INs have a role in developing health policy and in assessing the usability of devices for consumers and other healthcare professionals.

THE ROLES OF THE INFORMATICS NURSE AND INFORMATICS NURSE SPECIALIST

The ANA (2008) revised the language in its Scope of Nursing Informatics Practice statement to be consistent with that used to describe other clinical nurse specialists and to move away from job titles to role functions. The result led to a distinction between the **informatics nurse (IN)** and **informatics nurse specialist (INS)**. The IN refers to the RN who works in the area of informatics. This individual has experience or an interest in the area but no formal informatics preparation. In contrast the INS has advanced, graduate education in nursing informatics or a related field and may hold ANCC certification. Both the IN and the INS may work under a variety of different titles and in various settings. The IN employs strategies that transform data into information and information into knowledge and ensures that information is disseminated at appropriate times for appropriate uses in the healthcare continuum. The INS needs to play an active role in research and theory development and in the design and testing of information systems and the human-computer interface; he or she also needs to help shape policy and serve as an advocate for the design and use of informatics to serve other healthcare professionals and the public. Other facets of the INS role include responsibilities in administration, telehealth, education and professional development, compliance issues, and discovery in databases and analysis. The INS is prepared to assess work processes and subsequently design, select, implement, and evaluate data structures and suggested technology intended to improve productivity and contribute to the body of nursing knowledge. Both the IN and the INS must be aware of uniform language efforts and have a concept of the value of documentation from healthcare information systems.

APPLICATIONS OF NURSING INFORMATICS

Informatics offers many solutions to support the work of healthcare professionals and healthcare consumers as they seek self-help and care (Brennan 2006). Some examples of how informatics and computers support the various areas of nursing and consumer health follow:

Nursing Practice
- Worklists to remind staff of planned nursing interventions
- Computer-generated client documentation including discharge instructions and medication information
- Monitoring devices that record vital signs and other measurements directly into the client record
- Computer-generated nursing care plans and critical pathways
- Automatic billing for supplies or procedures with nursing documentation

- Reminders and prompts that appear during documentation to ensure comprehensive charting
- Quick access to computer-archived patient data from previous encounters
- Online drug information

Nursing Administration
- Automated staff scheduling
- Online bidding for unfilled shifts
- E-mail for improved communication
- Cost analysis and finding trends for budget purposes
- Quality assurance and outcomes analysis
- Patient tracking and placement for case management

Nursing Education
- Online completion of mandatory education requirements
- Online course registration and scheduling
- Computerized student tracking, testing, and grade management
- Course delivery and support for Web-based education
- Remote access to library and Internet resources
- Teleconferencing and Webcast capability
- Presentation software for preparing slides and handouts
- Online test administration
- Communication with students

Nursing Research
- Computerized literature searching
- The adoption of standardized language related to nursing terms
- The ability to find trends in aggregate data, which is data derived from large population groups
- Use of the Internet for obtaining data collection tools and conducting research
- Collaboration with other nurse researchers

These examples demonstrate the importance of information sharing. Nursing informatics, through the use of computers, can facilitate and speed information sharing in all practice areas. For this to be most effective, nurses must have a basic understanding of informatics.

Consumers turn to the Internet for health information and services as well. Additional consumer applications may include:

- Communication with healthcare providers via e-mail and instant messaging
- Remote monitoring and other telehealth services
- Support groups
- Online scheduling

BENEFITS FOR CONSUMERS AND OTHER HEALTHCARE PROFESSIONALS

Nursing informatics benefits nurses and other healthcare professionals and consumers, healthcare organizations, education planners, and resource managers (ANA 2008). For example, other providers can use data collected and documented by nurses using automated systems, thereby helping to eliminate silos of information typically amassed by each individual group. In addition, multidisciplinary critical pathways are used by nurses and providers to plan and document care for a client. The aggregate critical pathway data may be analyzed for trends related to overall effectiveness of client care.

Other healthcare disciplines may have information systems that use data collected by nursing systems. For example, pharmacy information systems make use of data collected by nursing information systems, such as current medications, allergies, client demographic information, and diagnosis. This feature eliminates redundant data collection by different professionals, saving them time. Laboratory information systems may also connect to nursing systems. When a laboratory test is ordered and entered into the computer on the hospital unit, the information is transferred to the laboratory computer system. This replaces handwritten paper requisitions, saving time and improving communication. Similarly, other hospital departments may receive requests for consults.

Other uses of automation within healthcare may also improve communication and increase profitability. One example is inventory control. Healthcare product suppliers use technology to decrease administrative costs and to attract customers with improved inventory control. Specifically, suppliers can more quickly fill orders, check hospital inventory, and allow customers to receive prices and place and confirm orders through information systems. Some suppliers provide the inventory system for customer use. Customers get a more accurate inventory, automatic replacement of supplies as they are used, and the ability to maintain a smaller inventory to reduce costs. This process is known as Web-based purchasing or e-procurement. Thus, client care and consumer demands drive the healthcare delivery system toward working smarter, which is often best accomplished through automation.

Many of the benefits of automation in healthcare are seen with the development of the electronic medical record, which is an electronic version of the client data found in the traditional paper record. Some specific benefits of electronic medical records include the following:

- *Improved access to information.* The electronic medical record can be accessed from several different locations simultaneously, as well as by different levels of providers.
- *Error reduction and improved communication.* Automation eliminates problems associated with illegible handwriting and provides a series of checks and balances.
- *Decreased redundancy of data entry.* For example, allergies and vital signs need be entered only once.
- *Convenience.* Diagnostic images are a part of the record and can be viewed from various locations.
- *Decreased time spent in medication administration and documentation.* Automation facilitates efficient medication administration and allows direct entry from monitoring equipment, as well as point-of-care data entry.
- *Increased time for client care.* More time is available for client care because less time is required for documentation and transcription of physician orders.
- *Facilitation of data collection for research.* Electronically stored client records provide quick access to clinical data for a large number of clients.
- *Improved quality of documentation.* Prompts help to ensure that key information is noted.
- *Improved compliance with regulatory requirements.* Automated systems can require information needed for regulatory bodies, ensuring that it is included in documentation.
- *Improved record security.* Access to the health record is limited to individuals with computer access.
- *Improved quality of care and patient satisfaction.* Built-in tools remind nurses to provide interventions appropriate for certain patient problems.
- *Decreased administrative costs for location and maintenance of client records.*
- *Creation of a lifetime clinical record facilitated by information systems.*

Other benefits of automation are related to decision-support software and computer programs that organize information to aid in decision making for client care or administrative issues. Some of the benefits that can be realized with these systems include the following:

- Decision-support tools as well as alerts and reminders notify the clinician of possible concerns or omissions. For example, the client states an allergy to penicillin, and this is documented in the computer system. The physician orders an antibiotic that is a variation of penicillin, and this order is entered into the computer system. An alert informs the clinician that a potential allergic reaction may result and asks for verification of the order.
- With access to reference databases, nurses can easily review information on medications, diseases, and treatments as part of the automated system.
- Effective data management and trend-finding include the ability to provide historical or current data reports.
- Extensive financial information can be collected and analyzed for trends. Information related to cost by diagnosis and treatment can be more easily tracked using computer systems. For example, one can determine the least expensive drug that is effective for a particular diagnosis.
- Data related to treatment such as inpatient length of stay and the lowest level of care provider required could be used to decrease costs.

EDUCATIONAL OPPORTUNITIES FOR NURSING INFORMATICS

Informatics programs have grown since the first recommendations for the education of healthcare professionals in the field in the 1970s. The Health and Medical Informatics Education workgroup of the IMIA (2000) developed recommendations for programs by level and discipline, with a particular focus on skills for information processing and communication technology as a foundation. This group defined learning outcomes for all health professionals as users of IT as well as learning outcomes for informatics specialists. The work of this group provided a framework for curriculum development. Informatics was first introduced into schools of nursing in the late 1970s with the State University of New York at Buffalo offering a course on computers and nursing (Tallberg, Saba, & Carr 2006). In subsequent years other groups offered conferences and training for nurses on the use of IT. The EDUCTRA project of the European Advanced Informatics in Medicine Programme and the IT-EDUCTRA project of the Telematics Applications Programme, Health Sector provided training materials and courses (Hasman 1998). The European Union funded the Nightingale Project during the 1990s (Mantas 1998). Professional groups also played a part in this process.

Graduate, doctoral, and certificate programs are now available in nursing informatics. Projections for the number of INs needed range from Gugerty's (2006) figure of 6,000 to 12,000 to estimates of 50,000. Nursing, healthcare, clinical informatics graduate programs and biomedical informatics programs collectively lag behind projected needs. This is due, in part, to a lack of sufficient numbers of qualified faculty.

Abundant continuing education opportunities exist to help bridge the gap between undergraduate and graduate programs and help nurses with preparation in the field up-to-date. The Health Information Technology Scholars Program (HITS 2007) is a year-long faculty development program first offered in 2008 as a result of a collaborative effort among the Universities of Kansas, Colorado, and Indiana and the NLN. The AMIA sought to provide 10,000 clinicians with training in applied health and medical informatics by the year 2010 (AMIA 2007). AMIA training continues with an internationally focused variation of the successful 10x10 program called i10x10 (AMIA 2011).

The HITECH Act provided additional funding for informatics education and training. These included:

- The establishment of Regional Extension Centers to provide information and assistance to providers striving to become meaningful users of EHRs
- Monies for institutions of higher education (or consortia) to support curriculum development in HIT
- Efforts to create or expand intense, nondegree Community College programs designed to be completed in 6 months or less
- A component of the Health IT Workforce Program designed to rapidly prepare persons to serve in designated HIT professional roles
- The establishment and initial administration of a set of health IT competency examinations (ONC 2011)

FUTURE DIRECTIONS

Nursing informatics has an important role to play in the improvement of health through its contributions to the development of standard languages, design and evaluation of IT, assisting peers to develop the competencies needed in an increasingly complex environment, facilitating consumer acceptance and use of technology, and contributions to nursing's scientific body of knowledge (Brennan 2006; Saranto et al. 2006; Strachan, Delaney, & Sensmeier 2006). IN specialists must serve as leaders to help drive the changes necessary to transform the healthcare delivery system, improve quality of services delivery, and improve safety. *Nursing Informatics: The scope and standards of practice* (ANA 2008) noted that the discipline is changing rapidly. Some of the competencies now associated with INs and specialists will transition downward to nurses in general practice. There will be a continued blur between nursing informatics and other health informatics with more interdisciplinary projects. New technologies will impact the practice of nursing informatics in ways that cannot be forecast at present. Nanotechnology, genomics, robotics, wearable monitoring devices, and new developments in educational technology represent some of these new technologies. New educational models are needed to incorporate informatics competencies, and new care models must be developed.

Emerging Trends

The drive for patient safety, transparency in healthcare, error reduction, increased efficiency, and additional requirements on the part of regulatory agencies will continue to shape healthcare delivery and informatics practice for many years to come. Consumers will assume a greater responsibility for their healthcare choices as they shoulder a larger portion of the costs.

Role Changes

As the practice of nursing informatics continues to evolve so will the roles of the IN and INS. This evolution will occur in response to the ongoing growth of the nursing profession, changes within the healthcare delivery system, and informatics in general. This process will result in additional differentiation between the levels of practice now seen. These changes will require the INS to actively work to keep aware and abreast of these developments.

Interactions with Consumers

Nursing informatics has been virtually invisible to healthcare consumers up to this point in time. This will change as more professionals specialize in this area of informatics practice either to help consumers to better manage their healthcare conditions through the design and testing of monitoring devices and human-computer interfaces or by helping consumers become more discriminating consumers of Web-based information, whether it represents comparable data on providers or details on specific conditions.

Issues

While the development of nursing informatics promises to deliver many benefits, it will not be without a few bumps along the way. There are many different informatics groups within healthcare. Ideally they present a united front and work together. Individuals are confronted with several choices for entry into the field both in area of focus and programs of study.

Visit nursing.pearsonhighered.com for additional cases, information, and weblinks.

CASE STUDY EXERCISE

A client arrives in the emergency department with shortness of breath and complaining of chest pain. Describe how informatics can help nurses and other healthcare providers to more efficiently help the client.

SUMMARY

- Data are a collection of numbers, characters, or facts that are gathered according to some perceived need or analysis and possibly for action at a later point in time.
- Data have little meaning alone, but a collection of data can be examined for patterns and structure that can be interpreted. At this point, data become information.
- Knowledge is the synthesis of information derived from several sources to produce a single concept or idea.
- Healthcare delivery systems are knowledge-intensive settings with nurses as the largest group of knowledge workers within those systems. Information technology offers several tools to support nurses and other healthcare workers in their knowledge work.
- Good information management ensures access to the right information at the right time to the people who need it. This is particularly important when the volume of information exceeds human processing capacity.
- Informatics is the application of computer and statistical techniques to the management of information.
- Nursing informatics is the use of information and computer technology as a tool to process information to support all areas of nursing, including practice, education, administration, and research. The definition of nursing informatics continues to evolve.
- A formal definition of nursing informatics serves to shape job descriptions and educational preparation for informatics practice.
- Nursing informatics is a necessity, not a luxury, in today's rapidly changing healthcare delivery system. All nurses need basic informatics skills.
- Computer technology facilitates the collection of data for analysis, which can be used to justify the efficacy of particular interventions and improve the quality of care.
- Other healthcare providers also benefit from nursing informatics.
- Nursing informatics allows nurses to have better control over data management.
- According to the American Nurses Association the informatics nurse specialist (INS) has advanced graduate education in nursing informatics or a related field and may hold ANCC certification in informatics whereas the informatics nurse is a nurse who works in informatics or has an interest in the area but does not have formal informatics preparation.

- Current educational programs fall short of providing the number of needed INSs.
- New technologies will impact the practice of nursing informatics in ways that cannot be forecast at present.
- Nursing informatics will continue to evolve with changes in the profession, the healthcare delivery system, and informatics in general.
- Consumer interactions will become an increasingly important part of nursing informatics practice.

REFERENCES

Aarts, J., & Koppel, R. (2009). Implementation of computerized physician order entry in seven countries. *Health Affairs (Project Hope), 28*(2), 404–414.

Abbott, P. A. (2002). Introducing nursing informatics. *Nursing, 32*(1), 14.

Academic Medical Publishing & CancerWEB. (1997). *On-line medical dictionary.* Retrieved December 28, 2002, from http://cancerweb.ncl.ac.uk/cgi-bin/omd?query=informatics&action=Search+OMD

Ackoff, R. (1989). From data to wisdom. *Journal of Applied Systems Analysis, 16,* 3–7.

Agency for Healthcare Research and Quality (AHRQ). (2006). *The Patient Safety and Quality Improvement Act of 2005, Overview.* Retrieved June 13, 2007, from http://www.ahrq.gov/qual/psoact.htm

Agency for Healthcare Research and Quality (AHRQ). (2010). *AHRQ study shows using bar-code technology with eMAR reduces medication administration and transcription errors.* Press Release, May 5, 2010. Agency for Healthcare Research and Quality, Rockville, MD. http://www.ahrq.gov/news/press/pr2010/emarpr.htm

Agency for Healthcare Research and Quality (AHRQ). (2011). Welcome to the PCMH Resource Center. Retrieved from http://www.pcmh.ahrq.gov/portal/server.pt/community/pcmh__home/1483

Agency for Healthcare Research and Quality (AHRQ). (n.d.). About the health care report card compendium. Retrieved October 31, 2011, from https://www.talkingquality.ahrq.gov/content/reportcard/about.aspx

Alliance for Health Reform. (2006, December). *Linking providers via health information networks.* Washington, DC: Alliance for Health Reform.

American Academy of Nursing. (2010). *Workforce commission.* Retrieved from http://www.aannet.org/i4a/pages/index.cfm?pageID=3293

American Association of Colleges of Nursing (AACN). (1996). *The essentials of master's education for advanced practice nursing.* Retrieved from http://www.aacn.nche.edu/Education/pdf/MasEssentials96.pdf

American Association of Colleges of Nursing (AACN). (1998). *Essentials of baccalaureate education for professional nursing practice.* Washington, DC: AACN.

American Association of Colleges of Nursing (AACN). (2006). *The essentials of doctoral education for advanced nursing practice.* Retrieved from http://www.aacn.nche.edu/publications/position/dnpessentials.pdf

American Association of Colleges of Nursing (AACN). (2008). *The essentials of baccalaureate education for professional nursing practice.* Retrieved from http://www.aacn.nche.edu/Education/pdf/BaccEssentials08.pdf

American Association of Colleges of Nursing (AACN). (2011a). *About AACN.* Retrieved from http://www.aacn.nche.edu/ContactUs/index.htm

American Association of Colleges of Nursing (AACN). (2011b). *The essentials of master's education in nursing.* Retrieved from http://www.aacn.nche.edu/Education/pdf/Master'sEssentials11.pdf

American Hospital Association. (2002). *In our hands: How hospital leaders can build a thriving workforce.* Washington, DC: Author.

American Medical Informatics Association (AMIA). (2007, July 25). AMIA 10x10™. Retrieved November 13, 2007, from http://www.amia.org/10x10/

American Medical Informatics Association (AMIA). (2011). 10x10 courses. Retrieved from http://www.amia.org/education/10x10-courses

American Nurses Association (ANA). (2001). *Scope and standards of nursing informatics practice.* Washington, DC: American Nurses Publishing.

American Nurses Association (ANA). (2006). *Essential nursing competencies and curricula guidelines for genetics and genomics.* Retrieved November 6, 2007, from http://www.genome.gov/Pages/Careers/HealthProfessionalEducation/geneticscompetency.pdf

American Nurses Association (ANA). (2008). *Nursing informatics: Scope and standards of practice.* Washington, DC: Nursesbooks.org.

American Nurses Association, Council on Computer Applications in Nursing. (1992). *Report on the designation of nursing informatics as a nursing specialty.* Congress of Nursing Practice unpublished report. Washington, DC: American Nurses Association.

American Nurses Credentialing Center (ANCC). (2001). *Computer based testing for ANCC certification.* Retrieved December 11, 2002, from http://www.nursingworld.org/ancc/certify/cert/catalogs/CBT.PDF

American Nurses Credentialing Center (ANCC). (2007). *Informatics nurse certification.* Retrieved June 19, 2007, from http://www.nursecredentialing.org/cert/eligibility/informatics.html

American Nurses Credentialing Center (ANCC). (2011). *Program overview.* Retrieved from http://www.nursecredentialing.org/Magnet/ProgramOverview.aspx

Anderson, S. (1992). *Computer literacy for health care professionals.* New York: Delmar.

Apoid, J., Daniels, T., & Sanneborn, M. (2006). Promoting collaboration and transparency in patient safety. *Journal on Quality and Patient Safety, 32*(12), 672–675.

Arnold, J. M. (1996). Nursing informatics educational needs. *Computers in Nursing, 14*(6), 333–339.

Association of College and Research Libraries (ACRL). (2002). *Information literacy competency standards for higher education.* Retrieved November 18, 2002, from http://www.ala.org/acrl/ilintro.html#ildef

Ayer, A. J. (1966). *The problem of knowledge.* Baltimore, MD: Penguin.

Ball, M. J., & Hannah, K. J. (1984). *Using computers in nursing.* Reston, VA: Reston Publishing.

Barton, A. J. (2005). Cultivating informatics competencies in a community of practice. *Nursing Administration Quarterly, 29*(4), 323–328.

Bauer, J. C. (2006). Patient safety: Getting it right by doing it backwards. *Journal of Healthcare Information Management, 20*(4), 5–7.

Bemmel, J. H., & Musen, M. A. (Eds.). (1997). *Handbook of medical informatics.* New York: Springer.

Bleich, M. R., Connolly, C., Davis, K., Hewlett, P. O., & Hill, K. S. (2006). In B. J. Hatcher (Ed.). *Wisdom at work: The importance of the older and experienced nurse in the workplace.* Princeton, NJ: The Robert Wood Johnson Foundation. Retrieved from http://www.rwjf.org/files/publications/other/wisdomatwork.pdf

Bolton, L. B., Gassert, C. A., & Cipriano, P. F. (2008). Smart technology, enduring solutions. *Journal of Healthcare Information Management, 22*(4), 24–30.

Booth, R. G. (2006). Educating the future ehealth professional nurse. *International Journal of Nursing Education Scholarship, 3*(1), 1–10.

Brennan, P. F. (2006). Nursing informatics and the NIH roadmap. In C. A. Weaver, C. W. Delaney, P. Weber, & R. L. Carr (Eds.), *Nursing and informatics for the 21st century: An international look at practice, trends, and the future.* Chicago: Healthcare Information and Management Systems Society, pp. 483–488.

Burroughs, T. E., Waterman, A. D., Gallagher, T. H., Waterman, B., Jeffe, D. B., Dunagan, W. C., . . . Fraser, V. J. (2007). Patients' concerns about medical errors during hospitalization. *Journal of Quality and Patient Safety, 33*(1), 5–14.

CDW Healthcare. (2011, March 8). *Elevated heart rates: EHR and IT security report.* Retrieved from http://webobjects.cdw.com/webobjects/media/pdf/Newsroom/CDW-Healthcare-Elevated-Heart-Rates-EHR-and-IT-Security-Report-0311.pdf

Centers for Medicare & Medicaid Services (CMS). (n.d.). *Eligible professional meaningful use table of contents core and menu set measures.* Retrieved from http://www.cms.gov/EHRIncentivePrograms/Downloads/EP-MU-TOC.pdf

Consumer Influence on Technology Investments. (2006). *Healthcare Financial Management, 60*(9), 153–154.

Courey, T., Benson-Soros, J., Deemer, K., & Zeller, R. A. (2006). The missing link: Information literacy and evidence-based practice as a new challenge for nurse educators. *Nursing Education Perspectives, 27*(6), 320–323.

Cousins, D. H., & Baker, M. (2004, May). The work of the National Patient Safety Agency to improve medication safety. *British Journal of General Practice, 332*–333.

Davenport, T. H., Thomas, R. J., & Cantrell, S. (2002). The mysterious art and science of knowledge worker performance. *MIT Sloan Management Review, 44*(1), 23. http://web.ebscohost.com/ehost/detail?vid =22&hid=22&sid=ed572e2cceb3–4e61–8144–2dbf9023e1ce%40sessionmgr2–bib4up#bib4up

Davidson, C., & Voss, P. (2002). *Knowledge management: An introduction to creating competitive advantage from intellectual capital.* Auckland: Tandem Press.

Desjardins, K. S., Cook, S. S., Jenkins, M., & Bakken, S. (2005). Effect of an informatics for evidence-based practice curriculum on nursing informatics competencies. *International Journal of Medical Informatics, 74*(11/12), 1012–1020.

Devine, E., Williams, E., Martin, D., Sittig, D., Tarczy-Hornoch, P., Payne, T., & Sullivan, S. (2010). Prescriber and staff perceptions of an electronic prescribing system in primary care: A qualitative assessment. *BMC Medical Informatics and Decision Making,* 1072.

DiCecco, K. L. (2005). Information literacy, part II: Knowledge and ability in the traditional resources. *Journal of Legal Nurse Consulting, 16*(4), 15–22.

Dodge, J. (2010). Data breach. *Health Data Management, 18*(9), 40.

Donley, R. (2005). Challenges for nursing in the 21st century. *Nursing Economics, 23*(6), 312–318.

Doucette, J. N. (2006).View from the cockpit: What the airline industry can teach us about patient safety. *Nursing, 36*(11), 50–53.

Dreher, M. C., & Miller, J. F. (2006). Information technology: The foundation for educating nurses as clinical leaders. In C. A. Weaver, C. W. Delaney, P. Weber, & R. L. Carr (Eds.), *Nursing and informatics for the 21st century: An international look at practice, trends, and the future.* Chicago: Healthcare Information and Management Systems Society, pp. 29–34.

Educational Testing Service. (2007). iSkills assessment. Retrieved June 1, 2007, from http://www. ets.org/portal/site/ets/menuitem.1488512ecfd5b8849a77b13bc3921509/?vgnextoid= fde9af5e44df4010VgnVCM10000022f95190RCRD&vgnextchannel=cd7314ee98459010 VgnVCM10000022f95190RCRD#WhatProficiency

EHR coming on strong, but so are security risks. (2011). *Healthcare Risk Management, 33*(3), 32–34.

Engelhardt, H. T., Jr. (1980). Knowing and valuing: Looking for common roots. In H. T. Engelhardt & D. Callahan (Eds.), *Knowing and valuing: The search for common roots* (Vol. 4, pp. 1–17). New York: Hastings Center.

Food and Drug Administration (FDA). (2004). *FDA issues bar code regulation.* Retrieved June 19, 2007, from http://www.fda.gov/oc/initiatives/barcodesadr/fs-barcode.html.

Garde, S., Harrison, D., & Hovenga, E. (2005). Skill needs for nurses in their role as health informatics professionals: A survey in the context of global health informatics education. *International Journal of Medical Informatics, 74*(11/12), 899–907.

Gaylin, D., Moiduddin, A., Mohamoud, S., Lundeen, K., & Kelly, J. (2011). Public attitudes about health information technology, and its relationship to health care quality, costs, and privacy. *Health Services Research, 46*(3), 920–938. doi:10.1111/j.1475-6773.2010.01233.x

Gluck, J., & Baltes, P. B. (2006). Using the concept of wisdom to enhance the expression of wisdom knowledge: Not the philosopher's dream but differential effects of developmental preparedness. *Psychology and Aging, 21*(4), 679–690.

Gooch, J. J. (2006, October 1). Providers and payers work to ease into e-prescribing. *Managed Healthcare Executive,* Retrieved November 13, 2007, from http://www.managedhealthcareexecutive .com/mhe/Technology/Providers-andpayers-work-to-ease-into-e-prescribi/ArticleStandard/ Article/detail/376826

Graves, J. R., & Corcoran, S. (1989). The study of nursing informatics. *Journal of Nursing Scholarship, 21,* 227–231.

Guenther, J. T., & Caruth, M. P. (2006). Mapping the literature of nursing informatics. *Journal of the Medical Library Association, 94*(2) Supplement, E92–E98.

Gugerty, B. (2006). The state of informatics training and education for nurses. *Journal of Healthcare Information Management, 20*(1), 23–24.

Haase-Herrick, K. S., & Herrin, D. M. (2007). The American Organization of Nurse Executives' Guiding Principles and American Association of Colleges of Nursing's Clinical Nurse Leader: A lesson in synergy. *Journal of Nursing Administration, 37*(2), 55–60.

Hannah, K. (1985). Current trends in nursing informatics: Implications for curriculum planning. In K. Hannah, E. Guillemin, & D. Conklin (Eds.), *Nursing uses of computer and information science.* Proceedings of the IFIP-IMIA International Symposium on Nursing Uses of Computers and Information Science. Amsterdam: Elsevier Science.

Harsanyi, B. E., Lehmkuhl, D., Hott, R., Myers, S., & McGeehan, L. (1994). Nursing informatics: The key to managing and evaluating quality. In S. J. Grobe & E. S. P. Puyter-Wenting (Eds.), *Nursing informatics: An international overview for nursing in a technological era.* Proceedings of the Fifth IMIA International Conference on Nursing Use of Computers and Information Science, San Antonio, TX, pp. 655–659.

Hart, K. A. (2007). The aging workforce: Implications for health care organizations. *Nursing Economics, 25*(2), 101–102.

Hasman, A. (1998). Education and training in health informatics: The IT-EDUCTRA project. *International Journal of Medical Informatics, 50*(1–3), 179–185.

Hatcher, B. J., (Ed.), Bleich, M. R., Connolly, C., Davis, K., Hewlett, P. O., & Hill, K. S. (2006). *Wisdom at work.* The Robert Wood Johnson Foundation.

Healthcare.gov. (2011). *Accountable care organizations: Improving care coordination for people with Medicare.* Retrieved from http://www.healthcare.gov/news/factsheets/accountablecare03312011a.html

Healthcare Information and Management Systems Society (HIMSS). (2002). *Using innovative technology to enhance patient care delivery.* A report delivered by the Improving Operational Efficiency through Elimination of Waste and Redundancy Work Group at the American Academy of Nursing Technology and Workforce Conference in Washington, DC. Retrieved January 1, 2003, from http://www.himss.org/content/files/AANNsgSummitHIMSSFINAL_18770.pdf

Hebert, M. (1999). *National Nursing Informatics Project discussion paper.* Retrieved June 24, 2003, from http://www.cna-nurses.ca/pages/resources/nni/nni_discussion_paper.doc

Heller, B. F., Oros, M. T., & Durney-Crowley, J. (2003, June 24). The future of nursing education: Ten trends to watch. *NLN Journal.* Retrieved June 24, 2003, from http://www.nln.org/nlnjournal/infotrends.htm

HHS.gov/Recovery. (2011). *Comparative effectiveness research funding.* Retrieved from http://www.hhs.gov/recovery/programs/cer/index.html

HIMSS Nursing Task Force. (2007). The TIGER update: Facilitating collaboration among participating organizations to achieve the TIGER vision. Retrieved June 27, 2007, from http://www.himss.org/handouts/TIGER_PhaseII_Collaboratives.pdf

HITS: Health Information Technology Scholars Program. (2007). Retrieved November 13, 2007, from http://www.hits-colab.org/index.htm

Hobbs, S. D. (2002). Measuring nurses' computer competency: An analysis of published instruments. *Computers, Informatics, Nursing, 20*(2), 63–73.

Hohenhaus, S., Powell, S., & Hohenhaus, J. T. (2006). Enhancing patient safety during hand-offs. *American Journal of Nursing, 106*(8), 72A–72D.

Holt, C. (2011). Emerging technologies: Web 2.0. *Health Information Management Journal, 40*(1), 33–35.

Hulford, P., Gough, K., & Krieger, M. (2007). Making business intelligence 'End-user friendly' with Cognos 8 Go! Search and the Google Search Appliance. A Ziff Davis Webcast sponsored by Cognos. Retrieved February 17, 2007 from www.eseminarslive.com

Informatics Education. (2000). *Recommendations of the IMIA on education in health and medical informatics.* Retrieved November 13, 2007, from http://www.imia.org/pubdocs/rec_english.pdf

Institute for Healthcare Improvement (IHI). (2007). *Protecting 5 million lives from harm.* Retrieved June 11, 2007, from http://www.ihi.org/IHI/Programs/Campaign/Campaign.htm?TabId=1

Institute for Healthcare Improvement (IHI). (2011). About IHI. Retrieved from http://www.ihi.org/IHI/About/aboutusindex.htm

Institute of Medicine (IOM). (1999). *To err is human: Building a safer health system.* Washington, DC: National Academies Press.

Institute of Medicine (IOM). (2001). *Crossing the quality chasm: A new health system for the 21st century.* Washington, DC: National Academies Press.

Institute of Medicine (IOM). (2004). *Keeping patients safe: Transforming the work environment of nurses.* Washington, DC: National Academies Press.

Institute of Medicine (IOM). (2006). *Rewarding provider performance: Aligning incentives in Medicare.* Washington, DC: National Academies Press.

Institute of Medicine (IOM). (2007). *The learning healthcare system: Workshop summary.* Washington, DC: National Academies Press.

International Council of Nurses. (2010). Pillars & programmes. Retrieved from http://www.icn.ch/pillarsprograms/pillars-a-programmes/

International Medical Informatics Association. (2003). The Special Interest Group on Nursing Informatics. Retrieved April 7, 2004, from http://www.IMIA. org/NI/

International Medical Informatics Association Working Group I: Health and Medical Informatics Education. (2000). *Recommendations of the IMIA on education in health and medical informatics.* Retrieved November 12, 2007, from http://www.imia.org/pubdocs/rec_english.pdf

Joint Commission for Accreditation of Healthcare Organizations (JCAHO). (2007). *About the Joint Commission.* Retrieved June 13, 2007, from http://www.jointcommission.org/AboutUs/

Joint Commission International Center for Patient Safety. (2007). *World Alliance for Patient Safety.* Retrieved June 11, 2007, from http://www.jcipatientsafety.org/14685

Kegley, J. (2010). Avoid being the next data-security-breach headline. *Health Management Technology, 31*(9), 18–19.

Khajouei, R., & Jaspers, M. (2008). CPOE system design aspects and their qualitative effect on usability. *Studies in Health Technology and Informatics,* 136309–136314.

Kim, C., Majka, D., & Sussman, J. H. (2011). Modeling the impact of healthcare reform. *Healthcare Financial Management, 65*(1), 50–60.

Kisilowska, M. (2006). Knowledge management prerequisites for building an information society in healthcare. *International Journal of Medical Informatics, 75*(Issue 3/4), 322–329.

Manno, M., Hogan, P., Heberlein, V., Nyakiti, J., & Mee, C. L. (2006). Patient-safety survey report. *Nursing, 36*(5), 54–63.

Mantas, J. (1998). Developing curriculum in nursing informatics in Europe. *International Journal of Medical Informatics, 50*(1–3), 123–132.

McBride, A. B. (2006). Informatics and the future of nursing practice. In C. A. Weaver, C. W. Delaney, P. Weber, & R. L. Carr (Eds). *Nursing and informatics for the 21st century: An international look at practice, trends, and the future.* Chicago: Healthcare Information and Management Systems Society, pp. 5–12.

McCoy, M. J. (2006). Advanced clinician order management—A superset of CPOE. *Journal of Healthcare Information Management, 19*(4), 11–13.

McDermott Will & Emery. (2009, February 20). *Economic stimulus package: Policy implications of the financial incentives to promote health IT and new privacy and security protections.* Retrieved from http://www.mwe.com/info/news/wp0209e.pdf

McDowell, D. E., & Ma, X. (2007). Computer literacy in baccalaureate nursing students during the last 8 years. *Computers, Informatics, Nursing, 25*(1), 30–36.

McNeil, B. J., Elfrink, V. L., Pierce, S. T., Beyea, S. C., Bickford, C. J., & Averill, C. (2005). *International Journal of Medical Informatics, 74*(Issue 11/12), 1021–1030.

Middleton, B. (2009). The clinical decision support consortium. *Studies in Health Technology and Informatics,* 15026–15030.

Miller, E. A., & West, D. M. (2009). Where's the Revolution? Digital technology and health care in the Internet age. *Journal of Health Politics, Policy and Law, 34*(2), doi: 10.1215/03616878-2008-046

Murray, A. J. (2000). Knowledge management and consciousness. *Advances in Mind–Body Medicine, 16*(3), 233(5p).

Nath, C. (2007). Literacy and diabetes self-management. *American Journal of Nursing, 107*(6 supplement), 43–49.

National Advisory Council on Nurse Education and Practice (NACNEP). (1997). *A national agenda for nursing education and practice.* Rockville, MD: U.S. Department of Health and Human Services, Health Resources and Services Administration.

National League for Nursing (NLN). (2007). *NLN News National League for Nursing issues call for faculty development and curricular initiatives in informatics.* Retrieved from http://www.nln.org/newsreleases/informatics_release_052908.htm

National League for Nursing (NLN). (2008). *Preparing the next generation of nurses to practice in a technology-rich environment: An informatics agenda.* Retrieved from http://www.nln.org/aboutnln/PositionStatements/informatics_052808.pdf

Newbold, S. K. (2002). FAQs about nursing informatics. *Nursing, 32*(3), 20.

Nugent, C., Wallace, J., Kernohan, G., McCreight, B., Mulvenna, M., & Martin, S. (2007). Using context awareness within the 'Smart home' environment to support social care for adults with dementia. *Technology & Disability, 19*(2/3), 143–152.

Nursing Informatics: Special Interest Group of the International Medical Informatics Association (IMIA-NI). (1998). Proceedings of the General Assembly Meeting, Seoul, Korea.

Office of the National Coordinator for Health Information Technology (ONC). (May 5, 2011). *HITECH and funding opportunities.* Retrieved from http://healthit.hhs.gov/portal/server.pt/community/healthit_hhs_gov__hitech_and_funding_opportunities/1310

Ornes, L. L., & Gassert, C. (2007). Computer competencies in a BSN program. *Journal of Nursing Education, 46*(2), 75–78.

Panniers, T. L., & Gassert, C. A. (1996). Standards of practice and preparation for certification. In M. E. Mills, C. A. Romano, & B. R. Heller (Eds.), *Information management in nursing and health care.* Springhouse, PA: Springhouse Corporation, pp. 280–297.

Pesut, D. J. (2006). 21st century nursing knowledge work: Reasoning into the future. In C. A. Weaver, C. W. Delaney, P. Weber, & R. L. Carr (Eds.), *Nursing and informatics for the 21st century: An international look at practice, trends, and the future.* Chicago: Healthcare Information and Management Systems Society, pp. 13–21.

Pike, G. (2008). VA data breach and the privacy act. *Information Today, 25*(2), 15.

Pravikoff, D. S., Tanner, A. B., & Pierce, S. T. (2005). Readiness of U.S. nurses for evidence-based practice. *American Journal of Nursing, 105*(9), 40–51.

Quality and Safety Education for Nurses (QSEN). (2011). *Project overview.* Retrieved from http://www.qsen.org/overview.php

Rabinowitz, A. B. K., Clarke, J. R., Marella, W., Johnston, J., Baker, L., & Doering, M. (2006). Translating patient safety legislation into health care practice. *Journal on Quality and Patient Safety, 32*(12), 676–681.

Rahimi, B., Timpka, T., Vimarlund, V., Uppugunduri, S., & Svensson, M. (2009). Organization-wide adoption of computerized provider order entry systems: A study based on diffusion of innovations theory. *BMC Medical Informatics and Decision Making*, 952.

Rath, P. (2011). Shhh! Patient safety includes keeping secrets. *ASRT Scanner, 43*(4), 23.

Rogers, G., Alper, E., Brunelle, D., Federico, F., Fenn, C. A., Leape, L. L., . . . Annas, C. L. (2006). *Joint Commission Journal on Quality and Patient Safety, 32*(1), 37–50.

Saba, V., & McCormick, K. (1996). *Essentials of computers for nurses.* New York: McGraw-Hill.

Saba, V. K. (2001). Nursing informatics: Yesterday, today and tomorrow. *International Nursing Review, 48*(3), 177.

Sandars, J., & Heller, R. (2006). Improving the implementation of evidence-based practice: A knowledge management perspective. *Journal of Evaluation in Clinical Practice, 12*(3), 341–346.

Saranto, K., Weber, P., Hayrinen, K., Kouri, P., Porrasmaa, J., Komulainen, J., . . . Jauhiainen, A. (2006). Citizen empowerment: Ehealth consumerism in Europe. In C. A. Weaver, C. W. Delaney, P. Weber, & R. L. Carr (Eds.), *Nursing and informatics for the 21st century: An international look at practice, trends, and the future.* Chicago: Healthcare Information and Management Systems Society, pp. 489–500.

Scholes, M., & Barber, B. (1980). Towards nursing informatics. In D. A. Lindberg & S. Kaihari (Eds.), *Medinfo, 80* (pp. 70–73). London: North-Holland.

Schwirian, P. (1986). The NI pyramid—A model for research in nursing informatics. *Computers in Nursing, 4*(3), 134–136.

Sensmeier, J. (2007). The future of IT? Aggressive educational reform. *Nursing Management, 38*(9—Supplement: IT Solutions), 2, 4, 6, 8.

Shendell-Falik, N., Feinson, M., & Mohr, B. J. (2007). Enhancing patient safety. *Journal of Nursing Administration, 37*(2), 95–104.

Sidlow, R., & Katz-Sidlow, R. J. (2006). Using a computerized sign-out system to improve physician–nurse communication. *Journal on Quality and Patient Safety, 32*(1), 32–33.

Simpson, R. (2006). Automation: The vanguard of EBN. *Nursing Management* (June), 13–14.

Simpson, R. (2007). Information technology: Building nursing intellectual capital for the information age. *Nursing Administration Quarterly, 31*(1), 84–88.

Simpson, R. L. (2005). Error reporting as a preventive force. *Nursing Management, 36*(6), 21–24, 56.

Singh, S. P., Hummel, J., & Walton, G. S. (2005). Consumer driven healthcare: Strategic, operational, and information technology implications for today's healthcare CIO. *Journal of Healthcare Information Management, 19*(4), 49–54.

Skiba, D. J. (2005). Preparing for evidence-based practice: Revisiting information literacy. *Nursing Education Perspectives, 26*(5), 310–311.

Smedley, A. (2005). The importance of informatics competencies in nursing: An Australian perspective. *CIN: Computers, Informatics, Nursing, 23*(2), 106–110.

Snyder-Halpern, R., Corcoran-Perry, S., & Narayan, S. (2001). Developing clinical practice environments supporting the knowledge work of nurses. *Computers in Nursing, 19*(1), 17–23.

Spurr, R. (2007). Portal to a golden age. *Health Management Technology, 28*(4), 44–43.

Staggers, N., Gassert, C. A., & Curran, C. (2001). Informatics competencies for nurses at four levels of practice. *Journal of Nursing Education, 40*(7), 303–316.

Staggers, N., & Thompson, C. B. (2002). The evolution of definitions for nursing informatics: A critical analysis and revised definition. *Journal of the American Medical Informatics Association, 9*(3), 255–261.

Steyn, G. M. (2004). Harnessing the power of knowledge in higher education. *Education, 124*(4), 615–630.

Strachan, H., Delaney, C. W., & Sensmeier, J. (2006). Looking to the future: Informatics and nursing's opportunities. In C. A. Weaver, C. W. Delaney, P. Weber, & R. L. Carr (Eds). *Nursing and informatics for the 21st century: An international look at practice, trends, and the future.* Chicago: Healthcare Information and Management Systems Society, pp. 507–516.

Styles, M. (1989). *On specialization in nursing: Toward a new empowerment.* Kansas City, MO: American Nurses Foundation.

Tallberg, M., Saba, V. K., & Carr, R. L. (2006). The international emergence of nursing informatics. In C. A. Weaver, C. W. Delaney, P. Weber, & R. L. Carr (Eds.), *Nursing and informatics for the 21st century: An international look at practice, trends, and the future.* Chicago: Healthcare Information and Management Systems Society, pp. 45–51.

Technology Informatics Guiding Education Reform (TIGER). (2007). *The TIGER Initiative.* Retrieved May 31, 2007, from www.tigersummit.com

Thompson, C. A. (2005, August 1). JCAHO views medication reconciliation as adverse-event prevention. *American Journal of Health-System Pharmacy, 62*, 1528, 1530, 1532.

Thomson Reuters. (2011a, March 28). *100 top hospitals: Study overview and research findings,* 18th ed. Retrieved from http://100tophospitals.com/assets/100%20Top%20Hospitals%20National%202011%20Abstract.pdf

Thomson Reuters. (2011b, August). *100 top hospitals: CEO insights: Keys to success and future challenges.* Retrieved from http://100tophospitals.com/assets/CEOInsightsResearchPaper.pdf

TIGER Initiative. (n.d.). *Collaborating to integrate evidence and informatics into nursing practice and education: An executive summary.* Retrieved from http://www.tigersummit.com/uploads/TIGER_Collaborative_Exec_Summary_040509.pdf

Trossman, S. (2006a). Staying power? Retaining mature RNs in the workforce. *American Journal of Nursing, 106*(7), 77–78.

Trossman, S. (2006b, November–December). Show us the data! NDNQI helps nurses link their care to quality. *The American Nurse, 1*, 6.

Turley, J. P. (1996). Toward a model of nursing informatics. *Image: Journal of Nursing Scholarship, 28*(1), 309–313.

VanVactor, J. D. (2008). RFID tags and healthcare supply chain management. *Healthcare Purchasing News, 32*(2), 54–55.

Walker, P. H. (2010). The TIGER Initiative: A call to accept and pass the baton. *Nursing Economics, 28*(5), 352–355.

Wang, H. (2009). Impact of the patient-centered medical home on stakeholders in the care management industry. *Journal of Management & Marketing in Healthcare, 2*(4), 343–354.

Warman, A. R. (1993). *Computer security within organizations*. London: Macmillan.

Watson, M. (2007). Knowledge management in health and social care. *Journal of Integrated Care, 15*(1), 27–33.

Wertenberger, S., Yerardi, R., Drake, A.C. , & Parlier, R. (2006). Veterans Health Administration Office of Nursing Services exploration of positive patient care synergies fueled by consumer demand: Care coordination, advanced clinic access, and patient self management. *Nursing Administration Quarterly, 30*(2), 137–146.

Wickham, V., Miedema, F., Gamerdinger, K., & DeGooyer, J. (2006). Bar-coded patient ID: Review an organizational approach to vendor selection. *Nursing Management, 37*(12), 22–26.

Wojcik, J. (2007). Electronic Rx program helps cut health care costs at General Motors. *Business Insurance, 41*(5), 6.

World Health Organization (WHO). (2007). *Patient safety*. Retrieved June 11, 2007, from http://www.who.int/patientsafety/solutions/patientsafety/en/index.html

World Health Organization (WHO). (2011). *Action on patient safety—High 5s*. Retrieved from http://www.who.int/patientsafety/implementation/solutions/high5s/en/index.html

Yang, M., Huang, H., & Huang, S. (2009). Connecting health and humans. Applying RFID systems to improve the correctness of newborn identity reconfirmation. Proceedings of NI2009: The 10th International Congress on Nursing Informatics. *Studies in Health Technology & Informatics*, 146805–146806.

Yee, C. C. (2002). Identifying information technology competencies needed in Singapore nursing education. *Computers, Informatics, Nursing, 20*(5), 209–214.

CHAPTER 2

Hardware, Software, and the Roles of Support Personnel

After completing this chapter, you should be able to:

1. Explain what computers are and how they work.
2. Describe the major hardware components of computers.
3. Understand what networks are and list the major types of network configurations.
4. Explain some considerations for choosing and using a computer system.
5. List the advantages and disadvantages of mainframe, client–server, and thin client technology.
6. Compare and contrast mobile and wireless devices, including personal digital assistants, cell phones, MP3 players, iPods, iPhones, and the BlackBerry in terms of basic technology and implications for use.
7. Understand the major types of software commonly used with computer systems.
8. Discuss the roles and responsibilities of various computer support personnel.

Acomputer is an electronic device that collects, stores, processes, and retrieves data. Information output is provided under the direction of stored sequences of instructions known as computer programs. The physical parts of a computer are frequently referred to as **hardware**, and the instructions, or programs, are collectively known as **software**. A computer system consists of the following components:

- Hardware
- Software
- Data that will be transformed into information
- Procedures or rules for the use of the system
- Users

Rapid advances in technology reshape computer capabilities and user expectations. Many changes have occurred since the introduction of the first computers in the 1940s. In general, computers have become smaller but more powerful and increasingly affordable. This is particularly evident with current notebook, tablet, personal digital assistant (PDA), and hybrid devices.

HARDWARE

Computer hardware is the physical part of the computer and its associated equipment. Computer hardware consists of many different parts, but the main elements are input devices, the central processing unit, primary and secondary storage devices, and output devices. These devices may be contained within one shell or may be separate but connected via cables or infrared technology. Figure 2–1 describes the relationship among these components.

Input Devices

Input devices allow the user to feed data into the computer. Common input devices include the keyboard, mouse and trackball, touch sensitive screen, stylus, microphone, bar code reader, fax modem card, joystick, image scanner, fingerprint scanner, digital camera, and Webcam.

Central Processing Unit

The **central processing unit (CPU)** is the "brain" of the computer. It has the electronic circuitry that actually executes computer instructions. The CPU can be divided into the following three components:

- The **arithmetic logic unit** executes instructions for the manipulation of numeric symbols.
- **Memory** is the temporary storage area in which programs and data reside during execution. Memory is subdivided into two categories: read-only memory and random access memory. **Read-only memory (ROM)** is permanent; it remains when the power is off. It typically

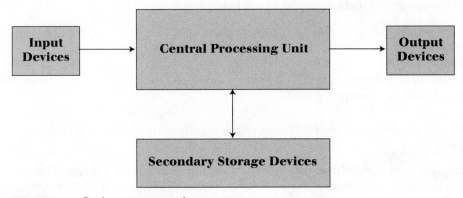

FIGURE 2–1 • Basic components of a computer

cannot be changed by the user unless additional memory is installed. Read-only memory contains start-up instructions that are executed each time the computer is turned on. (i.e., booted). **Random access memory (RAM)** is a temporary storage area that is active only while the computer is turned on. It provides storage for the program that is running as well as for the data that are being processed. Since RAM may be segmented, more than one program may be resident in memory. As an example, a personal computer (PC) may have a word processing program, a spreadsheet program, and a database program all in memory at the same time. Note, however, that only one of these programs is actually running at any point in time. This capability is referred to as multiprogramming and is implemented within the operating system.

- The **control unit** provides instructions to other parts of the computer, including input and output devices. It executes stored programs one instruction at a time and directs other computer parts to perform required tasks.

The CPU is located inside the system cabinet, which is the box that many people think of as "the computer." The CPU and memory are found on the main circuit board of the personal or desktop computer, which is known as the motherboard. The cabinet contains other components as well. Figure 2–4 will show some items that may be inside a computer cabinet.

Secondary Storage

Secondary storage provides permanent space to retain data in an area separate from the computer's memory after the computer is turned off. Common mechanisms for secondary storage include **hard disk drives**; **USB flash drives**; **digital versatile** or **video disks (DVDs)**; and **high-density optical disc format (HD-DVD)**, which is the successor to DVD. Hard disk drives store digitally encoded data on rotating platters with magnetic surfaces. USB flash drives are portable, fairly inexpensive devices slightly smaller than a cigarette lighter that plug in to a USB port and can easily be transported from one computer to another. Digital video disks resemble the CDs and are used to record and play music but offer a larger amount of storage. **Blu-ray** is a high-density optical format rival to HD-DVD. Some older machines may still have **compact discs (CDs), floppy drives** and **diskettes**, and **zip drive disks,** but these are not found on current computers. The CDs used for computers resemble those used for music. Floppy diskettes and zip diskettes come in square plastic cases. **Magnetic tape drives** are still used for some large computers. Their primary purpose is for the backup of data stored on magnetic disk.

Output Devices

Output devices allow the user to view and possibly hear processed data. Terminals or video monitor screens, projectors, printers, speakers, and fax modem boards are examples of output devices.

COMPUTER CATEGORIES

Computers vary in size, purpose, capacity, speed, and the number of users that can be accommodated simultaneously. The main categories of computers are:

- Supercomputers
- Mainframe computers
- Minicomputers
- Personal computers (also known as PCs or desktop computers)
- Laptop or notebook computers
- Tablet computers
- PDAs and other handheld combination devices such as the iPhone, iPod, iPad, and BlackBerry
- Embedded

The PDA has become a very popular device that is revolutionizing information access in healthcare. Table 2–1 provides a brief description of the various types of computers and some advantages and disadvantages associated with each.

TABLE 2–1 Types of Computers

Type	Description	Advantages	Disadvantages
Supercomputer	Designed and used for complex scientific calculations	Performs complex calculations very quickly	Expensive Limited functionality
Mainframe	Used to support organizational information systems Multiple processors Varies in size	High-speed transactions Supports many terminals and users simultaneously Large storage capacity	Expensive Software expensive and inflexible
Minicomputer	Smaller version of a mainframe Designed for multiple users Supports corporate computing for smaller organizations	Less expensive than a mainframe Supports many terminals and users simultaneously	Relatively expensive
Personal computer (PC) or desktop computer	A single- or dual-processor machine intended for one user	Inexpensive processing Can connect to other systems through a network, dial-up, cable, or wireless connection	High support costs Somewhat slower response with fewer capabilities than larger systems
Laptop or notebook computer	Streamlined, portable version of a PC or desktop system	Provides portable computer capability	Limited battery life More expensive than a comparably equipped PC Generally has a smaller keyboard than a PC
Tablet computer	Smaller than a notebook computer Weighs 2–3 pounds or less	Small size makes it easy to carry Generally accepts handwriting or keyboard input May receive and transmit data from and to other systems	Limited battery life Slightly more expensive than a desktop system Cannot receive transmissions in some areas known as deadzones
Handheld/personal digital assistant	Small special-use device	Small, lightweight Inexpensive Quick learning curve Easily taken to the point of care Increases access to information Can improve productivity May accept handwriting, voice, or keyed input May download data from information systems and transmit data to other service May incorporate the functionality of more than one device (i.e., PDA, e-mail terminal, cell phone)	Small screen size Offers less functionality than desktop and notebook computers Limited battery life Limited speed and processing ability May not hold up to rough use Synchrony with other computers may require special equipment E-mail connectivity/telephone service requires wireless systems Small size makes it easy to steal Information security concerns related to theft May not be able to receive transmissions in some areas known as deadzones
Hybrid Embedded	Small, multipurpose device Small, special purpose	Often combines telephone, text and/or e-mail messages, other Internet services, address book, and calendar functions Easily transportable Integral part of many appliances, automobiles, and other devices such as intravenous infusion pumps	Small screen and keys can be difficult to use Limited functionality

Supercomputers are the largest, most expensive type of computers. They are complex systems that can perform billions of instructions every second. Prohibitive cost limits their use primarily to government and academic settings.

Mainframes, which are large computers capable of processing several million instructions per second, are used for quickly processing large amounts of data and supporting large user communities. Mainframe computers support organizational functions and therefore were the traditional equipment in hospital environments until recently. Software for mainframes supports many customized functions, and this level of specialization results in its high cost.

A **minicomputer** is a scaled-down version of a mainframe computer. Minicomputers are slightly less costly than mainframes but are still capable of supporting multiple users as well as the computing needs of small businesses. Because they have become more powerful, minicomputers may be used in hospitals. Typically, minicomputers are used as servers in client–server systems.

Personal computers (PCs) are also known as desktop computers and were previously referred to as **microcomputers**. This computer category provides inexpensive processing power for an individual user. A PC may stand alone or be connected to other computer systems through a network, dial-up or wireless connection, or cable service. Personal computers connected via a network are sometimes referred to as clients, in client–server systems. Improved reliability, availability, manageability, and processing capabilities allow PCs to assume responsibilities once associated with mainframe computers. Some variations of the microcomputer are the notebook or laptop, tablet PC, and handheld computers. All these devices offer portable computer capability away from the office or desktop. The **notebook** or **laptop** computer is a streamlined version of the PC, using batteries or regular electric current. These devices are more expensive than comparable desktop computers. The **tablet PC** can be carried in one hand like a clipboard and is smaller and lighter than a notebook computer but rivals notebook capability. It not only accepts handwritten input via a stylus but also incorporates a keyboard and supports Windows-based applications. The stylus can be used like a mouse. Devices may also be configured to accept dictation. Handheld computers are special-use devices that offer portability and many of the features found in laptop and tablet PCs. Advances in technology add to the functionality of these devices. Some can accept handwriting and voice input, as well as send and receive data.

Personal digital assistants are a well-known type of handheld computer. These small devices were once used to keep appointment calendars, addresses, and telephone numbers. Advances in processing capability, memory, and design make PDAs attractive for a wide variety of functions, including many common software applications and data collection. Personal digital assistants can store extensive reference materials and can access patient information and transmit and receive information such as electronic prescriptions. These devices may be used for decision making at the point of care.

Hybrid or combination devices comprise another category of handheld devices. Hybrids may combine PDA capability with cell phones, MP3 players, or other functions. The BlackBerry, iPhone, and iPod are hybrid devices. An MP3 player is a small handheld digital music player. It received its name from the audio file extension that it supports. MP3, also known as MPEG audio layer 3, compresses audio signals without sacrificing sound quality, resulting in small, easily transferred files. MP3 players often support other file types as well. The iPod is a portable music player that supports MP3 and other file types. Its large capacity allows it to download, store, and play songs, movies, games, and photo slideshows from a computer or wireless connection. The iPod supports games, functions as a portable hard drive, and offers contact and calendar functions that can synchronize with PCs.

The iPhone is a multimedia, Internet-enabled mobile phone with touch screen and virtual keyboard and buttons. Functions include a camera, text messaging, visual voice mail, and a portable media player. The iPhone also supports the following Internet services: e-mail, Web browsing, and local Wi-Fi connectivity. The BlackBerry is a handheld device that supports wireless services that include a mobile telephone, push-mail, text messaging, Internet faxing, and Web browsing. It also supports address books and calendars.

Work is under way at several universities on a quantum computer, which will break away from the binary mold used for current digital computers. Quantum computers will harness the power of quantum states and encode information as qubits. A **qubit** is a measurement similar to the bit but allows for a superposition of both 1 and 0.

Another relatively new computing technology is called grid computing. Grid computing exploits the concept of distributed processing to solve certain classes of computing problems that cannot be solved within reasonable periods of time, even with the use of supercomputers. In healthcare research, one such class of problems is the identification of potentially effective drug treatments for certain diseases. Since the potentially effective drugs can number in the hundreds of millions, researches cannot look at each treatment individually. Grid computing allows for thousands of individual computers to be assigned this evaluation task, thereby reducing the elapsed time. Harnessing the computing power of these thousands of computers results in the creation of a computing grid. Today, the premier grid computing facility in the world is the World Community Grid. This grid is comprised of thousands of individual computers connected via the Internet. You personally can participate in the World Community Grid by making your own computer available as one of the problem-solving nodes. See Figure 2–2 for an example of grid computing toplogy. Visit www.worldcommunitygrid.org for more details on grid computing.

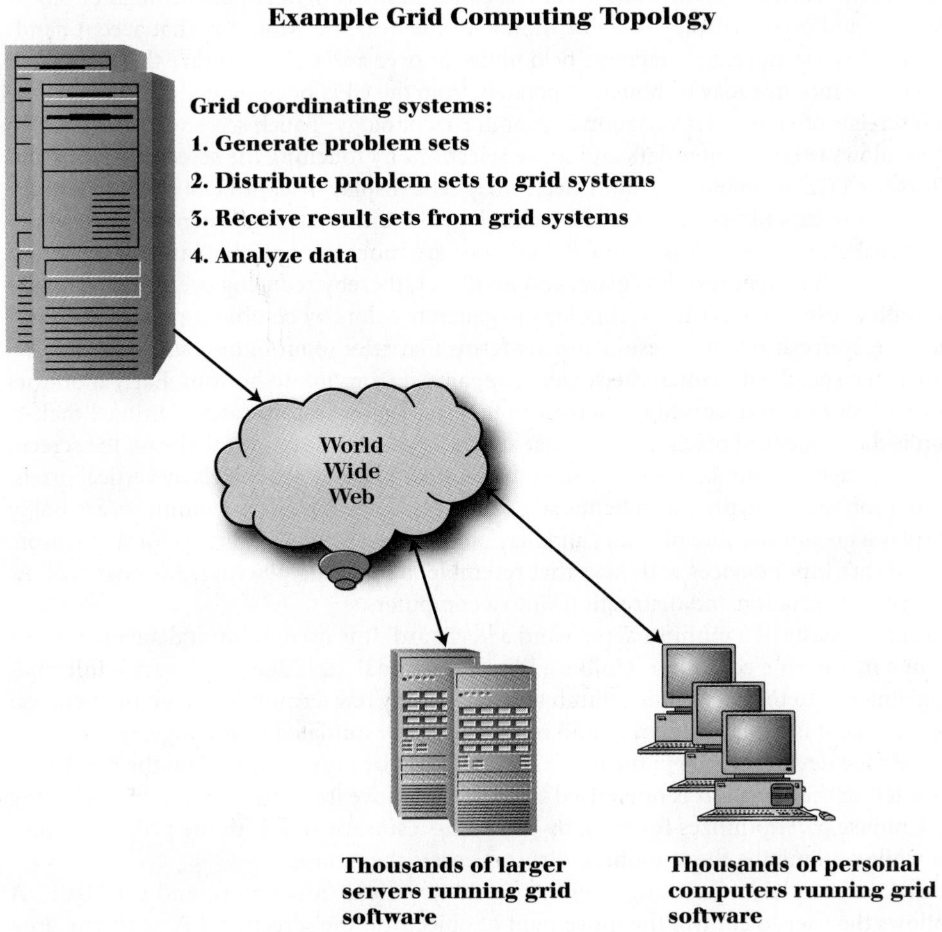

Example Grid Computing Topology

Grid coordinating systems:

1. Generate problem sets

2. Distribute problem sets to grid systems

3. Receive result sets from grid systems

4. Analyze data

World Wide Web

Thousands of larger servers running grid software

Thousands of personal computers running grid software

FIGURE 2–2 • Example grid computing topology

PERIPHERAL HARDWARE ITEMS

Peripheral hardware or, more simply, a **peripheral**, is any piece of hardware connected to a computer. Examples of peripheral devices include:

- Monitors
- Keyboards
- Terminals
- Mouse and other pointing devices such as trackballs and touchpads
- Secondary storage devices such as external CD and DVD drives and memory sticks
- Backup systems
- External modems
- Printers
- Scanners
- Digital and Web cameras (Webcams)
- Multifunction devices that combine functions such as printers that also scan, copy, and fax

The **monitor** is the screen that displays text and graphic images generated by the computer. Personal computer monitors use LCD or cathode ray tube (CRT) technology. **Liquid crystal display (LCD)** technology uses two sheets of polarizing material with a liquid crystal solution between them. An electric current sent through the liquid causes the crystals to align so that light cannot pass through them. Each crystal acts like a shutter, either allowing light to pass through or blocking the light. Liquid crystal displays may be monochrome or color. Monitors that accept handwriting via a stylus use an electromagnetic field under or over an LCD to capture the movement on the screen. The monitor may be housed separately from the CPU or contained within the same box. Touch screens offer another variation in monitor technology. Touch screens are sensitive to contact; this allows users to enter data and make selections by touching the screen. Laptops and flat monitors use LCD technology. Liquid electromagnetic display–backlit LCD panels are available but are a more expensive variant of the technology. Liquid crystal display monitors require less desktop real estate; weigh less than CRT devices; are more energy efficient; and provide a brighter picture with crisper text, less glare, and no flicker, thereby reducing eye strain. Cathode ray tube monitors use old television technology to generate colors by combining amounts of red, green, and blue. **Refresh rate** and **resolution** are terms that refer to monitor characteristics. The refresh rate is the speed with which the screen is repainted from top to bottom. Early monitors had a slow refresh rate that caused the screen to flicker. Higher refresh rates eliminate flicker. **Resolution** is the number of pixels, or dots, that appear horizontally and vertically on the screen, making up the image. Resolution is expressed as the number of horizontal pixels by vertical pixels. Higher resolution numbers provide a better screen image. Cathode ray tube monitors are bulky but can display a greater number of colors and may be preferred by graphic artists for that reason.

Keyboards are input devices with keys that resemble those of a typewriter. Keyboards allow the user to type information and instructions into a computer.

A **terminal** consists of a monitor screen and a keyboard. It is used to input data and receive output from a mainframe computer. Unlike a PC, the terminal itself does not process information, thus giving rise to the expression "dumb terminal." Very few terminals remain in operation due to the fact that it is expensive to find and replace parts for outdated technology.

The **mouse** is a device that fits in the user's hand and can be moved around on the desktop to direct a pointer on the screen. It is often used to select and move items by pressing and releasing a button. A mouse pad optimizes function by providing a surface area with the proper amount of friction while minimizing the amount of dirt that enters the mouse.

Some other examples of pointing devices include joysticks, touchpads, and trackballs. A **joystick** allows the user to control the movement of objects on the screen and is primarily used with games. A **touchpad** is a pressure- and motion-sensitive surface. When a user moves a finger across the touchpad, the on-screen pointer moves in the same direction. A **trackball** contains a ball that the user rolls to move the on-screen pointer. Touchpads and trackballs work well when available space is limited, as with laptop computers.

Secondary storage devices are generally provided via the hard disk drive, flash drive, or DVD or Blu-ray drives. Older computers and large mainframe computers may make use of technology that is not found on new PCs. The hard disk drive allows the user to retrieve and read data as well as save, or write, new data. Data are stored in the hard drive magnetically on a stack of rotating disks known as *platters*. The amount of information that can be stored on a disk is known as its *capacity*. Capacity is measured in bytes. Hard disk drives generally offer a larger capacity than do secondary storage devices. Home and office PCs offer hard disk drives with a capacity that is measured in gigabytes. One gigabyte is equivalent to 1,073,741,824 characters.

Unlike the CD drives that they replaced, DVD drives can read or play CDs as well as DVDs and access data more quickly. Most DVD drives now read and write data, storing up to seven times more data than a CD. A DVD is similar to a CD used to record music and is commonly used to store multimedia or full-length movies. A few older computers may still have floppy disk drives. A floppy disk is a thin plastic platter within a plastic cover. The amount of storage provided was small compared to a DVD. Digital versatile or video disk drives are generally located within the system cabinet but may also be external and connected using cables. Other options for secondary storage particularly on larger computers include optical disk drives, magnetic disk or tape drives, and RAID. **Optical disk drives** rely on laser technology to write data to a recording surface media and read it later. The advantage of this technology is its large storage capacity. A **tape drive** copies files from the computer to magnetic tape for storage or transfer to another machine. A file is a collection of related data stored and handled as a single entity by the computer. The concept of a file is more of a logical concept rather than a hardware concept. In a virtual tape system data is saved as if it were stored on tape, but it is actually stored on a hard drive or another storage medium. Virtual tape systems offer better backup and retrieval times at a lower operating cost. The tape drive uses tiny electromagnets to write data to a magnetic media by altering the surface. A **redundant array of independent disks (RAID)** is precisely what the name indicates: duplicate disks with mirror copies of data. Using RAID may be less costly than using one large disk drive. In the event that an individual disk fails, the remaining RAID would permit the computer to continue working uninterrupted.

Backup systems are devices that create copies of system and data files. These systems use secondary storage device technology or take advantage of online backup options. The copies are generally kept at a location separate from the computer. A backup system is an important measure for protection against computer failure or data loss.

A **modem** is a communication device that allows computers to transmit information over telephone or cable lines. Faster modems transfer information more quickly. This, in turn, saves time and telephone charges. Modem speed is measured by the number of bits that can be transferred in 1 second of time, or **bits per second (bps)**. A **bit** is the smallest unit of data that can be handled by the computer. In actuality, transfer occurs in thousands of bits per second, or **kilobits (kbps)**. Many PCs include modem and fax capabilities via a fax modem board. A **fax modem** board allows computers to transmit images of letters and drawings over telephone lines. **Wireless modems** allow users to send and receive information via access points provided with a subscription to wireless service. The **digital subscriber line (DSL) modem** allows users who have this service available to them both by virtue of location and subscription to access high-speed service via telephone lines.

A **printer** produces a paper copy of computer-generated documents. Several types of printers are available. Laser printers offer the highest quality print by transferring toner, a powdered ink, onto paper like a photocopier does. Ink-jet printers heat ink and spray it onto paper to provide a high-quality output. Dot matrix printers create letters and graphics through the use of a series of metal pins that strike a ribbon against paper. Color is an option with all three printer types. Prices vary according to quality and capability, with prices starting under $100 and ranging upward. Overall operating costs are based on purchase, supplies, and power consumption. Ink-jet printers were once considered cost effective, but ink costs over time make laser printers a viable option. Printers that also scan, copy, and fax are available. Users should base their selection on need. Laser printers are the office standard because they are quiet and provide a high-quality print. Ink-jet printers are suitable for some settings but can be slow, and ink may smear when exposed to moisture. Dot matrix printers are noisy, provide a poor-quality print, and are rarely found now.

The **scanner** is an input device that converts printed pages or graphic images into a file. The file can then be stored and revised using the computer. For example, a printed report can be scanned, stored in the computer, and sent electronically to another output device. **Digital cameras** offer a means to capture and input still images without film. Digital images may be downloaded to a computer, manipulated, and printed. A **Webcam** is a small camera used by a computer to send images over the Internet. **Multiple function devices** combine functions such as printers that also scan, copy, and fax.

NETWORKS

A **network** is a combination of hardware and software that allows communication and electronic transfer of information between computers. Hardware may be connected permanently by wire or cable, or temporarily through modems, telephone lines, or infrared signals. This arrangement allows sharing of resources, data, and software. For example, it may not be practical to have a printer for every PC in the house or office. Instead, several PCs are connected to one printer through a network. Common use of hardware requires consideration of overall needs, convenience of location, priority by user and job, and amount of use. Figure 2–3 depicts a network.

Networks range in size from **local area networks (LANs)**, with a handful of computers, printers, and other devices, to systems that link many small and large computers over a large geographic area. For example, some LANs provide support for **client/server** technology. In client–server technology, files are stored on a central computer known as the **server**. Any type of computer may act as a server, including mainframes, minicomputers, and PCs. One current trend is to combine servers by partitioning the hard drive to act as more than one server. This is known as a virtual server. **Client** computers can access information stored on the server. One major advantage of a LAN is that only one copy of a software program is needed for all users since it can be stored on the server. The client computers then access the server to use the software. This contrasts with the need to supply a separate copy of a software program for each PC user. The primary disadvantage to client–server technology is vulnerability. If the server fails, the network fails.

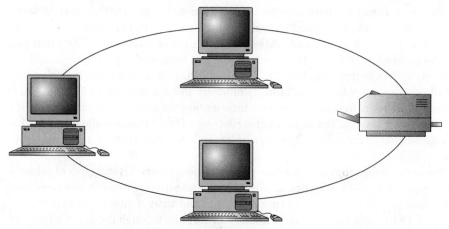

FIGURE 2–3 • Schematic representation of a network

Multiple servers circumvent this problem. Larger, more expansive systems are known as **wide area networks (WANs).**

Thin client technology, also known as **server-based computing**, represents another networking model that relies on highly efficient servers. All system processing occurs on the server, rather than on the client or local PC, as seen in traditional client–server technology. The thin client is primarily a display, keyboard, and mouse or other pointing device. It sends keystrokes and mouse movements to the server over the network, and the server sends back changes in the display. Any PC can serve as a thin client. The minimal hardware requirements for this model give rise to the name "thin client" as opposed to "fat client," as seen in traditional client–server technology. This model helps to reduce hardware costs; older equipment can be used longer, and new thin clients cost less than traditional PCs because no local drives or storage devices are required. The absence of local drives and storage also reduces maintenance and administrative costs and facilitates software upgrades. Software resides on the server requiring one upgrade at the server rather than a physical visit to each PC or client. Security is enhanced because users cannot run foreign disks locally that may contain a virus.

The largest and best known network in the world is the **Internet,** also known as the **Net.** The Internet actually consists of thousands of interconnected networks. The Internet was once limited to individuals affiliated with educational institutions and government agencies. Variations of Internet technology are available via intranets and extranets. Both intranets and extranets use software and programming languages designed for the Internet. **Intranets** are private company networks that are protected from outside access. **Extranets,** on the other hand, apply Internet technology to create a network outside the company system for use by customers or suppliers.

Like all computer technology, the Internet is evolving into what is being called Internet 2.0. This evolution will dramatically change the manner in which users will interact with each other. This next generation Internet will immerse users into a three-dimensional virtual world. Avatars will represent individual users, who will be able to meet, conduct business, and collaborate on ideas, all in virtual space. One of the more widely known implementations of the next generation Internet is Linden Lab's Second Life. Visit www.secondlife.com for details on how to participate in this new, evolving technology.

HOW COMPUTERS WORK

Computers receive, process, and store data. They use binary code to represent **alphanumeric** characters, which are numbers and alphabetic characters. **Binary code** is a series of 1s and 0s. All 1s are stored on the disk as magnetized areas, and 0s are stored as areas that have not been magnetized. Each 1 or 0 is called a **bit.** Eight bits make up one **byte.** The unique code for each character is eight bits long. In the code for numeric characters, each position corresponds to a specific power of 2. Box 2–1 provides a binary representation of the number 13.

BOX 2–1   Binary Representation of an Arabic Number

The Arabic number 13 is represented using the binary system as 00001101. Each bit (0 or 1) represents a particular power of 2, depending on its position. If the position is taken by a 0, then it has no value. If the position is taken by a 1, it has the value of the associated power of 2. The Arabic number represented is the total of the powers of 2 represented by the 0s and 1s.

Binary representation of 13	0		0		0		0		1		1a		0		1		
Powers of 2 by bit location	2^7		2^6		2^5		2^4		2^3		2^2		2^1		2^0		
Arabic value of position	128		64		32		16		8		4		2		1		
Actual value of bit	0	+	0	+	0	+	0	+	8	+	4	+	0	+	1	=	13

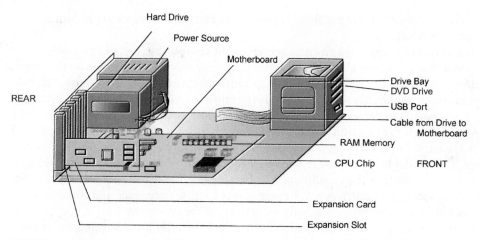

FIGURE 2–4 • Internal view of a PC

Computer programs, or software, use binary code to provide the instructions that direct the work computers do. Personal computers, notebooks, and PDAs differ slightly from supercomputers, mainframe computers, and minicomputers in the structure of their CPU. The CPU in larger computers is generally composed of one or more circuit boards, whereas smaller computers rely on a **microprocessor chip,** which contains the electronic circuits of the CPU etched on a silicon chip, mounted on a board, otherwise known as the **motherboard.** All electrical components, including the main memory, connect to this board. Figure 2–4 depicts the internal components of a PC. The motherboard also provides slots for network interface cards and peripheral device interface cards. The **network interface card** physically connects a computer to a network, controlling the flow of information between the two. Likewise, **peripheral device interface cards** connect equipment such as printers to the computer and control the exchange of information. The slot arrangement on motherboard allows users to change or add computer system components easily. Portable or laptop computers can be connected to networks or peripheral devices through the use of a **Personal Computer Memory Card International Association (PCMCIA) card.** These cards can be inserted into a slot, in the case of the laptop computer, to add increased functionality such as additional memory or network connections. The Personal Computer Memory Card International Association was founded to establish standards for integrated circuit cards and promote interchangeability among mobile computers (PCMIA 2007). The organization also promotes interchangeability in other devices that include cameras, cable television, and automobiles.

The processor speed on PCs is measured in **gigahertz.** A gigahertz (GHz) represents 1 billion cycles per second. The processor speed determines how rapidly instructions are handled. In general, each new PC model offers a faster CPU speed.

Whenever the power to a PC is turned on, the computer performs a start-up process. The program code for this test is stored in permanent memory and is known as **basic input/output system (BIOS).** The BIOS confirms that information about component parts is present and that this information coincides with existing hardware.

SELECTION CRITERIA

Equipment selection should be based on needs and expectations. When selecting a computer system and related hardware, it is important to consider the following:

- *The types of applications required. For example, some people use primarily word processing programs, whereas others need applications to perform numeric calculations.*

- *The program execution time and computer capacity needed to process jobs.* Complex jobs require higher processor speed and more memory for timely execution.
- *The number of workers who need computer access at any one time.* Single-user access demands can be met by a PC. Multiple demands for access may be better served by a network.
- *Storage capacity.* Storage needs are determined by the amount of information that must be kept and the length of time it must be retained.
- *Backup options.* When information stored and processed on computers is critical to conduct daily business, another copy should be available to restore normal services after a crash.
- *Budget considerations.* The cost of hardware and software for various options should be considered in relation to the benefits and limitations associated with each.
- *Maintenance considerations.* There are several issues related to maintenance. These include durability, battery life and time required for recharging batteries, and the ability to easily disinfect or clean equipment to minimize the chances of spreading infection (Neely & Sittig 2002). Infection control may be accomplished via placement of computer equipment in areas away from splatter, the use of hand washing and antimicrobial hand cleaners, keyboard skins, and designated cleaning procedures with periodic cultures of equipment.
- *Portability.* Not all users require portability but when it is called for, size, weight, and equivalent functions must be evaluated.

These factors will help determine which type of computer or network is the best option, as well as the required hardware features. Advance planning ensures that current and future computer needs are well served.

User Needs and Ergonomic Considerations

Human factors should be considered in every work environment. Human factors, otherwise known as **ergonomics,** involve the study and design of a work environment that maximizes productivity by reducing operator fatigue and discomfort. Ergonomics considers physical stresses placed on joints, muscles, nerves, and tendons as well as environmental factors that can affect hearing and vision. Poor setup of computer equipment leads to somatic complaints that include headaches, eye strain, irritation, stress, fatigue, and neck and back pain. Even though the number of reported occupational injury claims has declined, failure to consider ergonomics is costly in terms of lost productivity (Bernhart 2006; "Body Knowledge" 2007; Brewer et al. 2006; "Eye Strain" 2010; Imrhan 2006). Ergonomics should receive the same attention given to other workplace education particularly since workplace injuries do not always start in the workplace. Additional research is also needed on the efficacy of interventions performed given that few quality studies have been done in this area. Ergonomics is especially important for users of laptop computers because these devices are designed for portability rather than good ergonomics. The keyboard and screen are too close together causing eyestrain and poor hand position, and perching the computer on one's lap leads to poor posture (Gorman 2006; Holzer 2006; Tessler 2006). Whenever possible, plug-in keyboards and laptop stands should be used to foster good ergonomics. Two health problems associated with poor ergonomics include computer vision syndrome and repetitive motion disorders.

Computer vision syndrome (CVS) is a term the American Optometric Association uses to describe eye and vision problems that result from work done in proximity, such as when using a computer for long periods of time (Krader & Anshel 2010; Rosenfield, Gurevich, Wickware, & Lay 2010). Eye and vision problems comprise the most frequently reported health problems and do impact productivity but receive less attention than do the musculoskeletal disorders primarily because vision problems are largely symptomatic and fleeting. Special consideration must also be given to the needs of the aging employee in designing work spaces. Computer vision syndrome symptoms include eyestrain, headaches, blurred distance or near vision, dry or red eyes, neck and/or backache, double vision, and light sensitivity. Poor lighting conditions, poor posture, and existing refractive errors contribute to the development of CVS in up to 90% of all computer workers.

Repetitive motion disorders or repetitive stress injuries (RSIs) result from using the same muscle groups over and over again without rest (National Institute of Neurological Disorders and Stroke 2007). One well-known example of a repetitive motion injury is **carpal tunnel syndrome.** Carpal tunnel syndrome occurs when the median nerve is compressed as it passes through the wrist along the pathway to the hand. This compression results in sensory and motor changes to the thumb, index finger, third finger, and radial aspect of the ring finger. Other repetitive motion injuries may involve the neck and shoulders. Good ergonomics helps to avoid occupational injuries and keeps employees productive. Box 2–2 provides a checklist to ensure good ergonomic design when designing and working at computer workstations. Another aspect of ergonomics addresses worker concerns about alleged health risks associated with computer use. The list of alleged health risks includes, but is not limited to, the following: cataracts, conception problems, miscarriage, and/or birth defects. Research has not established any clear links between computer use and these risks. Table 2–2 lists several examples of commercially available ergonomic devices.

BOX 2–2 Measures to Ensure Good Ergonomics When Using a Computer Work Station

Determine how a workstation will be used. Choose optimal settings for the chair, desk, keyboard, and monitor for the person who will use the area or that can easily be adjusted for each user. Adjustments are appropriate when wrists are flat and elbow angle is 90 degrees or more to prevent nerve compression.

Determine the length of time the user will be at the workstation. Individual adjustments are less critical if use is occasional or for very brief periods.

Configure work areas for specific types of equipment. Most workstation desks are designed for PCs rather than notebooks. Use a docking station or plug-in keyboard and stand if needed to ensure proper monitor and keyboard height.

Select sturdy surfaces or furniture with sufficient workspace. Desks should have room to write and use a mouse.

Provide chairs with good lumbar support. Relaxed sitting requires chairs that allow a reclined posture of 100 to 110 degrees.

Educate all workers on the need for good body mechanics when working with computers. Good posture is essential to reduce physical strain whether the individual works from a standing or sitting position.

Position monitors just below eye level approximately one arm's length away. The monitor should be about 30 inches from eye to screen and 20–40 degrees below the line of sight. This will help to prevent neck strain, especially for bifocal wearers.

Adjust screen resolution, font size, and brightness as needed. Sharp screen images help to reduce eye strain.

Periodically look away from the monitor to distant objects. This helps to avoid eye-focusing problems.

Minimize screen glare. Purchase nonglare monitors or place monitors at right angles to windows. Provide blinds or draperies, or adjust area lighting as needed.

Take frequent breaks. Intersperse computer work with other activities to avoid RSIs.

Avoid noisy locations. Noise is distracting and stressful.

Place the workstation in a well-ventilated area. Fresh air and a comfortable temperature enhance working conditions.

Use ergonomic devices with caution. Select items that have been researched. Do not continue use if it remains uncomfortable after a trial period. Just because an item carries the label *ergonomic* does not mean that it is beneficial.

Use optical prescriptions designed for computer work. Everyday visual correction does not always work well for extended periods of computer work.

Provide lighting that can be adjusted to the needs of the individual. Older individuals need more light than younger persons to clearly view a task. Too little light contributes to eye fatigue and decreased productivity.

TABLE 2–2   Examples of Ergonomic Devices

Device	Purpose
Glare filter	Reduces eyestrain related to glare or light reflected from a monitor and may help make images appear sharper and text easier to read
Negative tilt keyboard	Tilts away from the user with the keyboard below elbow height to allow the user to rest arms, shoulders, neck, and back during pauses in typing
Document holder	Keeps documents at the same height and distance from the user as the monitor, limiting head and neck movement and tension
Ergonomic mouse	Various designs that aim to reduce wrist and hand pain
	No consistent research findings to support its use
Lumbar support	Maintains the natural curves of the back, minimizing back pain
Wrist rests	May actually increase carpal tunnel pressure unless a broad, flat, firm surface provides a place to rest the palm, not the wrist
Support braces/gloves	May relieve carpal tunnel symptoms when worn at night
	There are no consistent research findings to support use while typing
Ergonomic keyboards	Split keyboard designed to improve posture
	Research fails to support the benefit of this device
Foot rest	Encourages proper posture and supports the lower back to keep the pelvis properly tilted

Some controversy exists regarding the degree to which these devices benefit the user and prevent injury. Young (2006) suggested that organizations provide an area where employees can test ergonomic devices before bulk purchases are made. This would also be helpful for employees who need assistance to adapt to new types of devices (Armbrüster, Sutter, & Ziefle 2007).

Physical Constraints

Space is a chronic problem in healthcare settings. For this reason, workstation planning is less a function of good ergonomics and more a function of finding a place to put the equipment. Ergonomics rarely receives high priority in planning. Provisions should be made for adequate numbers of computers in the clinical setting, located in quiet areas such as conference rooms.

Another major constraint to the installation of computers and networks in any institution centers on wiring and cabling. Adding power lines and cables for network connections to a current work space may prove to be more expensive than building a new work area. This is one reason for the growing popularity of wireless systems.

MOBILE AND WIRELESS COMPUTING

The terms mobile and wireless are often used interchangeably but are not the same. A device can be mobile without being wireless. **Mobile computing** uses devices that can be carried or wheeled from place to place. These devices may or may not have the capability to transmit and receive information while they are mobile. When mobile devices do not have a wireless connection the user must re-establish a connection periodically to receive updated information or to send collected information to a large computer on the network. This connection may be achieved by plugging into a network port; docking port; or, in the case of some handheld devices, the use of a special cable to communicate with a computer that is connected to the network. Mobile devices may include desktop, specialized workstations or notebook computers on carts as well as some PDAs. **Wireless devices** are equipped with a special card enabling the broadcast and reception of signals that reach the network via access points. That network may be wireless or ultimately a traditional network connected by cable. Wireless devices are not tethered by a physical connection such as a cable or telephone line. Wireless devices can continually receive and transmit up-to-date information. Increasingly the term *mobile* is used to refer to wireless devices. Mobile and wireless computing offer the following advantages:

- *Both technologies bring computing to the bedside.* Point-of-care access allows healthcare providers and clients to view relevant information at the location where it is needed and eliminates the need to return to a workstation at the nurses' station, which might be in use.
- *Cost.* Mobile and wireless technology reduce the number of computers needed because the healthcare worker takes the device with him or her to where it will be used rather than require a device at a fixed location. Mobile and wireless systems also reduce the costs associated with connecting a traditional network with cables. Installing cable is labor intensive, disrupts care, and can be difficult to accomplish, particularly in older buildings.
- *Improved data collection.* Computers at the point of care facilitate data collection. Care providers collect and input data once rather than taking handwritten notes for later entry into a computer.
- *More efficient work processes.* Wireless technology and redesign of work processes enable healthcare professionals to work more efficiently. A graphic example is seen with online prescription of drugs where the physician or nurse practitioner quickly accesses allergy and drug interaction information and instantly sends prescriptions to the hospital or patient's pharmacy without problems with interpretation of handwriting.
- *Error reduction.* Wireless technology is hailed as a means to prevent errors because it can deliver up-to-date information, provide decision support, access reference materials, and even provide electronic prescription application access at the point of care.

Until recently, wireless technology was plagued by a lack of interoperability. This obstacle was removed by the adoption of a standard for wireless data transmission, making it possible for all wireless devices manufactured after the adoption of the standard to communicate. Recent advances in processing capability make the PDA particularly attractive because it is small, lightweight, and easy to use.

The advantages associated with mobile and wireless technology also raise concerns that include:

- *Theft and loss.* These devices are more subject to theft and easy to lose because they are mobile and small enough to carry away. This requires the implementation of safeguards to protect information contained on stolen devices.
- *Threats to data security.* The security of data may be compromised when devices are stolen. The technology used to protect data on wireless networks has been less secure than technology used to encrypt information on traditional, hardwired networks. Vendors have been working on this issue.
- *Battery life.* Battery life varies according to use patterns and processing demands. Around-the-clock use requires close attention to the use of charge units and/or spare batteries.
- *Data loss.* Mobile devices are used to collect and send information to another computer system. Damage to devices, theft, loss, or downtime related to dead batteries may lead to loss of data before it can be shared.
- *Memory limitations.* While advances continue to add to the capability of handheld devices, memory limitations remain an issue, particularly when users expect additional features and capabilities.
- *Limited ability to display and see information.* Small screen size limits the amount of information that can be viewed at one time.
- *Deadzones.* Wireless devices may not be able to transmit and receive information in certain locations.

- *Lack of a means to readily exchange data between hospital information systems and handheld devices.* Physicians typically want clinical information systems available to them on their PDAs. The ability to provide clinical data to handheld devices can be arduous and expensive to develop.

Another concern related to the use of PDAs is that organizations need to develop a comprehensive strategy for their use and support if they do not already have one in place. Many physicians and other healthcare providers are purchasing their own PDAs but cannot fully realize benefits associated with their use without organizational plans for PDA use and support. Purchase recommendations from Information Services staff can help to avert disappointment. Useful information related to PDA use and available applications and databases can be found through the publications and Web sites of professional organizations. *PDA Cortex was* an early online journal for mobile computing for healthcare professionals. The *PDA Cortex* web site remains available but has not been updated since 2005. There are now several journals that focus upon mobile computing and mobile computing in healthcare. Mobile computing now incorporates a wider variety of devices beyond PDAs.

SOFTWARE

Software is a set of instructions that tells the computer what to do. **Programs** and applications are forms of software. All software is written in **programming languages.** Each programming language provides a detailed set of rules for how to write instructions for the computer. Numerous programming languages exist. A few examples are listed here. Common Business Oriented Language (COBOL) remains popular for business applications. Massachusetts General Hospital Utility Multi-Programming System (MUMPS) has been used for healthcare applications. Ada is a high-level, general-purpose programming language originally developed for the defense department. Ada supports real-time applications. C is a flexible language that is particularly popular for PCs because it is compact. C++ is a descendent of C. Unlike its predecessor it supports object-oriented programming, which allows reuse of some instructions. C++ is favored for graphical applications in the Windows and Macintosh environments. Beginners All-Purpose Symbolic Instruction Code (BASIC) is widely found in home computing. Java is a popular language for the development of programs for use on the Internet. Visual Basic is a programming language used for the development of graphical user interfaces. Structured Query Language (SQL) is an example of a programming language that allows the user to query or search a database for specific information.

Several categories of software exist; each has a different purpose. Some major software categories include operating systems, application software, database management systems (DBMSs), and utility programs.

Operating Systems

The most essential type of software is the **operating system.** The operating system is a collection of programs that manage all of the computer's activities, including the control of hardware, execution of software, and management of information. Control of hardware refers to the ability of different parts of the computer to work together. Operating systems allow users to manage information through the retrieval, copying, movement, storage, and deletion of files.

The operating system also provides a user interface. The **user interface** is the means by which the individual interacts with the computer. For many years PC users had to enter specific text commands. Microsoft Windows provided a **graphical user interface (GUI)**. A GUI provides menus, windows, and other standard screen features intended to make using a computer as intuitive as possible. Graphical user interfaces decrease the amount of time required to learn new programs and eliminate the need to memorize commands. Work is under way on natural interfaces. The most natural user interface is the voice. Natural user interfaces are expected to free the user from conventional constraints such as mechanical keyboards, pointing devices, and GUIs, thereby making computers easier to use. Significant progress has occurred in recent years. An example of this progress may be seen in Apple's iPhone 4 with its integration of Siri, a voice-enabled personal assistant feature that allows users to converse with their phone (Ionescu 2011). Siri uses Apple applications on the iPhone 4 to find the information requested. Wireless technology, a highly mobile lifestyle, and advances in interactive voice recognition also contribute to the increased use of voice recognition in call centers and for dictation. Voice recognition will not replace keyed data for some time yet in general use. There are still limits to the number of words that are recognized, and it is necessary to create a model of the user's voice before use. There is also an issue with accuracy, which is less than 100%.

Operating systems exist for all categories of computers. Windows and Linux are operating systems for PCs. Windows has been through several versions. Current versions include XP, VISTA, and, most recently, Windows 7. **Macintosh computers**, or **Macs**, have their own operating systems. Macs are commercial computers that offer a graphical interface and are available for home and office use. Macs are produced by Apple Computer Incorporated. Fewer software programs are available for Macs, but adaptations are available that permit Macs to run PC software. UNIX is an operating environment developed in the 1970s that can run on virtually any hardware platform, from PCs to mainframe systems.

Application Software

Application software is a set of programs designed to accomplish a particular task such as word processing, financial management, or drawing. Application software builds on the foundation provided by the operating system. Box 2–3 lists some common types of software applications.

Another factor that facilitates computer use is the development of software tutorials and online help. Most software packages now offer tutorials for review before application use, making software much more accessible to first-time users. Help screens are available while the program is running.

BOX 2–3 Common Types of Software Applications

- **Word processing.** Allows the creation of documents, utilizing features such as spelling and grammar correction, thesaurus, and graphics or pictures.

- **Presentation graphics.** Supports the preparation of slides and handout materials.

- **Spreadsheet.** Performs calculations, analyzes data, and presents information in tabular format and graphical displays.

- **Database.** Helps to manage large collections of information, such as payroll information, phone directories, and product listing. Performs calculations and produces reports from the stored information. Allows the user to find specific information.

- **Desktop publishing.** Offers expanded features that may not be commonly found in word processing programs. Useful for the creation of newsletters and other publications.

- **Web design.** Allows the user to create or revise Web pages and content that can then be posted to a Web site.

- **Specialized software**

  Project management. Supports the management of projects with identification of tasks and time frames for completion, including program evaluation review technique (PERT) charts.

  Personal information managers. Enhance personal productivity with time management tools, including an appointment calendar, telephone directories, and reminder lists.

  Personnel scheduling. Automates the process of scheduling staff.

  Report software. Allows database use for queries and to discern trends without the need to write code in computer programming languages.

Examples of application software, which perform healthcare-specific functions, include the following:

- Patient Registration (ADT)
- Electronic Patient Record
- Patient Accounting
- Physician Order Entry/Results Reporting
- Quality Management

Software to perform these functions may either be purchased from one or more software vendors or be developed in-house by the healthcare organization. The decision to build or buy software is discussed in later chapters of this textbook.

Database Management Systems

A DBMS is a software application responsible for the creation, maintenance, and use of a database. A database is an integrated collection of data structured for multiple uses. Today, the most common database type is the relational database. A majority of the previously mentioned applications have, as their foundation, a relational database. Figure 2–5 is a partial example of a relational database design for an electronic health record application.

Utility Programs

Utility programs help to manage the computer and its data. Early operating systems offered few utility options such as optimization of the hard disk, system backup, or virus checks. To fill this need, a separate category of software evolved. Many utility programs are now included as part of the operating system. However, users may still choose to install and use utility programs that are independent of their operating systems.

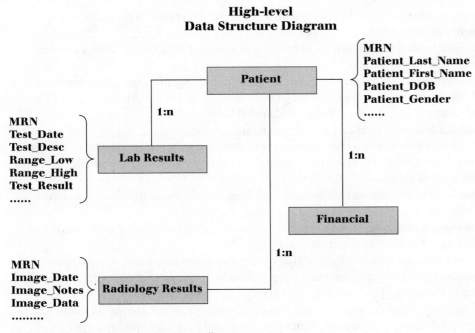

FIGURE 2–5 • High-level data structure diagram

FUTURE DIRECTIONS

Technology is a pervasive part of everyday life. It is an integral part of home appliances and found throughout the healthcare delivery system. It is frequently invisible to the user but does require a bevy of behind-the-scenes people to ensure both its ongoing and optimal use. Technology will continue to develop and evolve in ways that are difficult for us to imagine today. Devices will become smaller and easier to use. This process will extend the capabilities of providers and create new disciplines. One area that is expected to have a large impact in the near future is nanotechnology. **Nanotechnology** is the science and technology of engineering devices at the molecular level (Gulson & Wong 2006; "Health and Medicine" 2006; Knowles 2006; McCauley 2005). Nanotechnology is already used in cosmetics and sunscreens and other industries. Work is under way to create electrical circuits that would allow the development of smaller computers, design new monitoring technologies, and develop smart drug delivery systems. At this time the effects of nanotechnology on human health are not known and will need to be monitored over time.

CASE STUDY EXERCISE

You are appointed to the hospital's information technology committee as the representative for your nursing unit. The charges of the committee include the following:

- Identify PC software that is needed to accomplish unit work, such as word processing, spreadsheets, and databases.
- Determine criteria for the selection and placement of hardware on the units.

Discuss these issues and how they affect patient care and workflow.

SUMMARY

- Computers are machines that process data under the direction of a program, or stored sequence of instructions.
- The major hardware components of computers are input devices, the CPU, secondary storage, and output devices.
- The major categories of computers are supercomputers; mainframes; minicomputers; PCs or desktop systems; laptop or notebook computers; tablet computers; and handheld devices such as PDAs, the BlackBerry, iPod, and iPhone.
- Peripheral hardware items, such as the keyboard, mouse, monitor, modem, and printer, help the user put data into the computer, read output, and communicate with other users.
- Networks are linked systems of computers. Local area networks, WANs, and the Internet are all types of computer networks.
- Networks may use various technologies including cabling, radio signals, client–server, and thin client.
- In choosing a computer system, one must consider current and future information processing needs, budget, and human factors.
- Good ergonomics reduces physical discomforts and injury associated with computer use.
- Mobile and handheld computer technology provide the promise of efficiency, improvements in the safety of care delivery, cost savings, and work redesign.
- Software is the set of instructions that make a computer run and control its resources. Operating systems, applications, utility programs, and programming languages are all types of software.
- Support personnel are essential to help people use PCs and information systems effectively and to maintain and upgrade hardware and software.

REFERENCES

Armbrüster, C., Sutter, C., & Ziefle, M. (2007). Notebook input devices put to the age test: The usability of trackpoint and touchpad for middle-aged adults. *Ergonomics, 50*(3), 426–445. Retrieved December 27, 2007, from CINAHL with Full Text database.

Bernhart, H. (2006). Ergonomics offers preventive approach to musculoskeletal problems. *Employee Benefit News, 20*(13), 55–58. Retrieved December 27, 2007, from Business Source Elite database.

Body Knowledge: Improved Ergonomics = Improved Productivity. (2007, February). *Material handling management*. Retrieved December 27, 2007, from Business Source Elite database.

Brewer, S., Van Eerd, D., Amick, B., Irvin, E., Daum, K., Gerr, F., . . . Rempel, D. (2006). Workplace interventions to prevent musculoskeletal and visual symptoms and disorders among computer users: A systematic review. *Journal of Occupational Rehabilitation, 16*(3), 325–358. Retrieved December 27, 2007, from CINAHL with Full Text database.

Eye strain no longer limited to hours of computer viewing. (2010). *EHS Today, 3*(9), 22. Retrieved from http://ehstoday.com/health/news/eye-strain-hours-computer-viewing-6321/

Gorman, R. (2006, January). Pain relief for laptop-lovers: Notebook computers are easy to adore—But hard on your body. Here are 5 easy fixes. *Health, 20*(1), 97–98. Retrieved December 27, 2007, from CINAHL with Full Text database.

Grove, T., & Demster, B. (2007, January). *HIMSS Toolkit: Managing information privacy & security in healthcare administrative requirements for privacy*. Healthcare Information and Management Systems Society. Retrieved December 31, 2007, from http://www.himss.org/content/files/CPRIToolkit/version6/v6%20pdf/D73_Admin_Requirements.pdf

Gulson, B., & Wong, H. (2006). Stable isotopic tracing: A way forward for nanotechnology. *Environmental Health Perspectives, 114*(10), 1486–1488.

Hall, M. (2006, May 8). A focus on "proper" ergonomics. . . . *Computerworld, 40*(19), 10. Retrieved December 27, 2007, from Business Source Elite database.

Health alert: Never overlook ergonomics. (2006, April). *Quill*. Retrieved December 27, 2007, from Business Source Elite database.

Health and medicine. (2006). *Futurist, 40*(6), Special section pp. 4–5.

Holzer, L. (2006, April). *Good piano technique: The key to healthy computer keyboarding*. Positive Health. Retrieved December 27, 2007, from CINAHL with Full Text database.

Imrhan, S. (2006). Health alert: Never overlook ergonomics. *Quill, 94*(3), 40.

Ionescu, D. (2011, October 5). Siri: FAQs about the iPhone 4s personal assistant. *PCWorld*, Retrieved November 6, 2011, from http://www.pcworld.com/article/241171/siri_faqs_about_the_iphone_4s_personal_assistant.html

Kane, C. (2007). Trends in IT outsourcing. *Associations Now, 3*(10), Special section pp. 8–9.

Knowles, III, E. E. (2006). Nanotechnology. *Professional Safety, 51*(3), 20–27.

Krader, C., & Anshel, J. (2010). Computer use can lead to vision complaints. *Optometry Times, 2*(9), 47. Retrieved from EBSCOhost.

Laptop use spurs ergonomic pain. (2007). *New Orleans CityBusiness (1994 to 2008), 27*(45), 23–24. Retrieved from EBSCOhost.

McCauley, L. A. (2005). Nanotechnology: Are occupational health nurses ready? *AAOHN Journal, 53*(12), 517–521.

National Institute of Neurological Disorders and Stroke. (2007, February 14). *NINDS repetitive motion disorders information page*. Retrieved December 29, 2007, from http://www.ninds.nih.gov/disorders/repetitive_motion/repetitive_motion.htm

Neely, A. N., & Sittig, D. F. (2002, July 23). Basic microbiologic and infection control information to reduce the potential transmission of pathogens to patients via computer hardware. *Journal of the American Medical Informatics Association, 9*, 500–508.

Personal Computer Memory Card International Association (PCMCIA). (2007, December 29). *About PCMCIA*. Retrieved December 29, 2007, from http://www.pcmcia.org/about.htm

Rosenfield, M., Gurevich, R., Wickware, E., & Lay, M. (2010). Computer vision syndrome: Accomodative & vergence facility. *Journal of Behavioral Optometry, 21*(5), 119–122. Retrieved from EBSCOhost.

Tessler, F. (2006, January). Laptop ergonomics. *Macworld, 23*(1), 85–86. Retrieved December 27, 2007, from Business Source Elite database.

Versage, B. (2006). The clinical information analyst. *Pennsylvania Nurse, 61*(2), 15.

Young, W. (2006). You're invited to an ergo room. *Journal of Accountancy, 202*(6), 39. Retrieved December 27, 2007, from Business Source Elite database.

CHAPTER 3

Ensuring the Quality and Best Use of Information

After completing this chapter, you should be able to:

1. Define *data integrity* and its relevance for healthcare.

2. Discuss the relevance of data management for data integrity.

3. Identify strategies to ensure the accuracy of data.

4. Differentiate between online and offline data storage.

5. Explain how storage conditions can affect data integrity.

6. Debate the relative merits of outsourcing data storage.

7. Discuss factors that should be addressed when planning for data retrieval.

8. Identify characteristics associated with quality information.

9. Discuss the significance of data cleansing for data warehousing and data mining.

10. Define *data mining* and recognize its uses within healthcare.

11. Examine the relationship between data mining, knowledge discovery in databases, and evidence-based practice.

12. Explore the role of the nurse with knowledge discovery in databases.

Data functions as the theoretical constructs in knowledge development. As the building blocks for knowledge, it is crucial to comprehend aspects for ensuring data integrity in addition to characteristics of quality information, quality data and database management, data mining, and knowledge discovery in databases (KDD). According to Nicolini, Powell, Conville, and Martinez-Solano (2008), to best manage knowledge in a new era of evidence-based practice, meaningful information will need to be accessed for Meaningful Use in order to transform nursing science to best practice. This process, however, requires the collection of the right information in its entirety, no compromises to the quality of collected data and special analysis using statistics, artificial intelligence, and machine learning technologies to provide useful information about patterns and relationships that might not otherwise be obvious. Figure 3–1 depicts the characteristics of quality information.

According to de Lusignan (2009), high-quality information is needed by healthcare providers to best inform quality decision making. In addition, quality information supports best practice in the translation of nursing science to the point of care by providing high-quality and cost-effective care. The characteristics summarized in Box 3–1 can be attributed to quality information (Rao, Fung, & Rosales 2011).

According to Li, Bheemavaram, and Zhang (2010), quality is threatened whenever data is manipulated whether by storage variance, format variance, transfer, or extraction. Format variations can accentuate inaccuracies and erode data quality, particularly as the number of databases and the age of the stored data increase. For example, a client may have been registered and treated at one hospital a number of times, using a slightly different version of the client's name for each registration. One registration may have been created using the client's legal name, another using a nickname, and another omitting a middle initial. There also may have been a change in address during this period. It can be difficult in this instance to verify that all records belong to the same person; until recently, each record had to be examined

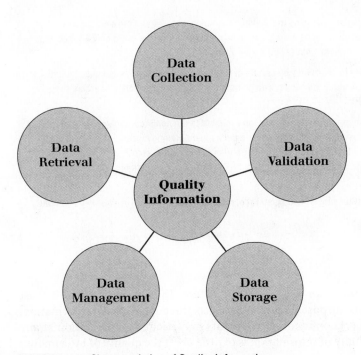

FIGURE 3–1 • Characteristics of Quality Information

BOX 3–1 Attributes of Quality Information

- **Timely.** Information is available when it is needed. The ability to access the client's insurance information at the time of an outpatient visit allows timely verification of coverage for specified procedures.

- **Precise.** Each detail is complete and clear. An example of a lack of precision is the client's report of previous *abdominal surgery*. Precise data would be the identification of the specific surgical procedure, such as appendectomy.

- **Accurate.** Information is without error. An example of inaccurate data is documentation of the wrong leg in a below-the-knee amputation.

- **Numerically quantifiable.** The ability to measure data improves quality. An example is seen with the ability to measure and stage a decubitus ulcer, which aids the subsequent assessment of its status by other professionals.

- **Verifiable by independent means.** Two different people can make the same observation and report the same result. If two people listen to a client's apical heart rate simultaneously, both of them should report the same rate.

- **Rapidly and easily available.** For example, the nurse can quickly retrieve a client's allergies from a past medical record stored in the computer system when a critically ill patient arrives in the emergency department.

- **Free from bias, or modification with the intent to influence recipients.** Data should be based on objective rather than subjective evaluation. Documenting that a client is depressed represents subjective interpretation. A better approach is to document observations about the client's activity level and interactions with others. These are quality data.

- **Comprehensive.** Required information is present. When a nurse asks a client for a list of current medications, the list should include medication name, dosage, and frequency taken.

- **Appropriate to the user's needs.** Different users have different data needs. The appropriate data must be available for each user. For example, the nurse must be able to access data related to a client's previous diabetic teaching.

- **Clear.** Information is free from ambiguity, reducing the likelihood of treatment errors. An example is seen in the client's report of an allergy to eggs. On questioning, the nurse determines that the client only dislikes eggs and does not wish to be served them but has never had a truly allergic response.

- **Reliable regardless of who collects it.** There may be certain data that multiple professionals collect. Client allergies may be documented by the nurse, physician, and pharmacist. All documentation of allergies should agree.

- **Current.** All files should contain the most current information available to the healthcare team. For information to be kept current, a regular system for updating must be put in place. Having current information available on the computer will help avoid errors that could be harmful to clients. For example, data retrieved at an outpatient setting should include all recent inpatient data that is pertinent, not just the most recent outpatient data.

- **In a convenient form for interpretation, classification, storage, retrieval, and updates.** The user must be able to access and use the data without difficulty.

individually for error. Software tools can now perform this task. The data source that is most likely to be correct is used for this purpose. Figure 3–2 depicts three requisites of information: (a) quality, (b) availability, and (c) confidentiality. Threats may occur to information at any point in this continuum. Availability of information is of little use if the quality of information is poor. Likewise confidentiality is contingent upon quality information that is available when needed.

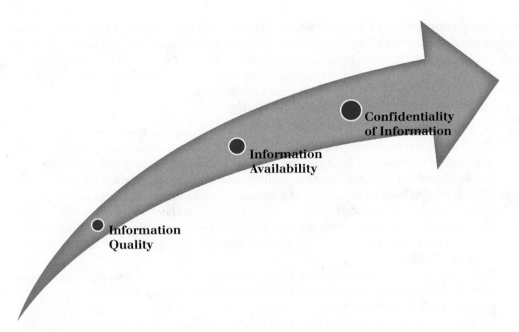

FIGURE 3–2 • Information Requisites

DATA INTEGRITY

Data integrity is a comprehensive term that encompasses the notion of wholeness when data is collected, stored, and retrieved by the authorized user. For data to be complete and orderly, systematicity must exist so that data integrity is preserved to ensure a state of current and correct form. Data integrity is crucial in the healthcare environment because data serves as a driving force in treatment decision making. Information technology must ensure that decisions derived from healthcare data are based on authentic data. If the quality of data is somehow flawed or incorrect, treatment outcomes are adversely impacted. For example, if data is faulty or incomplete, the quality of derived information may be poor, resulting in decisions that may be inappropriate and possibly harmful to clients. For example, if the nurse interviewing a client collects data related to allergies but fails to document all reported allergies, the client may be given drugs that cause an allergic reaction. In this case, the data were collected but not stored properly.

Ensuring Correct Data Collection and Entry

Computer systems facilitate data collection but may increase the potential for entry of incorrect data through input errors. These errors may include hitting the wrong key on a computer keyboard, selecting the wrong item from a screen using touch or a mouse, or failing to enter all data collected. Several measures can be taken to decrease the likelihood of input errors, including educating personnel, conducting system checks, and verifying data.

Educating Personnel Staff who are proficient in the use of the input device and computer system are less likely to make data collection and entry errors. Research by Haller, Haller, Courvoisier, and Lovis (2009) found that text entry on handheld versus laptop computers poses potential error that should be anticipated. All personnel should attend classes that emphasize appropriate system access, input device use, potential harmful effects associated with incorrect data, data verification techniques, and error correction. On the completion of classes, all employees should demonstrate competence in system use. Even after competence is demonstrated by personnel, continuing education should occur on a routine basis and as indicated by problems such as increase in data errors.

Ensuring Accuracy and Completeness Data entry systems should be easy to use and should provide periodic checks to ascertain that data are correct and complete. A **system check** is a mechanism provided by the computer system to assist users by prompting them to complete a task, verify information, or prevent entry of inappropriate information. Computer systems facilitate data collection and verification in several ways. Examples of computer system safeguards and generated prompts include the following:

a. *Data cleansing technology.* Information technology can help an organization to derive improved information and generate knowledge from data stored on different information systems (Liu & Chen 2009; Lorenzi & Riley 2010). Originally software was developed to eliminate variations in name and address information for direct mail campaigns used by businesses as a means to avoid multiple mailings for the same party. Used at the point of data entry, it serves to prevent data input errors. This is best illustrated when the system asks the user to confirm whether there is a match already in the database for a patient, thereby eliminating duplicate entries with several variants in name or address.

b. *Requesting information about a client's allergies when no entry has been made regarding allergies.* In the absence of an entry regarding allergies, the system may not accept medication and radiology orders.

c. *Informing the user that an order already exists when the user attempts to enter a duplicate order.* The system requests verification before processing the duplicate order. This can prevent unintentional repetition of expensive diagnostic tests. For example, a physician previously ordered a complete blood count (CBC) to be drawn on the current day. Another physician has ordered a hemoglobin and hematocrit (H&H), also to be drawn on the current day. When the order for the H&H is entered into the computer, the system will alert the user that this is a duplicate order, because the H&H is part of the CBC.

d. *Producing printouts alerting the nurse that a prescribed medication has not been documented as given.* This improves the quality of client care and documentation.

Data Verification Techniques According to Clarke et al. (2008), and Pakhomov, Jacobsen, Chute, and Roger (2008), another means to ensure data accuracy is to have clients verify data that are collected during the admission and assessment processes. The active participation of the client in the data verification process remains a relatively new concept in relation to healthcare computer systems. This verification may be accomplished through one of the following methods:

a. Verbal confirmation
b. Asking clients to review data on selected screens
c. Asking clients to review printouts of entered data

Each of these methods has potential problems. For example, with verbal confirmation clients may answer *yes* without actually hearing or understanding what was said to them. Screen review is difficult for the visually impaired or may be done too quickly for the client to scan all information. Finally, reading printouts is impractical for the visually impaired or illiterate. It also creates the additional problem of papers that must be disposed of with consideration for their confidential nature. All methods may be problematic for the individual who does not speak English.

Although the initial data collection and entry process provides an excellent opportunity to verify data accuracy and completeness, it should not be the only time that this is done. Healthcare consumers should be able to review their records at any time and furnish additional information that they believe is important to their care or to dispute portions of their record with which they do not agree. Privacy-preserving data processes are ensured through federal legislation (Fung, Wang, Fu, & Yu 2010).

Minimizing Fraudulent Information

Another concern in the concept of data integrity is the entry of fraudulent information. Fraudulent information can lead to financial loss to the provider and third-party payer as well as sully the credit rating of an innocent victim whose identity and insurance information were used. It may also result in treatment errors. At present, admitting clerks and physician office staff ask for the client's insurance card at the time of treatment. This request should also include proof of identification, preferably photograph identification, as a means to decrease claims filed under another person's identity. Clients should be informed of the purpose of this request and sign a statement indicating that they are aware that insurance fraud is a criminal act and that use of another person's insurance data may result in bodily harm secondary to treatment decisions based on someone else's health record.

DATA MANAGEMENT

The changing healthcare delivery system provides the driving force for improved data management. **Data management** is the process of controlling the collection, storage, retrieval, and use of data to optimize accuracy and utility while safeguarding integrity. Computers are an essential tool in this process. Good data management is essential for organizational decision making and is sometimes referred to as *business intelligence* (Hristidis 2009; Lorenzi & Riley 2010). One important part of decision making is the distribution of information via reports. Good data management involves knowing who needs report information, what reports are generated and what they are called, and when reports are available (Kudyba 2010).

Several levels of personnel are involved in data management. Personnel at the point of data entry include employees and, in some cases, clients. System analysts help the users to specify the data that are to be collected and how data collection will be accomplished. Programmers create the computer instructions, or program, that will collect the required data. They also build the **database,** a file structure that supports the storage of data in an organized fashion and allows data retrieval as meaningful information. Some facilities may also employ a **database administrator**, who is responsible for overseeing all activities related to maintaining the database and optimizing its use.

A **relational database** is one that is devised using tabulated data. In healthcare, such an approach can be more easily manipulated in order to quickly answer clinical questions. A **data warehouse** offers a more robust application for data management by serving as a data repository for storage and retrieval (Bhansali 2009). A data warehouse is a repository for storing data from several different databases so that it can be combined and manipulated to provide answers to various questions.

Costs and benefits are additional considerations in the management of data. Storage and management of paper and film records are labor intensive and expensive. Retrieval of paper and film records must be done manually, and information may not be available when and where it is needed. Physical records are also subject to loss. One current solution is **document imaging,** which involves scanning paper records onto computer disks or other media to facilitate electronic storage and handling. Converting paper records to other storage media may facilitate management, but a better solution is to move away from paper, with data entered directly to automated records. Although automated solutions may also be costly, they provide increased efficiency and improved access.

Automation of healthcare records creates new issues related to data storage and retrieval. Recent estimates project that personal computer, network, and mainframe storage requirements will grow 50% per year. Along with an increase in volume and types of materials for storage, data storage and retrieval require special conditions to ensure data integrity.

Data Storage

There are two basic types of data storage: online and offline. **Online storage** provides access to current data. Online storage is rapid, using high-speed hard disk drives or storage space allocated on the network. **Offline storage** is used for data that are needed less frequently, or for long-term

---

BOX 3–2   Data Storage Considerations

- **Environmental conditions and physical hazards.** These include temperature, humidity, shock, dust control, and protection from damage by fire, water, or electromagnetic fields. Some media are more sensitive to environmental factors than others. Strict environmental controls protect the storage media and the data they contain. In general, temperatures in the 10°C range in conjunction with ideal environmental conditions help to maximize the shelf life for media.

- **Control of equipment and media.** This refers to who may access computer equipment and data and is supported through a combination of physical and logical restrictions. Physical restrictions maintain a secure locked environment for the computer hardware and operations areas. Logical restrictions limit data access to only those staff who require this information. For example, admission clerks might be restricted from accessing clinical information such as test results but might be able to access demographic and insurance information.

- **Contingency planning.** A secondary or backup copy of the data is created as a safeguard in the event of loss or damage to the primary data. This backup copy should be stored at another location separate from the computer, reducing the danger that a disaster will affect both the computer and the storage area.

- **Storage period for each record type.** The minimum length of time that client records must be stored is dictated by state laws. An organization may choose to retain records indefinitely, but cost and physical storage constraints must be considered.

- **Plans to transfer data to new media before degradation occurs.** For example, data stored on magnetic tape may degrade after 1 to 50 years, depending on storage conditions. If the organization intends to retain records indefinitely, the data must be transferred to other media.

- **Recognition that most electronic media will be threatened by the obsolescence of the hardware and software needed to access them.** Rapid advances in technology lead to the discontinuation of formats and media as more efficient storage modalities are introduced.

- **Maintenance of access devices.** Problems with access devices are one of the most common causes of damage to magnetic storage media. Consideration should be given to writing and reading archive copies from different devices as a means to protect against data loss from malfunctioning devices.

---

data storage, as may occur with old client records. Offline storage can be done on any secondary storage device. Access to data stored offline is slower than that with online storage. Immediacy of need for particular data is a key factor in determining whether it is stored online or offline.

According to Shreeves and Cragin (2008), to protect computerized information, institutions need a storage strategy that addresses unique data storage conditions. The considerations summarized in Box 3–2 address these conditions.

Outsourcing Data Management and Storage

Internal data storage is costly in terms of human resources and space that can be allocated for other purposes. Storage costs include the purchase price for devices and the costs of media, maintenance, and environmental control. These costs may consume a significant portion of the information services budget. Storage can be handled internally or outsourced. **Outsourcing** is the process by which an organization contracts with outside agencies for services. Outsourcing provides a means to cut costs that would otherwise be required for the physical space, special conditions, and support personnel needed to maintain storage media and data.

Outsourcing companies specialize in all aspects of data management for multiple customers, providing services at a lower cost than if the customers performed the tasks themselves. It is important to review the contract to ensure that the outsourcing company can meet all of the institution's requirements for data storage and retrieval.

Data Retrieval

Data retrieval is a process that allows the user to access previously collected and stored data. Data retrieval most commonly occurs as a function of a software application in conjunction with secondary storage media. Recent developments in technology have cut storage costs and improved access and capacity. In addition to new options in storage media, a variety of automated devices are available that provide access to stored data. Automated magnetic tape has been used to archive healthcare data for many years.

The significance of data retrieval may be seen in the development of an automated client record that covers the client's life span. Although these advances are critical to the development of a birth-to-death health record, many providers are still in the first phase of developing systems for each client visit and have limited archival access. Furthermore, present hospital data storage systems save data but often lack the ability to manipulate data to demonstrate patterns. For example, it should be possible to easily extract demographic data on the population served, individual and aggregate responses to specific treatment modalities, or abnormal laboratory values for a given client.

The following factors should be considered when planning for data retrieval:

a. *Performance. Performance* refers to the ability of the system to respond to user requests for data retrieval. Some of the specific factors that define performance include acceptable retrieval response time and the ability to accommodate numerous simultaneous requests for data.

b. *Capacity.* Capacity is the number and size of records that can be stored and retrieved.

c. *Data security.* Data must be protected against unauthorized access and retrieval.

d. *Cost.* The costs include hardware, software, and support personnel. Data storage and retrieval costs overlap in many cases.

Retrieval needs are frequently underestimated. For example, some systems sharply limit the amount of archival data available to users and may impede treatment. Determination of system performance requirements helps data management personnel and administrators choose storage and retrieval strategies for user needs. Generally, record demand is highest soon after data are collected, with the number of access requests and need for rapid retrieval diminishing with the passage of time.

Data Exchange

In the past, data retrieval was primarily performed for use within a single institution. Changes in the healthcare delivery system now mandate exchange of client information between institutions. For example, a client may have surgery at a major medical center but have follow-up appointments at a satellite location. The client's record must be accessible to clinicians at both sites. Several other factors contribute to the need to send client records in a timely fashion from one provider to another and to submit reimbursement claims in a timely fashion. These factors include, but are not limited to, a highly mobile population and consumer demands for efficiency. **Electronic data interchange (EDI)** streamlines the flow of clinical and financial data from one location to another. Electronic data interchange is the communication of data in binary code from one computer to another. As the number of automated client record systems increases, so does the need to establish standard record structure and identifiers for individual data items to facilitate data exchange.

Although EDI facilitates record exchange, there are problems associated with it. A major problem is that different computer systems use different formats for data. The data format from the sending system may not be understood by the receiving system. One solution to this problem is the development of a standard data format for EDI. At the present, no agreement exists among healthcare groups in the United States regarding a common EDI standard. Several groups are currently working toward a common standard.

Data Cleansing

The first step in data cleansing is determining the extent of the problem. This can help users to decide where to focus their efforts for quality improvement for the input of new data as well as data that have already been collected. Manual review and correction of poor-quality data are extremely labor intensive. **Data cleansing** or **scrubbing** is a procedure that uses software to improve the quality of data to ensure that it is accurate enough for use in data mining and warehousing. It uses technology to reconcile data inconsistencies that arise from different systems as well as duplicate entries in one system. These inconsistencies may include typographical errors, misspellings, and various abbreviations as well as address changes. According to Sox and Rennie (2006), data errors have accounted for a variety of legal precedents. The fact that abbreviations can have totally different meanings in different systems becomes a major problem with data warehousing. Another problem is the use of automatic defaults, which fill in blanks with information that is not accurate. One example is seen when the name of the ordering physician is "defaulted in" for the primary physician when it is not the same. Data cleansing is essential to data warehousing. Data inconsistencies that did not pose problems for daily operations do create a problem for data warehousing because it requires a higher-quality data.

According to Liu, Zhang, Cen, Ru, and Ma (2007), the use of Internet technology for data entry by employees as well as clients serves to minimize some problems but accentuate others. This is because employees can be trained in data entry and can be called back for additional training if problems are noted. Clients have not had the benefit of system training to know what constitutes acceptable entries, and they may not have the incentive to correct errors in some cases. The use of data cleansing technology was once limited by its high costs and difficulties in implementation, but improvements in the quality of data can provide safety and save money through elimination of duplication.

Data Disposal

Appropriate disposal of electronic and print data that are no longer required is an important aspect of data management (Wickramasinghe, Bali, Gibbons, & Schaffer 2008). Print media can be discarded in special receptacles designated for confidential materials. Data destruction may be achieved through physical destruction and software destruction. Physical destruction may be accomplished by deforming storage media or using a magnet to destroy contents. Special equipment is available to destroy hard drives. Commercial software may be used to overwrite data by filling the hard drive with zeros. Destruction may be done internally or outsourced. Factors in the selection of vendor services should include:

a. Procedures used to determine that destruction has occurred as planned
b. Vendor security to protect data and/or equipment
c. Errors and omissions insurance in the event that some data are accidentally disclosed

It is important to ensure that disposal occurs as planned to avoid violating legislation intended to safeguard patient privacy.

DATA MINING

Data mining is a knowledge management tool that engages software to uncover inter-relationships within large data sets (Nicolini et al. 2008). It uses artificial intelligence, statistical computation, and computerization to drill down through the large data sets in order to identify potential inter-relationships. Data mining has long been utilized in marketing and politics to determine buying and voting trends within society and has more recently been applied to healthcare organizations in order to determine a variety of healthcare outcomes. It is prominently featured in epidemiological applications such as biosurveillance as well as related public health applications.

Data mining has also been used extensively in primary care, healthcare performance initiatives, and ongoing quality improvement (Curcin, Bottle, Molokhia, Millett, & Majeed 2010). It is used in healthcare for health resource planning, research, and surveillance, and to identify successful standardized treatments for specific diseases and pay-for-performance, track performance, chart quality improvement, and determine clinical system usage (Neubauer & Heurix 2011; Zheng, Mei, & Hanauer 2011). Increasingly complex data mining applications offer high-quality and cost-effective benefits by identifying referral patterns of healthcare providers and other related data trends (Stankovski et al. 2008). For example, the DataMiningGrid is one such application that "integrates a diverse set of programs and application scenarios within a single framework" (p. 69) to sort and compare data in many different ways to discover relationships. The driving factor of such an application is that it can offer a cost-effective approach that features scalability, flexible extensibility, and sophisticated support. Such grid computing possibilities make data mining an essential ingredient in organizational structure. Although data mining is now more accessible, the lack of increased application of standardized clinical language continues to function as a barrier to accessing clean data that is necessary for effective mining. Data mining naturally leads to the KDD paradigm.

KNOWLEDGE DISCOVERY IN DATABASES

According to Serrant-Green (2008), in nursing and healthcare, "data discovery underpins all our research work" (p. 3). Accordingly, **knowledge discovery in databases (KDD)** can be defined as the development of skills, understandings, and integrative abilities derived from data. Data mining provides trended patterns that can then be transformed into useful data (Bonchi & Ferrari 2010). Clinical databases hold huge amounts of information about patients and their medical conditions. The potential to discern patterns and relationships within those databases that would contribute to new knowledge was recognized some time ago, but efforts were hampered by the paucity of methods to discover useful information until recently (Brown 2008; Lyman, Scully, & Harrison 2008). New tools offer the capability to expand research. Clinical repositories are now available for research and utilization purposes. According to Nicolini et al. (2008), knowledge management is particularly suited for the healthcare sector. Certainly healthcare providers, and in particular, nurses, are in the best position to deliver high-quality and cost-effective care that is dependent upon their ability to translate knowledge (evidence) into practice. Such translational science will require access to data trends that can be mined from large data sets and then used to answer clinical questions in order to deliver best practice through interprofessional collaboration and further research.

FUTURE DIRECTIONS

The future offers unprecedented change in knowledge discovery and management, data mining, and translational science. Standard data exchange models will foster translation science as investigators achieve interoperability through increased database engagement if roadblocks to data mining tool access are overcome (Ash, Anderson, & Tarczy-Hornoch 2008). Roadblocks to data mining tool access include financial barriers and the lack of organizational support. Increased database engagement means translation science can be improved. Data mining and KDD will promote translational science, further contributing to evidence-based practice, and translational informatics tools and related research systems implementation. According to Gama (2010), KDD could be used to generate nursing knowledge by creating models that identified clients at risk for falling using minimum data set data. In addition, the development of data mining algorithms will further contribute to the body of evidence supporting care (Bakken, Stone, & Larson 2008) as the United States moves toward electronic health record adoption as a part of its national healthcare agenda (Bahensky, Jaana, & Ward 2008).

CASE STUDY EXERCISE

Agnes Gibbons was admitted through the hospital's emergency department with congestive heart failure. During her admission she was asked to verbally acknowledge whether her demographic data were correct. Ms. Gibbons did so. Extensive diagnostic tests were done, including radiology studies. It was later discovered that all of Ms. Gibbons' information had been entered into another client's file. How would you correct this situation? What departments, or other agencies, would need to be informed of this situation?

SUMMARY

- Quality information is essential to the delivery of appropriate client care.
- Data can be managed using a database application.
- A data warehouse is a collection of several databases that can be manipulated to provide complex data analysis.
- Information quality is ensured when measures to protect it are an integral part of its collection, use, storage, retrieval, and exchange.
- Data integrity strategies should provide safeguards against data manipulation or deletion, and entry of fraudulent facts.
- Data storage measures should provide safe, accessible storage to authorized persons through a plan that considers provider, client, and third-party payer needs; physical threats to information and media; performance requirements; pros and cons of on-site versus off-site storage; technological advancements; and future needs.
- Performance, capacity, data security, and cost should be considered when planning for data retrieval.
- Electronic data interchange standards provide timely access to providers at distant sites and computer systems.
- Data cleansing uses software to improve the quality of data to ensure that it is suitable for all purposes including data mining and warehousing.
- Data mining uses software to look for hidden patterns and relationships in large groups of data such as performance information and successful treatments for specific diseases. It allows users to sort and compare data in many different ways to discover relationships.
- Knowledge discovery in databases uses data mining to derive knowledge from trends and patterns discovered in data mining.
- Nurses are well-situated to make good use of knowledge discovered in databases.

REFERENCES

Ash, J. S., Anderson, N. R., & Tarczy-Hornoch, P. (2008). People and organizational issues in research systems implementation. *Journal of the American Medical Informatics Association, 15*(3), 283–289.

Bahensky, J. A., Jaana, M., & Ward, M. M. (2008). Healthcare information technology in rural America: Electronic health record adoption status in meeting the national agenda. *Journal of Rural Health, 24*(2), 101–105.

Bakken, S., Stone, P. W., & Larson, E. L. (2008). A nursing informatics research agenda for 2008-18: Contextual influences and key components. *Nursing Outlook, 56*(5), 206–214.

Bhansali, N. (2009). *Strategic data warehousing: Achieving alignment with business.* Boca Raton, FL: Chapman & Hall.

Bonchi, F., & Ferrari, E. (2010). *Privacy-aware knowledge discovery: Novel applications and new techniques*. Boca Raton, FL: Chapman & Hall.

Brown, D. E. (2008). Introduction to data mining for medical informatics. *Clinics in Laboratory Medicine, 28*(1), 9–35.

Clarke, D., Breen, L., Jacobs, M., Franklin, R., Tobota, Z., Maruszewski, B., & Jacobs, J. P. (2008). Verification of data in congenital cardiac surgery. *Cardiology in the Young, 18*(2), 177–187.

Curcin, V., Bottle, A., Molokhia, M., Millett, C., & Majeed, A. (2010). Towards a scientific workflow methodology for primary care database studies. *Statistical Methods in Medical Research, 19*(4), 378–393.

de Lusignan, S. (2009). Usability: A neglected theme in informatics. *Informatics in Primary Care, 17*(4), 199–200.

Fung, B. C. M., Wang, K., Fu, A., & Yu, P. S. (2010). *Introduction to privacy-preserving data publishing: Concepts and techniques*. Boca Raton, FL: Chapman & Hall.

Gama, J. (2010). *Knowledge discovery from data streams*. Boca Raton, FL: Chapman & Hall.

Haller, G., Haller, D. M., Courvoisier, D. S., & Lovis, D. (2009). Handheld vs. laptop computers for electronic data collection in clinical research: A crossover randomized trial. *Journal of the American Medical Informatics Association, 16*, 651–659.

Hristidis, V. (2009). *Information discovery on electronic health records*. Boca Raton, FL: Chapman & Hall.

Kudyba, S. P. (2010). *Healthcare informatics: Improving efficiency and productivity*. Boca Raton, FL: Chapman & Hall.

Li, W. N., Bheemavaram, R., & Zhang, X. (2010). Transitive closure of data records: Application and computation. *Data Engineering: International Series in Operations Research & Management Science, 132*, 39–75.

Liu, S. S., & Chen, J. (2009). Using data mining to segment healthcare markets from patients' perspectives. *International Journal of Healthcare Quality Assurance, 22*(2), 117–134.

Liu, Y., Zhang, M., Cen, R., Ru, L., & Ma, S. (2007). Data cleansing for web information retrieval using query independent features. *Journal of the American Society for Information Science and Technology, 58*(12), 1884–1898.

Lorenzi, N. M., & Riley, R. T. (2010). *Managing technological change: Organizational aspects of health informatics*. New York: Springer.

Lyman, J. A., Scully, K., & Harrison, J. H. (2008). The development of healthcare data warehouses to support data mining. *Clinics in Laboratory Medicine, 28*(1), 55–71.

Neubauer, T., & Heurix, J. (2011). A methodology for the pseudonymization of medical data. *International Journal of Medical Informatics, 80*(3), 190–204.

Nicolini, D., Powell, J., Conville, P., & Martinez-Solano, L. (2008). Managing knowledge in the healthcare sector: A review. *International Journal of Management Reviews, 10*(3), 245–263.

Pakhomov, S., Jacobsen, S. J., Chute, C. G., & Roger, V. L. (2008). Agreement between patient-reported symptoms and their documentation in the medical record. *American Journal of Managed Care, 14*(8), 530–539.

Rao, R. B., Fung, G., & Rosales, R. (2011). *Knowledge-driven medicine: A machine learning approach*. Boca Raton, FL: Chapman & Hall.

Serrant-Green, L. (2008). Data discovery underpins all our research work. *Nurse Researcher, 15*(4), 3.

Shreeves, S. L., & Cragin, M. H. (2008). Institutional repositories: Current state and future. *Library Trends, 57*(2), 168–190.

Sox, H., & Rennie, D. (2006). Research misconduct, retraction, and cleansing the medical literature: Lessons from the Poehlman case. *Annals of Internal Medicine, 144*(8), 609–613.

Stankovski, V., Swain, M., Kravtsov, V., Niessen, T., Wegener, D., Rohm, M., . . . Dubitzky, W. (2008). Digging deep into the data mine with datamininggrid. *Internet Computing, 12*(6), 69–76.

White, K., & Dudley-Brown, S. (2011). *Translation of evidence into nursing and healthcare practice*. New York: Springer.

Wickramasinghe, N., Bali, R. K., Gibbons, M. C., & Schaffer, J. (2008). Realising the knowledge spiral in healthcare: The role of data mining and knowledge management. *Studies in Health Technology Information, 137*, 147–162.

Zheng, K., Mei, Q., & Hanauer, D. A. (2011). Collaborative search in electronic health records. *Journal of the American Medical Informatics Association, 18*, 282–291.

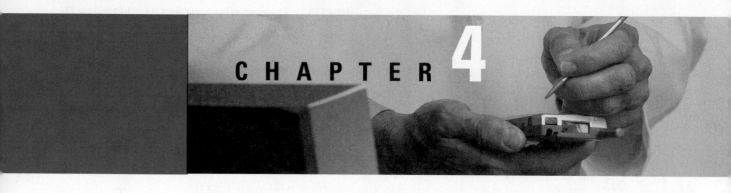

CHAPTER 4

The Internet and the World Wide Web: An Overview

After completing this chapter, you should be able to:

1. Define *electronic communication* and compare and contrast e-mail, instant messaging, and text messaging.

2. Differentiate between the Internet and the World Wide Web.

3. Identify the process required to access both the Internet and the World Wide Web.

4. Discuss services available on the Internet and the World Wide Web.

5. Relate the advantages and disadvantages that the Internet and the World Wide Web have over traditional means of communicating information.

6. Compare and contrast a Web *page,* a Web *portal,* a *blog*, and a *wiki.*

7. Discuss the terms *search index, search engine,* and *search unifier.*

8. Evaluate the quality of information for a Web site.

9. Compare and contrast the purpose and use of intranets and extranets to the purpose and use of the Internet.

10. Discuss the advantages and disadvantages of the Internet as a platform for healthcare applications.

he Internet, also popularly referred to as "**the Net**," is a global network that connects millions of computers. The origins of the Internet began in the early 1960s with the development of **ARPANET (Advanced Research Projects Agency Network)** by the U.S. Defense Department. ARPANET was a test bed for new networking technologies and encouraged researchers at different governmental and academic sites to share their findings. From modest beginnings, the Internet has evolved tremendously and now links government, universities, commercial institutions, and individual users. The Internet can now be accessed at many places by a variety of means, including mobile Internet devices, such as cell phones, netbooks, laptops, PDAs (personal digital assistants), and more.

Today, content and information exchanged on the Internet are relatively free from the control of any government or single organization, although several nations would prefer more local jurisdiction and China actually limits what its citizens can access (Governmental delegations 2005). Leaders at the United Nations (UN) and the European Union proposed that Internet control go to the UN Working Group on Internet Governance (WGIG), noting that the present system unfairly favors the United States. WGIG identified the following areas of concern: rights of nations to control Internet assets; the desire for developing nations to have a voice in the work of international bodies; control over the Internet domains; spam and Internet crime (The need for global policies 2005; UN to control 2005). Still others propose that that Internet administration occur under a multilateral treaty (Cukier 2005). The United States has provided oversight and coordination of the Internet in four critical areas: domain names, Internet protocol numbers, root servers, and technical standards. The U.S. government established the nonprofit Internet Corporation for Assigned Names and Numbers (ICANN) in 1998. The ICANN allocates top-level domain names and settles domain name disputes (Cukier 2005; McCarthy 2006). ICANN also assigns Internet protocol numbers that are needed by every machine on the network for recognition by other machines. In 2009 oversight of the ICANN was placed in the hands of the world and the ICANN Board approved a fast-track process for international top-level domain names (ICANN 2010).

Governments are looking at jurisdictional problems created by the Internet and ways to harmonize laws related to hacking, fraud, and child pornography. The Council of Europe drafted the Cybercrime Treaty in an attempt to provide common definitions. The U.S. Senate ratified this treaty in 2006 joining 40 other nations in fighting crimes committed via the Internet (Senate ratifies treaty 2006). Acceptance has not been unanimous (Newly nasty 2007). The 14 nations of the South African Development Community (SADC) have also been working to harmonize their cybercrime laws to make it easier to prosecute criminals across boundaries (Malakata 2005).

The Internet Society (ISOC) has the greatest overall influence on the Internet. This nonprofit, professional organization provides direction when issues arise that can impact the Internet. The Internet Society also serves as a home for groups responsible for the promulgation of Internet infrastructure standards. These groups include the Internet Engineering Task Force (IETF) and the Internet Architecture Board (IAB). The IAB is chartered both as a committee of the IETF and as an advisory body of the ISOC. Its responsibilities include architectural oversight of IETF activities and Internet Standards Process oversight and appeal.

The Internet Society serves as a global clearinghouse for information about the Internet and facilitates and coordinates Internet-related initiatives. The Society sponsors several events, including the annual International Networking (INET) conference as well as training workshops, tutorials, research, publications, public policy, and trade activities for the benefit of people throughout the world (Internet Society, n.d.).

The Internet expands the range of available healthcare information through e-mail, discussion lists, blogs, wikis, file transfer protocol (FTP), Telnet, and World Wide Web resources. Many materials are no longer published on paper but are available only electronically. Some examples include research reports, journals, practice guidelines, educational materials, and conference proceedings.

The Internet is the largest, best-known wide area network in the world. Its exact size is difficult to estimate because of its rapid growth, but its users number in the millions. One major factor in the growth of the Internet is the development of companies known as **Internet service providers (ISPs)** that furnish Internet access for a fee to small business and home users. Some well-known examples of ISPs include America Online (AOL), Microsoft Network (MSN), and EarthLink. In addition, cable and telephone companies often bundle Internet services with their primary services. Internet access through an ISP requires computer access, a modem, and communication software. Several variations for connectivity exist, including telephone dial-up, wireless, or high-speed access through digital subscriber line (DSL), cable, fiber optic, or satellite. Dial-up is slow, but may be the only option available to some customers. DSL uses existing copper telephone wires, but differs from the traditional dial-up connections in that it requires a special modem and is always "on." DSL is limited to customers who fall within a certain distance of the telephone switching station. Cable service has relied on coaxial cable to transmit television signals. Cable service also requires a special modem. Fiber optic cable service can be used for high-speed Internet service as well as an alternative cable television service. While fiber optic may be used in combination with cable, it can also be provided all the way into the client's home or business for speeds several times faster than standard cable or DSL (Fiber: Friend or foe 2007; Hesseldahl 2007). Satellite service has been plagued with a reputation of difficult and expensive installations, poor service, and suspect performance. For these reasons it is less common except in areas where neither DSL nor cable is available. Other options for connectivity that are in various stages of development include the use of the existing electrical power grids and encoded light transmissions (Dunn 2006; Kavehrad 2007).

ISPs provide software and directions on how to access the Internet and a special account that provides Internet and World Wide Web access. Customers generally pay their ISP a monthly fee; in some cases there is an additional charge for access time. Some hotels, coffee shops, parks, hospitals, and even communities provide free Internet connections for their customers. Most ISPs provide a local telephone number for customer use.

The Internet offers many types of services and resources, including the following:

- *Electronic mail or e-mail.* **E-mail** is the use of computers to transmit messages to one or more persons. Delivery can be almost instantaneous. While e-mail was originally developed for sending simple text messages, many e-mail applications support e-mail messages, which include color, formatted text, and pictures. E-mail attachments are files that are sent along with the e-mail message. E-mail can be sent anywhere in the world as long as the individual has an Internet address. Internet addresses are based upon a domain name which is based on the type of institution or ISP provider. For example Jane Doe, a nurse at St. Francis Medical Center, might have jdoe@stfrancismc.edu as her work e-mail address. Jane Doe can check her e-mail while at work or may be able to log on to her e-mail account from outside locations on her days off to check for announcements of upcoming meetings and new procedures and other pertinent messages.
- *Instant messaging (IM).* **IM** is real-time text-based discussions that may take place on computers or other devices using a software client. Most IM services are free and provide their own software or browser-based client to the users. IM has given rise to its own language or set of abbreviations as a means to allow communication in an expeditious manner. IM has gained some acceptance in the workplace, but does not replace formal communication. Early instant messaging was known as *Internet relay chat (IRC)*.
- *File transfer.* File transfer allows users to move files from one location to another directly over a network. The benefit of file transfer is that users can capture, view, edit, or use work developed by others rather than starting anew. It is particularly useful for large files that exceed the size allowed by e-mail systems, such as a procedure manual or student handbook.

- *Database searches.* This feature allows users to conduct comprehensive literature searches online in a shorter period of time than could be accomplished manually. Access to database searches is obtained through universities, public libraries, or on a subscription basis using an Internet connection. Previously searches were done via hardcopy manuals or periodic database increments on disc. In addition to literature databases, there are databases that contain information about particular patient populations such as cancer patients, those who had cardiothoracic surgery, and many more groups.
- *Remote log-on.* This feature allows users to access computer resources, such as directories, files, and databases at other locations. Most systems, such as the Virginia Henderson International Nursing Library, require an account, identification, and a password for **remote log-on**.
- *Discussion and news groups.* The Internet provides a place where specialty interest groups can address concerns, discuss solutions, and exchange information in a timely fashion. One example of an international resource for student nurses is SNURSE-L. Groups provide specific instructions on how to participate and can be found through professional publications, conferences, word of mouth or a Web search.

INTERNET SERVICES

E-mail and Instant Messaging

E-mail is one of the most frequently used Internet applications. It is commonly found in private organizations, colleges, universities, corporations, hospitals, and private homes. It is a powerful connectivity tool and often is the feature that first attracts users to the Internet. E-mail encourages networking among peers, yields helpful tips and shared resources, and saves time and money that would otherwise be spent on printing and postage and individual problem solving. E-mail is a convenient way to contact employees, colleagues, students, and recruiters. It allows users to participate in educational offerings and send announcements and resumes. Box 4–1 lists some advantages and disadvantages associated with e-mail and IM. The next few paragraphs explain the composition and management of e-mail.

An e-mail application is a computer program that assists the user to send, receive, and manage e-mail messages. Most have basic text editing and spell-checking capability. Popular commercial e-mail applications include Microsoft Outlook, Lotus Notes, Thunderbird, and Eudora. Individuals who work in an environment supported by large mainframe computers may use other e-mail programs. Despite its popularity, some healthcare workers still do not have e-mail accounts. E-mail applications may reside locally on the user's computer or are Web based. Many organizations and ISPs allow users to access their accounts via a Web page affording them the opportunity to check their messages from almost any location. There are also Web sites such as Gmail, Hotmail, Yahoo! Mail, and others that supply free e-mail accounts.

As e-mail popularity grows, so do concerns related to its use. These concerns include threats to data integrity and security, confidentiality, verification that messages emanate from the identified source, spam, and HIPAA (Health Insurance Portability and Accountability Act) compliance. Data integrity may be threatened by **computer viruses** and other malicious software, known as malware. Viruses are malicious programs that can disrupt or destroy data and sometimes overwhelm networks with traffic. Viruses are not transmitted via e-mail messages themselves, but may be found as file attachments sent with messages or launched when infected files are opened. The best way to minimize the threat of viruses is to scan all attached files with the latest version of antivirus software before opening. One can also delete e-mail and attachments from unknown sources at the risk of deleting wanted materials. When content needs to be kept secure and confidential, **encryption** is recommended. Encryption uses mathematical

BOX 4–1 E-mail and Instant Messaging: Advantages and Disadvantages	
E-mail Advantages	**Instant Messaging Advantages**
Eliminates phone tag. Provides the ability to contact someone whose phone is busy or to leave a written message.	**Bypasses phone use.** Allows instant communication without wasted time for trivial communication.
Convenient. Can be sent or retrieved from multiple locations, including work, home, or while traveling. Can be used on a 24-hour basis.	**Convenient.** Can be sent or retrieved from multiple locations, including work, home, or while traveling. Can be used on a 24-hour basis.
Easy to prepare and send. Requires less effort to prepare and send than the traditional means of written communication.	**Easy to prepare and send.** Requires less effort to prepare and send than the e-mail and traditional means of written communication.
Saves time and money. Eliminates postage and paper expenses.	**Saves time and money.** Direct, short messages encourage the elimination of unnecessary information. Provides immediate responses.
Delivery can eliminate the time lag associated with traditional mail.	**Presence technology.** Shows whether the desired recipient is online.
Time- and date-stamped. Messages are time and date stamped providing documentation of the actual time of the mail transaction. Can also provide a log of when the message was received, read, and answered. Messages are searchable.	**Time- and date-stamped.** Messages are time and date stamped. May also provide a log of conversation. Can save copy of IM conversation as a log.
E-Mail Disadvantages	**Instant Messaging Disadvantages**
Interpretation of messages without the benefit of voice inflection or facial expression.	**Interpretation of messages without the benefit of voice inflection or facial expression.**
High volume of messages sent and received. E-mail's popularity and ease of use make it easy to generate large numbers of messages, including copies, forwarded messages, and "junk mail."	**Message sent and received in an abbreviated language.**
Malware contamination can occur via attached files. Attached files that contain a virus or worm or other malware may contaminate the recipient's computer.	**Malware contamination can occur via attached files.** Attached files that contain a virus or worm or other malware may contaminate the recipient's computer.
Security concerns related to maintaining confidentiality. Message may be intercepted and read by unintended parties. Employers may read all messages on company systems. Employees may read messages not intended for their eyes. Deleted messages may be retrieved during system backups.	**Security concerns related to maintaining confidentiality.** Message may be intercepted and read by unintended parties. Employers may read all messages on company systems. Employees may read messages not intended for their eyes. Deleted messages may be retrieved during system backups.

formulas to code messages. Message recipients decode content with special software known as an encryption key. Encryption may be done at the desktop or at the server level. Many e-mail applications provide the option to encrypt a message. Encryption serves to protect both the individual computer and its network.

Methods to validate e-mail author identity include **public key infrastructure (PKI)** and digital credentialing. PKI provides a unique code for each user that is imbedded into a storage device. User information is stored in a database by the organization that created the code. Identity is confirmed when the storage device and a password or other form of identification match information stored in the database. A simpler alternative to PKI is the **digital signature** or credential. The digital signature is a unique identifier issued to the individual that can be verified against the sender's public key. Intel and the American Medical Association worked collaboratively to develop digital credentialing for physicians. Physician digital credentials are routed through a firewall to the Intel Internet Authentication Service (ITAS) to validate user identity and create an audit trail. This same process is available for other healthcare workers. Although the digital credential does not require biometric measures to verify identity, there is increased interest in the use of biometric measures as a means to ensure that only authorized users access private health information.

Another issue that has been raised about the security of health information transmitted via e-mail is the security of the mail server, or the computer on which e-mail messages reside, both incoming and outgoing messages. Use of the health provider's e-mail for nonwork purposes can open up the server to viruses and hackers. Secure e-mail applications ensure that all information remains available to enterprise servers when it is needed. The use of a secure e-mail service provider is likened to using a private postal carrier, which helps to maintain data integrity, as well as provide audit trails and proof of receipt. This arrangement usually requires that servers on both ends are registered, so it is best suited for organizations that communicate regularly. Yet another safeguard of confidentiality is the ability to screen outgoing messages for appropriate content and to block messages sent to unknown or suspect addresses.

Other issues surrounding e-mail focus on its increasing volume: the time required to sift through e-mail messages; unwanted or "junk" e-mail, also known as **spam**; accurate interpretation of messages; and HIPAA compliance. The number of legitimate e-mail messages has grown exponentially, but so has the number of unwanted messages. A significant portion of all e-mail traffic is now spam. Spam is a problem because thousands of messages may be sent at one time. Spam spreads advertisements and may be used to collect personal and credit card information. Spam is constantly evolving to use new approaches to avoid filters. Spammers forge return e-mail addresses and domain names, making it difficult to track and prosecute them when they engage in fraudulent claims and illegal activity. Efforts to block spam include lawsuits, state and federal legislation, industry initiatives, establishing separate e-mail accounts for different purposes, e-mail rules for incoming mail and filtering software, and challenge response tools. Additional proposals for dealing with spam have called for the establishment of a "do not e-mail" list, limiting the number of messages that can be sent out per day via free e-mail accounts, and a requirement that advertisements be labeled. Spam is costly in terms of user time to delete unwanted messages, costs for filtering and challenge software, and higher costs for ISP service.

Challenge response software works by asking the e-mail sender to answer a question or complete a task that requires human intervention. No e-mail is accepted unless its validity has been confirmed by a human being. Challenge response software is sometimes referred to as **CAPTCHAS**, which stands for **C**ompletely **A**utomatic **P**ublic **T**uring Test to Tell Computers and **H**umans **A**part. Challenge response tools are effective in filtering out spam, but they create additional network traffic. Box 4–2 provides some informal rules to guide e-mail and IM use.

Like other Internet services, e-mail is based on a client/server system. In client/server technology, files are stored on a central computer known as a **server**. In this case, the server receives mail from other Internet sites and stores it until it is read, answered, or deleted. The client computer requests mail access from the server and generates new mail that will be handled by the server.

Components of an E-mail message Every e-mail message has several standard components. These components include a header, body, attachments, and possibly a signature. The ***header*** lists who sent the message, when, to whom, and a subject line. Message copies may also be copied to others through either a "cc," which stands for carbon copy or "bc," which stands for blind carbon or blind carbon copy. Persons designated to receive a bc will not have

BOX 4–2   Informal Rules for E-mail and Instant Messaging (IM) Use

- Change passwords for e-mail access immediately upon assignment and frequently thereafter.
- Limit e-mail copies to the people who need the information. This keeps the number of messages manageable. When sending a copy to the boss, list his or her name first if the e-mail package permits this action, some applications automatically alphabetize all recipients.
- Choose an accurate description for the e-mail subject line. This practice helps recipients to determine which messages should be read first.
- Avoid the use of blind copy (bc). It is considered unethical in many circles.
- Do not use e-mail or IM as a means to criticize or insult anyone.
- Use e-mail priority status and read receipts sparingly. Misuse may be found insulting.
- Check the e-mail list of recipients before pressing "send" to be certain that it is appropriate.
- Give e-mail and IM the same consideration given to business correspondence. Messages may be seen by parties other than intended recipients. Write nothing that would not otherwise be said or posted publicly. Consider how your message might be interpreted before sending it.
- Make messages clear, short, and to the point. Include original messages, or a portion, with your reply to provide context.
- Avoid the use of all capital letters. All capitals are difficult to read, and may be perceived as shouting, according to e-mail etiquette.
- Limit abbreviations to those that are easily understood.
- Read mail, file messages in categories, and delete messages no longer needed on a regular basis. This frees storage space and helps to optimize system function, as well as makes it easier to find and retrieve messages later.
- Try to reply to e-mail within 24 hours.
- Consider using mechanisms to prevent unwanted e-mail.
- Limit the use of emoticons in professional communication.
- Do not reply to messages that do not require a reply unless adding relevant information.

their names displayed on the e-mail copies sent to either the primary recipient or individuals receiving carbon copies. The subject line allows a brief phrase to describe the subject of the e-mail. While it is possible to send a message without completing the subject line, many recipients will not bother to read such a message. The **body** of the e-mail contains the main contents of the message as typed by the sender. Most e-mail systems allow the sender to create a standard ending for all messages, which is known as the signature and typically includes the sender's name, address, and other contact or identifying information. E-mail software allows the sender to send messages with files. The attached files are known as **attachments** and are considered an easy way to share files.

Designated recipients of e-mail are listed in the to:, cc:, and bc: fields by their e-mail addresses. The user may see either the address or the person's name because it is stored along with that address in the e-mail system. E-mail addresses are created using a standard format that includes a user's name followed by the @ symbol and the location or computer where that person's e-mail account can be found. In the example thebda@chamberlain.edu the user is found at Chamberlain College. Additional information may be included to identify a subdivision within an organization. General information is listed first followed by more specific information separated by periods or back slashes. The last portion of an e-mail address indicates the type of organization and is known as the domain. Box 4–3 lists some common e-mail organizational domains.

BOX 4–3   E-Mail Organizational Domains

The last portion of an e-mail address indicates the type of organization that provides the e-mail service used by the addressee. For example, *thebda@chamberlain.edu* indicates that a user named thebda is located at an educational organization. Country codes are two characters. Following is a partial list of some common organizational domains.

.com   commercial organization

.edu   educational organization

.gov   government

.mil   military

.net   networking organization

.org   nonprofit organization

.ca   Canada

.th   Thailand

.uk   United Kingdom

E-mail can be composed online or in advance. In this case, "online" refers to the period that one computer is actively connected to another. Composing messages ahead of time can decrease costs for connection time and improve the organization of expressed thoughts. E-mail prepared in advance may be saved in e-mail draft form or done in another application and later pasted into an e-mail message. Mail received may be read while online or downloaded to the recipient's computer for later review.

Suggested Use and Netiquette E-mail is now a widely accepted form of communication; it is both fast and convenient. It should not be used in lieu of face-to-face meetings to convey unpleasant news such as work lay-offs or a bad diagnosis. It has evolved its own set of conventions and abbreviations. The appropriate and courteous use of e-mail is known as **netiquette**. The following list contains general standards for online communication.

- *Do not make assumptions.* Avoid one-word responses. Do not assume that the recipient remembers the original question or statement. Avoid abbreviations that are not commonly known.
- *Do not be judgmental.* Be professional and careful in what is written. E-mail is easily forwarded to others and can be printed. Instant messages may be shown to other people as well. Word statements carefully to prevent misinterpretation. Flaming is the use of angry and insulting language directed at a particular person or group.
- *Proofread messages.* Poor grammar and spelling reflect badly on the sender.
- *Reply in a timely fashion.* This is simple courtesy.
- *Use attachments wisely.* Check with recipients before sending a file to determine if they have the software to access it. For example, large files may take a long time to download and the recipient may prefer to receive this information in a compressed format. Special software is required by the sender to compress a file. The recipient must use the same software to restore the file for use. The process to attach a file is the same whether it is compressed or not.
- *Make postings brief and to the point.* Recipients may not read lengthy e-mail messages or postings.
- *Use online communication appropriately.* Do not send chain letters. Mass mailing of unsolicited "junk" mail is annoying for recipients and uses network resources. Do not copy or forward mail unless there is a "need-to-know."

- *Avoid the use of all capital letters.* This is known as shouting and is considered rude.
- *Respect others.* Read the frequently asked questions before participating in listserv or other group discussions to avoid unnecessary repetition.

Managing E-mail Because e-mail is popular, it is easy to become inundated with incoming mail. For this reason it is wise to develop some strategies for handling e-mail. The subject line should describe the contents in the subject line to help the reader evaluate its urgency and decide whether to read it or delete it unread. E-mail should be read frequently to prevent large numbers of messages accumulating. Once read, messages should be deleted or organized into electronic folders for future reference. Most ISPs and e-mail applications include features to limit the number of spam messages, block messages from unwanted senders, and automatically delete some messages. It is important to consider whether recipients really want to receive copies or forwarded mail. Some organizations automatically delete e-mail after a specified time.

E-mail software programs allow users to develop lists of recipients for mailing and to set their preferences for how incoming mail is displayed. These preferences can include chronological or reverse chronological order, by sender or date. Read messages may appear differently than unread messages. It is also possible to search e-mail to find particular content, subjects, or senders.

The large number of e-mail messages can decrease productivity rather than enhance it if users are not careful to set limits. It has extended the workday for many persons who feel compelled to check messages before leaving for work, after coming home, and on weekends and holidays. Some work places now forbid the use of e-mail one day a week and encourage telephone calls and face-to-face meetings as a means to foster productivity. Another management strategy is to turn off new e-mail alerts and limit the number of times per day that one checks for new messages to once or twice a day. Recipients may not receive all of their messages if their message box is full.

Instant Messaging (IM)

IM requires a connection to the Internet, an account with one of the IM services, and IM client software. IM services offer the capability for one-on-one or multiparty text chat and file transfer. IM operates on a real-time basis, sending a text message immediately to the intended recipient. Users can limit access to a select few individuals or a larger community. Voice and videoconference may also be supported. IM relies upon presence technology to determine whether the recipient is available and informs users of their status. No time is wasted trying to communicate with persons who are not there. Public IM systems do not capture transcripts of messages. IM first entered into the workplace through free public networks such as AOL's Instant Messenger, MSN's Live Messenger, and Yahoo! Messenger. It is easier to use than e-mail because it is not necessary to type an address and is widely perceived as more time-efficient than either telephone or face-to-face conversations, because it eliminates social chit chat and provides almost immediate responses. Disadvantages associated with the public versions include privacy concerns, the possibility that messages may be intercepted, lack of central administration, and **SPIM.** SPIM refers to unsolicited messages often containing a link to a Web site that the spimmer is attempting to market. Secure versions are available for corporate use at a cost. Commercial IM requires central administration. Both free and commercial versions may distract employees, waste time, and may spread malware via file transfer (How malware sneaks 2010; Khan, Sher, Rasid, & Rahim 2009). On the other hand, IM readily lends itself to use for virtual office hours, class discussion, guest lectures, and mentoring. IM can take place between two or multiple participants and may actually boost productivity (McCullough 2010). Earlier IM software was not interoperable, meaning that users could not communicate without anyone having different software; however, that situation has changed in recent times.

Text messaging is similar in many ways to instant messaging, but exhibits some differences. Text messaging is the popular term for **Short Message Service (SMS),** which originated as a means to send short messages to and from mobile phones and handheld devices. Original messages were limited to 160 characters, giving rise to text messaging's heavy reliance upon abbreviations. Text messaging is private, less intrusive than a phone call, and supports automatic messages without typing each one individually. Recipients may respond in real time or at their leisure. Text messages are less expensive than regular phone calls and less prone to spam than e-mail. Messages are stored and may be reread. Text messages can support all languages and support binary data, ring tones, pictures, and even animation. Recipients may not receive all of their messages if their message box is full.

Database Searches

This feature allows users to conduct comprehensive literature searches over a shorter period of time than could be accomplished via a manual approach. Most universities and public libraries offer online databases for review. In this instance, "online" refers to databases that are available through Internet connections.

File Transfer

File transfer is the ability to move files from one location to another across the Internet. Users may download archived files that they find interesting or give their files to others. Transferred files can include graphics, text, or shareware applications. One means to achieve the actual movement of data is through the **file transfer protocol (FTP).** FTP is a set of instructions that controls both the physical transfer of data across the network and its appearance on the receiving end. The benefit of file transfer is that users can preview work developed by others rather than starting anew. FTP may be available with World Wide Web software. Internet etiquette traditionally calls for the transfer of large files after peak business hours to prevent slow response times.

Listservs

A **Listserv** is actually an e-mail subscription list. A mailing list program copies and distributes all e-mail messages to subscribers. All mail goes through a central computer that acts as the server for the list. Some groups have a moderator who first screens messages for relevance. Listservs are sometimes referred to as *discussion groups, mailing lists,* or *electronic conferences.* Listservs provide information on thousands of topics. Subscription may be open to anyone with an e-mail addressed or restricted. A comprehensive list of listservs may be obtained by visiting the Tile.net site (http://www.tile.net) or Catalist (http://www.lsoft.com).

To subscribe to a listserv, individuals must send the e-mail message "sub" or "subscribe," followed by their first and last names. Exact commands may vary slightly. Most listservs provide help and instructions on request. Subscribers may participate in discussions or just monitor them. Listserv participants should read their mail frequently and skim messages for subjects of interest to keep up with discussions. Subscribers may terminate their participation at any time by sending an "unsubscribe" message.

Newsgroups

Usenet news groups are another available Internet feature. Usenet groups are similar to listservs in content and diversity; however, users do not subscribe to these groups, nor do they receive individual messages. Instead, the Usenet is more of a bulletin board system, in which participants may use at any time free of charge. These groups provide a forum where any user can post messages for discussion and reply. More than 100,000 discussion groups exist, each dedicated to a different topic. ISPs do not carry every news group. ISP administrators decide which news groups will be available to their customers and how long messages will be stored. Only messages that are currently stored on the user's ISP computer may be read. Some ISPs restrict access to Usenet groups or restrict the length of time that messages are saved. It may be necessary to subscribe to a Usenet service to view older postings. Special browser programs called **news reader software** are needed by the individual users to read messages posted on the news group. Many different news readers are available. News readers often come bundled with Web browsers, such as Internet Explorer. A list of Usenet groups may also be found at the Tile.net site (http://www.tile.net) or on Google Groups (http://www.groups.google.com/). Some examples of nursing Usenet groups are the following:

- *sci.med.nursing.* This is a general forum for the discussion of all types of nursing issues. A review of discussion topics reveals current concerns in the profession by country and practice area. Individual nurses may request assistance with particular problems and receive help from people across the globe.
- *bit.listserv.snurse-l.* This is a group for international nursing students.

No single person is in charge of universal Usenet procedures, but informal rules and etiquette for participants have developed. The first rule is that all new users should read the **frequently asked questions (FAQ)** document before sending any messages of their own. The FAQ file serves to introduce the group, update new users on recent discussions, and eliminate repetition of questions. Additional Usenet guidelines call for:

- *Short postings.* This helps to maintain interest while preventing any individual or subgroup from monopolizing the group.
- *No sensationalism.* The intent of Usenet groups is the sharing of information, not gossip.
- *No outright sales.* Usenet originated in academia and relies on a cooperative environment. Advertising, by custom, is kept at a minimum.
- *Respect for the group focus.* Posting messages that are not relevant wastes time and resources.

News groups may be discovered through any of the following methods: searching the Web by topic, word of mouth from individuals with like interests, conferences, professional publications, or searching through lists of all available news groups. If no news group exists for a given topic, instructions on how to start one can be found on the Internet. Some groups that started as Usenet groups may now be accessed through a Web address.

Bulletin Board Services

Bulletin board systems (BBSs) started out as a computerized dial-in meeting and announcement system for users to make statements, share files, and conduct limited discussions. The original BBS did not require Internet access, just a computer and modem. Some BBS were free, while others required a subscription fee. The term *BBS* is sometimes used to refer to any online forum or message board. These sites may have moderators who determine what messages will be posted.

Remote Access

This feature allows individuals to use their computer to access directories, files, and databases housed on a distant computer via a secure connection or virtual private network. This type of access requires an account, identification, and a password. Typically users go to the home Web page of their company or school then follow the links.

THE WORLD WIDE WEB

The **World Wide Web (WWW) or "the Web"** is a system of linked documents accessed through the Internet. The *Web* is not synonymous with the *Internet*; rather it is a part of the Internet. The Web supports a multimedia approach that includes text, images, audio, and links to other documents. Most users access Web content through an application called a **Web browser**. The easy-to-use **graphical user interface (GUI)** makes it simple to learn and use. Users may search by specific words or move from one link to another. Links are displayed by highlighted keywords, text, or images. Selection of information in highlighted areas is accomplished through a click of the mouse button. The Web was first developed at the European Center for Nuclear Research (CERN) in Geneva by Tim Berners-Lee and Robert Cailliau for scientists to publish documents while linked via the Internet. The Web provides a forum for the exchange of ideas, free marketing, and public relations. It now serves as a platform for a growing number of businesses. Box 4–4 lists advantages and disadvantages associated with using the World Wide Web.

Web pages frequently change as content is revised and new technologies are incorporated. This results in a different appearance for the page the next time the user accesses it. The use of new technology and software in Web page design may leave some users unable to access certain features or content. Periodic browser updates and the use of additional applications that can be downloaded from the Web or purchased in stores help to address this situation. It may also be necessary to evaluate, upgrade, and replace hardware and software to access and use desired Web features and applications.

BOX 4–4   The World Wide Web: Advantages and Disadvantages

Advantages

- Browser software is available for all types of computers.
- Browser software is easy to use.
- Text, pictures, video, and audio are supported.
- The amount of information available on the Web is constantly expanding.
- Internet overload is decreased because it links to other documents instead of including them as attachments.
- The need to hold a line open while a document is read is eliminated because the document is transferred to the host computer and the connection is terminated.
- Document transfer is facilitated.
- Voice communications can be supported.
- Information is available in real time.

Disadvantages

- No one person or group controls the Web, just as no one controls the Internet.
- The quality of available information varies widely.
- Documents may not supply sufficient depth in content.
- Not all Web pages display a date of authorship or credentials of the source.
- Web sites may change without providing a "forwarding address."
- The Web is vulnerable to hacker attacks.
- The large amount of available information may be overwhelming.
- Excessive company time spent exploring sites that are nonwork related.
- Obsolete information may be out there.

One particularly popular Web feature is the home page, which is the first page seen at a particular Web location. The home page presents general information about a topic, a person, or an organization. Pages are written in hypertext markup language (HTML) or extensible markup language (XML). Markup languages include text as well as special instructions known as *tags* for the display of text and other media. Web browsers interpret HTML tags, displaying them in a graphical way to the user. Tags specify formatting information, such as the type of heading, font size, and alignment of type. Tags also indicate the location of other media such as graphics or even music. HTML can include links to other documents and may incorporate text, graphics or video, and sound files. Despite the fact that HTML is considered a standard, some variations exist to allow information to be displayed on PDAs, and other devices. XML is one such variation developed by the World Wide Web Consortium. The Consortium is a group of companies dedicated to the development of open standards to ensure the development of the Web.

Links, are words, phrases, or images distinguished from the remainder of the document through the use of highlighting or a different screen color. Links allow users to skip from point to point within or among documents, escaping conventional linear format. Clicking on links with the mouse establishes a TCP/IP (transmission control protocol/Internet protocol) connection between the client and server, which sends a request in the form of a HTTP command. The TCP/IP connection is closed after the information is sent, while the user is seamlessly transported to another area of the document or another Web site.

HTTP supports hypermedia information systems, including the Web. The initial portion of Web site addresses, "http," refers to this protocol. Links are associated with a **uniform resource locator (URL)**, a string of characters similar to a postal address. The URL identifies the document's Web location and the type of server on which it resides, such as HTTP or other Web server, FTP, or news server. Addresses that include an "s" (https) indicate secured sites, such as those that request entry and submission of credit card numbers.

Box 4–5 lists some steps required to create, post, and maintain a Web site. Web sites may consist of a single page or hundreds of pages of information. They vary in complexity from simple text to sites with elaborate graphics, sound, and videos. The person responsible for putting a Web site together and maintaining it is known as the Web editor. In the past, the process of creating a basic Web site was involved. A Web editor needed to know HTML, how to use a Web editing program, how to access the Web server, and more. In recent years, the evolution of the Web and new **Web 2.0** tools has made creating Web sites more accessible to the average user. The term *Web 2.0* refers to the second generation of the Web. Also known as the "Read/Write Web," Web 2.0 tools center on the ability for people to collaborate and share information. Blogs and wikis are examples of Web 2.0 applications. Box 4–6 lists examples of Web 1.0 and Web 2.0.

A **blog** is an abbreviation for *Web* and *log* (Anderberg 2007; Schloman 2006). The blog provides a forum for individuals to maintain an online journal on the Internet. Entries are time stamped. Simple blogs are regularly updated Web pages with the most recent entries appearing at the top of the page. Content varies widely from personal diaries, requests for contributions, and special interest blogs organized by topics. Blogs may not display credentials. Many blogs function as monologs, but may also serve as a discussion forum, news digest, classroom tool, and promotional device. Blogs can support text, images, MP3 files, and other media files. MP3 files are compressed without sacrificing quality for users. MP3 is primarily used to facilitate the exchange of music over the Internet.

Another Web 2.0 application is a **wiki** (Fichter 2005). Wikis are sites created with a Web application that allows anyone to collaboratively write and edit documents without any special technical knowledge. Ideally, a wiki is a collaboration space where the content is constantly changing or being updated by more than one person. Wikipedia, the free online encyclopedia,

BOX 4–5 Steps in Creating, Posting, and Maintaining a Web Site

Content and Design Considerations

- **Determine purpose, intended audience, and content.** A well-designed Web page starts with good planning.

- **Select a Web developer or an authoring tool.** A Web developer can help ensure the success of a site. A variety of tools, including word processors, browsers, and dedicated Web-authoring tools, can be used to create Web pages. The complexity of design, user comfort, and experience are factors in tool selection. Basic knowledge of HTML markup commands is helpful but not essential.

- **Determine page layout.** Do not crowd pages with information and images. Limit introductory page information so that essential data are visible without scrolling. Review existing Web pages for pleasing appearance and useful features.

- **Read easily.** Use high-contrast backgrounds for easy reading, such as black print on white. Dark backgrounds can cause fatigue. Use 12-point fonts or larger.

- **Choose links.** Links can make the site more interesting and useful. Organize links to help users find what they are looking for. Use specific link references rather than the phrase, *click here*.

- **Include contact information.** Contact information, such as name, organization, credentials, an e-mail link, and a postal address, provides the appearance of credibility and a means to establish contact.

- **Update/revision information.** A date helps the user to determine whether posted information and links are current. Updates and revisions also maintain interest, giving users a reason to come back. Consider the addition of icons to identify new or recently revised materials.

- **Downloads quickly.** Lengthy download times can frustrate users, causing them to move to other sites.

- **Check the page for errors.** Spelling, grammar, and content errors reflect poorly on the author or site. Review all materials prior to posting.

- **Do not include a counter.** Visitors do not need to know how many people visited a site.

- **Consider including activities for users.** Users want more than just information.

- **Consider copyright issues.** Request permission prior to using work developed by others. Register original work with the U.S. Copyright office and place a copyright notice with year next to protected material. Develop a written agreement that identifies copyright ownership when working with a Web developer.

Posting and Maintenance Considerations

- **Test the page before posting**. Ensure that it looks and performs as conceived. Use different browsers to view results. Pages that do not load properly or that have a sloppy appearance make a poor impression.

- **Gather information on ISPs and Web servers**. Compare service, cost, and support when selecting an ISP and home for Web pages.

- **Establish Internet access**. Internet access is essential for periodic review of Web materials and to receive mail generated by the site.

- **Find a Web server**. Many ISPs and Web sites offer space for home pages. Determine which service provider can best meet the requirements for the page being posted.

- **Obtain a Web or domain sites**. An address provides a location to post pages. A domain name refers to one or more IP addresses. Domain names are used in URLs. Suffixes provide information about the type of affiliation. Memorable names help users to find and return to pages. Initial cost to obtain a domain name may be minimal unless it presents a commercial interest.

- **Review and revision procedures**. To remain timely, pages should include review or revision dates.

- **Security issues.** Use mechanisms to protect against unauthorized changes in posted materials.

BOX 4–6   Some Examples of Web 1.0 and Web 2.0 Applications

Web 1.0 Examples

Personal Web page. A static page with personal or professional information listed

Online encyclopedia. Encyclopedia produced by a company, e.g., Encyclopedia Britannica (http://www.britannica.com)

Browser favorites/bookmarks. Web sites saved in a Web browser by a user, e.g., Internet Explorer favorites or Firefox bookmarks

Software application. Software that is installed locally on a computer, e.g., Microsoft Office Suite

Web 2.0 Examples

Blogs and wikis. A dynamic Web page that allows comments from other online users

Online wiki. An online encyclopedia produced by the users of the Web e.g., Wikipedia (http://www.wikipedia.com)

Online bookmarks. Web sites that are saved to an online bookmarking service, e.g., Delicious (http://www.delicious.com), Diigo (http://www.diigo.com), or Google Bookmarks

Online software. Software that is used on the Internet instead software installed on the computer, e.g., Google Docs (docs.google.com)

---

is an example of a wiki. In the past, the open editing capability raises concerns about misuse, abuse, and reliability of information. Wikis work best in an environment with a high level of trust when control can be delegated to the users. Like blogs, the security levels in most wiki software can be set to be public or private. Also like blogs, wikis can support text, images, audio, and other media files. Wikis are particularly valuable as an online workspace, allowing individuals to contribute knowledge and pertinent comments. Wikis can also be used in organizations to foster collaboration where access is restricted to internal use. Wikis are well suited for the storage of committee work and meeting minutes, as a log book of complaints and actions. While there is usually no indication of who is currently online, wikis do have a history section, which displays a list of page changes. This history page lists the author, date, and time the page was updated. In addition, an author or editor of the wiki can revert to a previous version of a page or compare/contrast changes that have been made.

Many blog and wiki software is free or **open-source**. Open-source generally refers to software that can be downloaded by the general public free of charge. The software can be modified and installed to run on a personal or company servers. Open-source software is typically created and updated by a community of users. If users or organizations don't have the resources or knowledge to support open-source software, there are many free online services that provide blogs and wikis to the public. Popular free blog services include Wordpress (wordpress.org), Google Blogger (http://www.blogger.com), and Live Journal (http://www.livejournal.com). Some popular free wiki services include PBworks (pbworks.com), Wikispaces (http://www.wikispaces.com), and Wetpaint (http://www.wetpaintcentral.com). Most of these companies offer free services to educational and nonprofit organizations. Often services can be upgraded for a small monthly or annual fee for additional features and services.

A **Bliki,** sometimes known as a WikiLog, Wog, WikiWeblog, Wikiblog, or Bloki, combines the concepts of Web-based collaboration and publishing from blogs and wikis. It incorporates posts or articles in reverse chronological order but allows editing in wiki style with a version history for each page. Permission to edit is at the discretion of the administrator(s). The Bliki aims to make the blogging experience more interactive while promoting quality and accuracy of posts. Blikis may be adopted by organizations to internal information centrally and is a format that is always accessible.

Really Simple Syndication (RSS) is a markup language for the delivery of syndicated Web content to users. In other words, it is the behind-the-scene code that brings users updates from the news and many other Web sites, blogs, and wikis. Users use an RSS reader or aggregator, such as Google Reader or FeedDemon to collect updates from various Web sites. For example, a user can subscribe to updates from CNN and Nurse.com. Its use is well suited for rapidly changing online newsletters. Blogging software and providers are available to help create and maintain blogs. Many blogs have been abandoned in recent years as their creators tire of the work associated with their blogs' ongoing maintenance.

Browsers

A **browser or Web browser** is a retrieval program that allows access to hypertext and hypermedia documents on the Web by using HTTP. The computer, acting as server, interprets the client's HTTP request and sends back the requested document for display. Browsers can also use Telnet FTP protocols. Browsers may be obtained from an ISP or downloaded for free over the Internet. The National Center for Supercomputing Applications (NCSA) developed Mosaic, the first Web browser. Web use greatly increased after the introduction of Mosaic. Examples of popular browsers include Microsoft's Internet Explorer (IE), Apple's Safari, Mozilla's Firefox, and the alternative browsers such as Opera and Google's Chrome. Internet Explorer has dominated the market, but alternative browsers are increasing in popularity. Browsers use the URL to request a document from the server.

Browsers are available for many types of systems and frequently offer features that extend their utility. However, there are still some things that browsers do not do. **Helper programs** and **plug-in programs** evolved to fill this void. Helper and plug-in programs are computer applications that have been designed to perform tasks such as view graphics, construct Web pages, play sounds, or even remotely control another PC over the Internet. The main difference between helper and plug-in programs is that the first does not require the browser to be running to function, while the second does require the browser to be running. Both are typically available on the Web at no cost and are often written in **Java**. Java is a programming language that enables the display of moving text, animation, and musical excerpts on Web pages. Java is popular for the following reasons:

- Applications will run on any Java-enabled browser.
- Actual code can reside on the server until it is downloaded to the client computer as it is needed.
- Java reduces the need to purchase, install, and maintain on-site software.

An alternative to Java for the development of Internet-enabled tools and technologies is Microsoft's ActiveX.

Search Tools

The overwhelming amount of data available on the Web requires the use of tools to locate specific information. Several types of search tools are available to help users find information on the Web. Most users are familiar with Google, Yahoo! and MSN but there are other many other tools and techniques that are less well known (Hawkins 2005; Notess 2007; Pike 2007). Knowledge workers, persons who primarily earn a living by developing or using knowledge, spend an estimated 9.5 hours per week, searching for information. This makes awareness of different tools and search techniques important. There is great variety in how search engines and search directories organize information. Some sites, such as Yahoo!, index links by broad subject categories. **Search indexes** are appropriate when general information is requested. **Search engines** use automated programs, such as robots or "bots" to search the Web, compiling a list of links to sites relevant to keywords supplied by the user. The search may also include Usenet discussions. Search engines are indicated when it is necessary to find a specific topic. Google and AltaVista are examples of search engines. Each search tool maintains its own list of information on the Web and uses its own method to organize materials. Because of this variation in organization, searches conducted with different engines yield different results. Although subtle differences exist among each, all permit the user to enter a search word or phrase. Web sites that contain the search item are then displayed. Since new sites are constantly being indexed, the number of hits or Web sites that contain the searched word or phrase varies according to the search engine used and when the search is done. Search engines also weight or rank pages. Weighting is designed to display the most useful links first. There are several ways to weight pages, but the best-known method is based on the popularity of each site as is represented by the number of other sites that link to it. Google uses this strategy, so the top results in Google are usually the most popular Web sites. Enclosing key phrases in quotation marks is recommended as a way to obtain better results (e.g., "nursing education"). Many search engines recognize this search strategy, but not all. Help pages and advanced search options are available to aid the user in conducting searches. Box 4–7 explains some commonly used search techniques and their corresponding search engines. Search engine strategies are constantly changing and improving, so be sure to read the Advanced Search section for the most up-to-date information.

It may also be necessary to use more than one tool for the best results, as search engines have their strengths and weakness. NoodleQuest (http://www.noodletools.com/noodlequest/) is a Web site that helps users identify the best search engine for the need. The newer browsers, search tools, and several Web sites make it easier to switch from one tool to another. Often results contain links that advertisers have paid the search engine to display; usually these links are labeled but not always. Consumer groups have asked the Federal Trade Commission to look at this issue. For scholarly work, a helpful place to start searching is Google Scholar. It helps users to locate scholarly works on the Internet. While it may be suitable as a starting point, users still need to resort to major database services for a thorough review of refereed scholarly works (Kent 2005).

Despite the success of search engines, important information is frequently missed; this occurs for several reasons. Search engines have interfaces in the major languages but may miss results that are not in any of those languages. Another reason that information is missed is that it is password-protected or stored in formats that are not indexed. Yet another reason that information is missed is that the incorporation of multiple concepts makes indexing difficult. There

---

BOX 4–7   Commonly Used Search Techniques for Specific Engines

Search Technique	Search Engines
Phrase Searching (e.g., "nursing education") Results will include only sites where both terms appear side-by-side as written.	Google (http://www.google.com) Yahoo! (http://search.yahoo.com) Bing (http://www.bing.com)
+Requires/-Excludes (e.g., +nursing -education) The "+" and "-" will force the search engine to include or exclude a term, so *nursing* will be in the search results, but *education* will not.	Google (http://www.google.com) Yahoo! (http://search.yahoo.com) Alta Vista (http://www.altavista.com)
Boolen Logic AND, OR, NOT (e.g., nursing AND education) Results will include Web sites on both *nursing* and *education*. OR will include results either or (i.e., nursing OR education). NOT will exclude a term (e.g., nursing NOT education).	Yahoo! (http://search.yahoo.com) Bing (http://www.bing.com)
Truncation (e.g., **nurse*) The asterisk (*) symbol will get results with alternate spellings for the word. For example *nurse will get results for "nurse," "nursing," "nurses."	Google (http://www.google.com) Yahoo! (http://search.yahoo.com)

are also problems with filters designed to block pornography that may block access to health information sites.

Metasearch engines can shorten search time by searching several engines at one time. Some examples of metasearch engines are include Dogpile (http://www.dogpile.com), Search (http://www.search.com), and Metacrawler (http://www.metacrawler.com). Users should try several search tools to determine what provides the best results for their needs.

OmniMedicalSearch (http://www.omnimedicalsearch.com) was created to bring the best sources of medical information together in one easy-to-use platform for consumers and healthcare professionals. It selects sources deemed as reliable. Medical World Search (http://www.mwsearch.com) is a search tool for selected medical sites that requires a subscription fee. It uses indexing and a thesaurus of uniform healthcare terms, which users can view before conducting a search.

Portals, Intranets, and Extranets

The terms *portal, intranet,* and *extranet* received considerable attention when they were first introduced, while the concepts remain viable, the terms themselves are used less frequently.

Portals A **portal** or "Web portal" refers to a Web site that offers services such as a search engine, e-mail, discussion forum, links to current news, shopping, and more. Portals often require registration and collect information from the user that can be used to personalize features for individual users. Portals organize data with different formats from multiple sources into a single, easy-to-use menu. AOL and Yahoo! were some of the first portal sites. Personalized start pages, such as iGoogle, MSN, and Bing have evolved from portals. Specialty portal, such as The Nursing Portal (http://www.nursing-portal.com) and Nurses.info (nurses.info), can offer specific information to a targeted audience. Physician's Briefing, WebMD, HealthAtoZ.com, Healthfinder.gov, and HealthCentral provide services for physicians, consumers, nurses, and office managers. CVS and other commercial pharmacies also have portal sites that provide information for consumers and allow prescriptions to be filled online. A portal for a health organization typically contains links to individual member organizations, physicians, educational material, and possibly scheduling capability for consumers with separate links for employees to online continuing education, policies, internal phone numbers, and other relevant information. Employees can access this information independently at times convenient for them to complete required education. Other uses for portal technology include providing secure Web access to patient care systems or information contained within these systems. This includes making results available to physicians, as well as digital images and monitor strips, and the opportunity for electronic review and sign-off of medical records. Basic portals furnish information in a static fashion. More sophisticated sites are interactive, allowing users to complete and submit forms online, complete health assessments, schedule appointments, and perform other activities. There are variations on the portal theme. Active portals focus on a specific topic and use a customized search agent that automatically updates searches. Enterprise portals provide access to information quickly and easily, extending user access across departments and organizations.

Intranets *Intranets* are private computer networks that are accessible only by an organization's members or employees. They were first developed in response to concerns over slowdowns, security breaches, and fears of Internet collapse. An intranet Web site may look like any other Web site, but it sits behind firewalls or other barriers and may not normally be available to people outside its organization. In some cases authorized users may be able to access content from remote sites.

Intranets allow integration of disparate information systems. Intranets can save money by providing an easy-to-use, familiar interface that is intuitive and therefore requires little training.

Most organizations use the corporate intranet first for publication of internal documents. This cuts down on paper and distribution costs, and makes materials available more quickly and widely. It also provides a mechanism to ensure that all parties view the most recent document, which does not always occur when hard copies are distributed. This type of intranet application may be used to distribute policy and procedure manuals or other reference materials. It also acclimates employees to using the intranet as the single source of information. Additional features may include the ability for employees to view and enroll in benefits, request vacation days, and apply for internal jobs. Intranets are also an effective tool for marketing and advertising. Intranets in healthcare enterprises may also be used for mail and messaging, conferencing, and access to clinical data once the infrastructure is in place to bring together clinical systems and authenticate authorized users. In some cases, clients may be able to view their own health information, schedule appointments, and register for the hospital online. The concerns associated with intranet use mirror those discussed earlier; these include data security, the need to develop and implement strong organizational policies on appropriate intranet use, and the development of the infrastructure to support an intranet. Remote access may present additional issues for users because intranet content is generally designed to take advantage of fast network connections.

Extranets *Extranets* are networks that sit outside the protected internal network of an organization and use Internet software and communication protocols for electronic commerce and use by outside suppliers or customers. In essence, an extranet is a partially accessible intranet. Extranets are more private than a Web site that is open to the public but are more open than an intranet, which can be accessed only by employees. Many extranets offer information that is a by-product of the organization's main business either gratis or for a fee. Customers benefit because information is available 24 hours a day. For example, a vendor may develop an extranet that customers can use to obtain prices and place orders for merchandise. Security measures can be used to restrict access and secure information, making extranets more private than the Internet. Extranets may be subject to viruses, worms, and hacker attacks. One example of an extranet in use is the U.S. Navy Medical Information Management Center's initiative to share medical and benefit information, newsletters, and e-mails with more than 100,000 users worldwide (Simpkins 2003). Hospitals and physician offices also use extranets to share data (Silkey 2004).

Social Media and Social Networking

Social media is a term often used to describe Web-based programs and technologies that allow people to interact socially with each other online (Webopedia 2010a). **Social networking** is a term used to describe Web sites that allows users to create a profile within the site and interact with other users of the site (Webopedia 2010b). Some common examples of social media and social networking sites are blogs, wikis, YouTube, Facebook, Twitter, and many more. A central thread among social media sites is **user-generated content** or UGC. UGC basically refers to any content such as blogs posts, discussion comments, audio, video, digital images, etc. that have been created by a user of a Web site. This content is usually publically available for other users to see and interact. Web sites that incorporate social media have become enormously popular and many businesses, educational institution, nonprofit, and healthcare organizations are using it to connect with their audiences. Social media tools specifically designed around healthcare are often informally referred to as "Health 2.0" or "Medicine 2.0" (Van De Belt et al. 2010). Patients Like Me (http://www.patientslikeme.com) and ShareCare (http://www.sharecare.com) are examples of healthcare related Web sites that incorporate social media.

Social media and Web 2.0 tools are also being used more frequently in both medical and nursing schools. Lemley and Burnham (2009) found that "a greater percentage of nursing schools than medical schools currently use Web 2.0 tools in their curricula, although a larger number of respondents from medical schools make greater personal use of the tools than do nursing school respondents." Blogs, wikis, videocasts, and podcasts seemed to be the most popular social media tools used (Lemley & Burnham 2009).

Wikipedia

Social media is a central component of Web 2.0 Web sites; a well-known example is Wikipedia (http://www.wikipedia.com). Wikipedia began as a free, Web-based encyclopedia project in 2001. The initial idea was to create a collaborative space where users of the Internet could contribute content to the online encyclopedia. Users can add content anonymously, under a pseudonym, or real name. Since its creation, it has grown tremendously with nearly 78 million visitors monthly (Wikipedia 2010a). Since Google search results are based on popularity, Wikipedia is often listed in the top 10 to 20 search results. Wikipedia states it operates under five pillars: It is an online encyclopedia; it has a neutral point of view; it is free content; users should interact in a respectful and civil manner; and it does not have firm rules (Wikipedia 2010b). While the majority of the content is open for users to edit, there are certain cases where editing is restricted to prevent vandalism; however, this is the exception rather than the rule. In addition to occasional vandalism, by far the largest criticism of Wikipedia is reliability and accuracy. While this remains a concern for many, a recent review by medical and scientific professionals reported that "against professional and peer reviewed sources found that Wikipedia's depth and coverage were of a very high standard, often comparable in coverage to physician databases" (Rajagopalan et al. 2010; Wikipedia 2010a). While several studies have supported the accuracy of Wikipedia, in most professional, academic, and medical settings, it is not considered an acceptable reference.

Twitter, Facebook, and LinkedIn

Twitter, Facebook, and LinkedIn are other popular social networking Web sites. Twitter (http://www.twitter.com) is a social messaging tool that allows users to post comments in 140 characters or fewer (Webopedia 2010c). Initially Twitter was based on the answer to the question, "What are you doing?" While early posts on the site were mostly mundane, Twitter is now being used by professionals to exchange useful Web resources and information. Professional organizations are also using Twitter to share news and updates to their members. In addition, Twitter is becoming a useful tool at professional conferences and associations. It can be used during a conference as a form of "backchannel" communication or way participants can share information in real time with each other during a keynote presentation or talk. There have even been instances where surgeons have "tweeted" from the operating room, allowing medical students and others to receive live updates as the surgery progresses. As with most social media tools, Twitter can be accessed through a Web site, desktop software, or a mobile device, making it easy and convenient to use.

Facebook (http://www.facebook.com) is another extremely popular social media and networking Web site. It is a space where users can connect with friends, family, and colleagues. Users can post status updates, pictures, videos, Web links and more. Many people use Facebook personally to connect with friends and family; however, some use it professionally to create professional pages and groups. Organizations also use Facebook to share information with members as it has more places to post information, events, and resources than Twitter. Regardless of how one uses Facebook, it is important to read and understand the privacy policies. Many social media and networking Web sites frequently change and update their settings and policies. There have been many cases where a user of a Web site posted information he or she thought was private, but turned out to be accessible by others. Consult Chapter 5 for additional information on professional use of electronic resources.

BOX 4–8 Advantages and Disadvantages of Social Media Web sites	
Advantages	**Disadvantages**
Community of users building knowledge together creates a wider depth and breadth of knowledge.	Some professionals see social media tools as trivial, unscholarly, and unprofessional. Information can be inconsistent and inaccurate.
Appeals to a wide-range and diverse group of people. Creates a space where disparate groups can build community and connections.	The use of social media among different ages groups, demographics, and social economic backgrounds varies widely, so the effective use of it as a communication tool will also vary.
Most tools are free and easy to use.	Lack of anonymity can foster polarization and harassment.
Creates a space to keep in touch with colleagues, friends, and family.	Can be time consuming and contributes to a feeling of "information overload."
Creates a space to develop an online professional presence.	Employers may look down on employees sharing too much personal/professional information online.

LinkedIn (http://www.linkedin.com) is a Web-based social networking space designed specially for professionals. Users can post their resumes, work experience, educational background, affiliations, and more. Users can also create "connections" with colleagues and seek out additional connections with people who share the same professional interest. In addition, LinkedIn provides a space for users to post recommendation or endorsements, as well as seek out job openings. Oftentimes employers use LinkedIn to search for information on a prospective employee. Box 4–8 notes some advantages and disadvantages of social media Web sites.

CONCERNS RELATED TO THE USE OF THE INTERNET AND WORLD WIDE WEB

There are a variety of concerns related to use of the Internet and the World Wide Web. One of the largest concerns for the average user is the quality of online information. Other concerns include security of client data, collection of personal information, worries over slowdown, the ability to transact business smoothly, viral contamination, and a lack of adherence to Internet standards, among some products.

Quality of Online Information

The Internet offers unprecedented access to healthcare information. While reports of the numbers of persons who access the Internet for information vary, Harrison and Lee (2006) noted that almost 90% of people with Internet access have used it to search for health information at some point. Unfortunately, the accuracy, readability, depth, diversity, and presentation of this content vary greatly from site to site. Some online information can even be harmful. The lack of a controlling body over the Internet makes it impossible to regulate the quality of information before posting. For this reason, healthcare professionals and consumers must be wary.

Evaluating Online Information

As the number of consumers who independently access health information online increases, it is essential that all healthcare professionals critically evaluate the quality of online materials and assist consumers to judge what they find. Many consumers do not examine the quality of

---

BOX 4–9   Evaluating Information Quality for Online Resources.

- **Source credentials.** Are they listed? Are they reputable? Does the expertise qualify them to speak authoritatively on the subject?
- **Ability to validate information.** Are original sources noted or can they be contacted?
- **Accuracy.** Is information provided to determine whether information is factual?
- **Comprehensive.** Does the site provide a well-balanced view or just a narrow focus?
- **Currency.** Are dates for posting, review, and revision obvious?
- **Sponsorship or bias?** Does the site sell products or have reason to provide a balanced view?
- Easy to use.
- States who the intended audience is.
- Includes a privacy policy and/or disclaimers.
- Demonstrates evidence of accreditation for quality of information.

---

information that they locate, while others rely upon their provider to help them find credible sources (Doctors now writing "Info" Prescriptions 2005; Fox 2006). Box 4–9 provides a summary of criteria to evaluate the quality of information on a Web site.

- *Credentials of the source.* Large professional associations, such as hospitals, universities, government, and official health organizations, tend to have the most reliable sites. The source may not readily apparent. For example, it is important to consider whether the information provided mirrors the focus of professional education and expertise. One way to check the credentials of a Web site is to use EasyWhois (http://www.easywhois.com). Go to EasyWhois and type in the address of a Web site (i.e., http://www.chatham.edu) and the results will show the name, person, or organization that has registered the domain or URL. This will give a user some indication of who is associated with the Web site.
- *Ability to validate information.* Validation of information can be difficult unless the source can be traced back to a reputable university or other agency. Many messages and Web sites identify a person or persons to contact for further information. When facts and studies are cited, the original source should be stated so users can review it and draw their own conclusions. It should also be possible to corroborate information from independent sources.
- *Accuracy.* Because no single person controls information that is placed on the Internet, the mere existence of information does not indicate that it is accurate. Postings should identify contact persons or cite references that may be checked to allow evaluation of posted information.
- *Comprehensiveness of information.* If the site professes to provide information about medications, it should discuss indications, contraindications, protocols, and dosages. If the user must go elsewhere to find relevant information, the site is not comprehensive. Sites with broad generalizations or poorly referenced research should be considered suspicious. The user should continue to use caution because the information could be biased.
- *Date of issue or revision.* One problem with the Internet and World Wide Web is that not all pages contain dates indicating when material was written, revised, or reviewed, making it difficult to determine whether information is current. Publication, review, and revision dates help the user to determine if material is current or outdated.
- *Bias or sponsorship.* Commercial uses of the Internet are growing daily. The consumer must consider whether information is biased in favor of a particular product or commercial service. One means to consider bias is to look for a funding and advertising policy.
- *Ease of navigation.* Content should be well organized with the appropriate use of hyperlinks. All links should be to current Web pages and load easily.

- *Intended purpose and audience.* Sites should indicate the intended audience and use terminology and a reading level appropriate to that population.
- *Disclaimers.* Sites that express individual opinions should contain a statement to that effect to help users distinguish between fact and opinion.
- *Site accreditation.* Several groups have been working to ensure the quality of information found on health-related Web sites. As a consequence of these efforts, some sites display a "seal" that indicates that their sites meet a set of predetermined standards for the quality of information posted. Compliance is purely voluntary.
- *Privacy policies.* Sites that collect personal information need to identify how that information may be used so that visitors can determine whether they choose to disclose information.

Organizations

A number of groups are concerned with the quality of posted materials, including most professional organizations, the Health Internet Ethics (Hi-Ethics) Alliance, the Health on the Net Foundation (HON), HealthWeb, Healthfinder, the Healthcare Coalition, the American Accreditation Health Care Commission (URAC), the European Council, and the World Health Organization. None of these groups impose mandatory controls over quality. Hi-Ethics published a set of 14 principles in 2000 that forms the basis for URAC accreditation. Sites that have URAC accreditation display a seal. The seal indicates that the site meets more than 50 standards that include disclosure, site policies and structure, content currency and accuracy, linking, privacy, security, and accountability. The accreditation process is one way to quickly identify posted content that meets quality standards. Accreditation can also foster trust. URAC accreditation also considers HIPAA security accreditation standards (Kohn 2003).The European Union has also developed criteria for evaluation of Web content that largely mirror those already defined by URAC (Commission of the European Communities 2002). HON has partnered with Google to provide data on each accredited site (Google Co-op 2006). When the user types in a broad disease condition, Google allows the user to refine his or her search by treatment, symptoms, and other appropriate areas. Results from accredited sites show that they are labeled by HON. Sites may receive approval from other partners as well.

Overload

The Internet consists of many interconnected networks. Actual collapse is improbable, although vendor and facility outages and problems will likely continue as the number of users increases. Many first-time providers are undercapitalized or have poorly trained staff, so periodic overload or slow service can be expected. These problems raise interesting questions about maintaining data availability and integrity for the healthcare institution that uses the Internet to transport health data.

The majority of overload and collapse problems result from technical problems, such as traffic jams, transmission difficulties, attacks by malware, and poor Web site design. These problems may occur on the user's network or an outside network. The popularity of the Internet makes it difficult to accommodate the needs of all of the users. Two initiatives that emerged to address these concerns were Internet2 and the Next Generation Internet. Internet2 (Internet2 2007; Matlis 2006) is a collaborative effort of universities, government, industry, and various research and educational groups. The purpose of the Internet2 effort is to build and operate a research network capable of enhancing delivery of education and other services, including healthcare. This includes the development and support of advanced applications and standards. The National Science Foundation Next Generation Internet project was launched by the Clinton administration (Rapoza 2002). This program conducted research but did not actually build a secure, newer Internet.

Security

Most organizations focus security efforts on their internal networks, for the obvious reason that any disruption in computer operation affects service. As a consequence of this action, Web sites traditionally received less attention. Web sites are also vulnerable to attack and subsequent disruption can affect business operations. Hacker changes to Web pages may prove embarrassing, endanger consumers who follow altered advice, and/or result in libel charges. This recognition brings with it a heightened awareness of the need to safeguard Web sites as well as internal networks. At the same time, Webmasters are being encouraged to put their organizations on the Web so the world can access them, but they must also protect the organization from intruders.

The following measures can protect Web sites and their information:

- *Construct a separate firewall for the Web server.* Firewalls provide the same level of protection for Web servers as they do for private networks with Internet access. Some, if not all, hacker attacks can be prevented with a firewall for each Web server.
- *Limit access to Web page content or configuration.* The risk of internal attacks or accidental damage is directly related to the number of persons with authority to change Web information or setup.
- *Isolate Web servers.* Web servers should not have direct connections to other agency systems, nor should they be located at a site subject to attack. This action minimizes the chance of Web site damage.
- *Heed security advisories.* Updates on hacker attacks and warnings on new breach techniques are posted by several sites on the Web, including the WWW Security FAQ and commercial sites such as Symantec.com. Webmasters should anticipate attack and take proactive measures.
- *Keep antivirus systems up-to-date and install intrusion detection systems to hail attacks.* Webmasters or network administrators need to maintain up-to-date virus detection to avoid having their site(s) being brought down by the latest virus or worm. Alarms and tracking mechanisms alert administrators or Webmasters to attacks early so that action can be taken to minimize Web site damage.

Contamination by Viruses, Worms, and Other Malware

Viruses can be spread when files are imported for use without subjecting them to a viral scan. The danger of contamination cannot be eliminated, but it can be reduced through the following measures:

- *Strict policies on Internet use.* These policies should include scanning all files before use, including FTP files, and deletion of files with unfamiliar file extensions. Viruses may be included in materials available for public consumption. Consider deleting all attachments with unfamiliar file extensions.
- *Use the latest version of antiviral software.* New viruses are created daily. Older releases of antiviral software cannot recognize new viruses; therefore, it is important to frequently update the virus files for antiviral software. This can usually be done using downloads from a Web site and may or may not require a fee.
- *Download and install software security patches.* Security patches for operating systems and applications are available from the vendor once problems have been identified.
- *Install or enable a computer firewall.* Some operating systems come with a firewall. A firewall provides a barrier against outsiders infiltrating a computer or network.
- *Use security features that come with software.* Word and Excel documents may contain macros that open automatically. This can be controlled by setting the security level to "high."

Firewalls

The open design of the Internet invites security abuse, particularly for private networks with Internet access. Most organizations with an Internet connection are under continuous attack by human attackers and automated software applications. Any of these attacks have the potential to pose a serious security breach or a launching pad for large-scale attacks on other computers. For this reason, private networks need a gateway to intercept and examine Internet messages before they are permitted to enter the private network. A **gateway** is a combination of hardware and software used to connect local area networks with larger networks. A **firewall** is a type of gateway designed to protect private network resources from outside hackers, network damage, and theft or misuse of information. It consists of hardware and software that can use one of several mechanisms to protect data. A firewall should be transparent to users. A firewall does not preclude the need for a security plan or periodic security testing; outside intruders may still be able to penetrate firewall protection.

Not all threats to a network arise from outside sources; firewalls alone do not protect against internal attacks or prevent viral contamination. Strong security policies for employees can minimize these threats as long as users are aware of the policies, their responsibilities, and the implications for policy violations. Another key factor in network protection is knowledge. Network administrators must educate themselves about attacks on Internet sites and protective measures recommended by the federally funded Computer Emergency Response Team (CERT) Coordination Center and Usenet groups. Subsequent work by a coalition of federal and private organizations produced a set of security configurations entitled "Consensus Baseline Security Settings." This effort was geared toward the protection of government Windows-based workstations from external and internal attacks, but it is expected to help other systems administrators to protect their systems and provide guidance for the future development of network protocols and systems.

Institutional Policies

All organizations with an Internet connection need policies that address the following areas:

- *Privacy.* The organization has the legal right to read employee electronic communication unless stated otherwise. Employees should be aware of their organization's policy. Some organizations may permit a limited amount of personal messages.
- *Encryption.* Potentially sensitive data should be coded or encrypted to prevent unauthorized people from reading it. Any client data are sensitive and should be encrypted for transmittal over the Internet.
- *Transmission of employee data or photographs.* Employers should obtain consent before the transmittal of employee pictures or personal data over the Internet.
- *Intellectual ownership.* Guidelines should establish how issues of intellectual ownership are determined for network postings and other communications. In other words, it is important to resolve who owns the information: the employee who developed it or the employer.
- *Free speech.* The organization's stance on ideas or images that it considers offensive or inappropriate should be plainly delineated. This helps to protect the organization from liability for inappropriate statements made by employees. Pornographic or sexually explicit or otherwise offensive materials are not acceptable.
- *Acceptable Internet uses in the workplace.* Permissible Internet uses must be identified and communicated to employees. Violations of accepted use may constitute grounds for dismissal. One example of unacceptable use is the downloading of pirated music or software. One means to enforce this policy is the inclusion of a section on acceptable Internet use in the employee's annual performance evaluation.
- *Citation of sources and verification of information downloaded from the Internet/Web.* Authors of materials on the Internet and Web deserve the same recognition as authors of any

other media. Failure to cite sources is plagiarism. Guidelines for the citation of online resources can be found at the American Psychological Association and the Modern Language Association Web sites as well as at most college and university sites.

- *Monitoring policies.* Employees need to be aware that e-mail and Internet use may be monitored and that inappropriate use can be cause for dismissal.
- *Acknowledgment of receipt of Internet policies.* Employees should sign a statement that they have read and understand the organization's Internet policies at the time of hire and on yearly review.

FUTURE DIRECTIONS

Electronic communication is here to stay. Its impact upon healthcare will continue to increase and evolve. As more consumers become connected and Internet savvy, more e-health applications will be seen. Nurses have an obligation to prepare for these changes and to assist healthcare consumers along in this journey.

Visit nursing.pearsonhighered.com for additional cases, information, and weblinks.

CASE STUDY EXERCISE

As the representative for your medical center's Better Care Initiative, a project with the purpose of identifying ways that services can be delivered in a more efficient manner, you have suggested that the Internet be made available to clinicians at the point of care. Develop a report listing both the potential uses as well as potential problems of using the Internet.

SUMMARY

- The Internet is a network of networks, connecting computers worldwide. It offers a wealth of information about many topics, and can be extremely useful for the exchange of healthcare information.
- Access to the Internet is provided through businesses known as Internet service providers (ISPs) via several methods that include existing telephone lines for either dial-up or high-speed digital subscriber line (DSL) access, or via cable, fiber optic, wireless or satellite options.
- The Internet offers a variety of services including e-mail and instant messaging. There are advantages and disadvantages associated with e-mail and instant messaging as well as accepted rules for use known as netiquette.
- Electronic mail, or e-mail, is the use of computer technology to transmit messages from one person to another. Delivery can be almost instantaneous. The Internet allows e-mail to be sent anywhere in the world, as long as the recipient has an Internet address.
- File transfer is the ability to move files from one location to another across a network.
- Other forms of electronic communication include instant messaging (IM), blogs, wikis, listservs (electronic mailing lists), and Usenet groups (message discussion groups). These forums provide information and support.
- The World Wide Web (Web or WWW), a popular Internet feature, allows users to find information more easily by conducting word searches using browser software or locating a specific Web site or address. It is characterized by a GUI that makes it easy to use.
- A popular Web feature is the home page, the first page seen at a particular Web location. The home page provides general information about a topic, a person, or an organization.

- Links are words, phrases, or pictures that are distinguished from other parts of a WWW home page, usually by color, and enable users to move directly to another Web location.
- The overwhelming amount of data available on the Web requires the use of tools to locate specific information. Several types of search tools are available to help users find information on the Web.
- *Social media* is a term used to describe Web-based programs that allow people to interact socially.
- Web 2.0 refers to the second generation of the Web. Web 2.0 applications allow people to collaborate and share information. Blogs and wikis are examples of Web 2.0 applications.
- Social media and Web 2.0 tools are also being used more frequently in both medical and nursing schools.
- Evaluation of online information entails consideration of the source of the information, validation, accuracy and depth, dates for publication or review and revision, possible bias or sponsorship, organization and linkage, intended audience, presence of disclaimers and privacy policies, and accreditation or sponsorship by reputable organizations.
- Security is a major concern surrounding the use of the Internet and electronic communication. Firewalls and encryption are two prevalent strategies for safeguarding information.
- Internet technology is used internally in an organization in systems known as intranets, or external to the organization in systems known as extranets. Increasingly, these applications are referred to as Web portals.

REFERENCES

Anderberg, K. (2007, February). Patience is OK. *Communication News,* p. 4.

Anonymous. (2010). How malware sneaks into your business. *NZ Business, 24*(5), 53.

Commission of the European Communities. (2002). eEurope 2002: Quality criteria for health related Websites. *Journal of Medical Internet Research, 4*(3), e15.

Cukier, K. N. (2005, November/December). Who will control the Internet? *Foreign Affairs.* Retrieved from http://www.foreignaffairs.org/20051101facomment84602/kenneth-neil-cukier/who-will-control-the-internet.html

Doctors now writing "info" prescriptions. (2005, February 1). *USA Today Magazine, 133*(2717), 4.

Dunn, D. (2006, May 22). Power line broadband expands. *InformationWeek,* 1090, 19.

Fiber: Friend or foe to DSL? (2007, March 29). *Electronic Design, 55*(7), 55.

Fichter, D. (2005). Intranets, wikis, blikis, and collaborative working. *Online, 29*(5), 47–50.

Fox, S. (2006, October 29). *Online health search 2006.* Washington, DC: Pew Internet & American Life Project. Retrieved from http://www.pewinternet.org/pdfs/PIP_Online_Health_2006.pdf

Google Co-op. (2006, November 10). Retrieved from http://www.hon.ch/Project/GoogleCoop/

Governmental delegations to watch in Tunis. (2005, November). *Information Today,* p. 49.

Griffiths, K. M., & Christensen, H. (2005). Website quality indicators for consumers. *Journal of Medical Internet Research, 7*(5), e55.

Harrison, J. P., & Lee, A. (2006). The role of e-health in the changing health care environment. *Nursing Economics, 24*(6), 283–289.

Hawkins, D. T. (2005). The latest on search engines. *Information Today, 22*(6), 37–38.

Hesseldahl, A. (2007, May 30). More bandwidth than you can use? *Business Week Online,* 26.

ICANN. (2010). *One world. One internet: 2010 annual report.* Retrieved from http://www.icann.org/en/annualreport/annual-report-2010-en.pdf

Institute of Medicine. (2001). *Crossing the quality chasm: A new health system for the 21st century.* Washington, DC: National Academies Press.

Internet Society. (n.d.). *Introduction to ISOC.* Retrieved from http://www.isoc.org/isoc/

Internet2. (2007). *Internet2 network.* Retrieved from http://www.internet2.edu/network/

Kavehrad, M. (2007). Broadband room service by light. *Scientific American, 297*(1), 82–87.

Kent, M. L. (2005, Winter). Conducting better research: Google Scholar and the future of search technology. *Public Relations Quarterly, 50*(4), 35–40.

Khan, Z. S., Sher, M., Rashid, K., & Rahim, A. (2009). A three-layer secure architecture for IP multi-media subsystem-based instant messaging. *Information Security Journal: A Global Perspective, 18*(3), 139–148. doi:10.1080/19393550902926046

Kohn, C. (2003, June 2). URAC board approves HIPAA security accreditation standards. *Managed Care Weekly*, 25.

Lemley, T., & Burnham, J. F. (2009, January). Web 2.0 tools in medical and nursing school curricula. *Journal of the Medical Library Association, 97*(1), 50–52.

Malakata, M. (2005, May 16). South African nations to standardize cyberlaws. *Computerworld*, 14.

Matlis, J. (2006, August 28). Quick study: Internet 2. *Computerworld, 40*(35), 30.

McCarthy, K. (2006, August 16). ICANN awarded net administration until 2011. *The Register*. Retrieved from http://www.theregister.co.uk/2006/08/16/icann_awarded_iana/

McCullough, M. (2010, September 13). Ending the Ebola death sentence. *Canadian Business, 83*(13/14), 73.

Newly nasty. (2007, May 26). *Economist, 383*(8530), 63–64.

Notess, G. R. (2007, June). Switching your search engines. *Online, 31*(3), 44–46.

Pike, S. (2007). Use a colon. *PC Magazine, 26*(13), 107.

Rajagopalan, M. S., Khanna, V., Stott, M., Leiter, Y., Showalter, T. N., Dicker, A., & Lawrence, Y. R. (2010). Accuracy of cancer information on the Internet: A comparison of a Wiki with a professionally maintained database. *Journal of Clinical Oncology, 28*(7). Retrieved from http://meeting.ascopubs.org/cgi/content/abstract/28/15_suppl/6058

Rapoza, J. (2002, July 15). It's time for next Internet. *EWeek, 19*(28), 58.

Schloman, B. F. (2006, October 20). Is it time to visit the blogosphere? *Online Journal of Issues in Nursing*. Retrieved from http://www.nursingworld.org/ojin/infocol/info_21.htm

Senate ratifies treaty on cybercrimes. (2006, August 4). *Congress Daily*, 8.

Silkey, R. C. (2004). Extranet helps practices keep their business connected. *Ophthalmology Times, 29*(19), 31–32.

Simpkins, A. (2003, February). Navy secures healthcare network. *Communications News, 40*(2), 20.

The need for global policies. (2005, November 1). *Information Today*. Retrieved from http://www.allbusiness.com/technology/telecommunications/948099-1.html

U.N. to control use of Internet. (2005, February 22). *WorldNetDaily*. Retrieved from http://www.worldnetdaily.com/news/article.asp?ARTICLE_ID=42982.

Van De Belt, T. H., Engelen, L. J., Berben, S. A., & Schoonhoven, L. (2010). Definition of health 2.0 and medicine 2.0: A systematic review. *Journal of Medical Internet Research, 12*(2), e18.

Webopedia. (2010a, October). *Social media*. Retrieved October 24, 2010, from http://www.webopedia.com/TERM/S/social_media.html

Webopedia. (2010b, October). *Social networking site*. Retrieved October 24, 2010, from http://www.webopedia.com/TERM/S/social_networking_site.html

Webopedia. (2010c, October). *Twitter*. Retrieved October 24, 2010, from http://www.webopedia.com/TERM/T/Twitter.html

Wikipedia. (2010a, October 22). *Reliability of Wikipedia*. Retrieved October 23, 2010, from http://en.wikipedia.org/wiki/Reliability_of_Wikipedia#Science_and_medicine_peer_reviewed_data

Wikipedia. (2010b, October 21). *Wikipedia: Five pillars*. Retrieved October 23, 2010, from http://en.wikipedia.org/wiki/Wikipedia:Five_pillars

CHAPTER 5

Professional Use of Electronic Resources

After completing this chapter, you should be able to:

1. Identify examples of online sources for healthcare information and services useful to healthcare professionals.

2. Discuss typical resources found on a professional organization's Web site

3. Describe basic aspects of e-learning.

4. Relate how wikis and Web logs might be used in online learning.

5. Explain the use of Web-based learning objects.

6. Discuss possible roles of virtual worlds in educating healthcare professionals.

7. Identify specific kinds of online services available to healthcare professionals.

8. Name specific online publications for healthcare professionals.

9. Describe typical marketing services useful to healthcare professionals.

10. Discuss selected technology and techniques for managing information.

This chapter presents brief discussions on the many electronic resources available to healthcare professionals and how these services might best be used. Topics include healthcare information and services, professional organizations, educational opportunities, online services, online publications and journals, marketing services, appropriate use and policies for Web 2.0 applications, and the use of technology to organize and use information.

HEALTHCARE INFORMATION AND SERVICES

The Internet offers a wealth of information on nearly any topic of interest. Sorting through the numerous offerings can be daunting and time-consuming. This section presents some Web sites of general interest to most nurses, and potentially to other healthcare practitioners. These Web sites are available to individuals; Web sites with services only to organizations are not included. Web resources are listed in alphabetical order, and much of the content is drawn directly from the Web sites.

The Agency for Healthcare Research and Quality (AHRQ) is the part of the Department of Health and Human Services (DHHS) and is responsible for improving the quality, safety, efficiency, and effectiveness of healthcare for all Americans (http://www.ahrq.gov). AHRQ supports health-services research in these areas and provides information for practitioners on areas such as disaster preparedness, quality and patient safety, datasets, and related research findings. Of particular interest is a listing of AHRQ resources for nurses (http://www.ahrq.gov/about/nursing/nrslinks.htm).

The American Nurses Credentialing Center (ANCC) (http://www.nursecredentialing.org) is a subsidiary of the American Nurses Association (ANA). ANCC focuses on making available to individual registered nurses and organizations practice resources for pursuing excellence in practice. ANCC credentials individual nurses in various nursing specializations. The Magnet Recognition Program and the Pathway to Excellence Program promote safe, positive work environments for nurses. ANCC also accredits providers of continuing education for nurses.

BioMed Central (http://www.biomedcentral.com/home/) is a publisher using an open access publishing model. All of its published research articles are permanently accessible online, for free, at publication. All research articles in BioMed Central's 206 journals are peer reviewed. *BMC Nursing* (http://www.biomedcentral.com/bmcnurs/) publishes original, peer-reviewed research articles in all aspects of nursing research, training, education, and practice.

The Centers for Disease Control and Prevention (CDC) works to protect the health of individuals and communities through health promotion, prevention of disease, injury and disability, and preparedness for new health threats. The Web site provides users with access to numerous health and safety topics, data and statistics, publications, and multimedia presentations. An A-to-Z topic index is provided to facilitate searching the site (http://www.cdc.gov).

The DHHS has a well-organized and comprehensive Web site with numerous resources for healthcare professionals. Main sections of the Web site are HHS Secretary, News, Jobs, Grants/Funding, Families, Prevention, Diseases, Regulations, and Preparedness. Many subtopics are found within each of these main sections (http://www.hhs.gov/). Some specific agencies within DHHS are included in this section as these are organizations that impact on healthcare professionals. These agencies are National Institutes of Health (NIH), AHQR, Food and Drug Administration (FDA), and the CDC.

The FDA, an agency within the DHHS, is comprised of six product centers, one research center, and two offices. The FDA is responsible for the safety, effectiveness, and security of human and veterinary drugs, medical devices, food, cosmetics, dietary supplements, and products emitting radiation. FDA also regulates tobacco products and helps speed up product innovations that can protect public health. Its Web site has many informational resources specifically developed for health professionals (http://www.fda.gov).

A metadirectory is a directory of directories. Hardin Meta Directory of Internet Health Sources (Hardin MD) is one of the best and most complete directories for medical and health-related links: a prime "starting point" for finding Web medical information. Created and maintained at the University of Iowa's Hardin Library, Hardin MD provides access to the best resource sites in 37 medical disciplines. Link checking is used as a quality-control method for the Web resources provided in Hardin MD. Hardin MD offers a huge, up-to-date collection of medical images and information. Some examples of subject clusters are AIDS; cancer; children's diseases; flu (including bird flu); heart disease; infectious diseases; the nervous, respiratory, and skeletal systems; skin diseases; and women's health (http://www.lib.uiowa.edu/hardin/md/index.html).

The Health Resources and Services Administration (HRSA), an agency of the DHHS, is responsible for improving access to healthcare services for people who are uninsured, isolated, or medically vulnerable. One of its major activities is providing leadership and financial support to healthcare practitioners in every state and U.S. territory. HRSA provides grants to organizations for training health professionals and improving systems of care in rural communities. This agency also oversees organ, bone marrow, and cord blood donation; supports programs that prepare against bioterrorism; compensates individuals harmed by vaccination; and maintains databases that protect against healthcare malpractice and healthcare waste, fraud, and abuse (http://www.hrsa.gov/index.html).

The Interagency Council on Information Resources in Nursing (ICIRN) is a voluntary group of agencies and organizations concerned with providing library and informational resources for nursing and improving access to library services for all nurses. The ICIRN's mission is to advance the profession of nursing by establishing an effective system of information resources. ICIRN publishes *Essential Nursing Resources,* a compendium of important and helpful references to support nurses and the librarians who support nursing research (Interagency Council on Information Resources in Nursing 2010). Both a PDF and HTML version of this publication are available from the ICIRN's Web site (http://www.icirn.org).

The NIH, a part of the DHHS, is the nation's medical and nursing research agency that focuses upon discoveries that improve health and healthcare, and save lives. NIH encompasses 27 research institutes and centers, each with its own Web site. In addition to these specific Web sites, the NIH site provides information on health topics; grants and funding; news items; and research, training, and scientific resources (http://www.nih.gov/).

The National Institute of Nursing Research (NINR) is one of the 27 institutes within NIH. NINR funds nursing research and research training, with a mission to improve and promote health among individuals, families, communities, and larger populations. This mission is accomplished through support of research in a number of science areas. Current areas of research are chronic and acute diseases, health promotion and maintenance, symptom management, health disparities, care giving, self-management, and the end of life (http://www.ninr.nih.gov/). NINR has a page of online links to federal government health resources, nursing organizations, and some other helpful resources (http://www.ninr.nih.gov/Footer/Links.htm).

The National Library of Medicine (NLM) is part of NIH. NLM collects, organizes, and makes available biomedical science information to scientists, healthcare professionals, and the public. The NLM's Web-based bibliographic databases, including PubMed/Medline and MedlinePlus, are used around the world. The NLM Gateway (http://gateway.nlm.nih.gov/gw/Cmd) provides Web-based access to the incredible wealth of information resources in the library. Users can search simultaneously in multiple retrieval systems, from one Web interface.

PROFESSIONAL ORGANIZATIONS

Today, a professional organization that wants to thrive must have a Web site. Organizations that embrace and use the applications of Web 2.0 are most likely to catch and keep emerging practitioners (Pettit 2009). The quality and usefulness of the site will vary from organization to organization. It is safe to say that membership and impact of any organization will depend on continual assessment and improvement of its Web site. A presence on the Internet facilitates access to organizational information for members and interested potential members, alike.

Typically, a professional organization's site will have information about the organization; membership; educational opportunities; certification; past, present, and future conferences; resources; purchase of organizational memorabilia and attire; policy work; and a career center for assistance in finding employment. Often, a news feed or news center is available for updates on current organizational and/or healthcare issues. Increasingly, a section on research is provided (e.g., American Holistic Nursing Association, American Physical Therapy Association).

Organizations with different membership groups usually provide online sections dedicated to those groups. For example, the American Society for Clinical Pathology (ASCP) has sections for pathologists, laboratory professionals, students, and program directors.

The use of social media (described in more detail in a following section) is prevalent. A professional organization may use social media, such as Twitter, Facebook, LinkedIn, and YouTube. Often, an organization has an online community message board or listserv, where members can develop and contribute to discussions on many different topics.

Podcasts and Webinars are educational resources used by many professional organizations. These online presentations are available initially as live broadcasts, then retained for later access. Members usually have free access, and others might have access after payment of a fee. Many organizations provide continuing education credits for viewing podcasts and Webinars.

E-LEARNING

Computers and the Internet are increasingly popular resources for life-long learning. Basic and graduate-level academic preparation and continuing-education opportunities are available online for health professionals. Several different terms are used to denote learning that uses the Internet: *e-learning, Web-based learning, Internet-based training, advanced distributed learning, courseware and Web-based instruction, computer-based or computer-assisted learning, online learning,* and *open/flexible learning* (to name the most common). *Distributed learning* or *hybrid learning* usually means a course that combines elements of an online classroom with an in-person classroom (sometimes called "bricks-and-mortar").

Blake (2009) noted that e-learning overcomes many of the traditional barriers to education and offers many advantages. For example, asynchronous teaching-learning enables learners and teachers to connect to virtual classrooms at different times; this flexibility supports a work environment where learners have different shifts and workdays. Further, time is not spent commuting to and from a physical classroom. Online library resources are available when needed and when the seeker has time to search the literature. Learners acquire skills and confidence in using information technology.

Web-based learning assumes that students are self-directed and able to judge their learning needs (Kowlowitz, Davenport, & Palmer 2009). Students take on responsibilities for seeking assistance and clarifying content. Sometimes, online students experience a sense of isolation and a lack of connection with faculty and/or other students. Online courses can be more time-consuming and more work, as most courses require all the learners to participate in the classroom more than once a week.

A good online learning environment provides high levels of interactivity from learners and instructors. Required participation in discussions is one method of fostering interactivity and community among students. Virtual discussion boards, problem-based learning situations, collaborative workspaces, interactive lectures, videos, and chat rooms, along with written assignments, can be used to foster connectivity and critical thinking. Most e-learning platforms (the software that organizes and manages the learning environment) provide cafes or lounges where students can meet online to discuss assignments or talk about various topics of interest.

A good online learning setting also includes ease of access, new knowledge that is useful to the learner, and content developed by subject-matter experts. The curriculum needs to be presented at the appropriate learning level of the targeted students. The e-learning platform should be user-friendly and intuitive. A method for tracking what the student has learned (e.g., content) is useful for the learner, the teacher, and managers (if a continuing-education course is provided by an employer).

Wikis for Education

A wiki is "the simplest online database that could possibly work" (WikiWikiWeb 2002). Put simply, a wiki is a Web site where users not only read the content but can add to or edit the content. Even more simply, a wiki is a shared online resource. Wikis allow knowledge to be disseminated quickly to an audience.

Wikis can be classified as open or closed. In an open wiki, the information can be edited by anyone with access to the wiki. A closed wiki restricts editing to a select group. The information on a wiki may also be restricted to a particular group or be available to anyone (Younger 2010).

Wikipedia (http://www.wikipedia.org), "the free encyclopedia that anyone can edit," is an open wiki available since 2001. It probably is the best-known example of a wiki. *WikiWiki,* the name of the first wiki, is Hawaiian for *quick* (WikiWikiWeb 2010). While Wikipedia is intended to be a broad-based information resource, specialized-subject wikis also exist.

Wikis used in education can foster and facilitate collaboration among learners. With geographically distributed learner populations working in different time zones and different shifts, an asynchronous method for collaborative learning is essential. Wikis can be used to disseminate learning resources and provide links to other resources, such as emerging clinical practices. Students can use wikis to share learning experiences. A class project may include compilation of one or more wikibooks. (A wikibook, logically, is a collection of writings (documents) brought together by one or more writers for a specific purpose.) A wiki may serve as a content-management system for one online course or an entire program, such as an MSN-degree program.

Web-Based Learning Objects

If you are designing a Web-based educational offering, you may encounter the idea of Web-based learning objects. A **learning object** is an entity or learning event that can stand alone without losing meaning, usually addressing only one or two learning objectives (Jesse, Taleff, Payne, Cox, & Steele 2006). A teacher can select from a collection of learning objects, organize them into unique learning tools or lessons, and reuse them in the same or different constructions. Thus, a learning object also is known as a reusable learning object (RLO). An RLO is believed to enhance learning by chunking down complex material into smaller packets.

The World Wide Web enhances the development and use of RLOs by increasing the possible levels of interactivity and supporting the embedding of learning materials such as video and audio clips, text, applications, or animations. Jesse et al. (2006) note several benefits of Web-based learning objects: consistency, enhancement of collaboration, improvement of faculty and student satisfaction, efficient use of resources, and increased access for student learning.

Repositories of nursing-oriented Web-based RLOs are increasing. Think of these repositories as a library of already-developed lesson materials. In publicly available repositories, nursing educators find individual objects with learning activities developed and tested by content experts. Look for an RLO with learning outcomes, enough content to enable a learner to reach those outcomes, one or more activities in which the learner must apply the content (practice component), and a method for assessing learning (Billings 2010). Repositories may offer RLOs for free or require payment.

NEAT is a learning object repository developed in partnership with the University of Texas Medical Branch (UTMB) (http://webcls.utmb.edu/neat/). MERLOT (Multimedia Educational Resource for Learning and Online Teaching) provides free access to learning resources for many disciplines (http://www.merlot.org/). Universities and schools or colleges within a university may develop their own repositories.

Web Logs (Blogs)

A Web log or blog is an online document that grows sequentially, in chronological order. A single individual or a group of bloggers contribute to the main content. The contents of a blog can be read by anyone who has reading access. Readers can register and post comments to any entry. The main entry cannot be edited. A blog entry can be written content only or can include audio or video clips, as well as other Web-available media.

Educators may use blogs to supplement coursework, providing a discussion forum for learners and a place for additional content to which students can respond. In continuing education, a blog might provide an environment for new nurses to reflect on the orientation experience, all staff to report issues with new equipment or practice changes, feedback from preceptors, or updates on clinical practice topics (Billings 2009).

Virtual Worlds

Virtual worlds are online simulated environments in which multiple users interact. The simulated environment may reflect contemporary life, a setting found in works of fiction, or a setting unique to a virtual world–developer's imagination. Other terms for virtual worlds include *digital worlds, simulated worlds, multiuser virtual environments (MUVE),* and *massively multiplayer online games (MMOGs).*

Virtual worlds share some common features: Many users may participate at the same time; the game space is visual, ranging from two to three dimensions; interaction is in real time (immediate); players can modify the world; the world exists even if no one is logged in; social groups and communities are encouraged within the world (Virtual Worlds Review n.d.).

Although originally created for commercial game playing, virtual worlds are being used for many different purposes, and those uses are growing, along with the number of virtual worlds. Commercial virtual worlds focused on community building and socializing can be found. The use of virtual worlds for education is increasing. Education worlds usually are sponsored by educational and nonprofit entities. However, some corporations sponsor educational worlds. Active Worlds Educational Universe encompasses over 1,000 3D virtual-reality worlds. MobileKids, sponsored by Daimler, focuses on road safety for children. Different ways of governing and expressing political will are explored in virtual worlds such as AgoraXchange. The U.S. military and groups that train military personnel use virtual worlds as well. Second Life (SL), launched in 2003 by Linden Lab, is one of the largest, oldest, and best-known virtual worlds. In Second Life, each user is a resident of a specific world. Each resident is represented by an avatar (animal, icon, person, character, etc.). Second Life is not a single place on the Internet with a specific use in its design. Rather, SL provides a gathering place where residents build their worlds, developing societies, living places, adventures, and experiences.

Skiba (2007) describes the importance of SL to higher education, whether academic or professional development. SL provides an immersive environment; is dependent on content generated by the users, fostering creativity and a sense of contribution to the world; and it fosters social interaction (Skiba 2007). Three schools using Second Life for educating nurses are Tacoma Community College in Washington, the University of Kansas School of Nursing, and the University of Wisconsin Oshkosh College of Nursing (Skiba 2009). A tour through Second Life reveals numerous communities related to health and healthcare: Mayo Clinic, CDC Island, USF Health, Ann Meyers Medical Center, and many more.

ONLINE SERVICES FOR HEALTHCARE PROFESSIONALS

Among the plethora of resources and services provided by the HRSA is a section on cultural competence (http://www.hrsa.gov/culturalcompetence/). In this section, nurses and others may take advantage of assessment tools for cultural and linguistic competence. Educational content on general aspects of cultural competence as well as content on specific groups is available.

Healthlink is a free Web site for healthcare professionals and consumers. The primary focus of this site is assisting users with accessing medical and healthcare information, products, resources, services, and practitioners on the World Wide Web (WWW). Healthlink also provides a series of free online forums for healthcare discussions, a free area for classified advertisements, and a listing of doctors, dentists, and hospitals. The searchable database has over 256,000 links and is growing steadily. All links in the directory are visited and reviewed for content, professionalism, and validity (http://www.healthlinks.net/index.html).

An example of a commercial online source providing services is Healthcare Providers Service Organization (HPSO), a division of Affinity Insurance Services, Inc. The core service from HPSO is insurance, especially professional liability insurance and risk-management information. In addition to insurance information, the Web site provides a variety of information to assist a healthcare practitioner in understanding circumstances that place practitioners at risk. This information includes studies of claims against healthcare practitioners, articles on risk management, legal case studies, a newsletter, and presentations (http://www.hpso.com/about-us/index.jsp). Other insurance providers have similar content on their Web sites.

Online continuing education is another service available to healthcare professionals. Numerous organizations provide educational opportunities through home study, live seminars, and online study. For health professionals in states that have mandated courses, most of these continuing-education organizations provide those courses. When selecting a continuing-education provider, make sure that the provider is credentialed by the appropriate credentialing body (e.g., a state board of nursing, American Psychological Association, or National Association of Alcohol and Drug Abuse Counselors).

State professional licensing agencies now allow many professionals to manage their licenses online. Professionals can submit an application for initial licensure, renew a current license, check on the status of the application or renewal, and explore additional services. Many licensing agencies now offer licensees, employers, and the general public the opportunity to conduct searches of licensed professionals via a secure Web site.

Online Publication and Journals

Fully online journals for nursing and other healthcare professions are growing in number. A fully online journal is one that is not printed on paper. Some professional publications are available in both online format and print format, with subscribers selecting one format; sometimes print subscribers also have access to the online format. Articles in most professional publications are now available in full text when retrieved from a bibliographic database such as the Cumulative Index to Nursing and Allied Health Literature (CINAHL).

The shift to online publication, while not complete, is a steadily growing movement. Online publishing offers advantages over paper-based publishing:

- *Time frame between writing and publishing is shorter.* As soon as content is written or as soon as it is approved, the content can be posted to the Internet. Using electronic communication to distribute manuscripts for peer review and obtain the completed reviews shortens that cycle immensely. In the print publication environment, the time from submission to publication can be quite lengthy, reducing the timeliness of the information.
- *Reduced costs.* In an online environment, there are no final printing costs. Distribution costs are minimal, since a posting to a Web site makes the document immediately available to all who have access to that site.
- *Collaboration is enhanced.* Electronic communication, the use of shared document sites, or online collaboration sites (e.g., SharePoint, Google Docs) enable authors from distant locations to collaborate on manuscripts.
- *Multimedia can be included.* Text articles can be enhanced by still pictures, moving images, audio, and interactive segments.

- *Increased access.* The Internet eliminates delays of distance and time for accessing published materials.
- *Searching is supported.* Readers can search for similar documents and search within a document for specific words or phrases.
- *Space savings.* Libraries and readers do not have to store print documents, reducing storage requirements and maintenance costs.

Launched in June 1996, the *Online Journal of Issues in Nursing (OJIN) is* the first totally electronic journal in nursing. *OJIN* is a peer-reviewed publication that provides a forum for discussion of the issues inherent in current topics of interest to nurses and other healthcare professionals. The intent of this free journal is to present different views on issues that affect nursing research, education, and practice, thus enabling readers to understand the full complexity of a topic. The interactive format of the journal encourages a dynamic dialog resulting in a comprehensive discussion of the topic, thereby building up the body of nursing knowledge and suggesting policy implications that enhance the health of the public. The journal is indexed by Medline, CINAHL, and Scopus (http://www.nursingworld.org/ojin/).

The *Online Journal of Nursing Informatics (OJNI)* began publishing in 1996, as well. It is the longest-running journal dedicated to nursing informatics. *OJNI* is published every four months and is launched at the end of February, June, and October. *OJNI* is a free, international, professional, refereed publication that focuses on nursing informatics in all practice settings. *OJNI* is committed to addressing the theoretical and practical aspects of nursing informatics as it relates to the art of nursing. CINAHL indexes the journal (http://ojni.org/index.html).

Other online journals discovered through a limited search of the Internet, using the term *online journal* are *Online Journal of Rural Nursing and Health Care, Dermatology Online Journal,* and *Southern Online Journal of Nursing Research (SOJNR).*

Questia is an online library that provides 24/7 access to the world's largest online collection of books and journal articles in the humanities and social sciences, plus magazine and newspaper articles. Users can search by individual words, phrase, title, author, or subject through the entire online collection of books and articles. Every title can be read online. Multiple users can read the same book at the same time. A search of Questia, using the term *nurse,* resulted in 74,094 hits: 25,011 books, 9068 journal articles, 7,558 magazine articles, 32,423 newspaper articles, and 34 encyclopedia articles. A free trial is available before subscribing (http://www.questia.com/Index.jsp).

Marketing Services

Marketing is a process of creating interest in a company's goods or services. Companies use marketing to generate sales, develop their business, build customer relationships, and create value for customers. Traditional marketing activities include public relations; media relations; advertising in print, radio, television, and outdoor formats; and event planning.

The rise of the Internet and Web 2.0 has included the development of online marketing services and numerous organizations to provide these services. These services might be categorized as Internet, computer, social media, and advertising.

Internet-related services may include securing domain names for a business, arranging for e-mail addresses, establishing the ability to conduct electronic commerce, hosting one or more Web sites, designing and maintaining company Web sites, content management systems (CMS), and customer relationship management (CRM). For computer-related services, an online service organization might purchase a company's computers and related hardware and set up internal and external networks. Social media services can include setting up and running a Twitter account, one or more Facebook pages, and a blog. Starting online social media is not hard. The hard work comes in keeping the content updated. Using a marketing service saves a professional time and resources.

Some specific examples of marketing services are the following:

- *Job postings*. Openings can be posted online, and applicants can respond online. Some services support posting of résumés online for searching by employers.
- *Virtual tours*. An organization or school might compile a video or photographic tour of the facility, with or without narration.
- *Advertisements*. Organizations or individual healthcare professionals may provide information about services, facilities, prices, and staff.
- *Product information*. Healthcare-related vendors and manufacturers use their Web sites to disseminate information about product lines, research that supports the products, information on finding distributors, and related educational content.

WEB 2.0 APPLICATIONS

At the heart of Web 2.0 applications are two ideas: Users are in charge and information is to be shared. Social media are the main applications of Web 2.0, including Facebook, Twitter, eBay, Craigslist, and LinkedIn. Chapter 4 discusses Web 2.0 in some detail. This section addresses the appropriate use of social media by healthcare professionals and the response of organizations to employee use.

Appropriate Use

Healthcare professionals who use social network sites need to be careful. Putting information about one's practice along with personally identifiable information can impact practitioner–patient relationships. Be careful about text, photographs, videos, or audio content that could be linked to a specific patient or group of patients. Avoid critical remarks about co-workers, patients, or employers. Remember that employers are using social network sites to check up on applicants and existing employees. Keep in mind the constraints of HIPAA and the Family Educational Rights and Privacy Act.

Accepting a patient or former patient as a social network friend impacts the professional boundaries expected of healthcare professionals. Work-related communications, even through Facebook, Twitter, or a blog, need to remain professional (e.g., avoid emoticons). Using these very public venues requires critical thinking and caution. If someone asks for health advice, it is best to refer the person to his or her regular healthcare provider. Liability insurance does not cover this use of social media.

Using search engines to locate a patient on Facebook could be a violation of professional ethics. For example, the American Psychiatric Association does consider such behavior an ethical violation, if found information does not directly promote care for a patient (Luo 2009). Even if such information does promote patient care, consider the violation of autonomy, dignity, and trust that searching for such information engenders.

Social media sites are not secure. Content of these sites can be used as evidence in legal actions.

Institutional Policies

Personal information on social-network sites becomes public information. Privacy is nearly nonexistent. Because of privacy issues, most employers now ban the use of Internet-based social networks. Use of social network Web sites via an organization's portal to the Internet has actual and potential risks for employers and employees:

- Negative impact on organization's information system performance
- Potential for harming employers' reputation
- Reduction in employee productivity

- Liability of employer for employee actions on a social network site
- Violation of organizational policies
- Breach of employee–employer contract
- Violation of professional practice codes

Many healthcare organizations use electronic barriers to limit access to social sites, including Facebook, Twitter, and MySpace. These organizations cite confidentiality and privacy issues as well as patient safety as their rationales. Other facilities have written policies on the use of such sites and rely on staff education to ensure compliance. Most policies set an age limit (e.g., over 18 years) and warn against posting any patient-related information. Instead of blocking access, David Scott advises all organizations to write a social media use policy and create formal guidelines (Scott 2010). He notes that the guidelines used by IBM can serve as one example (http://www.ibm.com/blogs/zz/en/guidelines.html).

USING TECHNOLOGY TO ORGANIZE AND USE INFORMATION EFFECTIVELY

Bradford Eden writes that information users have "the power to arrange, classify, find, order, deconstruct, and reconstruct information and knowledge in any fashion he or she wishes" (Eden 2008, 50). Along with this power comes the need for tools (technology). This section explores some of the software applications and techniques that can support this power. The *Wall Street Journal* points out professionals are exposed to an average of 1.6 gigabytes of information every day, through the multiple communication technologies found in the workplace and at home (Coombes 2009).

E-Mail

Simple techniques are available to manage the daily flood of e-mails. These techniques include schedules, priorities, sorts, filters, folders, deletes, politeness, highlights, and conciseness.

- *Schedules.* Allocate specific times during the day to work on e-mails and avoid working on e-mails at any other time. Remove all alerts related to incoming e-mails.
- *Priorities.* Scan e-mails to see if the task or needed action is readily apparent. If not, ask. When sending an e-mail, be clear in the first two sentences about what actions are needed—or if no action is needed.
- *Filters.* Filters work; use them. Junk mail takes time to review and process. Spam filters are inexpensive and effective.
- *Sort.* Sort the inbox by sender. This sorting can allow one e-mail response to be sent that addresses many action items. Sometimes, a requested task is cancelled in a later e-mail and sorting by sender can prevent unnecessary work.
- *Folders.* Use e-mail folders and e-mail rules to sort messages from specific people or groups into specific folders. This sorting technique helps in working on priorities. Subfolders can help further organize messages and work.
- *Deletion.* Frequently, e-mail inboxes and folders contain multiple e-mails with each e-mail having one more reply in a long thread of replies. Deleting all but the most recent posting in the thread will retain the information but reduce the clutter.
- *Politeness.* Do not send "thank–you" e-mails automatically.
- *Highlights.* Create rules to have messages from managers and important stakeholders marked with different colors.
- *Conciseness.* Write short e-mails with clear subject lines. Brevity helps avoid overloading the recipients.

RSS Feeds

RSS (Really Simple Syndication) feeds allow you to subscribe to content eliminating the need to manually search for new information on sites that offer the RSS option. Typically the content is of a nature that is frequently updated such as newsletters, podcasts, professional journals, or government Web sites. Special software, known as reader software, checks for updates and helps you to organize the content into folders that appear under the RSS category in your e-mail application. Unlike regular e-mail, however, these updates are not visible unless you choose to open the folder. The individual "feed" messages can be used to link to the update. Individual feed messages can be shared, prioritized, categorized, or deleted. Subscription is as easy. First you must have or obtain a reader. Readers are often combined with browsers. Next look for a button labeled "RSS" and follow the instructions to subscribe.

Spreadsheets

Many people use electronic spreadsheets to organize data, especially data in the form of lists. Building work schedules for a group of people or a list of customer orders are common uses of spreadsheets. The familiar look of a spreadsheet, the sorting function, and the ease of entering data are part of the attraction. If the number of data rows (records) on the spreadsheet is small (less than 2,000) and the relationships between data are simple, a spreadsheet may work well for simple data storage and manipulation.

Databases

Spreadsheet functions are simpler in nature than those same functions in a database. For example, sorting in a spreadsheet is limited to one column of data at a time (e.g., the last name or assigned work shift). A sort lists everyone (or everything) on the list in ascending or descending order, according to values in one column. To find information using a database, a query is used. A query can include more than one value, such as the names of people and a specific shift on a specific day. The amount of information presented is reduced and is more precise. Databases enable more control over data integrity, allowing restrictions to be placed on the values entered for each data item.

Social Media

Facebook and Twitter (and their counterparts) are fun, innovative, and useful applications. Along with the positive side of these social tools comes a need to manage friends, followers, and one's own postings. Naturally, a wealth of tools and tips are available to manage these applications and all the associated information. It is beyond the scope of this section to collect and/or comment on all the tools available. And, each tool has its promoters and detractors. A few observations may provide ideas for searching the Internet to find tools useful to each person.

Facebook Friends Keeping track of a large number of friends can be challenging. Facebook allows subscribers to create lists of different friends and allows a user to control or block information made available to different lists. A list can be used to send a group e-mail and to link friends to specific groups or events. For users with a lot of friends, some caution and planning are necessary when creating friend lists. Facebook does not support merging or connecting lists, so a large number of lists could become cumbersome. Before launching into list making, write down a few categories or names and begin slowly. Typical themes for lists include context (where or how you met someone: via friends, travel, shopping, or vacation) and affiliation (groups such as work, sports, or associations). Once lists are created, privacy settings can be adjusted to control how much information is presented to list members.

Twitter Favorites Regular Twitter users often read updates that they want to save or read later. For these situations, Twitter offers the function of favorites. This function allows a particular tweet to be marked for follow-up. Putting the cursor over the tweet reveals a star (*). Clicking on the star saves the tweet to the favorites area. These collections of saved tweets are available for review by anyone who is an approved follower of the original author's account (http://support.twitter.com/articles/221312). Third-party applications are available that allow better manipulation of favorites than does the Twitter software.

FUTURE DIRECTIONS

The rapid growth of social media, smart phones, and mobile computing applications points to a healthcare environment where rapid, responsive communication is expected and possible. Healthcare professionals and healthcare organizations need to be familiar with and adaptive to the many different methods of communication and the communication expectations that different healthcare consumers bring to healthcare encounters.

Visit nursing.pearsonhighered.com for additional cases, information, and weblinks.

CASE STUDY EXERCISE

Someone who has been seen by you for healthcare services contacts you online, asking to be your Facebook friend. How should you respond to this request? Explain your reasoning.

SUMMARY

- There are abundant online sources for healthcare information and services useful to healthcare professionals. These include but are not limited to government agencies, professional organizations, and publishers.
- Establishing a presence on the Web is critical for professional organizations. Content typically includes background information, links to news, current issues, conferences, publications, and special members-only sections.
- E-learning provides a popular option for both formal study and continuing education. Other terms for learning that uses the Internet include Web-based learning, Internet-based training, advanced distributed learning, courseware and Web-based instruction, computer-based or computer-assisted learning, online learning, and open/flexible learning.
- Distributed learning or hybrid learning usually means a course that combines elements of an online classroom with an in-person classroom. A good online learning environment provides high levels of interactivity from learners and instructors as well as ease of access, new knowledge that is useful to the learner, and content developed by subject matter experts.
- Wikis used in education can foster and facilitate collaboration among learners.
- Reusable learning objects (RLOs) are learning events that can stand alone and address one or two learning objectives.
- The World Wide Web enhances the development and use of RLOs by increasing the possible levels of interactivity and supporting the use of learning materials such as video and audio clips.
- Libraries of nursing-oriented Web-based RLOs with developed learning activities and content tested by experts exist that can be used by others to facilitate learning. Examples include NEAT and MERLOT.

- Blogs may be used to supplement coursework, providing a discussion forum for learners and a place for additional content to which students can respond.
- Virtual worlds are online simulated environments in which multiple users interact. Second Life (SL) is an example of a commercially available virtual world that has been used for educating nurses.
- An increasing number of professional publications and journals are now available either entirely or partly online.
- Additional online services of interest to professionals include the ability to view job posting and post résumés online.
- Social media, or Web 2.0, applications such as Facebook, Twitter, and LinkedIn can be useful, but healthcare professionals who use social network sites need to be careful about the nature of information they post and aware of policies their employers have on social media use.
- Technology can be used to help organize and effectively access information via e-mail setup, use of RSS Feeds, spreadsheets, databases, and social media.

REFERENCES

Billings, D. M. (2009). Wikis and blogs: Consider the possibilities for continuing nursing education. *Journal of Continuing Education in Nursing, 40*(12), 534–535. doi: 10.3928/00220124-20091119-10

Billings, D. M. (2010). Using reusable learning objects. *Journal of Continuing Education in Nursing, 41*(2), 54–55. doi: 10.3928/00220124-20100126-08

Blake, H. (2009). Staff perceptions of e-learning for teaching delivery in healthcare. *Learning in Health and Social Care, 8*, 223–234. doi: 10.1111/j.1473-6861.2009.00213.x

Coombes, A. (2009, May 17). Don't you dare email this story. Retrieved from http://online.wsj.com/article/SB124252211780027326.html

Eden, B. L. (2008). Technology: Dispatches from the field. Ending the status quo: The future of information organization. *American Libraries, 39*(3), 38.

Interagency Council on Information Resources in Nursing. (2010). Interagency council on information resources in nursing: Promoting information literacy for nursing. Retrieved from http://www.icirn.org

Jesse, D. E., Taleff, J., Payne, P., Cox, R., & Steele, L. L. (2006). Reusable learning units: An innovative teaching strategy for online nursing education. *International Journal of Nursing Education Scholarship, 3*(1), 14.

Kowlowitz, V., Davenport, C. S., & Palmer, M. H. (2009). Development and dissemination of Web-based clinical simulations for continuing geriatric nursing education. *Journal of Gerontological Nursing, 35*(4), 37–43.

Luo, J. S. (2009). The Facebook phenomenon: Boundaries and controversies. *Primary Psychiatry, 16*(11), 19–21.

Pettit, S. L. (2009). Cyberspace and connectivity: The new fabric of life and learning [Opinion]. *Delta Kappa Gamma Bulletin, 76*(2), 39–42.

Scott, D. M. (2010). Let them communicate. *EContent, 33*(3), 40.

Skiba, D. J. (2007). Nursing education 2.0: Second life. *Nursing Education Perspectives, 28*(3), 156–157.

Skiba, D. J. (2009). Nursing education 2.0: A second look at second life. *Nursing Education Perspectives, 30*(2), 129–131.

Virtual Worlds Review. (n.d.). What is a virtual world? Retrieved from http://www.virtualworldsreview.com/info/whatis.shtml

WikiWikiWeb. (2002, June 22). What is Wiki? Retrieved September 10, 2010, from http://www.wiki.org/wiki.cgi?WhatIsWiki

WikiWikiWeb. (2010). Retrieved from http://c2.com/cgi-bin/wiki?WikiWikiWeb

Younger, P. (2010). Using wikis as an online health information resource. *Nursing Standard, 24*(36), 49–56.

CHAPTER 6

Healthcare Information Systems

After completing this chapter, you should be able to:

1. Identify the various types of information systems used within healthcare institutions.

2. Define the terms *healthcare information system, hospital information system, clinical information system, nursing information system, physician practice management system, long-term care information system, home care information system,* and *administrative information system.*

3. Explain the functions of a nursing information system.

4. Differentiate between the nursing process and critical pathways/protocol approaches to the design of a nursing system.

5. Review the key features and impacts on nursing and other healthcare professionals associated with order entry, laboratory, radiology, and pharmacy information systems.

6. Describe the functions of client registration and scheduling, and coding systems.

7. Explain the purpose of decision support and expert systems.

8. Identify ways that mobile devices such as personal digital assistants, tablet computers, and iPods can improve the utility of healthcare information systems.

An **information system** can be defined as the use of computer hardware and software to process data into information to solve a problem. The terms **healthcare information system** and **hospital information system (HIS)** both refer to a group of systems used within a hospital or enterprise that support and enhance healthcare. The HIS comprises two major types of information systems: clinical information systems and administrative information systems. **Clinical information systems (CISs)** are large, computerized database management systems that support several types of activities that may include provider order entry, result retrieval, documentation, and decision support across distributed locations.

Clinicians use these systems to access client data that are used to plan, implement, and evaluate care. CISs may also be referred to as *client care information systems*. Some examples of CISs include nursing, laboratory, pharmacy, radiology, medical information systems, emergency department systems, physician practice management systems, and long-term and home care information systems. **Administrative information systems** support client care by managing financial and demographic information and providing reporting capabilities. This category includes client management, financial, payroll and human resources, and quality assurance systems. Coding systems use clinical information to generate charges for care. Figure 6–1 shows the relationships between various components of a hospital information system.

Clinical and administrative information systems may be designed to meet the needs of one or more departments or functions within the organization. In recent years the trend has been to adopt vendor-based solutions with little, if any, customization, allowing implementation to occur more quickly. Either clinical or administrative systems can be implemented as standalone systems, or they may work with other systems to provide information sharing and seamless functionality for the users. Any one healthcare enterprise may use one or several of the clinical and administrative systems but may not use all of them. Increasingly, organizations are looking at the need to improve productivity, improve safety, increase the quality of care, meet regulatory and reimbursement requirements, and reduce costs across the enterprise. Information technology is seen as the means to achieve these ends through the application of evidence-based care, improved work flow, and better management of resources. Patient safety initiatives also require facilities to establish a culture of safety in which problem areas are identified, the culture is measured periodically, findings are shared, and feedback for change is solicited (Smetzer & Navarra 2007, p. 136).

CLINICAL INFORMATION SYSTEMS

Although many CISs are designed for use within one hospital department, clinicians and researchers from several areas use the data collected by each system. For example, the nurse documents client allergies in the initial assessment. The physician, the pharmacist, the dietician, and the radiologist can then use these data during the client's hospital stay. The goal of CISs is to allow clinicians to quickly and safely access information, order appropriate medications and treatments, and implement cost-effective, evidence-based care while avoiding duplicate services. Several tools help clinicians to achieve these goals. These include electronic health records, clinical decision support systems, bedside medication administration using positive patient identification, computerized provider order entry (CPOE), patient surveillance, and the clinical data warehouse (CDW). While large teaching hospitals generally have more monies to invest in the information technology, all healthcare providers are now looking at information technology solutions in order to meet Meaningful Use requirements and realize HIT benefits. Mobile and wireless technology used with CISs allow information entry and retrieval at the point of care or wherever it is needed by the healthcare professional. This is best seen by the healthcare professional who can view client lab results while walking or at the point of care which enhances worker productivity because it eliminates the need to walk back to a central location to view test results, and it improves client service because

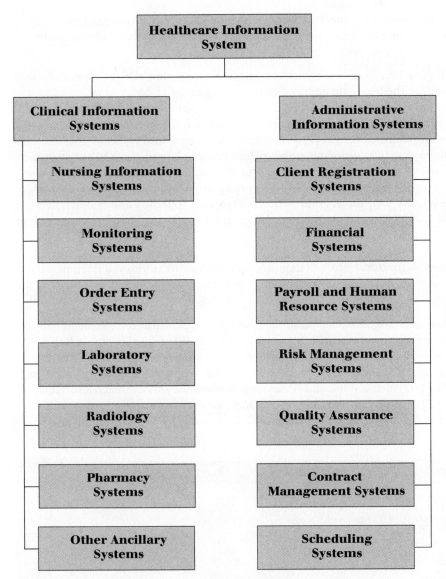

FIGURE 6–1 • Relationship of the healthcare information system components

treatments can be ordered and initiated in a more timely fashion. Internet technology also changes the way that users interact with CISs. This capability allows physicians to view client test results from home, office, the golf course, or at the mall. Despite the fact that the technology exists to permit this type of access, not all facilities can provide it at this time. The following descriptions of CISs address those that are most frequently seen in the hospital setting.

Nursing Information Systems

According to Hendrickson (1993) a **nursing information system** supports the use and documentation of nursing processes and activities, and provides tools for managing the delivery of nursing care. An effective nursing information system must accomplish two goals:

- Support the way that nurses function, allowing them to view data, collect necessary information, provide quality client care, and document the client's condition and the care that was given.

- Support and enhance nursing practice through improved access to information and tools such as online literature databases, drug information, and hospital policy and procedure guidelines.

Consideration of these two goals in the selection and implementation of a system ensures that it will benefit nursing. The two main approaches to nursing care and documentation using automated information systems have been the *nursing process approach* and the *critical pathway,* or *protocols,* approach. The traditional nursing process approach allows documentation of nursing care using well-established formats such as admission assessments, problem lists, and care plans. Ideally this approach incorporates **standardized nursing languages (SNLs)** accepted by the American Nurses Association because SNLs provide a common language across the discipline of nursing that allows all nurses to describe nursing problems, treatments, and outcomes in a manner that is universally understood. SNLs facilitate data collection and research that can be replicated and shared across all of nursing. The advantages of using an information system are listed in Box 6–1.

Nursing Process Approach The nursing process approach to automated documentation often uses the nursing diagnosis and traditional paper processes long used by nurses as the organizational framework. Components in this approach include:

- *Documentation of nursing admission assessment and discharge instructions.* A menu-driven approach ensures capture of essential information. A **menu** lists related commands that can be selected from a computer screen to accomplish a task. For example, the menu may include selections such as past medical history, advanced directives, organ donation status, psychosocial history, medications, and review of body systems. This approach also helps to ensure that all necessary information is covered in the client's discharge instructions, including follow-up appointments and diagnostic studies; diet and activity restrictions;

BOX 6–1   Advantages of an Information System

- Better access to information
- Enhanced quality of documentation through prompts
- Improved quality of client care
- Increased productivity
- Improved communications
- Reduced errors of omission
- Reduced hospital costs
- Increased employee satisfaction
- Compliance with agency regulations
- Common clinical database
- Improved client perception of care
- Enhanced ability to track records
- Enhanced ability to recruit/retain staff
- Improved hospital image
- Improved mandatory reporting capability

wound care; and medication information such as drug names, instructions for administration, and common side effects that the client should report. The system should generate printed copies of these instructions for clients to review on discharge and for their use at home, as well as for use by the Home Health staff.

- *Generation of a nursing worklist that indicates routine scheduled activities related to the care of each client.* These activities can be grouped according to scheduled time or skill level.
- *Documentation of discrete data or activities such as vital signs, weight, and intake and output measurements.* The automation of this type of data promotes accuracy and allows the data to be readily available to all care providers at any time.
- *Documentation of routine aspects of client care, such as bathing, positioning, blood glucose measurements, notation of dietary intake, and/or wound care in a flowsheet format.*
- *Standardized care plans that the nurse can individualize for clients as needed.* This feature saves time yet allows flexibility to address the client's needs while promoting quality care.
- *Documentation of nursing care in a progress note format.* The nurse may accomplish this through narrative charting, charting by exception, or flowsheet charting. Regardless of the method used, automated documentation can improve the overall quality of charting by prompting the nurse with predefined selections. Box 6–2 describes three of these traditional formats and some typical automation approaches.
- *Documentation of medication administration.* This multistep feature may be performed through the information system, but increasingly it is done via a separate medication administration application. Worklists associated with this feature specify administration times and medications for each patient; the nurse can use the worklist for preparation and administration of medications with subsequent documentation through the system.

Recent initiatives to improve patient safety and decrease medication errors call for the use of barcode medication administration systems. While these are not considered to be a part of a nursing documentation system, barcode systems are designed to prevent common medication administration errors at the bedside, document medication administration, and capture

---

BOX 6–2   Automation of Traditional Nursing Documentation Methods

Many forms of nursing documentation have been automated by various nursing information systems. Some of these formats are listed next.

- **Narrative charting.** Traditionally, nurses complete charts using narrative text. In a nursing information system, this may be accomplished using free text entry or menu selections.

- **Charting by exception.** Client-specific documentation addresses only the client's exceptions to normal conditions or ranges. Automated documentation should provide all normal standards and allow the nurse to easily document any exception observed. This may involve menu selections or free text entry.

- **Flowsheet charting.** Routine aspects of care are documented in tabular form. This format is most effective when presented in a personal computer–based graphical user interface. A pointing device such as a mouse is used to make menu selections or text entries. One form of flowsheet charting is the automation of medication administration records.

- **Standardized nursing languages.** This approach uses NANDA nursing diagnoses as well as the Nursing Interventions Classification and Nursing Outcomes Classification languages. It removes the ambiguity of meaning found in other documentation systems.

charges. These systems require a nurse to scan the barcodes found on his or her identification, the patient's identification bracelet, and on all prescription medications during the medication administration process. These systems are designed to help the busy nurse to ensure that the right medication is given in the correct dosage and form at the correct time for the right patient. Barcoding systems often include warnings for high-risk drugs, medications with sound-alike names, dosage discrepancies, and maximum dosages.

Critical Pathway or Protocols The critical pathway or protocol approach to nursing documentation is the second approach used in automated nursing information systems and it is often used in a multidisciplinary manner, with many types of care providers accessing the system for information and to document care. Nurses, nursing or patient care assistants, dietitians, social workers, respiratory therapists, physical and occupational therapists, case managers, and physicians all use these systems for documentation. Critical pathway systems include the following features:

- *The nurse, or other care provider, can select one or more appropriate critical pathways for the client.* If more than one path is selected, the system should merge the paths to create one "master" path or protocol.
- *Interaction with physician orders.* Standard physician order sets can be included with each critical pathway and may be automatically processed by the system.
- *Tracking of protocol variances.* The system should identify variances to the anticipated outcomes as they are charted and provide aggregate variance data for analysis by the providers. This information can be used to fine-tune and improve the critical pathways, thereby contributing to improved client outcomes.

Despite the many reasons to establish a nursing information system and the fact that nurses constitute the majority of workers in healthcare, most systems today are designed for use by all clinicians and incorporate features discussed here.

Monitoring Systems

Monitoring systems are devices that automatically monitor biometric measurements in critical care and specialty areas, such as cardiology and obstetrics. These devices may send information to the nursing documentation system. For example, a monitoring system would directly enter measurements such as blood pressures, eliminating the need for the nurse to enter these data manually. Another example may be seen with blood glucose monitors that send client readings to the laboratory system for display with other laboratory tests. Box 6–3 describes some additional features of monitoring systems.

BOX 6–3   Some Common Features of Monitoring

- **Alarms alerting the nurse of significant abnormal findings.** Sophisticated systems provide different alarms indicating various abnormalities. For example, the nurse may be able to hear a specific alarm sound that indicates which cardiac arrhythmia the client is experiencing.

- **Portable monitoring systems.** These systems allow easy transportation of the client throughout the facility without loss of data or functionality.

- **Records of past abnormal findings.** The system maintains a record of all past abnormal findings during this monitoring episode. The system allows the user to find trends in data using graphical displays and to focus on specific details.

- **Download capabilities.** The system may be able to transfer patient data to a separate system in another facility to provide a continuous patient record.

Order Entry Systems

With **order entry systems**, orders for medications and treatments are entered into the computer and are directly transmitted to the appropriate areas such as the pharmacy, laboratory, radiology, social service, or another area. The preferred method is direct entry of orders by the physician, nurse practitioner, physical therapist, or other provider because this eliminates issues related to illegible handwriting and transcription errors, checks orders for accuracy and completeness, speeds the implementation of ordered diagnostic tests and treatment modalities, decreases adverse drug events, enhances staff productivity, saves money, promotes safety, and improves outcomes when used in conjunction with evidence-based practices (Dentzer 2009; Leapfrog hospital survey results 2009; Powell 2011; Standardize order sets for improved care 2010). This process is known as computerized physician, provider, or prescriber order entry (CPOE). CPOE represented a major initiative on the part of the Institute of Medicine and Leapfrog Group to improve the quality of care and reduce medication errors (Conn 2007). While most CPOE is found in inpatient settings, its benefits apply to outpatient and ambulatory settings as well, where it also plays a critical role in the prevention of prescription errors. The safety of CPOE systems is enhanced through the incorporation of built-in reminders and alerts that help the prescriber to select the most appropriate diagnostic test or medication for a particular patient as well as the appropriate dose and form. Challenges to the implementation of CPOE include buy-in by busy clinicians, significant changes to work processes, difficult system sign-on, limited system access or response time, funding constraints, inadequate access to clinical data to support the expert decision-making features of CPOE, and the perception by many physicians that CPOE affords them few advantages. Successful CPOE implementation requires significant expertise in healthcare processes, information technology, and change management, as well as careful planning and building that includes input from nurses, pharmacists, and other stakeholders. At present Meaningful Use requirements for hospitals constitute a major driver for the adoption of CPOE (CMS 2010). In some settings, transcription of physician orders into the clinical information system is still done by a nurse or by ancillary personnel. When entries are made by ancillary personnel, nurses are responsible for ensuring that entries are correct.

Entry of an order into a clinical information or order entry system alerts all departments to carry out orders. For example, when a physician orders a barium enema, the order entry system can automatically notify the dietary department to hold the client's breakfast, the pharmacy to send the appropriate medications, and the radiology department to schedule the test. These systems prompt the clinician to provide the information necessary for carrying out the order.

Another feature of an order entry system is duplicate checking. When an order is entered, the system checks to see if a similar order has been placed within a specified time frame. If this is the case, the system can alert the user with a message, or automatically combine the two orders, permitting only one execution of the order.

The order entry system can reflect the current status of each order. For example, the status may be listed as pending, complete, or canceled. This allows the user to see a comprehensive list of the client's orders at any point in time. It can also afford a mechanism for the entry of charges for a procedure once it has been completed.

One mechanism that is used in some order entry systems uses rules-based or knowledge-based programming. Rules provide guidelines to assist physicians to select the preferred and most cost-effective medication along with the best route and dose for a particular patient problem. Rules can also provide prompts for when patients should be seen next and diagnostic tests that should be performed. These automated reminders help to improve the quality of care by reducing reliance upon memory, providing evidence-based practice guidelines, and informing the prescriber when a more cost-effective oral medication is available in lieu of an intravenous form (Chazard et al, 2009; Matsuura & Weeks 2009).

Despite the many advantages associated with CPOE, it may also introduce new problems and errors related to new work processes (Ash et al. 2007; Bradley, Steltenkamp, & Hite 2006;

Cornish, Etchells, & Knowles, 2006; Moniz 2009; Weant, Cook, & Armistead 2007). These unintended consequences may include an increase in medication errors even if the level of harm related to errors does not increase. Pharmacists can help identify potential problem areas and needed modifications prior to implementation. Some examples include reminders or alerts to:

- Prescribe laxatives for patients prescribed opioids
- Order drug levels for therapeutic levels
- Avoid lapses in medications
- Avoid prescribing drugs that are contraindicated for certain medical conditions such as impaired renal function

Pre-implementation planning should address unintended consequences. It is important not to underestimate the time required for training or the impact of CPOE on nursing practice as nurses are called upon both to assist physicians struggling to learn the system and to execute more verbal orders by physicians unwilling to use the system. Verbal orders are subject to errors, defeating the safety checks built into CPOE. Nursing leaders must provide sufficient resources to manage the additional workload as staff and physicians make the transition to CPOE and ensure that no verbal orders will be accepted except during emergency situations.

Laboratory Systems

Laboratory information systems (LISs) can provide many benefits, including a shorter turnaround time for results; prevention of duplicate testing; decreased likelihood of human error; and identification of abnormal results according to age, sex, and hospital standards. Systems have the capability to alert providers when new or stat test results are back or values are critical (Goedert 2007). Additional features can include the automatic entry of repeating tests at the time of the original order. An example might include the order "troponins x3," which would automatically schedule the first troponin level, with the second 8 hours later and the third level 8 hours after the second and which would subsequently bundle serial tests into one claim for reimbursement. Systems may also allow providers to enter orders without leaving the patient's electronic record. In addition, microbiology culture and sensitivity testing can provide treatment suggestions for the physician.

Automatic generation of specimen labels should occur when an order is placed either directly into an LIS or passed to an order entry system. Labels may include client demographic identifiers, the name of laboratory studies to be performed, and any special instruction for handling, such as "place on ice." Labels may be configured to print immediately at the client location for stat or nurse-collected specimens or in the laboratory in batch mode for laboratory-collected specimens. Batch mode allows the labels to be printed in groups for standard collection times, either on demand or at predefined times.

When specimens are processed by the laboratory instrumentation, the results are automatically transmitted to the LIS. The results can be viewed directly from the LIS or transmitted to another information system, such as the nursing or medical information system. Laboratory values are available immediately on completion of the testing process. If desired, printed paper copies of the results may be produced immediately at predefined locations, such as the nursing unit or physician's office, or can be printed in cumulative format for permanent chart copies.

Another feature of many laboratory systems is automatic client billing for tests completed. This information may be communicated to the client billing system.

Yet another feature seen in many laboratory systems is the ability to integrate results collected at the bedside using portable devices. This is seen with the performance of blood glucose monitor tests in the clinical area. Results are then sent to the laboratory system immediately or sent when the blood glucose monitor is docked. This affords clinicians an integrated view of patient results and the ability to compare glucose readings taken at the bedside with glucose readings from blood specimens sent to the laboratory. While this feature is widely used and appreciated more commonly, the demand is to have LIS results available at the bedside or via mobile devices such as personal digital assistants (PDAs) in which results are passed either through the laboratory or clinical information system to the PDA for review.

Another feature of some laboratory systems is the ability to use rules-based testing. A **rule** is a predefined function that generates a clinical alert or reminder. **Arden syntax** is the standard language used in the healthcare industry for writing rules. A rules-based LIS could automatically order a second test based on the results of an initial test. For example, if a client has an abnormal complete blood cell count value, the system will perform a differential, which is a more specific second test. Rules-based testing could also eliminate unnecessary testing after several consecutive normal results have been obtained, as when physicians order daily laboratory work. These measures save costs and the staff time of assessing the need for and performing the tests. The incorporation of rules-based technology may require the user to enter all of the information needed for specific tests. An example is weight for a creatinine clearance test to determine whether the client's renal function falls within the normal range. Another example of rules-based technology is seen when labels are printed with collection instructions such as tube color, amount needed, and directions such as "place on ice." Rules can also be used to limit tests to those covered by Medicare or other third-party payers or to determine how and where test results will be sent (Rogoski 2003).

Laboratory systems also have the potential to provide more meaningful information such as genetic predisposition toward certain diseases based on information that already exists in the hospital or laboratory database, information that can be useful in the diagnosis and procurement of payment from third-party payers (Rogoski 2003).

One traditionally weak area in the collection and processing of laboratory results is patient identification. Handwritten labels may be illegible for reasons of poor handwriting or spills. The use of barcoding in conjunction with an LIS to track specimens helps to eliminate this type of problem. Barcodes are either printed directly onto collection labels or affixed at the time of processing to help improve specimen tracking. This process results in improved patient safety and productivity.

Although many institutions are moving toward a paperless record, it has been common practice for staff and students to print out copies of laboratory findings for their personal reference and to communicate to other staff. The ability to send results directly to secure mobile devices helps to ensure the privacy of health information because it eliminates the need for large numbers of printouts and the need to fax sensitive information.

Radiology Systems

A **radiology information system (RIS)** provides scheduling of diagnostic tests, communication of clinical information, generation of client instructions and preparation procedures, transcription of results and impressions, and file room management such as tracking of film location. Orders may be entered directly into the radiology system or transmitted from an order entry system. Radiology clerical staff use order information to schedule patients for testing. Once the test is complete, the radiologist interprets the findings and dictates a report. This report can be transcribed using the radiology system or a separate transcription system. The radiology system generates billing information that can be sent to the billing system. The reports are then stored within the radiology system. They may also be faxed to the physician's office or viewed through the clinical or nursing information systems.

One example of how a radiology system might be used is seen with magnetic resonance imaging (MRI) orders. As the first step in placing an MRI order, the system generates a questionnaire that asks questions pertinent to the MRI procedure. For example, it asks whether the client is cooperative or claustrophobic, and if there are any metal foreign bodies related to previous surgeries or injuries. The nurse reviews these questions with the client, then enters the answers to each question and the order requested into the system. A radiologist reviews the order request and the questionnaire answers, and determines if the client is appropriate for testing. This procedure allows scheduling of appropriate clients only, and eliminates the time-consuming and costly scheduling and attempted testing of inappropriate clients.

More recent developments in RIS include digital, filmless images as a replacement for traditional radiology films. These **picture archiving and communications systems (PACS)** allow images to be electronically transmitted and viewed using sophisticated, high-resolution monitors. The enhanced quality of these images over traditional films may result in fewer repeat procedures and improved diagnostic capability. Digital filmless imaging is also an integral component in the evolution of the electronic client record. The use of this technology may allow hospitals to do away with radiology images captured on film. This reduces or eliminates the large expense of radiology films, as well as handling and storage of the x-rays. In addition, PACS allows the physician to view the image on a computer screen within seconds after the completion of a procedure. Another benefit of a PACS is that more than one physician can view an image simultaneously in multiple locations. While special workstations are available for PACS, images can be viewed on any computer albeit the resolution may not be as good.

Other benefits of this technology are seen when these images are transmitted to high-acuity areas, such as emergency departments and intensive care units, where quick turnaround and immediate availability of images are critical to providing optimum client care. The use of this technology can facilitate client care in remote rural healthcare facilities where a radiologist may not be on-site. Images can be transmitted to a major medical center for evaluation by radiologists and other physicians. Benefits are realized in terms of cost, because it is not necessary to staff a radiologist, and improved client care when a radiologist is on staff but not available.

Implementation of a PACS system should include consideration of the following issues:

- *Ability to exchange data with the RIS.*
- *Systems standards base.* The system should be operable without proprietary software that makes it difficult to use or upgrade.
- *Access to previous studies.* On-demand access to all prior client studies is preferable.
- *Required infrastructure.* Can the system be used with existing computers and the electronic medical record system?
- *System performance.* Are records available quickly and of sufficient quality for diagnostic purposes?

Pharmacy Applications and Systems

The inpatient pharmacy process is complex and the source of many medication errors given the large number of drugs on the market, sound-alike names, high patient acuity levels, and large number of medication orders processed. The National Coordinating Council for Medication Error Reporting and Prevention (2005, p. 4), a group comprised of more than 20 national organizations, including the Food and Drug Administration (FDA), defined a medication error as "any preventable event that may cause or lead to inappropriate medication use or patient harm while the medication is in the control of the healthcare professional, patient, or consumer." Several other groups have also worked on strategies to reduce errors. In 2001 the Patient Safety Task Force was formed under the Department of Health and Human Services' Quality Improvement Initiative to improve data collection on patient safety. The lead agencies in the Patient Safety Task Force included:

- FDA
- Centers for Disease Control and Prevention
- Centers for Medicare & Medicaid Services
- Agency for Healthcare Research and Quality

The FDA also reviews reports that come from drug manufacturers through the agency's safety information and adverse event reporting program, MedWatch. The FDA now rejects all applications for similar drug names by using a computer program that searches for similar sounding names. The Institute for Safe Medication Practices accepts reports from consumers and health professionals using collected information to publish a consumer newsletter on medication errors. Hospitals report medication errors via the national MedMARX error-reporting program.

Combining pharmacy information systems with barcode technology, as described in Box 6–4, can drastically reduce medication errors. Information systems can provide checkpoints at each phase of the medication ordering and administration process using evidence-based medication selection and dosing guidelines. Other checkpoints may include alphabetizing drugs by chemical name; decreasing the amount of floor stock so that staff are less likely to accidentally choose the wrong drug, dose, or form for administration; improved unit dose availability from the pharmaceutical companies; final preparation of drug admixtures such as antibiotics in the pharmacy, thereby eliminating drug errors and compatibility problems with the admixture solution; availability of online drug references; delivery of only one dose at a time; and delivery of single-dose packages.

BOX 6–4 Using Information Systems to Reduce Medication Errors

Order entry, pharmacy, and BCMA systems, along with automated medication supply management systems, can be used to assist healthcare providers in reducing the occurrence of medication errors. These systems interact to provide checks and alerts throughout the medication ordering and administration process, as directed in the following examples:

1. A physician enters a medication order into the order entry system.
2. The information is automatically transmitted to the pharmacy system.
3. The pharmacy system integrates laboratory values and uses rules to ask the physician if he or she chooses to change or add medications based on laboratory values or dose for patient size or age.
4. The pharmacy system checks the patient's history and alerts the physician to any drug interactions or allergies. The physician can change the order at this time, if indicated.
5. The pharmacy system issues a warning when sound-alike medications are ordered, forcing the physician and caregiver to consider which drug the patient is actually to receive.
6. The order creates a requisition in the pharmacy that contains a barcode indicating the correct medication, as well as a barcode identifying the patient.
7. A robot in the pharmacy fills the medication order by matching the medication barcode on the requisition to the barcode on the medication. The medication is transported to the nursing unit.
8. The nurse scans the barcode on the patient's identification band and the barcode on the medication, administers the medication only if there is a match, and documents medications given in the barcode medication administration system. A warning will appear if insufficient time has passed since the drug was last administered.
9. The system prompts the nurse to enter pain scale, blood pressures, and pulses where appropriate.
10. The system automatically adds the nurse's electronic signature.
11. The barcode medication administration system can generate the following reports:

    - A medication due list, showing medications that need to be administered within specific time parameters, including one-time, on-call, continuous, PRN orders, and regularly scheduled medications
    - PRN effectiveness list that prompts the nurse to record the effectiveness of PRN medications
    - Medication administration history, which records nurse initials and times for medications given in a traditional medication administration record format
    - Missing dose report—prints in pharmacy to alert staff when a dose needs to be reissued; done at the time the nurse was administering meds with essentially no disruption in work flow
    - Medications not given report—lists all missed doses according to the documentation on the medication administration record
    - Variance log—captures meds given more than 30 minutes early or late

Integration of the various clinical information systems with subsequent exchange of information decreases medication errors and improves therapeutic drug monitoring in patients with compromised renal function and those receiving drugs with narrow therapeutic ranges through the use of clinical decision support (CDS) alerts. Pharmacy systems offer many benefits that promote cost containment, improve the quality of care, and decrease medication errors. These systems can be used by a variety of healthcare professionals who perform activities related to the ordering, dispensing, and administration of medications. A hospital pharmacy may use an information system to access client data such as demographics, health history and diagnosis, medication history, client allergies, laboratory results, renal function, and potential drug interactions. Traditionally, pharmacists reviewed each client's medication profile, laboratory values, medical history, and progress notes manually to monitor medication disbursement and effectiveness. This is a time-intensive, laborious process that is no longer feasible. Automated systems pull in laboratory results and client information from the HISs more quickly and accurately than a manual process identifying allergy and interaction problems. This integration of information allows pharmacists to recommend changes in parenteral nutrition formula based on laboratory abnormalities, verify that medication dosages are appropriate based on serum drug levels, avoid drugs that may impair renal function, and monitor laboratory values for possible drug toxicity. Pharmacy systems can also provide automatic alerts that can save lives. Automation of previously manual processes also can reduce costs. Kuiper, McCreadie, Mitchell, & Stevenson (2007) noted that the successful use of technology reduced the potential for error by automating tasks that require high levels of accuracy and repetition. An example of this may be seen with the integration of intravenous administration pumps with pharmacy systems (Breland 2010; Sullivan 2010).

Another benefit offered by pharmacy systems is the tracking of medication use, costs, and billing information. Automation of these functions generally improves accuracy and is more cost-effective than manual methods. In addition, this information can be manipulated and analyzed more easily for executive decision making when it is available as a computer file.

Physicians and other direct care providers may also use pharmacy systems. These systems provide online access to client and drug information that is critical in the drug prescription process. Pharmacy systems can provide easy access to clients' health and medication history, as well as their allergies and demographic information. Access to formulary information and online drug reference information helps physicians determine the most effective drug and the appropriate doses for clients. In addition, these systems can provide comparisons of costs and drug effectiveness, particularly important in the managed care arena. Pharmacy information systems provide data for barcode medication administration (BCMA) systems.

Creating a culture of safety is a critical first step to making changes needed to reduce medication errors. There are many opportunities to use technology to prevent medication errors but the implementation of some of these applications has been delayed (Schneider 2007). The Institutes of Medicine recommends the use of pharmacy systems, BCMA, smart infusion pumps, and decision support software to improve safety (IOM 1999, 2001, 2007).

Pharmacy Dispensing Systems

Pharmacy systems can automatically dispense each client's medications in unit dose format, creating labels for each dose with the client's name and other demographic identifiers. The actual dispensing of the medications may be accomplished either with or without the intervention of the pharmacist. Some systems automatically dispense ordered medications in unit dose packages, which the pharmacy staff place in the client's medication drawer. This process can be streamlined by using robotic systems, which collect the appropriate medications and place them in the drawers. Robotic dispensing systems are seen as a mechanism to prevent medication errors as well as reduce inventory and labor costs (Lin, Huang, Punches, & Chen 2007). These systems serve to support rather than supplant the pharmacist.

Unit-Based Dispensing Cabinets Another aspect of pharmacy systems is the use of automatic dispensing systems for use by the nurse. These systems provide a medication dispensing unit in the clinical area, generally for use by nurses who administer medications. The system is usually secured by requiring a user ID and password or biometric measure for access to the system and the actual medications. Features include menu-driven prompts for identifying the client, medication, dose, and number of unit doses removed. The user can also be prompted to count the current number of doses on hand when removing narcotics or other controlled substances. Automatic dispensing systems provide accurate records of medicines given in terms of what was taken from the unit and the date, time, and user who performed this activity. These records can be accessed centrally in the pharmacy to determine when supplies in the clinical area dispensing units must be replenished. In addition, this information can be used to efficiently and accurately bill clients for medications used. Nurses must recognize that there are limitations to these safety devices and still carefully check medications before removing them from the cabinet, avoid returning unused doses, take only one dose for a single patient when it is needed, and avoid unsafe practices such as overriding the system (McCartney 2006).

Barcode and RFID Medication Administration Applications Bar-Code Medication Administration is a quality initiative identified by the Leapfrog Group and the Veterans Administration's National Center for Patient Safety (Educating patients 2007; Schneider, Bagby, & Carlson 2008, p. 1614). BCMA is a system that uses the barcode found on the unit-dose medication package and on a patient's identification bracelet to ensure that nurses administer the right drug to the right patient in the right dose at the right time and by the right route (Rivish & Moneda 2010). It prevents errors at the point of care, where they can do the most harm. It also helps hospitals comply with the Joint Commission standards and patient safety goals. Specifically, it helps hospitals meet requirements to verify orders and patients before medication administration. The reductions in medication errors provide a return on investment (ROI) (Elganzouri, Standish, & Androwich 2009). BCMA systems may exist as stand-alone systems or as a part of a complete hospital information system. Typically the nurse uses a portable scanner to scan a barcode on his or her identification badge to log on to the software application. Next the patient's identification bracelet is scanned. The system displays a list of the patient's medication orders and times for administration. Medications due for administration are scanned as the nurse checks them. Documentation is automated with the process. Successful BCMA implementation eliminates loopholes that allow nurses to bypass key features such as scanning the patient's identification bracelet. The extent of the benefits accrued from BCMA will be influenced by several factors, including adherence to standardized dispensing practices and human factors such as ergonomics associated with the medication cards (Mills, Neily, Mims, Burkhardt, & Bagian 2006). When discussing the prevention of medication errors, Manno (2006, p. 60) noted that technology that is used to enhance health and delivery systems "should be designed to make it easy to do the right thing and hard to do the wrong thing." Pairing BCMA with CPOE further decreases errors (Comeaux, Smith, & Stem 2006). Adding CDS to the combination drastically lowers mortality and the harm rate associated with adverse drug reactions and errors (Reifsteck, Swanson, & Dallas 2006). Additional features, such as prompts when pain assessments are past due, improve documentation. Other BCMA benefits include more consistent patient identification, fewer missed medication doses, and fewer adverse effects since system alerts warn the nurse of allergies and possible drug interactions (Mills et al. 2006). Radio Frequency Identification (RFID) technology offers the same benefits. It is slightly more expensive but is not subject to read errors with smudges or obscured visibility. The disadvantages associated with BCMA include poorly functioning scanners, identification bracelets that do not read consistently, and the need to transport equipment (McCartney 2006). Smart IV pumps that contain special drug error reduction software can be integrated with BCMA.

E-Prescribing E-prescribing is a process that allows the physician to enter a prescription into an information system. This information is electronically communicated to the client's pharmacy. This may be done using a variety of devices, including personal digital assistants (PDAs), wireless computers, or other handheld devices that allow prescriptions to be easily sent from the physician's exam room or the patient's bedside. Electronic prescriptions provide the following benefits:

- Elimination of telephone authorization for refills
- Review of clients' drug histories before ordering drugs
- Reminders to order home medications for the hospitalized client
- Alerts about drug interactions
- Checking of formulary compliance and reimbursement
- Provision of a longitudinal prescription record

Electronic prescriptions require direct links between physician offices, hospitals, pharmacies, and third-party payers. E-prescribing functionality is required for Meaningful Use reimbursement for physicians so adoption rates are expected to increase exponentially (Conn 2011).

Physician Practice Management Systems

A survey (Mattocks et al. 2007) revealed that practice management systems comprised the most commonly used type of technology in physician offices. Features typically include the ability to capture some demographic information, schedule appointments, maintain lists of insurance payers, perform billing tasks, track outcomes, and generate reports. There may, or may not, be a connection to electronic patient records although this will no doubt change as more practices adopt electronic health records (EHR) systems to qualify for Meaningful Use monies. Patient records in paper format are expensive to maintain and unwieldy to handle, making it difficult to locate information quickly which contributes to the overall fragmentation of individual health records. Some physician offices accepted hardware and software supplied by local hospitals in order to use their information systems and reap the associated benefits of a unified record. Automation of physician office records helps to maintain client confidentiality and HIPAA compliance because health information is contained within the information system rather than loose papers that can easily be viewed by unauthorized clinical and nonclinical office staff.

Long-Term Health Information Systems

The adoption of information technology (IT) has been slow in long-term care for many reasons, including fragmentation among facilities, limited operating budgets, high implementation costs, and multiple providers in one facility. This situation is beginning to change ("Information technology: Is Long-Term Care Leading the Way?" 2009). The integration of clinical information systems in this area is imperative for the improvement of quality of care, better management of the complex needs of the population, and a decrease in adverse drug effects (Alexander, Rantz, Flesner, Diekemper, & Siem 2007; Brandeis, Hogan, Murphy, & Murray 2007; Gillespie 2007; Shugarman, Nishita, & Wilber 2006; Subramanian et al. 2007). The adoption of information systems is also critical to the business survival of long-term health facilities given the constantly changing financial and reimbursement system (Nahm, Mills, & Feege 2006). Integration must extend beyond the walls of a single long-term care facility to best serve the needs of the patients. Boston Medical Center and University Geriatric Services partnered with nursing homes in several areas to provide the hardware and software that subsequently improved communication between providers, hospital, and nursing home staff. This was particularly important given the fact that many nursing home patients have multiple transfers from one facility and set of providers to another. Long-term care information systems include documentation and financial information. Ideally, features include order entry, results retrieval, and medication administration.

One particular example of improved communication is the use of the electronic record to document patient preferences about advanced directives. Lindner, Davoren, Vollmer, Williams, & Landefeld (2007) noted that modification of admission orders at a Veterans Affairs nursing home improved the completion of resuscitation status by physicians. IT also promises to ease the heavy burden of paper-based documentation in this setting. While doubts have been voiced about the acceptance of computerized documentation in long-term care, Yu, Qiu, and Crookes (2006) found that the majority of workers surveyed in nursing homes were willing to adopt electronic documentation. The cost of widespread adoption of IT in long-term healthcare must be carefully considered. The reality is that costs must be borne by facilities and physicians. Financial incentives may be required to encourage and expedite the use of technology in this arena (Subramanian et al. 2007).

Ambulatory Care Information Systems

Integration of technology into ambulatory care settings has been sporadic with some clinic settings having access to order entry and results retrieval from the affiliated hospital systems but still using paper for documentation. Medicare and Medicaid incentive payments are now in place for the adoption of certified EHR systems and demonstration of Meaningful Use (Collins, Wise, & HIMSS 2010). The Meaningful Use incentive arose from the expectation that EHRs would serve as the key to improve quality and efficiency in healthcare (HIMSS n.d.).

Home Care Information Systems

Braunstein (1994) noted that home care nurses were ideally situated to be early adopters of electronic systems because of their mobility, frontline role in the healthcare system, their lack of a support structure at the point of care, and the excessive demands for documentation. McBride (2006) noted that systems could be tailored to streamline the work of nurses, improve quality of care delivery, and improve payment for services because billing personnel can find needed information more quickly, allowing them to send out bills earlier. The adoption of technology for home care will increasingly make use of monitoring technology integrated into information systems as a way to care for an aging population at home (Cheek, Nikpour, & Nowlin 2005). At best, home care systems will communicate with hospital information systems for access to test results, medication lists and allergy information, and possibly order entry. Home care is expected to explode within the next few years given that it is more cost-effective than hospital care. A commensurate level of growth is expected in the acquisition and use of home care information systems (Homecare Information Software 2010).

Other Clinical Systems

A number of other clinical systems address the needs of specific departments within the healthcare setting. Box 6–5 lists some of these systems. The rapidly changing healthcare environment has resulted in several requirements on the part of the clinical information system vendor.

BOX 6–5 Other Common Clinical Systems

- Medical records/abstracting systems facilitate the abstracting, or coding, of diagnoses and chart management processes. Client records may also be stored on optical disk.
- Operating room systems may be used to schedule procedures, manage equipment setup for individual physicians, facilitate inventory control, and provide client billing.
- Emergency department systems provide ready access to independent systems such as poison control. They also provide tracking capability, alerts, and the capability to print specific discharge and follow-up instructions based on the client's diagnosis.

The vendor's initial support services and ability to provide ongoing support are critical success factors as the healthcare paradigm continues to shift.

Westbrook (2005) summarized research that found that the successful implementation of clinical information systems was determined by the complex interaction between the technical features of the system and human, social, and organizational factors that determine whether the system will be used and whether it will prove to be safe and effective.

ADMINISTRATIVE SYSTEMS

Various administrative systems may be used in healthcare organizations to support the process of providing client care. Box 6–6 provides a brief review of many of these systems.

Registration Systems

The client registration system is critical to the effective operation of many other systems within the healthcare setting. This system is used to collect and store client identification and demographic data that are verified and updated at the time of each visit. For this reason, these may also be known as admission/discharge/transfer (ADT) systems. CISs use these data for the management of client care and billing purposes. The information is shared with those clinical systems that communicate directly with the registration system.

An important aspect of a registration system used in a multi-entity health system network is the development of a unique client identifier. This number or identification code is used to identify the client in all information systems across the organization and across all entities. This enables accurate client identification, supporting the development of a longitudinal client record that contains all clinical information available for the client.

Scheduling Systems

A scheduling system allows a healthcare organization to schedule clients and resources efficiently. Client demographic information must be available in the system either by direct entry or through electronic communication with a registration system. For the system to be used to

---

BOX 6–6   Administrative Information Systems Used in the Healthcare Setting

- Financial systems provide the facility with accounting functions. Accurate tracking of financial data is critical for enabling the organization to receive reimbursement for services.

- Payroll and human resource systems track employee time and attendance, credentials, performance evaluations, and payroll compensation information.

- Contract management systems manage contracts with third-party payers.

- Risk management systems track and plan prevention of unusual occurrences or incidents.

- Quality assurance systems monitor outcomes and produce reports that are used to guide quality improvement initiatives.

- Physician management systems support patient registration, scheduling, coding, and billing in the physician's office and may support results retrieval. These systems also provide better protection of patient privacy than paper records.

- Executive information systems provide administrators with easy access to summarized information related to the financial and clinical operations of the organization.

- Materials management systems facilitate inventory control and charging of supplies.

schedule patient appointments, it must contain information regarding available resources. This resource information may include the following:

- Referral and authorization by patients' insurance
- Department
- Equipment
- Dates and times
- Room
- Staff
- Permits and preps
- Charging and billing information

The system uses predetermined rules for determining how resource and client information should be used to schedule a particular type of appointment. This provides the capability to schedule a patient in one location. In addition, scheduling across all facilities in an enterprise can be accomplished using one system. The benefits associated with using a scheduling system include increased staff productivity, increased client satisfaction, and cost savings to the organization.

Contract Management Systems

Contract management (CM) software provides invaluable assistance to organizations to better manage their resources and improve efficiency. Healthcare institutions typically have multiple contracts with third-party payers as well as with vendors and various suppliers. CM software provides the visibility and control that allow organizations to negotiate better contracts, ensure that suppliers meet their contractual obligations, track compliance, save money, and accelerate the cycle times from sourcing through contract (Avery 2006). Anthes (2006) noted that, traditionally, organizations focus efforts to maximize profits on cutting costs and boosting sales. Pricing is based upon competitors' prices and production costs, plus a standard markup fee or value pricing, which segments buyers and sets prices based on each segment. Value pricing requires good use of data mining and modeling capabilities. Value pricing reflects different levels of charges set by sellers of services for patients in accordance with their insurance plan. CM software features support contract creation, report capability, e-procurement, alerts, and notifications on key business events, and can even support automation of the entire contract process.

Financial Systems

Financial systems were generally the first information systems found in healthcare delivery organizations. Integration with registration systems ensured that patient demographic data and insurance information could be accessed to charge for services provided and receive reimbursement. As the sophistication of technology increased, it became possible to charge patients automatically once a clinical service was completed. For this reason all other information systems were typically built around financial systems.

Risk Management Systems

This type of system enhances an organization's ability to identify potential risks and develop strategies to deal with them inclusive of the ability to cross reference and compare losses using different variables and examine the impact at different levels of detail (Pozzi 2009). Losses can be tracked back to the point of origin to pinpoint and address specific liabilities. Both small and large organizations can benefit from risk management systems. Increasingly features include dashboard views; regular e-mailing of reports; and the ability to manage policies, claims, litigation, and other insurable risk information.

Decision Support and Expert Systems

Decision support and expert systems use data from both the clinical and the administrative information systems, and can provide information related to clinical and administrative users. According to Turley (1993), little agreement exists on the definition of the terms *decision support systems* and *expert systems* except for the distinction of how much authority is placed in the computer system.

Decision support systems aid in and strengthen the selection of viable options using the information of an organization or a field to facilitate decision making and overall efficiency. Decision support software organizes information to fit new environments. It provides analysis and advice to support a choice. The final decision rests with the practitioner. Software can be off-the-shelf or homegrown. Off-the-shelf software is commercially available. The advantage to the consumer is that someone else has borne the cost for its development and testing. It is, however, geared to a general market and may not meet the needs of a particular party. Homegrown software has been developed by the consumer to meet specific needs usually because no suitable commercial package is available. The customer bears the cost of its development, testing, and communication with other software applications. Decision support software can provide a competitive edge and facilitate the move to managed care.

Clinical decision support provides clinicians with knowledge or specific information that is intelligently filtered, or presented at appropriate times, to enhance health and healthcare (Mangalampalli, Chakravarthy, Raja, Jain, & Parinam 2006; Osheroff et al. 2007). Tools may include clinical practice guidelines, alerts and reminders, order sets, patient data reports and dashboards, diagnostic support, workflow tools, and financial applications. CDS is effective in all phases of the clinical process. CPOE with CDS has been shown to decrease medication errors by as much as 80% (Cornish et al. 2006). An example of a decision support application is a program that assists nurses performing a skin assessment to review available alternatives, from which the best may be selected to maintain skin integrity. CDS is best used when available at the point of care. Access is facilitated through the use of wireless devices such as PDAs, tablet computers, and iPhones, which are easily transported and with the practitioner at the point of care. While CDS has been proven effective in improving outcomes at many sites, it is not universally available or available at the same level at all locations (Simon, Rundall, & Shortell 2007). Strong external drivers are expected to change this situation. The American Medical Informatics Association has presented a roadmap for national action that calls for improved CDS capabilities and increased use throughout the U.S. health sector. Financial rewards for improved outcomes are expected to accelerate adoption of order entry with CDS.

Expert systems use artificial intelligence to model a decision that experts in the field would make. Unlike decision support systems that provide several options from which the user may choose, expert systems convey the concept that the computer has made the best decision based on criteria that experts would use.

KNOWLEDGE REPRESENTATION (DASHBOARD DISPLAY)

Information is often distributed across several different information systems, making it difficult to piece all of the relevant information together to see important trends or make appropriate decisions. The concept of a dashboard display is intended to address this situation bringing together important information from various systems on one screen. The significance of this capability is even greater when this display reflects real-time data. Dashboard displays may bring together key performance indicators for business decisions (Schrage 2007) or clinical data from several systems into a clinical dashboard. It is imperative that the persons using the dashboard have input into the identification of the indicators used and design of the actual display. There are a number of conceivable dashboard applications in clinical areas that include workload management, syndromic surveillance for trends, and individual clinical data.

BOX 6–7   Smart Technology

Carol Curio Scholle, Marcia McCaw, Toni Morrison, Darlene Lovasik

The Problem

On the cusp of healthcare reform the quest to improve quality, safety, and efficiency in patient care delivery is generating the opportunities for the creative use of technology. Healthcare reform is challenging organizations to increase quality standards while holding costs down. Regulatory organizations are not only asking for outcomes measurements but for proof of specific actions taken to achieve quality outcomes. Examples include documentation that every eligible patient receives flu and pneumonia vaccines, indwelling urinary catheters are removed at the earliest time, and all patients undergoing surgery receive their antibiotic within 60 minutes of incision. Nosocomial events such as pressure ulcers, injury from falling, and infections are no longer reimbursed by insurance payers thereby having a direct negative effect on organizational profitability. Accurate documentation by clinical staff is more important than ever not only to maintain patient safety but to meet organizational goals.

In response to these increasingly rigorous expectations, medical device and information technology companies have developed "smart" features in their products in an effort to provide safer, and more effective care options. A clinician of today may be responsible for operating and retrieving information from multiple devices which all offer essential clinical information but require him or her to manage and move this information to the right place. Such information might need to be documented in the electronic medical record (EMR), referenced and acted upon, or communicated to another provider. In any event manipulation of information requires additional time, attention, and actions by the clinician. The goal of Smart technology is to eliminate these extra steps.

What Is "Smart" Technology?

Smart technology is a system that optimizes workflow efficiency by solving real problems and ties multiple electronic solutions together to create seamless workflow for the clinician at the point of care. Smart technology enhances quality by reducing opportunity for error, prioritizing and reminding caregivers of tasks that need to be completed, and allows real-time documentation of tasks at the point of care. Real-time documentation also reduces steps for staff by eliminating the need for movement from the patient room to a computer. This documentation model also eliminates the opportunity for transcription error when clinicians enter information into the EMR which may be noted on a piece of paper at the point of care.

Benefits for Clinicians

This real-time documentation and point of care information display creates transparent communication between clinicians. For example, vital signs that are done and documented in the room by the nursing assistant are immediately available to the nurse who may be able to save steps by going to the medication room to get the antihypertensive medication to treat the elevated blood pressure prior to entering the patient room thereby saving time and steps. It also minimizes interruptions in care delivery, which have been proven to be opportunities for errors, particularly errors of omission, to occur. Ultimately, clinical staff are able to work in a more efficient manner. Reduced costs related to unanticipated overtime from rework, repeating steps, and batch documentation may be realized. Errors of omission, such as not consistently providing every two-hour change in position for an immobile patient, may result in pressure ulcers. In our current environment, in addition to the pain, suffering, and potential long-term adverse outcome to which the patient may be exposed, treatment related to this type of nosocomial event would not be reimbursed by payers. Smart technology puts reminders for this type of routine care at the point of care, making it difficult to omit by analyzing patient information and using clinical intelligence to determine priorities. Telemedicine systems may also be interfaced through smart technology. Physicians who practice from multiple locations have the opportunity to examine and interview their patients via a high-resolution video even when off-site. This feature supports continuity in care and allows the treatment plan to progress without interruption or delay.

Benefits for Patients and Families

Patients and families may also reap the benefits of smart technology. Systems may allow the patient to make nonurgent requests such as requesting a blanket, water, toiletries, or nutrition electronically and send the request directly to the person who can deliver the service. So instead of the patient calling out to the unit secretary via a call light system to request a fresh water pitcher and the secretary calling the nursing assistant to

(continued)

BOX 6–7 (*continued*)

fulfill the request, the request can be sent directly to the nursing assistant, reducing response time and improving patient satisfaction and comfort.

The technology can also be used for education of patient and family-related education related to conditions and procedures. Documentation of the education can be interfaced with the EMR. The education can be designed interactively with learning customized for a particular patient's needs, the ability to answer questions regarding understanding of materials presented, and the ability to document questions that the patient might want to ask of the caregiver for clarification.

The daily plan of care can be displayed for patients so that they know what to anticipate for the day. Goals for discharge can be made available to keep the patient, family, and entire care team on track with the plan.

The system may also include distractions for patients such as relaxation videos, electronic games, and e-mail availability. Patients who are in the hospital for a particularly long stay appreciate the ability to receive pictures and messages from their family and friends electronically and have pictures displayed in a slide show fashion if they desire.

Current State of "Smart Technology"

Currently there are a very limited number of systems that offer the benefits of smart technology. UPMC, a hospital system in Pittsburgh, Pennsylvania, developed a "smart" system following the identification of staff need to have information available at the point of care. UPMC is currently working in partnership with IBM to commercialize the SmartRoom workflow optimization system. Using real-time location system (RTLS) technology the system then authenticates the staff member and calls up real-time information and tasks from key clinical systems, such as the pharmacy and laboratory, on the display screen based on role. The underlying workflow module of the SmartRoom prioritizes tasks based on algorithms derived from optimal nursing workflow model. The clinician then calls up the task on the display screen and documents completion via touch screen with automatic updating of the appropriate portion of the patient's electronic medical record. The information is immediately available in the EMR for view by all care providers. The system may also pull up clinical information for reference during routine physician and nursing rounds and for patient teaching and plan of care discussions with the patient and family. The initial design and ongoing development and customization of the product include active and ongoing input and feedback from the end users, the clinicians at the bedside.

In the test environment the system demonstrated an 82% reduction in the time associated with documentation of vital signs, 57% reduction time associated with documentation of tasks, and 69% reduction in time associated with the documentation of activities of daily living (ADL). The SmartRoom system weighs tasks based on the relevance to patient safety; so a request for a blanket is prioritized lower than need for postprocedure vital signs, directing the staff to the place of the most urgent need. Tasks that, if omitted or delayed, could cause harm or a risk to patient safety are pushed to the top of the clinician's "to do" list. This prioritization helps to reduce missed care.

Opportunities for Future Development

Throughout the development and implementation of SmartRoom at UPMC, input on additional features that might be added to improve the patient experience and clinician workflow included:

- Full interface with the physical assessment documentation in the EMR
- Point-of-care lab label printing
- Physician order entry
- Telemedicine ability
- Direct integration with devices that have smart features such as:
  - Smart pumps
  - Vital sign monitors
  - Electronically controlled beds
  - Smart phones
  - Barcode scanning devices for:
    - Medications
    - Glucose meters
    - Blood products

BOX 6–7   (*continued*)

The list of enhancements that have been requested and are being explored to enhance the patient experience includes:

- Ability to view and review tests and procedures with the care team
- Electronic "just in time" dietary menu options
- Ability to order personal items from the hospital gift shop
- Survey of patient experience

Obstacles

As with development, implementation, and adoption of any new technology, obstacles appear along the way. Much of the technology that is currently in operation in today's hospitals is operating off the platform HL7, which has been in existence since the 1980s. Because of the age of this operating system, its capabilities are limited, if not challenging, to adapt into our current environment. Clinicians who use laptops, smart phones, and computers that work at lightning speed do not easily tolerate cumbersome systems that may still exist in the hospital environment. Systems often do not have the inherent ability to "talk" to each other. Smart technology needs to be able to crack the code, so to speak, to allow for translation of information from system to system thereby integrating the systems. This can be a significant challenge to overcome, depending on the systems.

As technology has evolved, many large or even not so large healthcare facilities have many, many different electronic systems. Some may even have more than one system to accomplish the same function in the same building. These systems not only need to be able to listen and understand all of the data coming in and have the ability to push data out, but need to be able to process and display the information in a format that is retrievable and usable for the front-line staff. These systems include those used for:

- Laboratory processing and reporting
- Pharmacy services
- Clinical documentation
- Data reporting
- Patient imaging
- Supply chain management
- Nutrition systems

Expense

There are capital expenses related to installation and implementation of this new type of technology which may not have easily quantifiable value to those who may be responsible for allocating funds to support this type of system. Smart technology is a tool to integrate existing technologies and it is not in and of itself a technology that will necessarily provide new or essential function. Demonstrating the value of the system requires looking carefully at roles, workflow, time studies of work, and costs associated with errors in transcription of information or errors of omission. In short it requires building a case for making the investment and demonstration of ROI. As with all technology, in addition to initial hardware, software, and infrastructure costs, system support and maintenance needs must be factored into the equation.

Adaption to Adoption

Adaption is when a form or structure is modified to fit a changed environment.

Adoption is to take over an idea or practice as if it were one's own.

Initial adaptation to new technology, despite the ultimate enhancement to workflow or work quality, is always a challenge since it requires people to change their routine and behaviors. Education and support during the implementation is a key element associated with success. This support will allow staff to adapt to the new tool. Adoption is quite another matter. Adoption happens when the new tool or technology becomes part of the new workflow and routine. Adoption is hardwired when staff find it difficult to work without the new tool.

(*continued*)

> **BOX 6–7** (*continued*)
>
> Adoption happens at different rates for different people. Background, exposure, experience, and generation have a significant impact on how willingly or quickly people adopt new ideas, practices, or workflow. A key element of a successful piece of smart technology is it is simple and intuitive to use for all. Baby-Boomers and generation Xers should be able to easily learn how, or just instinctively know how, to use the technology. Reducing steps and the time that it takes to do the work is an invaluable feature for any technology. If the technology is also simple to use, requires little education or reinforcement for people to remain competent in use of the system, adoption is facilitated and the change may become hardwired into workflow.

FUTURE DIRECTIONS

Information technology applications will become more commonplace, be easier to use, and offer additional features from this point forward. The drivers for this trend will include concerns for safety, worker retention, the need to expand evidence for evidence-based practice, reimbursement, and cost containment. McCartney (2006) noted that technology "can promote a safe environment for nursing practice by reducing negative exposure to risk and liability." Electronic databases offer the potential to facilitate retrospective analysis of errors.

CASE STUDY EXERCISE

You are a nurse participating in the customization and implementation of a barcode medication administration system. Analyze how the process will change from the current manual process. Include potential problem areas and solutions.

SUMMARY

- A hospital or healthcare information system consists of clinical and administrative systems.
- Well-designed clinical information systems can improve the quality of client care.
- Clinical information systems can extend the capabilities of healthcare providers.
- A nursing information system using the nursing process approach should support the use and documentation of nursing processes and provide tools for managing the delivery of nursing care.
- The use of standardized nursing languages such as NANDA, NIC, and NOC supports automation of nursing documentation and expands the utility of collected information.
- The critical pathway/protocol approach to nursing information systems provides a multidisciplinary format for planning and documenting client care.
- Other clinical systems, including order entry, radiology, laboratory, pharmacy systems, and physician management systems, give the nurse and other healthcare providers the support and tools to more effectively care for clients.
- Administrative systems support the process of client care by managing nonclinical, client-related information, including demographics, codes for procedures, and insurance.
- Information systems enable decision makers to examine trends and make informed choices during these times of healthcare reform.
- Federal initiatives for patient safety call for the implementation of computerized physician order entry and barcode medication administration as methods to reduce error.
- Personal device assistants and wireless technology further enhance the capability of information systems to support the work of clinicians.

REFERENCES

Alexander, G. L., Rantz, M., Flesner, M., Diekemper, M., & Siem, C. (2007). Clinical information systems in nursing homes: An evaluation of initial implementation strategies. *Computers Informatics Nursing, 25*(4), 189–197.

Anthes, G. (2006). The price point. *Computerworld, 40*(30), 33–35.

Ash, J. S., Sittig, D. F., Poon, E. G., Guappone, K. G., Campbell, E., & Dykstra, R. H. (2007). The extent and importance of unintended consequences related to computerized provider order entry. *Journal of the American Medical Informatics Association, 14*(4), 415–423.

Avery, S. (2005). How to use software to manage contracts. *Purchasing, Electronics & Technology, 134*(11), 39–41.

Bradley, V. B., Steltenkamp, C. L., & Hite, K. B. (2006). Evaluation of reported medication errors before and after implementation of computerized practitioner order entry. *Journal of Healthcare Information Management, 20*(4), 46–53.

Brandeis, G. H., Hogan, M., Murphy, M., & Murray, S. (2007). Electronic health record implementation in community nursing homes. *Journal of the American Medical Directors Association, 8*(1), 31–34.

Braunstein, M. L. (1994). Electronic patient records for homecare nursing. *Computers in Nursing, 12*(5), 232–238.

Breland, B. D. (2010). Practice report. Continuous quality improvement using intelligent infusion pump data analysis. *American Journal of Health-System Pharmacy, 67*(17), 1446–1455.

Centers for Medicare & Medicaid Services (CMS). (2010, July 28). Electronic health record incentive program final rule. *Federal Register, 75*(144), 44313–44588. Retrieved November 13, 2011, from http://edocket.access.gpo.gov/2010/pdf/2010-17207.pdf

Chazard, E., Ficheur, G., Merlin, B., Serrot, E., Beuscart, R., et al. (2009). Detection and prevention of adverse drug events: Information technologies and human factors. Adverse drug events prevention rules: Multi-site evaluation of rules from various sources. *Studies in Health Technology & Informatics, 148*, 102–111.

Cheek, P., Nikpour, L., & Nowlin, H. D. (2005). Aging well with smart technology. *Nursing Administration Quarterly, 29*(4), 329–338.

Collins, D. A., Wise, P. B., & Healthcare Information and Management Systems Society (HIMSS). (2010, December). *Meaningful use: Lessons learned on the path to EHR excellence in ambulatory care.* Retrieved November 13, 2011, from http://www.chcf.org/publications/2010/12/meaningful-use-lessons-learned

Comeaux, K., Smith, M. E., & Stem, L. G. (2006). Tech update. Improve PRN effectiveness documentation. *Nursing Management, 37*(9), 58.

Conn, J. (2007). More moving to entry level. CPOE adoption slowly gains ground, with larger number expecting installations. *Modern Healthcare, 37*(9), 41.

Conn, J. (2011, May 5). Study outlines docs' eRx barriers. *Modern Healthcare.* Retrieved November 13, 2011, from http://www.modernhealthcare.com/article/20110505/NEWS/305059989/&template=printpicart

Cornish, P. E., Etchells, E. E., & Knowles, S. R. (2006). Pharmacists' role in assessing potential value of CPOE. *American Journal of Health-System Pharmacy, 63*(22), 2182–2184.

Dentzer, S. (2009). Health information technology: On the fast track at last? *Health Affairs, 28*(2), 320–321.

Educating patients. (2007). *Hospitals & Health Networks, 81*(9), 82.

Elganzouri, E., Standish, C., & Androwich, I. (2009). The mat study: Global insight into the medication administration process. *Studies in Health Technology and Informatics, 146*, 424–428. doi:10.3233/978-1-60750-024-7-424

Gillespie, G. (2007, April). Erickson health takes long view with technology. *Health Data Management.* Retrieved November 29, 2007, from Erickson Health Takes Long View with Technology: http://www.mywire.com/pubs/HealthDataManagement/2007/04/01/3178636?extID=10037&oliID=229

Goedert, J. (2007). A new battery of tests for lab systems. *Health Data Management, 15*(9), 40–46.

Healthcare Information Management and Systems Society (HIMSS). (n.d.). *Meaningful use for ambulatory practices.* Retrieved November 13, 2011, from http://www.himss.org/asp/topics_FocusDynamic.asp?faid=408

Hendrickson, M. (1993). The nurse engineer: A way to better nursing information systems. *Computers in Nursing, 11*(2), 67–71.

Homecare information software and services market shares, strategies, and forecasts, worldwide, 2010 to 2016. (2010, February 09). *M2pressWIRE.*

Information technology: Is long-term care leading the way? (2009). *Long-Term Living: For the Continuing Care Professional, 58*(6), 53–54. Retrieved November 13, 2011, from http://www.ltlmagazine.com/ME2/dirmod.asp?sid=9B6FFC446FF7486981EA3C0C3CCE4943&nm=All+Issues&type=Publishing&mod=Publications%3A%3AArticle&mid=8F3A7027421841978F18BE895F87F791&tier=4&id=38CB8893F2D54E5E9995BC16E0F4A644

Institute of Medicine (IOM). (1999). *To err is human: Building a safer health system.* Washington, DC: National Academies Press.

Institute of Medicine (IOM). (2001). *Crossing the quality chasm: A new health system for the 21st century.* Washington, DC: National Academies Press.

Institute of Medicine (IOM). (2007). *Preventing medication errors: Quality chasm series.* Washington, DC: National Academies Press.

Kuiper, S., McCreadie, S., Mitchell, J., & Stevenson, J. (2007, January 5). Medication errors in inpatient pharmacy operations and technologies for improvement. *American Journal of Health-System Pharmacy, 64*(9), 955–959. Retrieved November 19, 2007, from CINAHL.

Leapfrog hospital survey results 2008. (2009). *Medical Benefits, 26*(12), 4.

Lin, A. C., Huang, Y. C., Punches, G., & Chen, Y. (2007). Effect of a robotic prescription-filling system on pharmacy staff activities and prescription-filling time. *American Journal of Health-System Pharmacy: Official Journal of the American Society of Health-System Pharmacists, 64*(17), 1832–1839.

Lindner, S. A., Davoren, J. B., Vollmer, A., Williams, B., & Landefeld, C. S. (2007). An electronic medical record intervention increased nursing home advance directive orders and documentation. *Journal of the American Geriatrics Society, 55*(7), 1001–1006.

Mangalampalli, A., Chakravarthy, R., Raja, M., Jain, A., & Parinam, A. (2006). IT systems. Clinical systems: Using IT to improve care. *British Journal of Healthcare Management, 12*(9), 277–281. Retrieved November 19, 2007, from CINAHL with Full Text database.

Manno, M. (2006, March). Preventing adverse drug events. *Nursing, 36*(3), 56–62. Retrieved November 19, 2007, from CINAHL with Full Text database.

Matsuura, G. T., & Weeks, D. L. (2009). Use of pharmacy informatics resources by clinical pharmacy services in acute care hospitals. *American Journal of Health-System Pharmacy, 66*(21), 1934–1938.

Mattocks, K., Lalime, K., Tate, J. P., Giannotti, T. E., Carr, K., Carrabba, A., . . . Meehan, T. P. (2007). The state of physician office-based health information technology in Connecticut: Current use, barriers and future plans. *Connecticut Medicine, 71*(1), 27–31.

McBride, M. (2006). The home healthcare pot of gold. *Health Management Technology, 27*(5), 22–23.

McCartney, P. (2006). Using technology to promote perinatal patient safety. *Journal of Obstetric, Gynecologic, & Neonatal Nursing, 35*(3), 424–431.

Mills, P. D., Neily, J., Mims, E., Burkhardt, M. E., & Bagian, J. (2006). Improving the bar-coded medication administration system at the Department of Veterans Affairs. *American Journal of Health-System, 63*(15), 1442–1447.

Moniz, B. (2009). Examining the unintended consequences of computerized provider order entry system implementation. *Online Journal of Nursing Informatics, 13*(1), 1. Retrieved November 13, 2011, from http://ojni.org/13_1/moniz.pdf

Nahm, E. S., Mills, M. E., & Feege, B. (2006). Long-term care information systems: An overview of the selection process. *Journal of Gerontological Nursing, 32*(6), 32–38.

The National Coordinating Council for Medication Error Reporting and Prevention. (2005, December). *NCC MERP: The first ten years "defining the problem and developing solutions."* Retrieved from http://www.nccmerp.org/pdf/reportFinal2005-11-29.pdf

Osheroff, J. A., Teich, J. M., Middleton, B., Steen, E. B., Wright, A., & Detmer, D. E. (2007). A roadmap for national action on clinical decision support. *Journal of the American Medical Informatics Association, 14*(2), 141–145.

Powell, V. (2011). Finding the pulse of health technology. *Pharmaceutical Representative, 41*(2), 24–25.

Pozzi, S. R. (2009). Monitor, measure and manage ERM. *Best's Review, 110*(2), 84.

Reifsteck, M., Swanson, T., & Dallas, M. (2006). Driving out errors through tight integration between software and automation. *Journal of Healthcare Information Management, 20*(4), 35–39.

Rivish, V. O., & Moneda, M. D. (2010). Medication administration pre and post BCMA at the VA medical center. *Online Journal of Nursing Informatics, 14*(1), 1–21.

Rogoski, R. (2003). LIS and the enterprise. *Health Management Technology, 24*(2), 20–23.

Schneider, P. J. (2007). Opportunities for pharmacy. *American Journal of Health-System Pharmacy, 64*(14), S10–S16.

Schneider, R., Bagby, J., & Carlson, R. (2008). Bar-code medication administration: A systems perspective. *American Journal of Health-System Pharmacy, 65*(23), 2216–2219.

Schrage, M. (2007). *Business Finance, 13*(4), 64.

Shugarman, L. R., Nishita, C. M., & Wilber, K. H. (2006). Building integrated information systems for chronic care: The California experience. *Home Health Care Services Quarterly, 25*(3–4), 185–200.

Simon, J. S., Rundall, T. G., & Shortell, S. (2007). Adoption of order entry with decision support for chronic care by physician organizations. *Journal of the American Medical Informatics Association, 14*(4), 432–430.

Smetzer, J., & Navarra, M. B. (2007). Patient safety. Measuring change: A key component of building a culture of safety. *Nursing Economics, 25*(1), 49–51.

Standardize order sets for improved care. (2010). *Health Management Technology, 31*(2), 38–39.

Subramanian, S., Hoover, S., Gilman, B., Field, T., Mutter, R., & Gurwitz, J. (2007, September). Computerized physician order entry with clinical decision support in long-term care facilities: Costs and benefits to stakeholders. *Journal of the American Geriatrics Society, 55*(9), 1451–1457. Retrieved November 19, 2007, from Health Source: Nursing/Academic Edition database.

Sullivan, M. (2010). Improving patient safety with intelligent infusion devices. *American Journal of Health-System Pharmacy, 67*(17), 1415. doi:10.2146/ajhp100316

Turley, J. P. (1993, May). *The use of artificial intelligence in nursing information systems.* Retrieved from http://www.vicnet.net.au/vicnet/hisa/MAY93/MAY93-The.html

Weant, K., Cook, A., & Armistead, J. (2007, March 1). Medication-error reporting and pharmacy resident experience during implementation of computerized prescriber order entry. *American Journal of Health-System Pharmacy, 64*(5), 526–530. Retrieved November 19, 2007, from Health Source: Nursing/Academic Edition database.

Westbrook, J. (2005). Guest editorial: Exploring the interface between organisations and clinical information systems. *Health Information Management Journal, 4*, 102–103.

Yu, P., Qiu, Y., & Crookes, P. (2006). Computer-based nursing documentation in nursing homes: A feasibility study. In H. Park, P. Murray, & C. Delaney (Eds.). *Consumer-centered computer-supported care for healthy people—Proceedings of NI2006*, pp. 570–574.

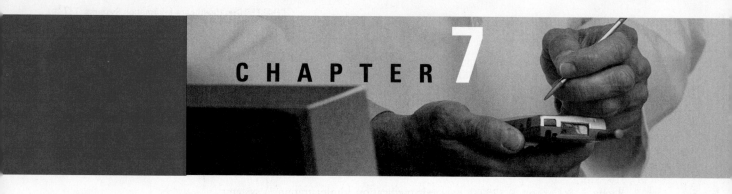

CHAPTER 7

Strategic Planning for Information Technology Projects

After completing this chapter, you should be able to:

1. Define strategic planning.
2. Describe how strategic planning is related to an organization's mission, scope, vision, goals, and objectives.
3. Identify the participants in the strategic planning process.
4. Understand the relationship between strategic planning for information systems and planning for the overall organization.
5. Explain the importance of assessing the internal and external environments during the planning process.
6. Discuss how potential solutions are derived from data analysis.
7. Review the benefits of using a weighted scoring tool when selecting a course of action.
8. Understand the importance of developing a timeline during the implementation phase of strategic planning.
9. List tools or processes that may be used to evaluate the outcome of and provide feedback to the planning process.
10. Discuss the relationship between strategic planning and information technology.

WHAT IS STRATEGIC PLANNING?

Strategic planning is very simply the process of determining what an organization wants to be in the future and planning how it will get there. Strategic planning is a management tool that allows an organization to consciously move toward a desired future while responding to dynamic internal and external environments. It is a process, not a one-time event, that is both creative and interactive. Strategic planning requires that choices be made about your organization's future, which will be driven by your organization's mission and vision, long-term goals, services to be offered, populations to be served, and the resources to be acquired. Strategic planning is the development of a comprehensive long-range plan for guiding the activities and operations of an organization (Brunke 2006; Crane 2007; Kaleba 2006). Zuckerman (2006) indicates that both planners and executives believe that strategic planning practices are effective and provide appropriate focus and direction for their organization. Strategic planning will become even more important as the healthcare reform legislation signed into law by President Obama in 2010 changes the way healthcare providers are paid, populations are insured, and organizations are retooled to become Accountable Care Organizations or Medical Homes.

Strategic planning is different from operational planning, which is generally short term; focuses on annual cycles; and requires the development of yearly objectives, tasks, and plans. The strategic planning process includes defining the corporate vision and mission, specifying achievable goals and objectives, developing strategies, and setting policy guidelines. This entails a determination of what products and services to offer and to what markets. This is particularly important in this time of change when most organizations have more potential markets than available resources or where there is a very competitive market. The organizational strategic plan should guide the planning for all areas within the organization, including information technology. Hospitals and healthcare enterprises face increasing regulatory challenges, pay-for-performance, consumer demands, and technological changes, and have mountains of data to analyze (Kaleba 2006). Typically organizations cut expenses in response to increased financial pressures, sometimes in the areas of personnel development or other areas that stifle creativity and development (Clarke 2006). All of these factors make good strategic planning even more critical for long-term survival.

For many businesses, including healthcare delivery, technology is transforming the strategic landscape and must be factored into the organization's strategic plan. Therefore, there should be an analogous information technology strategic plan that is informed by and aligned with the organization's strategic plan. This creates an environment whereby technology can help support the mission and vision. Moreover, technology facilitates the collection of data that will help administrators determine whether objectives and goals are met (Willging 2007).

Strategic planning is an outcome of strategic thinking. **Strategic thinking** is a broad process that an organization uses to determine what its future should look like. This is referred to as the vision of where the organization would like to find itself in (Willging 2006). Strategic planning provides the focus for how that vision will be achieved. Successful strategic plans require the identification of a single vision and a single mission that fits within that vision with all activities designed to meet the identified mission.

THE MISSION

The **mission** is the purpose or reason for the organization's existence and represents the fundamental and unique aspirations that differentiate the organization from others. The mission is often conveyed in the form of a mission statement that broadly declares what a business aspires to be by telling the organization's personnel and customers "who we are" and "what we do." The mission statement should incorporate meaningful and measurable criteria. The mission statement is an important tool when used to guide the planning process and should resonate with those involved with the organization. The mission statement should be one of the first things considered when evaluating a strategic decision. An example of a mission statement is seen in Box 7–1.

> **BOX 7–1   The Mission of St. Theresa Medical Center**
>
> The mission of St. Theresa Medical Center is the same as the mission of St. Theresa Health System which is:
>
> 1. To establish and maintain a hospital and other healthcare facilities for the care of persons with illnesses or disabilities that require that the patients receive hospital or long-term care, without distinction as to their religious beliefs, race, national origin, age, sex, disability, or economic status.
>
> 2. To carry on any educational activities related to rendering care to the sick and injured or the promotion of health which, in the opinion of the board of directors, may be justified by the facilities, personnel, funds, or other requirements that are or can be made available, including, but not being specifically limited to, the conduction of schools for the education of registered nurses and practical nurses with power to grant diplomas to graduates and residency programs for physicians in training.
>
> 3. To promote and carry on scientific research related to the care of the sick and injured insofar as, in the opinion of the board of directors, such research can be carried on in or in connection with the hospital.
>
> 4. To participate, as far as circumstances may warrant, in any activity designed and carried on to promote the general health of the community.
>
> In working toward the fulfillment of these objectives, as members of the healthcare team, we strive to give generously of our efforts and work harmoniously together for the love of God and of our neighbor. As a result, we find that our own lives and the lives of those with whom we come in contact are being enriched and blessed.
>
> The essence of our mission and philosophy is best depicted in our logo—St. Theresa and the words *healing body, mind,* and *spirit.*

The Scope

The **scope** of an organization's mission defines the type of activities and services it will perform. The scope should be clearly identified in the mission statement so that employees and customers understand which aspects of organizational operation are most important. For example, a broad scope for a healthcare enterprise might be to "provide healthcare." The problem with such a broad scope is that the target client population is not identified, nor are the types of services that will be provided. A narrower scope provides the amount of detail necessary to appropriately guide administrators and managers in decision making. In Box 7–1, the scope of the St. Theresa Medical Center is also seen in the mission statement, which states, "the patients receive hospital or long-term care, without distinction as to their religious beliefs, race, national origin, age, sex, disability or economic status." The medical center's commitment to caring for the indigent population is clearly described in the mission statement. This scope is the basis for the development of certain goals and objectives that guide the decision makers in strategic planning.

The Vision

The vision statement is a future-oriented, lofty view of what an organization would like to become. The vision statement is often the first consideration in strategic planning. St. Theresa Medical Center may craft a vision statement which reads:

St. Theresa Medical Center will strive to:

- Be the hospital of choice for patients, physicians, and employees in our area because of our preeminent patient care and teaching programs.
- Be well recognized as a technology leader in our region.
- Be the academic center of choice for residents and healthcare professionals.
- Be a prominent community member known for meeting the healthcare needs of the entire community through incomparable patient care and wellness programs.

TABLE 7–1 Areas of Potential Strategic Planning	
Goals and Objectives	**Strategy**
Meet federal mandates to increase reimbursement	Perform gap analysis of current data and reporting capabilities needed to meet mandate.
Ensure interoperable IT system to maximize internal and external data sharing	Create interfaces, develop warehouse, enhance reporting capabilities.
Improve organizational efficiency	Redesign work of processes so that tasks can be completed in fewer steps, more easily, and in a more cost-effective method.
Increase customer base	Target new populations within the already-defined geographic area as well as reach out to rural and outlying communities with new programs.
Maximize the use of existing resources	Cross-train workers so that they can perform several tasks.
Improve customer relationships	Create a Web site, or patient portal, that allows patients to find physicians, schedule appointments, e-mail providers, create and maintain a personal health record (PHR), access information on a variety of topics, and complete evaluations of services provided.

Goals and Objectives

Identification of an organization's goals and objectives is a critical factor in fulfilling the mission. The goals and objectives explain how the mission will be realized. A **goal** is an open-ended statement that describes in general terms what is to be accomplished. Examples of goals include maintaining quality client care while promoting cost-effective operations, striving to increase market share by attracting a larger percentage of clients than the competitor's, and broadening the scope of services offered. The ability to achieve defined goals is especially important in the rapidly changing healthcare environment as hospitals merge into large enterprises and services evolve to meet changing needs. Prior to writing goals and objectives, administrators need to communicate the vision and mission to employees in a manner that elicits understanding and buy-in (Willging 2006). Participant buy-in is critical to the success of the plan.

Objectives state how and when an organization will meet its goals. Some of the primary areas that goals and objectives may address are listed in Table 7–1. For example, objectives that support the goal of broadening the scope of services offered may include the following:

- *Development of clinics that support and promote wellness services.* Traditionally, clinics provide treatments for various medical problems. Expansion of these services to support wellness maintenance may attract a larger market share. Some additional services that may be offered are mammography, blood pressure, and cholesterol screening.
- *Creation of patient centered medical homes.* These services will expand comprehensive primary care by facilitating partnerships between individual patients, families, and providers to increase access, satisfaction, and safety while improving outcomes.

DEVELOPING STRATEGIES FOR SUCCESS

An organization's strategy is a comprehensive plan that states how its mission, goals, and objectives will be achieved (Breene, Nunes, & Shill 2007; Kaleba 2006; Willging 2006). An examination of the mission and goals will help to define the steps that are necessary to attain them. A clear understanding of the end point is critical to the effective development of the plan. It is also important to review current strengths, weaknesses, opportunities, and threats also called as SWOT analysis. This includes the presence of competition. The strategic position for the organization can be determined by its reputation for quality of service and innovation, its access, the scope of services provided, and the demographics of the population served. An analysis of the current position of the organization in relation to these factors will help to determine available options. It is then possible for management to select major initiatives to achieve their vision for the organization in light of available resources. Expediting the achievement of the mission and goals is the primary purpose of a strategic plan. It must be recognized, however, that strategy development is an ongoing task.

Strategic planning is led by members of the organization's upper management, including the board of directors and chief executive officer (CEO), who is ultimately responsible for the organization's strategic management (Breene et al. 2007; Strategy officers 2007). Day-to-day responsibilities faced by CEOs often prohibit them from managing the incremental progress of the strategic plan, giving rise to the emergence of the role of chief strategy officer (CSO). The CSO must clarify the vision created by the CEO and leadership team for his or her own benefit and for all managers and employees. It is then up to the CSO to drive change and monitor the timelines and progress toward realization of the strategic plan. CSOs may also face the potential challenge of conflict with the chief financial officer (CFO). Typically there is no clear career path or title for the CSOs although they share a wide skill set and prior experience in planning. Many organizations choose to bring in a dedicated project leader or manager instead, particularly when there is no margin for error, success is critical, and time constraints exist (Clark 2006; Kodjababian & Petty 2007). Dedicated project leaders generally have extensive experience working in multiple settings and are characterized by their ability to:

- Motivate a diverse group of staff to follow them
- Build consensus on important decisions
- Identify issues that must be dealt with by their team immediately to keep the project on track
- Anticipate and resolve interpersonal conflicts that can derail the best-managed projects
- Communicate progress to key executives
- Identify and manage project and business risks.

The next level of management, those who report to the CEO, such as vice presidents, are also major participants in strategic planning. They should include the chief information officer (CIO), the chief medical informatics officer (CMIO), and/or the chief nursing informatics officer (CNIO). The CIO is generally the senior team member, guiding technology acquisition, while the CMIO and CNIO guide the acquisition and use of information technology for those large groups of providers. A detailed description of the CNIO role is found later in this chapter. The CIO must ensure that executives understand the role that information technology plays in the organization as well as how information technology can be used to advance the goals of the organization, while the CMIO and CNIO ensure the effective and efficient use at the point of care. There must be a strong link between the organization's strategic plan and the information technology plan (Glaser 2006). It is the CIO's responsibility to see that upper management sees information technology as a tool to achieve organizational goals rather than just another cost center.

This involvement will help to provide direction for all information technology initiatives, establish priorities, eliminate the duplication of information systems, and ensure the wise use of information technology resources. Other lower-level managers within the organization, such as department heads, are responsible for supporting the planning process by providing information related to the current operations as well as insight into future needs of the organization. This information enables the planning team to balance the present reality against the future vision and goals. Changing economics, resources, and markets make planning more difficult, but a well-crafted strategic plan makes provisions for these changes as well as for the expenditure of time, money, and resources to carry out the plan. Consumer demands represent a major driver in the current market, forcing providers to analyze the actual costs for every service rendered, prepare for the scrutiny of comparison shopping, develop competitive prices, make prices and payment options available to consumers, and restructure billing statements for increased clarity (Bauer & Hagland 2006). These changes require extensive input from administrators, clinicians, and information services personnel.

STAKEHOLDERS

A stakeholder is defined as any group or individual who can affect or is affected by the achievements of the organization's objectives. The work of strategic planning cannot be limited to the board room and to executives who release copies of plans that seem to have little to do with everyday work. Today, organizations realize that their success comes largely from planning that is inclusive of the collaborative input of those directly and indirectly impacted by their services. The stakeholders are those internal or external individual customers, organizations, community members, and governing bodies that have a direct or indirect stake in the organization mission, scope, and goals. Stakeholders should be involved in strategic planning and all subsequent activities to reach goals through direct involvement, survey, or focus group in order to ensure responsiveness and relevancy of the plan.

STRATEGIC PLANNING FOR INFORMATION SYSTEMS

Although the broader scope of strategic planning concerns all areas of the healthcare institution, one important component is the plan for information systems. Without a plan that points information systems in the right direction and helps the organization use information systems to execute its business strategies, the organization will not be able to effectively meet its overall goals (Glaser 2006). The overall strategic plan used to guide an organization must have an analogous information technology strategic plan to support goals and objectives.

The strategic planning process is often initiated by other changes that are taking place within the organization. For example, suppose a healthcare enterprise plans to purchase a client monitoring system to be used throughout its facilities. Other organizational changes—such as plans for construction and unit relocation, and infrastructure upgrades, including computer wiring and cabling and updating the client care information systems in general—may have initiated the plans for obtaining the monitoring system. Once administrators realize the need for strategic planning for the monitoring system, they must identify the goals of the plan. These goals should be developed in accordance with the mission and goals of the organization.

External factors may also impact planning. In 2009, the $787 billion American Recovery and Reinvestment Act (ARRA) included $19.2 billion to increase the use of the electronic health record (EHR) by providers and hospitals through the Health Information Technology for Economic and Clinical Health Act (HITECH) through Medicare and Medicaid incentives. This has spurred tremendous energy toward the implementation of these information systems requiring extensive planning and rework of many healthcare organizations and their strategic plans.

Some of the goals of information systems strategic planning are discussed next. Each goal is followed by a brief explanation of how it applies to the previously described example of selecting a new client monitoring system.

- *To support business and clinical decisions.* Data management supports better decision making by providing timely and accurate information. In the example of planning for a new client monitoring system, a driving force behind these plans is the need to provide healthcare providers with accurate and complete data regarding the client's condition.

- *To make effective use of emerging technologies.* New technologies can create administrative efficiencies and attract providers and clients. A perfect example of this can be seen with the use of PDAs and other wireless devices to collect, view, and transmit patient information from the point of care. The Internet and e-health represent other developments that change the access to and delivery of healthcare because patient results can be made available online from any location, patients can become more connected to their healthcare, patient questions can be addressed, and decision making can be informed. These developments must be included in the strategic planning process as they can reconceptualize healthcare away from a known system to an unknown process.
- *To enhance the organization's image.* The effective use of information technologies enhances how the organization is perceived by providers, clients, the community, and other external groups. This is especially critical in these times of competitive healthcare. For example, achieving state-of-the-art technology for cardiac monitoring will provide efficient and effective client care. Patients are often looking for this latest technology when making healthcare choices.
- *To promote satisfaction of market and regulatory requirements.* Effective information systems strategic planning must include those issues related to meeting market and regulatory requirements, such as e-health, payer requirements, the Joint Commission guidelines, the National Quality Forum (NQF), client confidentiality, and data security. For example, when selecting a monitoring system, it is also important to determine that the system complies with safety regulations such as protection against damage from defibrillation.
- *To be cost-effective.* Cost-effectiveness is achieved when redundancies are eliminated. In the monitoring system example, this advantage is evident. If all of the critical care and monitored bed areas in the enterprise use the same monitoring system, training is cost-effective, because nurses need be trained on only one system to work in any monitored area of the hospital. Other cost benefits are seen in the need to maintain only one type of backup monitor for replacement of nonoperational equipment, as well as increased efficiency for the biomedical technicians who must maintain the monitoring equipment.
- *To provide a safer environment for patients.* There is strong initiative for patient safety at this time. A number of organizations, including government agencies, regulatory bodies, consumer groups, and professional organizations, are looking into ways to improve patient safety.

THE STRATEGIC PLANNING PROCESS

First there must be the realization that change is needed (Glaser 2006). This may be internally or externally driven. Then it is necessary to survey the changing internal environments of the organization with the goal to determine how each change affects the other. Each department in the organization should have its own long-range plan that fits within the larger organizational plan, and most departments within the organization are dependent on the management of information systems. As a result, each department comes to the information services department with its own requirements related to strategic planning. The IT strategic plan must support and enable the organization's goals. It is the responsibility of the CIO and information systems department to prioritize and merge these ideas together, helping to develop a master strategic plan for the organization. This task is complicated by the rapidly changing nature of information technology, consumer demands, and clinician expectations for information availability at the bedside whether that occurs via PDAs, BlackBerries, iPods, iPads, tablet computers, or other devices. The fast pace of evolving technology requires periodic review and revisions of both the organization's strategic plan and the information systems department's strategic plan.

The Role of Project Management

The CIO is ultimately responsible for information systems (IS) strategic planning. The need to create administrative efficiencies through e-commerce, mergers and acquisitions, and requests for outcomes reporting forces CIOs to look at ways that information technology can be used to achieve strategic and operational changes (Glaser 2006). The CIO generally selects a project manager or leader for each major project within the overall strategic plan if the organization does not have a dedicated project management office (PMO), which oversees all new projects.

Project management is a set of practices that, if executed well, will raise the likelihood that a project will succeed. Project management practices entail:

- Understanding the internal and external drivers of change
- Overseeing a detailed analysis and feasibility review
- Defining the scope of the project
- Determining the outcomes to be achieved
- Identifying the tasks within the project, when they must occur and any interdependencies
- Obtaining and organizing the human resources
- Defining who will be responsible for each task
- Establishing timelines for task and project completion
- Establishing how project decisions will be made
- Ensuring that stakeholders receive appropriate communication about the status of the project

The project manager may help to develop an advisory board or a strategic planning team. The strategic planning team is generally composed of top-level managers who devise the plan and present it to the CIO, who in turn presents it to the board of directors. One particularly important aspect of this process is the ability to prioritize all projects, particularly for next 2 to 5 years. This requires estimating benefits, resources, costs, and timelines for each and then reevaluating the priority of each as new developments come into play. Some developments that affect information technology in healthcare include legislation that involves patient privacy and billing as well as initiatives calling for the implementation of barcoding for medication administration, computerized physician order entry, a computerized patient record, concerns over bioterrorism, an emphasis upon customer relationship management, and consumer-driven demands (Bauer & Hagland 2006; Briggs 2003; Langer 2003; Magliore 2003; Young 2007). These developments impact information technology budgets. The IT plan should also include applications and systems that are under consideration, needed infrastructure changes, and any additional resources in the way of additional equipment, staff, or training.

Another level of strategic planning is performed by members of the project implementation team, which reports to the advisory board. This team is composed of representatives from the user departments, including managers and front-line employees who are most familiar with the activities of the department. The project implementation team looks at current workflows, designs the needed system, and implements the system changes. The project team needs the active involvement of end users to succeed. This is particularly true when nursing staff and other clinicians are ambiguous about change (Gillespie 2002). Stakeholders need to know the potential contributions as well as the limitations of new technology (Glaser 2006). Frequent communication between the advisory board and the implementation team is imperative for the ongoing success of the strategic plan. This plan generally addresses a time frame covering between 3 and 5 years into the future.

Strategic Planning Steps

Identification of Goals and Scope Once the strategic planning teams have been identified, the actual planning process can begin. Identifying the goals and scope is the second step in strategic planning. The goals of the project must meet the needs of the users as well as support the mission and goals of the institution. The identified goals will then provide the direction for the remainder of the planning process. The scope of the project is developed after initial analysis has been completed and provides a detailed description of the project, which includes what is in and what is out of the scope. In other words, it provides the boundaries around what can become a limitless project.

In the example of selecting a cardiac monitoring system for a healthcare enterprise, the goals and scope of the project might be to implement a one-vendor solution with integration to the clinical documentation system within the critical care areas only adding the emergency department in during a subsequent phase. This should result in the selection of a single system with the capability of direct interface of data into the documentation system that will meet the needs of the designated units in the organization. However, decisions should be made with input from key users and in collaboration with the enterprise technology group. Wagner and Piccoli (2007) indicate that to ensure implementation success, project teams must think creatively about how to foster end user active participation in development, going live, and maintenance activities. Good communication between information systems personnel and clinicians is critical to the success of any project. It is essential to elicit support from nurses and physicians in the selection of any system that they will use and to listen to their feedback (Gillespie 2002; Glaser 2006; Schuerenberg 2003). Nurses are resistant to change unless they see the potential benefits. Physicians will not use a system if it is not easy to access and use. More and more, that translates to the ability to access information at the bedside, office, or from home or other locations using a variety of devices, including traditional computers, PDAs, and other devices. No system should hinder clinical staff.

Scanning the External and Internal Environments The next step in the planning process is to **scan**, or gather information from, the external and internal environments. The **external environment** includes those interested parties and competitors who are outside of the healthcare institution, such as vendors, payers, competitors, clients, the community, and regulatory agencies. The **internal environment** includes employees of the institution, as well as physicians and members of the board of directors. The purpose of scanning the environment is twofold: to define the current situation and to identify areas of need. This step should also include surveying the changing internal environments of the organization with the goal to determine how each change affects the other.

Environment scanning is best accomplished by developing a detailed plan for collecting pertinent data. This step is often called the *needs assessment*. Information related to current trends in both healthcare and information technology should also be collected. Data may be collected from a variety of sources, including the following (McCormack 1996).

External Environment Scanning

- Published literature and reports
- Information from vendors
- Organizations such as HIMSS or KLAS
- Regulatory and accreditation requirements
- Information related to market trends

Internal Environment Scanning

- Interviews and questionnaires from managers and end users
- Observations of current technology and operations, as well as anticipated technological developments

When selecting a monitoring system, information regarding the technologies that are currently available may be obtained from vendors. All pertinent regulatory and accreditation requirements must also be investigated. A scan of the internal environment may include an inventory of equipment currently in use throughout the enterprise. Insufficient data comprises one of the pitfalls of strategic planning (Clark & Krentz 2006).

Data Analysis After data have been collected during the internal and external environmental scans, the project implementation team must perform analysis, identifying trends in the current operations as well as future needs and expectations, and determine feasibility from technical, financial, time, and resource perspectives. Current trends in healthcare should be identified when considering future needs and may be related to topics such as consumer-driven healthcare, managed care, and other financial healthcare coverage and reimbursement considerations. Some trends to consider include the merging of hospitals into large enterprises and the growing focus on care outside of the acute hospital setting, which has resulted in an increased number of services related to wellness promotion and home care. Information technology trends such as e-health, the Internet, telemedicine, client/server technologies, and the computerized client record must also be addressed.

In selecting a universal cardiac monitoring system, the features of each vendor's system, including the desirable and undesirable features of each, must be evaluated. For example, strengths may include an easy learning curve, vendor support, integration capability, transport monitor capabilities, and screen visibility. Weaknesses may include a large number of screens for each function, busy or hard-to-read screens, slow speed of initial data entry, and unsuitable cabling requirements.

Identification of Potential Solutions The next step in the planning process involves the identification of potential solutions, which may be in the form of system upgrades or replacements. At this point, the strategic planning team should be aware of the information system needs of the end users.

When identifying potential solutions, healthcare organizations must address many issues, including the following:

- *Hospitals with differing information systems may be merged together into one enterprise.* In this situation, either each organization continues to use its previous system or one system is chosen for use throughout the enterprise as a means to build a cohesive information systems strategy. Several factors influence the decision to retain or adopt an information system, including costs associated with the purchase and use of software and hardware; site licenses, consulting fees, contract negotiation, maintenance and support agreements, expenses associated with training personnel to use a new system, and the availability of support staff.
- *Many hospitals use mainframe* **legacy systems**, *older vendor-based systems that have often been highly individualized to meet customer specifications.* As it is necessary to upgrade or replace these systems, CEOs and CIOs must weigh the advantages and disadvantages of alternatives that may better meet the needs of the organization. These might include retaining current systems, providing a new look and easier access to legacy software via a Web interface, new versions of vendor software, client/server or thin client technologies, outsourcing services, or using an application service provider (ASP). Box 7–2 lists several information technology considerations related to strategic planning. Box 7–3 identifies pros and cons associated with the outsourcing of services.

Selecting a Course of Action Once all of the potential solutions have been identified, they must be analyzed and compared. If the organization decides to purchase a vendor built system, then a request for proposal (RFP) is developed that incorporates the detailed list of end user requirements. Vendors are then asked to reply and to identify their ability to meet the specific

BOX 7–2 Information Technology Considerations for Strategic Planning

- Does the system use open architecture?
- Is the system based on personal computer, client/server, thin client, or Internet technology?
- Does it support the use of PDAs, iPods, iPads, tablets, and other devices to retrieve data?
- Does it follow human–computer interaction design standards?
- Does the software comply with HL7 standards for interfaces?
- Does the database incorporate SNOMED, LOINC, and other terminology standards?
- Does the system sufficiently safeguard individual patient data from unauthorized users?
- Does the system allow the user to query aggregate data and produce online reports?
- Does it support performance measurement?
- Does it support a customized view or the ability to customize functions?
- Can it support expansion of features, increased numbers of users, and/or records?
- Does it allow the use of evolving technologies, such as smart cards, optical disks, interface engines, wireless technology, integrated services digital network (ISDN) communication, e-health or e-commerce, video conferencing, telemedicine, and fiberoptic networks?
- Does it support a paperless environment?
- How much will it cost for purchase, installation, training, and ongoing support?
- Have criteria been developed to measure successful implementation?

BOX 7–3 Pros and Cons Associated with the Outsourcing of Services

Pros

- Allows the organization to focus on its core competencies
- Can shorten the timeframe to implement new applications or technology
- Better compliance with project implementation dates
- Easier to budget and manage because costs for development and implementation are shifted to the outsourcing agency
- May improve customer satisfaction because services can be delivered at the same or at a higher level as in-house services but at a lower cost
- Provides leading-edge technical skills when skilled labor resources are not available in-house
- Contract negotiations aid definition of project scope

Cons

- Limited control over data security and confidentiality
- Lack of control over application maintenance and downtime
- Insufficient advance notice of downtime
- Lack of control over when updates are implemented
- Customization may not be available
- Promises may exceed ability to deliver
- Costs can be much higher than anticipated
- Identification and resolution of system problems may be delayed
- Ability to change outsourcing services may be limited

identified current and future end user requirements using a scale—perhaps on a 0 to 5 scale—that represents the functions currently present and in use in the system up to and including an acknowledgment of those functions which will not be developed in the near future. The organization then can create weighing criteria that take into account importance to organization process. For example, essential features may be given a weight factor of 5, and desirable but not essential features may be given a weight factor of 3. Weighing of each desirable system feature should be completed before the various systems are scored.

Implementation   The next phase in the strategic planning process is implementation of the chosen solution. The first step in the implementation process is to identify the working committee for the implementation phase. Development of a timeline is one of the initial tasks the committee will perform. Once all of the individual components of the timeline have been identified, the tasks can be assigned and initiated. Other tasks during this phase include budgeting, procedure development, and execution of the plan.

When implementing a universal cardiac monitoring system, the working committee may include representatives from the IS, purchasing, and staff development departments, as well as physicians and nurse managers. This group would first develop a timeline, prioritizing the order in which units would begin using the system. They would also be active in developing a procedure and a plan for educating staff in the use of the new equipment. Box 7–4 lists some measures to ensure a successful experience when services are outsourced.

Ongoing Evaluation and Feedback   Strategic planning is an ongoing process (Glaser 2006). Frequent evaluation of the current processes as well as the current and future needs must be performed. These plans need to be monitored continually and updated annually due

---

BOX 7–4   Measures to Ensure a Positive Outsourcing Experience

- Define information technology functions for possible outsourcing
- Research vendor availability and capabilities
- Establish outsourcing goals and objectives
- Select the vendor that meets the requirements
- Negotiate a contract that outlines the following:
  - Term of contract and provisions for termination and renewal
  - Management of the relationship
  - Vendor and client responsibilities
  - Liabilities
  - Warranties
  - Ownership issues regarding assets/intellectual property
  - Fee structure
  - The process for staff assignment
  - Performance measures
  - Resources key to success
  - Security safeguards
  - Back-up and disaster recovery measures
  - Service level agreements inclusive of availability, response times, service quality
- Develop and use oversight procedures
- Insure against losses related to poor work

to the rapidly changing healthcare environment. In this way, the organization is able to remain current with changing technology, regulatory requirements, reporting needs, and healthcare trends. The process of identifying evaluation tools can be difficult. Measures must be adjusted to environmental changes and competitor actions as a means to help ensure success of strategic plans. One particular type of measure is benchmarking.

Benchmarking is the continual process of measuring services and practices against the toughest competitors in the healthcare industry. An example of benchmarking is to compare the number of IS staff required to support the clinical applications for the enterprise to that of other healthcare providers with similar demographic and volume statistics. When needs are no longer met, or the organization falls far below the benchmark, the process of identifying potential solutions and selecting the best option is begun again. Clinical examples of benchmarks might include the organization's cost for open heart surgery or length of stay. Benchmarking has become widespread throughout the healthcare industry.

THE ROLE OF THE CHIEF NURSING INFORMATICS OFFICER

A few words about this relatively new role are needed. The role of the CNIO was mentioned as a key decision maker in the strategic planning process as well as the aligned information technology strategic planning activity. One of the newest and fastest-growing roles to emerge in recent years is that of the CNIO modeled on the CMIO role. What is a CNIO? The CNIO is the most senior informatics executive who functions as a bridge between nursing and the Information Technology (IT) department through critical relationships with the CIO, the CNO, and the CMIO. Depending on the needs and structure of an organization, the CNIO position may be one that is horizontal to the CNO and the CIO. In other organizations, the CNIO position has a dotted line linkage to the CNO or the CIO (Swindle & Bradley 2010).

The key responsibility of CNIOs is to capitalize on their nursing informatics knowledge and skills which encompass an understanding of computer, information, and nursing sciences, in order to lead strategically and operationally. The CNIO is focused on the design, selection, and implementation of health information systems and for managing the adoption of other supporting clinical initiatives (Swindle & Bradley 2010). This role will be one to watch as it matures over the next 10 years.

FUTURE DIRECTIONS

Strategic planning is an example of a process which has resurged in importance. In the 1970s, strategic planning was universal and mandated by Public Law 93-641, the National Health Planning and Resources Act of 1974. The act stipulated that any hospital desiring to make an investment in new technology had to have a plan that indicated how the investment met goals set forth in public policy by reducing cost, improving quality, or increasing access since the infusion of funds via Medicare and Medicaid in 1965 was seen as a conduit for investment and spending if not constrained by plans (Bauer 2005). In 1983, mandatory strategic planning was abandoned with the repeal of Public Law 93-641 under then President Reagan who favored deregulation as a policy to fight rising healthcare costs. Now in this current decade, with healthcare reform legislatively mandated, there is a great need for both strategic planning to achieve organization and population healthcare goals of accountable organizations and patient centered care and for information technology strategic planning to accomplish the Meaningful Use of systems. For the next few years, organizations will be focusing on increasing the infiltration of health information technology within the infrastructure. Organizations will be engaged in the implementation of the electronic health records, bar code medication administration, clinical documentation systems, data structures to participate in regional health information exchanges, and in the development of customer portals, patient health records, and other customer directed initiatives. Strategic planning for hospitals must address these needs.

CASE STUDY EXERCISE

You are a nurse manager in a hospital that has recently merged with two other hospitals, forming a large healthcare enterprise. Each of the three hospitals currently uses a different clinical information system. You are a member of the strategic planning committee, which is charged with the task of selecting which of the three systems will be used throughout the enterprise. Describe the process you would use to scan the internal and external environments, as well as the types of data you would collect.

SUMMARY

- Strategic planning is the development of a comprehensive long-range plan for guiding the activities and operations of an organization.
- Strategic planning is one of the most important factors in the selection, design, and implementation of information systems, because it can save valuable resources over time and ensure that the needs of the enterprise are met even as changes in reimbursement take effect.
- The strategic plan should support the mission, scope, vision, goals, and objectives of the organization.
- The mission is the purpose for the organization's existence and represents its unique aspects.
- Strategic planning is guided by upper-level administrators, including the CIO and CSO, but requires participation from other levels of management including the CMIO and/or the CNIO.
- Strategic planning involves the following steps: identification of the need for change, definition of goals and scope, scanning of external and internal environments, data analysis, identification of potential solutions, selection of a course of action, implementation, evaluation, and feedback.
- Project management is a process that can improve the likelihood of project success.
- Passage of the ARRA and the HITECH Act provides financial incentives for the adoption of health information technology.
- The CNIO should be a key decision maker in the strategic planning process.
- Strategic planning is an ongoing process.

REFERENCES

Bauer, J. C. (2005). Strategic planning and information technology: Back to the future all over again. *Journal of Healthcare Information Management, 19*(3), 9–11.

Bauer, J. C., & Hagland, M. (2006, July). Consumer-directed healthcare: What to expect and what to do. *Health Financial Management, 60*(7), 76–78, 80, 82.

Breene, R. T. S., Nunes, P. F., & Shill, W. E. (2007). The chief strategy officer. *Harvard Business Review, 85*(10), 84–93.

Briggs, B. (2003). Choose your battles wisely. *Health Data Management, 11*(4), 27–34.

Brunke, L. (2006). On reflection: Developing a strategic plan. *Nursing BC, 38*(2), 37.

Clark, C. S., & Krentz, S. E. (2006, November). Avoiding the pitfalls of strategic planning. *Healthcare Financial Management*. Retrieved December 1, 2007, from CINAHL with Full Text database.

Clark, F. C. (2006). IT homecoming. *ADVANCE for Health Information Executives, 10*(9), 47–48, 50–51.

Clarke, R. L. (2006). Managing the storm. *Healthcare Financial Management, 60*(7), 152.

Crane, A. (2007). The new era CFO. *Hospitals & Health Networks, 81*(6), 38–42.

Gillespie, G. (2002). IT a tough sell for nursing staff. *Health Data Management, 10*(4), 56–59.

Glaser, J. (2006, February). Wired for success. *Health Financial Management, 60*(2), 67–74.

Kaleba, R. (2006). Strategic planning getting from here to there. *Healthcare Financial Management, 60*(11), 74–78. Retrieved December 1, 2007, from CINAHL with Full Text database.

Kodjababian, J., & Petty, J. (2007). Dedicated project leadership helping organizations meet strategic goals. *Healthcare Financial Management, 61*(11), 130–134.

Langer, J. (2003). Prioritizing IT projects. *Healthcare Informatics, 20*(6), 110.

Magliore, M. (2003). Preparing business for biochemical attacks. *Contingency Planning and Management, 8*(4), 48–50.

McCormack, J. (1996). Strategic planning in changing times. *Health Data Management, 4*(12), 6–16.

Schuerenberg, B. (2003). Docs respond to group therapy. *Health Data Management, 11*(1), 34–38.

Strategy officers create new challenges for CFOs. (2007). *Financial Executive, 23*(9), 11.

Swindle, C. G., & Bradley, V. M. (2010). The newest O in the c-suite: CNIO. *Nurse Leader, 8*(3), 28–30.

Wagner, E. L., & Piccoli, G. (2007). Moving beyond user participation to achieve successful IS design. *Communications of the ACM, 50*(12), 51–55.

Willging, P. (2006). You can't get there without a road map. *Nursing Homes: Long Term Care Management, 55*(11), 14, 16–17.

Willging, P. (2007). Paul Willging says . . . You've got to construct your strategic plan. *Nursing Homes: Long Term Care Management, 56*(1), 18.

Young, T. (2007, October). Hospital CRM: Unexplored frontier of revenue growth? *Healthcare Financial Management, 61*(10), 86–90.

Zuckerman, A. M. (2006). Advancing the state of the art in healthcare strategic planning. *Frontiers in Health Services Management, 23*(2), 3–16.

CHAPTER 8

Selecting a Healthcare Information System

After completing this chapter, you should be able to:

1. Define the term *life cycle* as it relates to information systems.

2. List the phases of the life cycle of an information system.

3. Recognize the purpose of the needs assessment.

4. Identify the typical membership composition of the system selection steering committee.

5. Explain the importance of using the mission statement in determining the organization's information needs.

6. Identify several methods for analyzing the current system.

7. Discuss the value of using a weighted scoring tool during the selection phase.

8. Review the system criteria that should be addressed during the selection process.

9. Describe the request for information and request for proposal (RFP) documents.

10. Evaluate RFP responses from vendors.

11. Formulate a list of contract demands for a vendor once a system has been chosen.

At this writing healthcare information technology (IT) has risen to the top of national political agenda. With the signing into law of the American Recovery and Reinvestment Act (ARRA) on February 17, 2009, a portion of the law created the Health Information Technology for Economic and Clinical Health (HITECH) Act. The HITECH Act provided stimulus money to increase the use of electronic health records across the country in what many felt were aggressive timelines. The term "**Meaningful Use**" was created by both the Health Information Technology Policy and Standards Committees to determine how organizations would receive reimbursement for their implementation (Boyd, Funk, Schwartz, Kaplan, & Keenan 2010; Klein 2010). While debate continues on the details of the definition of "Meaningful Use," organizations have moved forward with plans to evaluate new systems and work with existing vendors to identify required enhancements. Strategic plans and business drivers should be used over the goal of getting stimulus money. "There needs to be an expectation that the organization will be different after implementation of advanced clinical systems, and both the clinical and business leadership of the organization need to be in agreement that this undertaking will affect every person in the health system"(Hoehn 2010, p. 11). For these reasons the selection and implementation processes are critical. Many options are available today, adding to the complexity of the task. No "right" solution exists for all facilities. The best starting point when considering the purchase or development of information technology is the organization's strategic plan, given that it sets goals and determines technology needs. From this point the selection and implementation of an information system occur through a well-defined process known as the **life cycle**. This term describes the ongoing process of developing and maintaining an information system. This cycle can be divided into four main phases that cover the life span of information systems. These four phases are:

Needs assessment

1. System selection
2. Implementation
3. Maintenance

Figure 8–1 illustrates the relationship of these phases as circular, because needs assessment and evaluation are ongoing processes. As needs change, the organization may find it necessary to upgrade information systems periodically. The first two phases, needs assessment and system selection, are discussed in this chapter. Details regarding system implementation and maintenance are covered in Chapter 9. It is essential to develop a timeline that delineates the major events or milestones when working through the various phases of the information system's life cycle. For example, while it is desirable to complete the needs assessment and selection processes in less than 1 year, it is necessary to recognize that the process may take 1 year to complete. Therefore, it is vital to organize responsibilities around a realistic timeframe. Figure 8–2 provides a template that may be used to develop a timeline or Gantt chart for the needs assessment and system selection phases of the information system's life cycle.

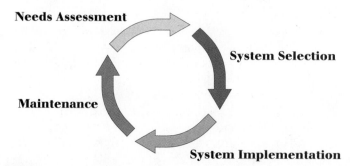

FIGURE 8–1 • The life cycle of an information system

Milestone	Person Responsible	Estimated Start Date	Completion Date
PHASE 1: NEEDS ASSESSMENT			
Develop steering committee			
Perform organizational needs assessment			
Identify system requirements and weighting of criteria			
Technical			
Administrative/general			
Registration			
Order entry/cope/results reporting			
Documentation/billing			
Medical records/printing			
Accounting			
Scheduling			
Reporting capabilities			
Inpatient vs. MD practice Specialty areas: ED, OB, Oncology, Cardiology, Anesthesia			
PHASE 2: SYSTEM SELECTION			
Develop the RFP			
Organization description			
System requirements			
Response evaluation procedures			
Evaluate RFP responses			
Conduct site visits			
Select the system for purchase			
Contract negotiations and contract signed			

FIGURE 8–2 • Sample template for developing a timeline or Gantt chart

NEEDS ASSESSMENT

Needs assessment is the first phase in the information life cycle (Costa & Marrone 2007; Jusinski 2007; Klein 2010; Teague 2007). The purpose of the needs assessment is to determine the gap between an organization's current state and the overall needs of the organization with consideration to the strategic plan. The process is usually initiated by a person or group with a vision of the future. Evaluation of the strengths and weaknesses of the organization related to efficiency, quality, and financial strengths should be considered. Understanding an organization's current state workflow process as well as long-term goals related to efficiency, quality, and financial outcomes by creating a gap analysis can assist the decision-making group. Long-term goals in today's environment include the patient needs within a clinical setting, getting feedback from patients to evaluate how they may use technology to connect with medical personnel for their healthcare needs. Use of systems for patients to self-schedule, entering data into daily logs for chronic illness, and Internet-enabled communication to their healthcare team are cogent considerations.

After the initial evaluation of the overall organization, it is appropriate to look at segments within an organization. A deficit in the current method of manual or automated information handling is often recognized by people from several different groups or disciplines, such as clinical and administrative personnel who use the information, as well as programmers and other technical staff who manage the information system. Once the deficit or need is realized, a more detailed understanding of the issues must be developed.

After the selection committee discusses the current deficits and needs, they brainstorm to generate a list of possible directions for action. These actions may include minor modifications to the current manual or automated system, major enhancements to the current system, or the purchase of a new automated information system. A preliminary scope document can be developed to list the overall goals and plan for the organization.

The analysis of identified possible actions and the decision-making process must be a collaborative effort, and is often performed by a committee that includes clinical users, information systems specialists, and administration or executive board representatives. In the age of patient-family–centered care it may be appropriate to have a board member who is also a voice for patients.

The Steering Committee

The steering committee is an essential component of the assessment and selection processes. Its membership should include board members to ensure that information technology is aligned with the organization's overall strategy (Marshall & Heffes 2007). Too often a disconnect exists between the expressed importance that board members assign to IT and budget allocations and actual IT applications. A general understanding of the capabilities of software and how electronic processes can impact business goals is imperative to the success of decision making within this group. Steering committee leadership may affect the success or failure of the project. The committee chairperson may be a manager, director of information services, or an informaticist, or have an administrative position elsewhere in the hospital, such as chief financial officer (CFO), chief nursing officer (CNO), or medical director. The committee membership must be multidisciplinary, including representation from all departments affected by the new system and incorporating the clinical, administrative, and information system divisions. This strategy is essential for identification of all pertinent issues and reduces the possibility of overlooking potential problems. In those healthcare organizations that include affiliations with other facilities, it is imperative that representation from these areas be included to address any additional needs. A general rule to follow is that any department or area that uses the information or is affected by it must have a voice in the selection process. Representation of the voice of the patient should be considered during the evaluative and/or decision-making process.

The structure of the steering committee must be defined early in the process. When designing the committee, it is important to consider the appropriate size of the group. The committee should be large enough to make a good decision but small enough to be effective and efficient. At this point, it is necessary to define who has the authority to make the final decisions. For example, decision-making power may be given to a particular department, shared among a group of administrators from various departments, or shared equally among all members of the steering committee.

One strategy that is effective in larger organizations is to develop a multilevel committee. The upper level or executive board of the committee is responsible for the final decisions regarding selection. This may be a small group of high-level executive chief officers, such as the chief executive officer(CEO), chief information officer(CIO), privacy officer, vice presidents responsible for major departments, medical staff leadership, or an informatics nurse specialist. This subcommittee is supported by a larger group of department managers and supervisors. Few guidelines exist for the selection of users to serve on the committee, but it should include some frontline employees who will actually be using the system (Jusinski 2007; Saleem, Jones, Van Tran, & Moses 2006). These are the people who will be responsible for doing most of the groundwork and investigation during the assessment and selection processes. There should also be representation from information services, risk management, patient registration, and financial services to ensure that related issues are addressed. Selected committee members must be able to devote the necessary time and energy to the project. Their managers must be willing to provide them with time away from their normal responsibilities and support their involvement in the project. This requirement can be difficult to meet given that the shortage of experienced nurses reduces time available to participate in the selection process (CDW Healthcare 2007). The CDW Healthcare second annual study of more than 1,000 nurses found that the involvement of an informatics nurse and nurses in information technology decisions can accelerate IT integration. In general an effective strategy is to assign tasks to individual members or subgroups based on their expertise and knowledge. Their findings are then presented to the larger committee for discussion and approval. The lack of guidelines for users to serve on the committee may result in a less than optimal membership. Front-end users should demonstrate functional expertise, good communication, and ideally a computing background.

Consultants Consultants may be hired for assistance in any phase of the selection process, including recommendations for the composition of the steering and selection committee, assessing the current information system, system planning, testing, security, policy and procedure development, and implementation (Hoch 2006; The future is now 2007). The effective use of consultants requires clear definition of the contractual relationship and expected outcomes, as well as good communication throughout the association. The consultant should be provided with all available data regarding the current system and identified needs. The consultant's role is to analyze this information and make recommendations for action. Box 8–1 lists some of the primary qualities of an effective consultant or consulting service. On occasion, problems arise with the use of consultants, including limited experience, and adequate knowledge of the needs of hardware and software applications under consideration. Also, there may be a lack of incentive to work toward the most useful and cost-effective solution, and failure to keep promises made to clients. A good consultant always acts in the best interest of the client (Czerniawska 2006).

Developing a Common Vision The needs assessment committee should start the process by examining the vision and mission statements of the organization as well as the strategic plan (Klein 2010; Wickham, Miedema, Gamerdinger, & DeGooyer 2006). This will guide the committee in looking to the future and determining the organization's information needs while continuing to support the mission. From this, goals should be developed to guide the work of the committee. These

---

BOX 8–1   Qualities of an Effective Consultant

- Experience, including longevity and diversity
- Knowledge and understanding of the healthcare industry
- Consulting skill and a proven methodology
- Verbal and written communication skills
- Good project management skills
- Clearly defined work plan and deliverables
- Advice that will result in cost savings
- Flexibility and availability
- A fit with the corporate culture
- Leadership in a team environment
- Ability to manage expectations rather than results
- Dedication to the project at hand
- Credibility
- Always acting in the best interest of the client

goals must reflect the organization's purpose, scope of services, and customers. The primary goal of the committee is to identify how healthcare delivery can be enhanced to provide optimum client care; this can be accomplished by providing more meaningful and accurate client data. Some additional expectations of an information system might be to save time, increase productivity, contain costs, promote quality improvement, enhance patient safety, and foster staff recruitment and retention. In addition, the system must be able meet and support regulatory guidelines such as those related to Health Insurance Portability and Accountability Act (HIPAA) requirements. The committee should consider using brainstorming techniques when defining the expectations of an information system. An open-minded and creative approach will facilitate comprehensive exploration of all possibilities.

Understanding the Current System A thorough understanding of how information is currently collected and processed is the starting point in performing a needs assessment. This is also known as assessing the internal environment. Methods for accomplishing this include questionnaires and observation of day-to-day activities (Saba & McCormick 1996). The goal is to determine what information is used, who uses it, and how it is used. Every data item used in the current paper or automated system should be analyzed. Some examples of data items include client name, sex, marital status, and diagnosis. Next, the committee must decide what information should be kept, what information is redundant, and what information is unnecessary. They should evaluate the strengths and weaknesses of the current manual or automated information system to determine the needs of the healthcare enterprise. How is data used between caregivers? Systems need to streamline the capture of data and present back as information that enables clinicians to coordinate care more easily and efficiently (Boyd et al. 2010).

Determining System Requirements To determine the appropriate course of action, the committee must first understand the organization's requirements for operation. One strategy for obtaining this information is to interview staff from each department or work area. The interviewer might ask what information is necessary to conduct business and what information is desired but not essential. These are often called the "musts" and the "wants." Some examples of essential information include client name, admitting physician, and insurance information. It is important to also consider those criteria that may not be necessary at the present time but might be important in the future, such as voice recognition technology. The information from numerous interviews is then compiled into a list of "musts" and "wants."

The next step is to prioritize or weight the list of "musts" and "wants" from high to low. To accomplish this task, selection committee members should develop a rating scale such as a 1 to 10 scale or rankings of low, medium, and high. Table 8–1 displays an example of some weighted "musts" and "wants" that could be identified when performing the needs assessment. The criteria should also be grouped into functional categories to present a comprehensive picture of the system requirements. Some of the common categories that may be considered are listed next.

Technical Criteria

Technical criteria include those hardware and software components necessary for the desired level of system performance. Areas to consider are the following:

- *Type of architecture.* **Architecture** refers to the structure of the central processing unit and its interrelated elements. An **open system** uses protocols and technology that follow publicly accepted conventions and are used by multiple vendors, so that various system components can work together.

    Examples of Criteria
    1. System maintains an open architecture environment that can continue to evolve as new technology becomes available
    2. Features ease of implementation and support of real-time integration to existing and future information systems

TABLE 8–1 Sample Weighting for Documentation Criteria		
Charting/Documentation Information Criteria	"Must" or "Want"	Weight
Is capable of multidisciplinary charting	M	10
Provides positive patient identification	M	10
Provides list of right medications and routes for the time	M	10
Automatically records medications during scanning process	M	10
Generates reminders of outstanding medications and pain assessments as due	M	10
Automatically totals fluid balance by shift and 24-hour period	W	6
Automatically calculates charted IV products into intake and output	W	7
Able to easily switch between functions (such as charting and entering orders)	W	5

*1–10, where 10 = most important.

- *Amount of downtime.* **Downtime** refers to the period of time when an information system is not operational or available for use. Some systems have daily scheduled downtimes, during which maintenance and backup procedures are performed.

  Examples of Criteria

  1. Provides 24-hour system availability with no scheduled daily downtime
  2. Does not have a history of prolonged or frequent unscheduled downtimes
  3. For open repository and comprehensive patient records, minimal downtime should be standard.
  4. Most system changes should be able to be made without bringing complete system down.

- *Connectivity standards.* These standards help to maximize the connectivity between application and information files, supporting system integration.

  Examples of Criteria

  1. Provides for HL7–compliant interfaces
  2. Includes the ability to interface from and to client care instruments such as monitors
  3. Many systems can also interface to pumps and handheld bar coding devices.
  4. If ancillary systems and specialty areas (e.g., cardiac cath lab, labor and delivery) have different vendor systems, interface of discrete data is preferred.
  5. Provides the ability for transmission of data for key regulatory reporting as in immunization registries
  6. Ability to hold bidirectional interface to outside medical labs to order and receive results

- *Test environment separate from live environment.* A separate environment for the development and testing of updates and changes to the system must be available, so that the actual system (live system) can continue to operate without interference during these activities.

  Examples of Criteria

  1. Provides the ability to update the test environment without impacting the live system
  2. Provides a training environment that is separate from the live and test environments

- *Response time.* **Response time** is the amount of time between a user action and the response from the information system. For example, after the user selects a laboratory test from a menu, the system requires a certain amount of processing time before that result can be viewed.

Examples of Criteria

1. Ensures acceptable response time for all online transactions (1 second or less)
2. Able to continuously track and monitor response time and provide reports containing this information
3. Log-on time is short, providing easy access to end users.

- *Support of electronic technologies.* The information system should support other technologies that will enhance client care and business operations.

Examples of Criteria

1. Supports various methods of data entry by the user, including touch screen entry and voice recognition
2. Allows the use of barcoding and scanning

Administrative/General Criteria

Administrative criteria describe how the system may be administratively controlled for appropriate and effective use of the information.

- *Security levels to comply with regulatory and legal requirements.* The Joint Commission, for example, regulates the confidentiality, security, and integrity of hospital systems. The HIPAA imposes requirements for the protection of patient data and penalties for noncompliance.

Examples of Criteria

1. Allows various levels of security to be defined for different user groups; each group should have access to only the information required for its client care or job duties
2. Provides an auditing utility to track and report what information has been accessed by which users

- *Data standards and data exchange.* The system must be ready to handle and work within the "standards" that are being used in the industry.

Examples of Criteria

1. HL7–clinical messaging
2. ICD-9 and CPT (coding), DICOM (imaging), and X12N (insurance claims)
3. Migration of ICD-9 to ICD-10 should be explored

- *Data storage options.* Organizations will need to determine if they want to have the ability to purge and restore data or have an open data repository to view patient data across visits for the life of the system. If the choice is to purge and restore, it is important to determine how long it is necessary to maintain online access to client data before sending it to other storage devices. Sometimes it becomes essential to restore these files for the purposes of audits, and the ease of performing these procedures must be considered. Advances such as the use of imaging technology to store diagnostic images and forms must be considered when purge criteria are defined.

Examples of Criteria

1. Includes a flexible client purge process, allowing both automatic and manual purge capabilities
2. Process for restoring data that have been purged to storage to be convenient and readily accessible
3. If a data repository option is chosen, discussions on architecture and hardware needed to support this over time should be discussed.
4. Cost of maintaining data in either method needs to be explored.
5. How vendors manage data in individual patient records during long length of stay to assure the system performance is optimal should be explored.

- *Report capabilities.* The system should provide a report-writing software component that allows specific types of information to be extracted from the database and presented in a report.

  Examples of Criteria
  1. Predefined reports to be produced automatically on a set schedule
  2. Users should be able to generate ad hoc reports on demand, with the capability to format them as desired.
  3. Reports should be available online, eliminating concerns related to printing costs, labor, distribution, storage, and disposal of confidential materials.
  4. Dashboard reporting capabilities are preferred for daily monitoring and management of patient care.

- *Ability to integrate with health information exchanges (HIEs).* The system should provide the ability to integrate with a regional health information exchange organization to provide more comprehensive patient data across regional areas.

  Examples of Criteria
  1. The ability to interface specific pieces of data to other systems such as a Regional Health Information Organization (RHIO)
  2. Audit capabilities to track who accessed the information

Registration Criteria

The registration criteria are essential for ensuring that the client is properly identified for all aspects of information management.

Examples of Criteria
1. Assigns each client a unique identifier across the organization
2. Supports multiple registration sites; clients may enter the health system at a number of points of service, including the physician's office, clinics, the emergency department, or the admissions office
3. Provides the ability to change or update registration information
4. Demonstrates the ability to track a client's location within the institution, as well as to track the use of system services
5. Prevents the user from omitting required data before completing a function
6. Has the ability to interface with other registration systems if integrating hospitals and/or office practices

Order Entry/CPOE/Results Reporting Criteria

These criteria ensure that accurate entry of physician orders is accomplished in a timely and efficient manner, resulting in improved client care.

Examples of Criteria
1. Able to indicate details of orders such as frequency (e.g., every six hours or daily) and priority (stat, routine, etc.)
2. Notifies the user when a duplicate order is entered, and requests verification before accepting the new order. For example, the client may have a previously ordered daily chest x-ray. If a new order for a chest x-ray is now entered, the system should alert the user and request verification that this additional test is necessary.
3. Through order entry and results reporting, produces an audit trail that identifies the person who entered the order, the date/time of order entry and execution, and the status of the order (such as pending or completed)
4. Supports documentation of medications and treatments, and relates this documentation to the appropriate order

5. Automatically generates client charges for specific orders or treatments as a result of entry or completion
6. Provides clinical decision support to end user at the time of order entry (e.g., dose range checking, drug allergy, drug-drug interaction alerts)
7. Displays appropriate results while ordering to assist end user in decision making
8. Supports e-prescribing functionality

Documentation/Billing Criteria

These criteria encompass a comprehensive architecture for documentation across the organization. Documentation should integrate key clinical events across ancillary, nursing, and physician documentation.

Examples of Criteria

1. The ability for key data fields to pull into physician documentation (e.g., results of cardiac catheterization report, pressure ulcer upon admission assessment, physical therapy recommendations)

Scheduling Criteria

These criteria should support the patient scheduling at many levels. Typically organizations utilize scheduling for appointments, procedures, and testing. Depending on the size of the organization, different scheduling systems exist.

Examples of Criteria

1. Integration of scheduling system with patient records
2. Ability to view upcoming schedules for patients
3. Ability to view office schedule while seeing patients with detail of patients in the waiting room
4. Ability to open patient chart from schedule view

Specialties Criteria

These criteria should be applied in organizations that intend to utilize the same vendor product across all venues for a best-of-breed approach. Best-in-class systems require integration. For large organizations that have many specialties, understanding the capabilities of the system as it applies to specialty documentation and workflow is key. To assure these features are covered, stakeholders from specialty areas should sit on the selection committee.

Examples of Criteria

1. Vendor has content and function for specialty areas
2. Specific function for areas in need (e.g., fetal monitoring for labor and delivery, workflow for emergency room triage, tracking, documentation and feedback to promote throughput)

Medical Records Criteria

The medical records criteria should support the storage of all pertinent client data obtained from various information systems, allowing the user to access a longitudinal record of all client activities and events or visits. The system should allow inquiry about clients, using various identifiers, including Social Security number, name, medical record, or account number.

Examples of Criteria

1. Provides support for automatic coding, including verification of codes entered with narrative description (e.g., ICD-9-CM and CPT-4 codes)
2. Translates diagnosis and procedure terminology into numeric code
3. Produces deficiency lists on demand for individual records and individual physicians

4. Produces a printed version of the patient's record which meets criteria of regulatory and risk management/legal reporting. Each episodic visit should produce a record which is not overwritten by subsequent visits.

Accounting Criteria

These criteria facilitate reimbursement for services rendered and help to ensure the financial stability of the enterprise.

Examples of Criteria

1. Generates summaries or detailed bills on demand
2. Allows the user to enter the client's insurance verification data, insurance plan, and charges at any time during the stay and to change the client's financial class
3. Supports physician billing and captures data for linkage to physician billing services

SYSTEM SELECTION

If the decision is made to purchase a new information system, the life cycle proceeds to Phase 2: system selection. This phase is critical to the success of the project. High cost for purchase, installation, and maintenance for new or upgraded technology mean that the decision must be made carefully. The information gathered during the needs assessment phase is the basis for the system selection process and decision. Because it has been determined that a new system must be purchased, further information must now be gathered. Box 8–2 identifies some system selection considerations. The selection committee should also be aware of the amount of money available for the purchase, installation, and maintenance of a new system, as this influence will guide their questions and impact available choices (Costa & Marrone 2007).

BOX 8–2 System Selection Criteria

- Overall costs
  Hardware, software, and network costs
  Implementation costs
  Support and maintenance costs

- Vendor characteristics
  CCHIT Certification
  Reputation
  Experienced staff and consultants
  Financial status

- Software features
  Ease of use
  Intuitive user interface, requiring minimal training
  Includes all functionality identified as "musts"
  Supports security requirements
  Supports interfaces with other applications
  Supports future growth options

- Environmental issues

- Energy consumption of equipment

- Recycling and e-waste options once equipment is outmoded

Additional Sources of Information

Trade shows and conferences are beneficial sources of information. Attendance at these events provides the opportunity to examine systems from various vendors in an informal atmosphere, to compare and contrast system capabilities, and to view demonstrations. The Certification Commission for Health Information Technology (CCHIT) (2010) has been certifying electronic health records since 2006; it developed the first practical definition of what capabilities are needed. A list of its certified vendors can be found on its Web site http://www.cchit.org.

Other potentially helpful sources of information include weekly publications, trade newspapers, and monthly journals that address information and technology and local user groups. Textbooks and reference books also provide discussions of system options. Published conference proceedings may provide insight into pertinent issues and solutions. Finally, communication via the Internet and World Wide Web can furnish additional information, including insights from other users of a given system. This avenue may provide the most current and candid responses to questions.

Request for Information

An information systems **vendor** is a company that designs, develops, sells, and supports systems. Consideration of vendor characteristics is crucial in choosing a system that will be responsive to current needs and unanticipated changes. Characteristics to examine include service, performance, and stability. A great deal of information can be gleaned from vendors who are eager to make a sale. The **request for information (RFI)** is often the initial contact with vendors. An RFI is a letter or brief document sent to vendors that explains the institution's plans for purchasing and installing an information system. The purpose of the RFI is to obtain essential information about the vendor and its systems to eliminate those vendors that cannot meet the organization's basic requirements. One method for obtaining names of appropriate vendors is to complete reader response cards following advertisements in professional journals.

The RFI should ask the vendor to provide a description of the system and its capabilities. Often the vendor responds to the request by sending written literature. More information can be obtained by asking additional specific questions of the vendor. Some topics to consider for questioning include:

1. The history and financial situation of the company, including the extent of its investment into research and development; this provides an indication of the company's commitment to enhancing and updating the product
2. The number of installed sites, including a list of several organizations that already use the product you are considering
3. System architecture, including the required hardware configuration
4. Use of state-of-the-art technology
5. Integration with other systems. Which other systems are currently integrated with the vendor's software in other hospital sites?
6. The methods of user support provided by the vendor during and after installation
7. Future healthcare provider development plans
8. Procedures for the distribution of software updates

Request for Proposal

At this point, the steering committee will probably be overwhelmed with information. The next step is to evaluate this information and prepare a formal document called the **request for proposal (RFP).** An RFP is a document sent to vendors that describes the requirements of a potential information system. The RFP prioritizes or ranks these requirements in order of their importance to the organization. Preparation of this document can be daunting. Its purpose is to solicit proposals from many vendors that describe their capabilities to meet the "wants" and "needs." The vendors' responses may then be used to narrow the number of competitors under consideration.

Strategies for a Successful RFP Because of the importance of the RFP, it must be structured to ensure successful system selection (Hoch 2006). All aspects of the document must be detailed and precise to facilitate an accurate response from the vendor. If questions are vague or poorly written, they could easily be misinterpreted by the vendor. For example, an ambiguous question might lead a vendor to indicate that the system meets a requirement when in fact it does not. It is advantageous to limit the number of requirements to those that are most important and to produce a simple and straightforward document. If an RFP is too lengthy, it will cost both the organization and the vendor a great deal of time and money to prepare and evaluate. It is difficult to evaluate a long document that is not focused on the important issues. Finally, a well-written RFP provides a framework that allows the steering committee to more accurately evaluate the vendor's proposal.

The format of RFP questions and answers may influence the authenticity of vendor responses. For example, for each question about a system feature, the RFP might offer four response choices, such as:

1. *"Yes."* If the vendor indicates that this functionality is currently available, then the vendor must also provide a written explanation of how the system performs this function.
2. *"Available with customization."* The vendor must provide an estimated cost of customization and time frame for availability.
3. *"Available in the future."* The vendor must provide an estimated time frame for availability.
4. *"No."* No further information is required.

RFP Design

Although the actual format of the RFP may vary from organization to organization, all RFPs must contain certain components that are essential for a complete and effective document. The RFP should include the following details:

- *Description of the organization.* The first objective of the RFP should be to familiarize the vendor with the organization. The RFP must describe the organization's overall environment, as well as the specific setting in which the system will function. The vendor needs to have enough information to facilitate proposal of appropriate systems and hardware configurations. The following information should be included:
  1. *Mission and goals.* The mission statement and any supporting documentation will provide the vendor with a view of the driving forces behind the selection process.
  2. *Structure of the organization.* The RFP should describe how the healthcare enterprise is structured, including all facilities and satellite areas that provide inpatient, outpatient, and home care services.
  3. *Type of healthcare facility.* The RFP should specify whether the facility is a profit or nonprofit organization and contain descriptors appropriate to the organization, such as community, university, government, or teaching facility.
  4. *Payer mix.* Additional information should quantify the proportion of clients for the various types of payers encountered. For example, the percentage of clients having private insurance, Medicare/Medicaid coverage, or health maintenance organization (HMO) membership should be indicated.
  5. *Volume statistics.* The RFP should provide volume statistics such as number of inpatient beds, average occupancy, annual outpatient visits, emergency department visits, volume of lab tests performed, number of operations annually, and number of various categories of staff, including physicians, nurses, and technicians and any plans for growth.

- *System requirements.* Following the description of the organization, the RFP should include a comprehensive list of the system requirements previously developed by the committee. One point to consider when defining system requirements is to avoid limiting the vendor to specific configurations, such as the type and number of devices, because the vendor may be able to suggest better solutions. The requirements should not necessitate the vendor to recreate a manual or current automated system. These limitations may prohibit the vendor from exploring improved methods of information use with the proposed technology (Metrick 2002).
- *Criteria for evaluation of responses.* Providing the vendor with an explanation of the RFP evaluation process may improve the quality of the vendor's response. If the vendors respond in the expected format, evaluating responses from multiple vendors can be more easily accomplished, and results more easily compared.
- *Deadline date.* Inform the vendor of the expected date of responses. Vendors who do not meet deadlines may be excluded.

Evaluation of RFP Responses

Once responses from various vendors have been received, the process of evaluation begins. Some initial considerations are related to how the vendor approached the RFP. For example, some questions to ask are:

- Was the response submitted by the deadline date?
- Does it represent the work of a professional team and company?
- Were the vendor representatives responsive and knowledgeable?
- Does the proposal address the requirements outlined in the RFP, or does it appear to be a standard bid?

Further evaluation is centered around the specific responses of the vendors to the requirements listed in the RFP. The prioritization and ranking of the requirements that were previously developed by the steering committee now are used to weight each item in the RFP. This produces an overall score for each vendor response. This score allows the vendors to be ranked objectively, based on their ability to meet the requirements. Vendors that are unable to meet all of the "musts" should be automatically eliminated.

The remaining vendors must now be evaluated in terms of benefits and costs. Examining the scores for the "wants" and discussing the vendor's proposed costs are components of the final decision-making process. It may be helpful to narrow the list to three finalists and then examine these more closely.

Hoch (2006) suggests that the committee might want to consider writing a **Request for Quote (RFQ)** instead, stating that the RFP invites vendors to focus on marketing hype. The RFQ is a statement of need that focuses upon pricing, service levels, and contract terms. It should be written in precise, technical but vendor-neutral language. When customers are unclear about needs in a particular area, they should request pricing for different solutions. The RFQ should ask for quotes based on present as well as projected levels of growth with consideration given to response times, stability, and monetary compensation for downtime and loss of business. Other issues for consideration include termination clauses and use of subcontractors.

Site Visits

The use of site visits is very helpful in selecting a system. Site visits allow the system to be seen in action at a location that is comparable in size and services provided. Comparison of site visit evaluations for the top three vendors may provide additional information that will facilitate decision making.

A successful site visit often begins with the preparation of a list of questions. Asking the same questions at each site visit helps the committee draw meaningful comparisons. It is helpful to request a demonstration of the live system. This will allow observations regarding the response

---

BOX 8–3   Questions to Ask During a Site Visit

- How reliable is the system?
- How much downtime do you experience?
- What is the response time?
- How is the system backup accomplished, and how frequently is this done?
- Are there any problems with information exchange with other information systems?
- How do customizations or enhancements get made to the system (in-house or by vendor)?
- How much training was required for users to learn the system?
- What do you like most about the system?
- What things would you like to change about the system?
- What features would you like to see added to the system?
- How is information access restricted, and how is security maintained?
- What have your experiences been with vendor support?
- Is it easy to generate reports, and can they be customized easily to meet user needs?
- What problems are you trying to solve?
- What would you do differently if you could go back in time?

---

time. It is also beneficial to examine reports and printed documentation produced by the system, and to interview people who are actually using the system. Often, more candid information can be obtained if the vendors are not present during the interview process. Box 8–3 lists several questions that may be used during a site visit.

In addition, the vendor should provide a contact list of users from other organizations who are willing to be interviewed by phone. Representatives from hospital departments may ask their counterparts in other organizations about the performance of the information system. This will provide insight into how the systems actually operate, as well as the support that the vendor provides.

Contract Negotiations

Once the decision has been made by the steering committee, the enterprise's legal and purchasing representatives carry out the actual contract negotiations. They may request the names of the three highest ranked vendors, as well as their RFP responses. In this way, the contract negotiations will be able to address issues not specifically included in the RFP responses, such as cost justification and expected implementation schedules. The end result will be the selection of one vendor and a system that will be implemented in the enterprise. After the contract is signed, the implementation phase begins.

FUTURE DIRECTIONS

As today's political healthcare IT agenda is pushed forward the demand for efficient and accurate system, selection has become increasingly important. The ability to select a system that meets the needs of an organization in all its complexity and remain affordable is the challenge. As organizations make these transitions, there will be much to learn from each of them as they move from manual or older systems to new platforms. The CCHIT organization is moving forward as the certifying organization for health information technology, vendors will be seeking certification if they have not already. Criteria on what "Meaningful Use" is will evolve which will require keeping up with the current requirements as well as standards and trends in the industry. There are many challenges with implementation that leave open research opportunities. System usability, integration across various platforms, and optimal training models have remained a challenge in many organizations and have not been fully identified at the time of system selection. Developing methods to measure and evaluate beyond system functionality leaves open opportunities. Selecting a system which has the criteria to meet organizational goals is only the first step.

CASE STUDY EXERCISE

You are a member of the committee that will select a clinical documentation system for nurses. Prepare a timeline for the needs assessment and system selection phases. These processes should be accomplished over a 6-month period.

SUMMARY

- The selection and implementation of an information system occur through a well-defined process called the life cycle of an information system.
- The four phases of the life cycle of an information system are needs assessment, system selection, implementation, and maintenance.
- The needs assessment process is often initiated when a deficit in the current method of manual or automated information handling is recognized.
- The system selection steering committee is an essential component of the assessment and selection processes, and leadership as well as membership of this group may impact the success or failure of the project.
- The needs assessment process should include an examination of the vision and mission statements of the organization, because these should guide the committee in looking to the future and determining the organization's information needs.
- A thorough understanding of how information is currently collected and processed is the starting point in performing a needs assessment.
- Determination of the system requirements should address criteria related to all aspects of system performance, including technical, administrative, registration, order entry, CPOE, results reporting, documentation, billing, scheduling, specialties, medical records, and accounting criteria.
- The request for information is a letter or brief document sent to vendors that explains the institution's plans for purchasing and installing an information system. The purpose of the RFI is to obtain essential information about the vendor and its system capabilities to eliminate those vendors that cannot meet the organization's basic requirements.
- The request for proposal is a document sent to vendors that describes the requirements of a potential information system. The purpose of this document is to solicit from many vendors proposals that describe the capabilities of their information systems and support services.
- A weighted scoring strategy will facilitate the evaluation of complicated request for proposal responses from vendors and will improve the ability of the steering committee to make an informed decision.

REFERENCES

Boyd, A. D., Funk, E. A., Schwartz, S. M., Kaplan, B., & Keenan, G. M. (2010). Top EHR challenges in light of the stimulus. Enabling effective interdisciplinary, intradisciplinary, and cross-setting communication. *Journal of Healthcare Information Management, 24*(1), 18–24.

CDW Healthcare. (2007). *Nurses Talk Tech 2007: The catch-22 of nursing and information technology*. Retrieved from http://webobjects.cdw.com/webobjects/docs/pdfs/healthcare/Nurses-Talk-Tech-2007.pdf

Certification Commission for Health Information Technology. (2010). About the Certification Commission for Health Information Technology. Retrieved from http://www.cchit.org/

Costa, M., & Marrone, B. (2007). What's the best approach to choosing IT? *Healthcare Financial Management: Journal of the Healthcare Financial Management Association, 61*(2), 108–112.

Czerniawska, F. (2006). Consultant: Good consulting firm: Bad. *Consulting to Management—C2M, 17*(2), 3–5.

Hoch, M. (2006, September). 3½ RFP rules. *Communications News, 43*(9), ISSN 0010-3632.

Hoehn, B. J. (2010). Meaningful use: What does it mean for healthcare organizations? *Journal of Healthcare Information Management, 24*(1), 10–12.

Jusinski, L. (2007). EHR selection suggestions. *ADVANCE for Health Information Professionals, 17*(10), 19.

Klein, K. (2010). So much to do, so little time. To accomplish the mandatory initiatives of ARRA, healthcare organizations will require significant and thoughtful planning, prioritization and execution. *Journal of Healthcare Information Management, 24*(1), 31–35.

Marshall, J., & Heffes, E. M. (2007). Most directors fail to link IT with strategy. *Financial Executive, 23*(6), 9.

Metrick, G. (2002). Selecting a product or services using the request for proposal process. *Scientific Computing and Instrumentation, 19*(12), L-8–L-12.

Saba, V. K., & McCormick, K. A. (1996). *Essentials of computers for nurses*. Philadelphia, PA: Lippincott.

Saleem, N., Jones, D. R., Van Tran, H., & Moses, B. (2006). Forming design teams to develop healthcare information systems. *Hospital Topics, 84*(1), 22–30.

Teague, P. E. (2007, March 1). 5 "musts" for justifying IT budgets. *Purchasing*, 41–42.

The future is now: Consultants spotlight. (2007, November 2). *Pharmaceutical Executive, 27*, 11–34.

Walker, J. M., Bieber, E. J., & Richards, F. (2005). *Implementing an electronic health record system*. London: Springer.

Wickham, V., Miedema, F., Gamerdinger, K., & DeGooyer, J. (2006). Bar-coded patient ID: Review an organizational approach to vendor selection. *Nursing Management, 37*(12), 22–26.

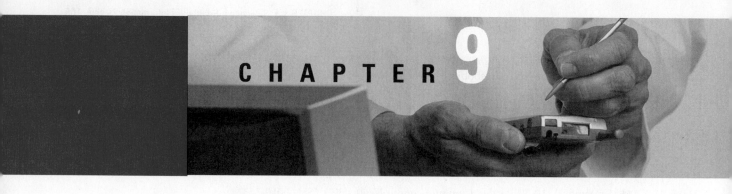

Improving the Usability of Health Informatics Applications

After completing this chapter, you should be able to:

1. Distinguish among the terms *human factors, ergonomics, human–computer interaction,* and *usability*.

2. Describe the goals of usability and its three axioms.

3. Identify the major components of human-computer interaction models.

4. Compare and contrast methods employed in usability studies.

5. Construct basic and advanced usability tests for health informatics applications.

We submit that usability is one of the major factors—possibly the most important factor—hindering widespread adoption of EMRs.

(GRAHAM ET AL. 2008)

Improved usability is critical for the adoption and use of health informatics products. All informaticists need a suite of skills to conduct usability tests, whether the focus of their work is design, development, implementation, use, or evaluation technologies. Concepts about usability and human–computer interaction (HCI) guide informaticists in creating and purchasing technologies that users find effective, efficient, and satisfying to use. This chapter presents definitions of major terms—*human factors, ergonomics, human–computer interaction,* and *usability*—along with usability goals and axioms. Examples of current usability issues are given and potential benefits are described. HCI frameworks are offered for guidance. Usability test construction and methods are explained in detail using rich examples of usability studies in health settings. After reading this chapter, health informaticists will be able to design and conduct usability tests to determine the effectiveness, efficiency, and/or satisfaction with health technologies.

INTRODUCTION TO USABILITY

The Current State of Usability in Health Informatics Applications

Usability issues in health information technology (IT) applications are a contemporary national concern (Armijo, McDonnell, & Werner 2009; HIMSS 2009; Stead & Linn 2009). Authors describe new errors in healthcare, uneven adoption of clinical applications, and unintended consequences of IT because of usability issues in clinical systems (Ash, Sittig, Dykstra, Campbell, & Guappone 2009; Ash, Sittig, Poon, Guappone, Campbell, & Dykstra 2007; Jha et al. 2009; Kuehn 2009). Beginning on January 25, 2010, the *New York Times* released a series of reports about fatal radiation doses and other grave errors affecting patients that were due to software usability and human factors problems in radiation oncology technology. The fielding of a worldwide ambulatory electronic health record (EHR) caused decreases in patient access to healthcare, severely reduced provider productivity, and created extreme frustration because of the lack of fit with provider workflow (Philpott 2006, 2009).

Usability principles and practices, while deemed critical for system adoption, have only slowly infused into healthcare (Armijo et al. 2009). Few studies document the usability of health informatics software or even evaluate the usability of major EHR systems provided by vendors (Armijo et al. 2009); yet, the United States is spending billions of dollars on the proliferation of health applications without having this kind of systematic evaluation. Stead and Lin (2009) more strongly stated that unless health IT applications better support the cognitive processes of system users, health IT could even worsen healthcare in the future.

The costs of unusable systems are substantial even without catastrophic events. Usability issues can result in decreases in productivity, errors, treatment delays, extreme user frustration, underutilization of applications, deinstallations, extra support personnel to install and maintain systems, covert and overt resistance to applications, and the need for substantial funding to redesign and remedy problems. Usability principles and practices can help prevent these costs to individuals and organizations.

Usability has a strong, often direct relationship with clinical productivity, error rate, user fatigue and user satisfaction—critical factors for EMR adoption.

(HIMSS 2009)

Potential Benefits of Expanding Usability in Health Informatics Applications

Well-designed systems can allow for improvements in patient safety, the number of errors, data entry, information displays, and information interpretation, and contribute to sound decision making. Other overall impacts include decreases in the time to complete tasks, user disruptions, training time, software rewrites, burden on support staff, and user frustration. Usability techniques allow informatics to identify issues with technology. More important, usability methods address *why* users are having those problems. Issues can then be addressed before technology is released.

Vendors may balk at incorporating usability into development processes because the time to market for new products may be lengthened. Yet, evidence is available that usability processes can reduce costs. In 1991 usability processes at IBM resulted in an average reduction of 9.6 minutes per task, a projected savings internally to IBM of $6.8 million. Karat (1990) also reported savings from usability engineering techniques at $41,700 for a small application used by 23,000 marketing personnel. Nielsen (2008) conducted a more recent survey and found an 83% decrease in key performance indicators such as time to complete common tasks after products were redesigned for usability.

Every health informaticist should be educated in usability techniques and promote more usable systems and technology applications. This chapter provides background material as well as the knowledge and skills to conduct usability tests.

DEFINITIONS OF TERMS AND INTERRELATIONSHIPS OF CONCEPTS

Human Factors

The term *human factors* is used to describe the interactions between humans and tools of all kinds. *Human factors* is a broad term that can include topics such as the design of motorcycle controls to fit human hands and feet or an evaluation of how work is performed within the layout of a hospital room in an intensive care unit. A most readable and classic text about the need for human factors in the design of common objects was written by Norman (1988).

The relationship of human factors terms is depicted in Figure 9–1. As may be seen, ergonomics, HCI, and usability are all embedded within the broader concepts of human factors. Usability overlaps both ergonomics and HCI.

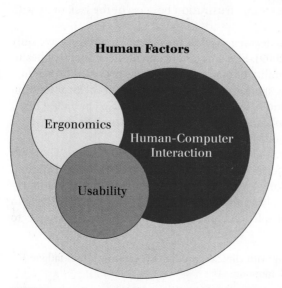

FIGURE 9–1 • The interrelationship of human factors terms
Source: Staggers N. (2003, August). Human factors: Imperative concepts for information systems in critical care. *AACN Clinical Issues, 14*(3), 310–319; quiz 397-318. Reprinted with permission.

Ergonomics

Ergonomics is concerned with human performance as it relates to the physical characteristics of tools, systems, and machines (Dix, Finlay, Abowd, & Beale 2004). Ergonomics focuses on designs for safety, comfort, and convenience (Langendoen & Costa 1994). The term *ergonomics* is often used interchangeably with *human factors* in Europe but less so in the United States. Examples of ergonomics issues include nurses complaining that a workstation on wheels is too bulky, heavy, and not convenient to take into a patient room. Ergonomics addresses the design of a cooking utensil to fit a human hand, the design of computer chairs to promote comfort and safety, and/or the intuitive operation of drinking fountains.

Human–Computer Interaction

Human–computer interaction is the study of how people design, implement, and evaluate interactive computer systems in the context of users' tasks and work (Dix et al. 2004). HCI blends psychology and/or cognitive science, applied work in computer science, sociology, and information science into the design, development, purchase, implementation, and evaluation of applications. Sample HCI topics include:

- The design and use of devices such as a mouse, or patient-controlled analgesia machine
- User satisfaction with a patient portal
- Users' perceptions of the effectiveness of the design of clinical documentation integrated with medication barcoding
- The meaning of icons
- The design and evaluation of applications or systems to support groups of people
- Principles of effective Web, graphical user interface (GUI), or adaptive interface design
- Social issues in computing such as dropping an individual from your virtual group
- Functional allocation of work between humans and computers
- User modeling such as cognitive analyses of users

Usability

Usability is a subset of HCI and one of its major components. The term *usability* is often used interchangeably with *HCI*. More formally, usability is the extent to which a product can be used by specific users in a specific context to achieve specific goals with effectiveness, efficiency, and satisfaction according to the International Standards Organization 9241-11, 2006. That is, a usable product is one that allows users to achieve specific goals with a product in a specific context (Rubin 2008). Usability is multidimensional, including topics such as:

- Using an application
- Learning to use a system
- Remembering interactions with technology after time has elapsed
- User satisfaction
- Efficiency
- Error-free/error-forgiving interactions
- Seamless fit of an information system to the task(s) at hand

Ease of use is a rather vague notion that can imply many factors, from having a suitable screen layout to easy navigation about a system to understanding what the system is doing during interactions to having appropriate language for users within a particular context. A health informaticist can assist in determining which aspects contribute to a usable product in particular settings.

The Goals of Usability

The broad goals of usability are promoting acceptance and use of systems through improved interactive systems and software, developing new kinds of applications to support specific work, and promoting job optimization with the use of information systems. A user interface can effectively disappear if a system is designed well. This allows users to focus only on the task at hand rather than tending to the technology itself.

Usability experts cite three main goals of HCI and usability, listed in Figure 9–2, which are effectiveness, efficiency, and user satisfaction. As may be seen, effectiveness is related to the usefulness of technology in completing desired goals. It includes completeness, accuracy, and flow of information; that is, how well the function matches a user's cognitive flow of information, the flow of information among a group of users, and/or the optimal allocation of functions between human and computer.

Of course, in life critical systems, such as a fetal-uterine monitor, the safety of the application is paramount. For example, the accurate transfer of physiological monitoring data to an information system in labor and delivery or the accurate display of patient medications in electronic medication administration records is critical.

The efficiency of systems deals with the expenditures of resources, where resources are time, productivity, error rates of users, or the costs of the system to the organization in terms of value of the product compared to the purchase price, little used options, or redesign of applications. Learnability is related to productivity because better designed systems can take less time to learn and remember.

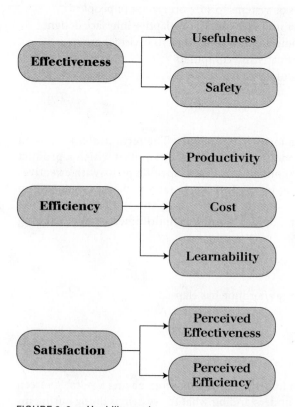

FIGURE 9–2 • Usability goals

Source: Adapted from Staggers, N. (2001). Human-computer interaction in health care organizations. In S. Englebardt & R. Nelson (Eds.), *Health care informatics: An interdisciplinary approach* (pp. 321–345). St. Louis: Mosby.

Last, user satisfaction can be assessed by measuring perceptions about the efficiency or effectiveness of interactions with the system. Users' perceptions about usability and the perceived benefits of using systems are components of satisfaction and can enhance application acceptance and use.

The Axioms of Usability

HCI authors agree on three axioms of usability (Dix et al. 2004; Rubin & Chisnell 2008):

- An early and central focus on users in the design and development of systems
- Iterative design of applications
- Systematic usability measures or observations of users and information systems

Gould and Lewis (1985) originally published these principles; 26 years later, they are still pertinent. An early and central focus on users means understanding users in depth (Rubin 2008). Informaticists will want direct contact with users early and often throughout a design or redesign process. Iterative design means having rounds of design and allowing users to evaluate prototypes to determine their effectiveness and efficiency. Nielsen (1993) claimed that one design is never adequate. Typically, three rounds of design or redesign are necessary. Users are central to requirements determination. Once a design is available, informaticists work with users to determine issues with effectiveness and efficiency. Major usability problems are then corrected by developers. Design and evaluation occurs in a recurring cycle. Authors stress the need for structured and systematic observations, even empirical assessments, of users as they interact with technology.

The usability and HCI literature has focused nearly exclusively on developing applications. However, these usability axioms apply to the selection, purchase, and customization of contemporary systems as well. Thus, informaticists can perform usability tests by understanding of local users, tasks, and environment. These can be critical to selecting an adequate system and subsequently customizing the new system to its intended environment.

HUMAN–COMPUTER INTERACTION FRAMEWORKS FOR HEALTH INFORMATICS

Human–computer interaction frameworks provide broad guidance for health informaticists to understand major elements of usability projects and usability testing. These frameworks guide health informaticists in completing user-centered design processes, usability tests, IT adoption evaluations, and usability research. The frameworks can guide advanced usability tests from a theoretical level. In this section, we will provide an overview of existing frameworks, describe an example of one framework—the Staggers Health Human–Computer Interaction Framework— and introduce a model for joint cognitive systems.

A Sample of Available Human–Computer Interaction Frameworks

In the past 5–10 years, authors created high-level representations of users and computer/technology interactions in frameworks and models (Ammenwerth, Iller, & Mahler 2006; Johnson, Johnson, & Zhang 2005; Staggers 2001; Yusof, Stergioulas, & Zugic 2007; Zhang & Butler 2007;). Constance Johnson and colleagues (Johnson et al. 2005) combined framework elements with associated usability methods to outline a framework for redesigning a fielded system. The redesign process and usability evaluation includes creating a prototype, conducting a heuristic evaluation, a small-scale usability study, and a comparison test of the previous and new versions.

The UFuRT (**U**ser, **F**unction, **R**epresentation, and **T**ask analysis) framework (Zhang & Butler 2007), the authors indicated, is based on work-centered research and distributed cognition.

This framework also combines both elements and usability processes. As such, it acknowledges multiple users, their expertise and cognitive characteristics, functional and tasks analysis to describe work, representational analysis to identify tasks, and steps in tasks and interactions. Technology is an implicit component of the UFuRT framework.

Usability is listed as a key component in recent IT adoption models. Despont-Gros and colleagues reviewed HCI models and created a combined adoption and HCI model (Despont-Gros, Mueller, & Lovis 2005). At the center of the model is a user interacting with a clinical information system. The user is contained within a context, workspace, and environment/organization. The model includes characteristics for major elements and a development process. An acceptance component is fed by many of the model elements.

The Fit between Individuals, Task, and Technology (FITT) framework (Ammenwerth et al. 2006) described the fit between an individual, tasks, and technology, having these three elements connected by "interactions and influences." The authors used the framework elements and interactions to guide an evaluation of IT adoption on four different patient care units in a German hospital.

Yusof and colleagues conducted a systematic review and subsequently created the **H**uman, **O**rganization, **T**echnology-fit (HOT-fit) (Yusof et al. 2007; Yusof, Kuljis, Papazafeiropoulou, & Stergioulas 2008). framework to describe IT adoption with central elements of system ease of use, user satisfaction, and system usefulness.

Existing frameworks are helpful but may be inadequate because they can be incomplete. Frequent missing elements include (1) interactions among disparate users, (2) the setting or context, and (3) a developmental time for interactions. The context is critical because designs for one unit, say a medical unit, will not fit work in labor and delivery. Authors need to consider the context of the interaction within a particular unit, profession, organizations, and/or social settings (Despont-Gros et al. 2005; Lindgaard 1992; Mantovani 1996) as well as broader concepts such as the design of work (Beuscart-Zephir, Brender, Beuscart, & Menager-Depreiester 1997; Zhang & Butler 2007). The developmental time element allows informaticists to consider designs for both inexperienced and expert users of a particular application (Despont-Gros et al. 2005; Staggers 2001). Usability methods can then be applied as appropriate. Critical elements for health informaticists to consider are a user or users in groups and their characteristics, interactions, tasks (work), information, technology and its characteristics, the context, and development over time. The following organizes these elements into a framework for health informatics.

Description of the Staggers Health Human–Computer Interaction Framework

The Staggers Human–Computer Interaction Framework, a sample HCI framework, is described in more detail in this section (see Figure 9–3). The current framework builds upon earlier work by Staggers and Parks (1992, 1993), outlining an interacting dyad of an individual and a computer. The early framework incorporated concepts from developmental psychology (development of the dyad over time) and typical elements of existing HCI frameworks of the early 1990s: a computer user, computer, interaction with information exchange, and a context or environment. The developmental timeline was a novel addition. An expanded HCI framework, published and described in 2001 (Staggers 2001), extended the framework to groups of providers, patients/health consumers, and provider/patient interactions, as well as single individuals working with computers. The framework is expanded again to indicate technology interactions, computers being only one example of available technologies.

The Health Human–Computer Interaction Framework in Figure 9–3 includes concepts from developmental psychology, consistent with the original work by Staggers and Parks. Concepts from developmental psychology indicate how to structure interactions between nonequivalent elements. Although psychology developmental frameworks are targeted to human exchanges,

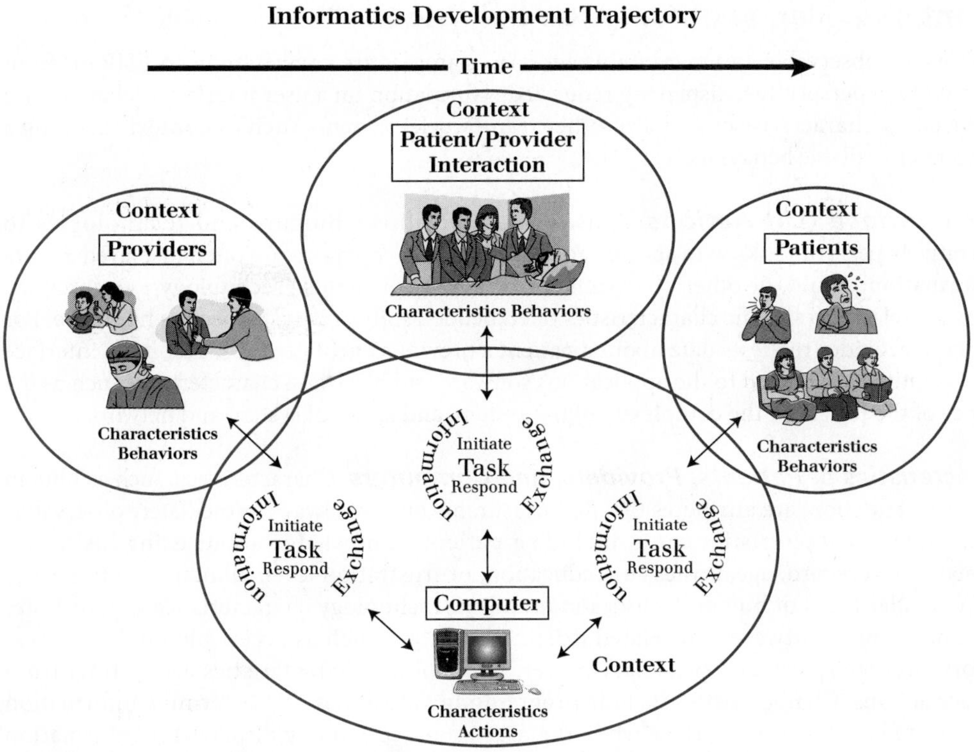

Informatics Development Trajectory

FIGURE 9–3 • Health human-technology interaction framework
Source: Staggers, N. (2001). Human-computer interaction in health care organizations. In S. Englebardt & R. Nelson (Eds.), *Health care informatics: An interdisciplinary approach* (pp. 321–345). St. Louis: Mosby.

these same concepts explain well humans interacting with intelligent technologies. Information is the currency of exchange or communication between elements. Interactions are defined in a system of mutual influences, with humans and technologies responding and acting from specific characteristics. All interactions are embedded in environment(s) or context(s). This means that any outcomes of interactions are distinct as defined by the single context or various contexts. Interactions mature and change over time; thus, outcomes of interactions are also defined by the length of time the interactions occur.

These concepts can be applied to provider–patient–technology interactions. Interactions are centered on information exchange among framework elements. All components act in a system of mutual influences of humans and technologies impacted by other framework elements of context and time. Provider, patient, and computer actions are a result of respective characteristics. Interactions occur within a context(s) and the interactions mature and change over time.

Humans or technologies can initiate interactions. The initiator sends information to the user interface for viewing, for example, sending an alert to a provider's mobile device about an abnormal laboratory result for a patient in a surgical unit. From the interface, the information is processed through either the technology according to its characteristics (software and hardware) or humans according to their characteristics (expertise, age, cognitive characteristics). The recipient then reacts to the information, for example, a provider would acknowledge the alert on the user interface and then access other functions and information to take action on the alert. The technologies or humans receive the new information and then process it according to their characteristics. As these iterative cycles continue, humans behave and computers act according to defined characteristics. Goals and planning are implicit in this framework.

Patient, Provider, and Computer Behaviors

Behaviors are observable and measurable actions. Examples are navigating in an EHR or, from the technology perspective, displaying requested information on a user interface. Behaviors are influenced by characteristics and also other framework elements such as context, defining a repertoire of available behaviors.

User Interface (UI) Actions A user interface allows humans and technologies to cooperatively perform tasks with specific goals. User interface actions are often displayed as data or information, sound, or other observable or detectable elements. Technology user interface actions are related to specific characteristics of embedded software and respective hardware. For instance, a provider requests data about a patient's previous encounter. The result, an interface action, is intimately related to the applications software and hardware characteristics such as the elegance of the program, the complexity of the system, and speed of system and network.

Characteristics of Patients, Providers, and Computers Characteristics, such as human memory or attention, are attributes that are measurable but not always immediately observable. Other human characteristics could include a patient's knowledge about using his or her personal health record, age, profession, education, or frustration level. Human characteristics are a particular focus of human factors and usability. Technology characteristics are attributes programmed into software and related existing hardware such as accessible random access memory, storage space, and processor power. Technology characteristics are distinct from interface actions. Characteristics include programming attributes that determine information to be directed to the user interface while the user interface actually displays the information according to the user interface and technology characteristics.

The Task Information Exchange Process Humans or technology begins the process by entering and retrieving information to complete a specific task. For example, providers may access the latest evidence about diabetes care from a highly rated Internet site. A nurse, pharmacist, and physician cooperate in completing a medication reconciliation process for a patient across inpatient and ambulatory records. Each task includes an explicit or implicit goal; even if the actions are to explore the system, a goal is still embedded in the process. Some behaviors and characteristics are outside any one particular task because each task accesses only a subset of all available behaviors and characteristics for elements in the framework.

Health Context Interactions are contained with a context. This environment may be an actual or virtual setting, for example, a conference room for change of shift report on an inpatient unit or virtual work space for a team of researchers in disparate locations. The context can include more abstract elements such as cultural or political contexts, norms or mores, and/or associated ergonomics features such as noise. Human–technology interactions are influenced by the characteristics of these contexts. Thus, clearly a handoff between two providers using an EHR on a quiet night shift is different than one on a busy unit with call bells, cell phones, and patient alarms interrupting the handoff.

Informatics

Developmental Trajectory The interactions of humans and technologies move along on a developmental trajectory over time. Progressing in this way allows the interactions and information exchange to change over time. New human and technology characteristics can influence the interaction because new information is displayed and exchanged as the process matures (or degrades) according the mutual influence of elements, characteristics, and behaviors. This component of the framework is critical for the health informaticist because it acknowledges the influence of human experience and practice with technology. The informaticist will assure that naïve users, those using technology for the first time, require distinct designs compared to users practiced with the application. Likewise, technology novices and experts need different features such as prompts and menus versus hot keys, respectively. Informatics will know that informants' initial responses to a particular design will be distinct from those practiced with it. Therefore, both perspectives are important to usability testing and design creation.

Joint Cognitive Systems

Since the early 1980s, Hollnagel and Woods (2005) promoted a concept called cognitive systems engineering. This notion grew from the realization that sociotechnical systems, that is, complex technologies embedded within social system, were increasingly complex, system failures were rampant, and simple HCI models did not account for the interacting issues. Instead of more traditional HCI models, these authors propose a cyclical model called contextual control model or CoCom. The model is based upon users' planning and action with feedback and feedforward loops. Users are part of the whole model and the influence of a context is direct. The distinctions of the CoCom model compared to others include that humans anticipate actions and human behavior is seen as a plan versus single actions. Joint cognitive systems may imply that information is shared or distributed among humans and technology.

The important point for this section is that using a theoretical structure can assist informaticists in thinking about health IT adoption, usability, and the conduct of usability studies. A theoretical structure also provides an organized way of thinking about how users interact with technology. This understanding could then be applied through greater involvement in systems selection, design, implementation, and evaluation.

USABILITY STUDIES

What is a usability study? What kinds of methods are used to conduct a usability test? When do you do one? Do you have to be an expert or a researcher to conduct a usability testing? Generally, usability tests are systematic and structured examinations of the effectiveness, efficiency, or satisfaction of any component or interactions in the HCI framework(s). For instance, a usability study could be done to describe the satisfaction and usability issues with a new computerized provider order entry (CPOE) application targeted to emergency room providers (Zafar, Gibson, Chiang, & Staggers 2010) Another usability test might evaluate the time and errors intensive care nurses make when they use a novel physiological monitoring screen compared to the traditional version. Errors could be analyzed to redesign the application to make it more usable or specific elements in the novel design could be evaluated for intuitiveness and redesigned for clarity. Biomedical informatics students could conduct a type of discount usability study, a heuristic evaluation, on an orders management module from a vendor before it is installed.

Usability studies can be informal or formal, simple or complex, and use a few individuals or a wide range of users. The exciting part of usability is that informaticists can derive rich details about user interface design using only a few participants. Likewise, usability researchers can design sophisticated studies combining usability precepts with traditional, experimental, or mixed methods research designs. The type of usability study an informaticist conducts is dependent upon a number of factors, including when the assessment is targeted within the systems life cycle, the desired outcome of the study, and available resources including time, people, and money.

Usability studies can be done at any point in the expanded systems life cycle (Thompson, Snyder-Halpern, & Staggers 1999), from clarifying users' requirements, to initial design or redesign using paper prototypes or simple computerized applications, to iterative prototype development, system selection, product customization, to evaluating the impact of a system during and after installation. Usability experts recommend usability tests early and often. Studies are divided in this section into basic and more advanced usability tests and include a discussion about usability methods. Informaticists can match these types of studies to the constraints of available resources, the position in an expanded systems life cycle, and outcomes needed.

Basic Usability Tests

In the early 1990s, Nielsen recommended a divergence away from large-scale usability studies to those with reduced numbers of users, early prototypes (even paper), and an evaluation inspection method done by experts. He titled these methods "discount usability methods." (Nielsen 1993, 1994a). These scaled-down studies and inspection methods can be completed by any health informaticist and offer economies of time, effort, and cost. They can be completed at any time during the systems life cycle even well after the technology is installed. Three types of discount usability studies are explained next.

Heuristic Evaluations or Heuristic Inspection Methods A heuristic is a rule of thumb. Heuristic evaluations compare applications against accepted guidelines or published usability principles. The broader term for these kinds of assessments is *usability inspection methods.* Heuristic evaluations can reveal both major and minor usability problems that concentrate on two of the three usability goals: efficiency and effectiveness. Heuristic evaluations are typically completed by usability experts, although any informaticist can complete a heuristic evaluation after modest training.

A number of usability heuristics are available to evaluate applications (Nielsen 1994a; Shneiderman & Plaisant 2005; Zhang, Johnson, Patel, Paige, & Kubose 2003). Guidelines were available as early as the mid-1980s; however, they were lengthy. Shorter and more often-used guidelines include Nielsen's 10 usability heuristics (Nielsen 1994a) with usability severity ratings (Nielsen 1994b) and Shneiderman's "eight golden rules" (Shneiderman & Plaisant 2005). Zhang et al. (2003) combined these into 14 heuristics, called the Nielsen-Shneiderman heuristics, and used them to evaluate medical devices. Once health informaticists understand the gist of each heuristic, they may evaluate a health application or technology for conformance to these rules of thumb. The 14 adapted heuristics and their definitions are in Table 9–1. Zhang and colleagues completed heuristic evaluations on two infusion pumps. They found 192 and 121 heuristic violations, respectively, and categorized them into 89 and 52 usability problems for pumps 1 and 2, respectively. They concluded that pump 1 could contribute to more medical errors.

Simplified Usability Tests Using Early Prototypes The second component of Nielsen's (1993) discount usability techniques includes the use of small numbers of users, typically an early prototype (even paper), and a specific method called "think aloud" protocols. Nielsen advocates the use of qualitative methods early and often during any design or redesign process. He recommends having five users talk aloud or "think aloud" as an observer watches them and records any issues. The process can detect as much as 60–80% of design errors (Nielsen 1994a). Later research confirms that as few as five to eight users are sufficient for most usability tests (Dumas & Fox 2008).

Cognitive Walkthrough This method is a type of usability inspection method or task analysis. It consists of a detailed review of a sequence of real or proposed actions to complete a task in a system (Dix et al. 2004). The method compares a developed user interface design (which is actually the designer's model of the tasks) to the users' understanding or model of the work to be done (Cockton, Woolrych, & Lavery 2008; Johnson et al. 2005) The method uses think aloud techniques to elicit users' thought processes while using an existing product. Users, experts, or even designers step through the actions in an application and check for potential usability

TABLE 9–1   Taxonomy of Usability Measures

Usability Focus	Usability Measures
User behaviors (performance)	Task times (speed, reaction times)
	Percentage of tasks completed
	Number and kinds of errors
	Percentage of tasks completed accurately
	Time, frequency spent in any one option
	Number of hits and amount of time spent on a Web site
	Training time
	Eye tracking
	Facial expressions
	Breadth and depth of application usage in actual settings
	Quality of completed tasks (e.g., quality of decisions)
	Users' comments (think aloud) as they interact with technology
	System setup or installation time, complexity of setup
	Model of tasks and user behaviors
	Description of problems when interacting with an application
User behaviors (cognitive)	Description of or system fit with cognitive information processing
	Retention of application knowledge over time
	Comprehension of system
	Fit with workflow
User behaviors (perceptions)	Usability ratings of products
	Perceptions about any aspect of technology—speed, effectiveness
	Comments during interviews
	Questionnaires and rating responses—workload, satisfaction
User behaviors (physiologic)	Heart rate
	EEG
	Galvanic skin response
	Brain-evoked potentials
User behaviors (perceptions about physiologic reactions)	Perceptions about anxiety, stress
User behavior (motivation)	Willingness to use system
	Enthusiasm
Expert evaluations (performance)	Model predictions for task performance times, learning, ease of understanding
	Observations of users as they use applications in a setting to determine fit with work
Expert evaluations (conformance to guidelines)	Level of adherence to guidelines, design criteria, usability principles (heuristic evaluation)
Expert evaluation (perception)	Ratings of technology, informal or formal comments
Context (organization)	Economic costs (increased full-time equivalent positions for the helpdesk for a new application)

(continued)

Usability Focus	Usability Measures
	Support staff, training staff for application or technology
	Observations about the fit with work design, workflow in departments, organizations, networks of institutions
Combined	Video- and audio-taping users as they interact with an application and capturing keystrokes. Can capture any combination of the above.

TABLE 9–1 (*continued*)

Adapted from Staggers (2001)

problems, such as the ease to learn the system through exploration versus formal training. Four questions are asked, according to Dix et al. (2004):

- Will the users be trying to produce whatever effect the action has?
- Will users be able to notice that the correct action is available?
- Once users find the correct action on the UI, will they know it is the right action for the effect they want?
- After the action is taken, will users understand the feedback they get?

A cognitive walk-through can include videotaping and audiotaping, allowing a structured evaluation for informaticists to record findings and track problems. Categorizing problems can help designers determine priorities for application changes, especially before product release. Informaticists can also better understand users' tasks by identifying specified task goals and actions. Cognitive walkthroughs are often used early in the systems life cycle to identify issues with prototypes and initial designs. They can also be used as an evaluation technique for established systems to identify usability problems and elements critical for technology redesign. For example, Kushniruk and Patel (1995) used cognitive walkthroughs and think aloud protocols to describe physicians' cognitive processing of information as they used information systems. They analyzed videotapes that included details about the physical settings, social context coupled with physicians' thought processes, searched for key words to determine frequencies of behaviors, problems in interpreting a UI, and/or describing tasks. Kushniruk, Patel, & Cimino (1997) have used this method to evaluate how physicians interact with a computer-based patient record as well as to identify UI "hot spots," or major usability problems in systems.

Types of Usability Tests

Usability studies can help determine or clarify users' requirements determination, assess the adequacy, or a design or redesign early in the systems life cycle. The latter uses concepts from Rubin and Chisnell (Rubin 2008).

Determining User Needs and Requirements This type of usability is typically conducted at the beginning of the systems life cycle or redesign cycle to elicit users' characteristics, task activities, work design, interactions among users and tasks in specific environments, and/or particular needs related to the context of interactions. Studies can be conducted with fairly limited resources but, depending upon the complexity of the elements, may consume a more substantial amount of time and effort. Assessments and exploratory work answer these kinds of questions:

- What are basic activities in this context?
- How do users cognitively process information and what information processing can be supported by technology?
- What special considerations should be made for users in this environment?
- What attributes need to be in place for an initial design?

An example is determining requirements for an application to support nurses during change of shift report. This cognitively intense time period includes determining information about the users (novice, expert; oncoming nurse or nurse giving report; whether nurses had the patient before), the interactions (what information is typically exchanged), the technology (paper, mobile, or stationary device), the context (the type of patients usually seen on this unit, the mandates from the organization such as the use of CPOE), and the developmental component (novice or expert clinical documentation user).

A health informaticist could observe nurses giving report, taking notes about the computer functions they access, if any; audiotape report and analyze information typically conveyed, and listen to nurses' responses to questions about whether shift report should be computerized. From this analysis preliminary requirements can be developed. Just such a study is available that analyzed the content and context of shift report for medical and surgical units (Staggers & Jennings 2009).

Exploratory Test This type of usability study is conducted early during development or redesign after very basic or preliminary designs are created. These can be paper based. Few resources would be committed to programming the function to derive the most benefit. The objective of an exploratory test is to evaluate the effectiveness of the emerging design concepts assessing (Rubin 2008):

- Is the basic functionality of value to users?
- Is basic navigation and information flow intuitive?
- How much computer experience does a user need to use this module?

Exploratory tests can be informal and require extensive interaction between informaticists and users. The major usability goal of interest is effectiveness. Informaticists have users perform common tasks with the prototype or step through paper mockups of the application. Informaticists strive to understand *why* users are behaving as they do with the application rather than how quickly the prototype completes a task. The informaticist is interested in finding cognitive disconnects with basic functions, finding missing information or steps, and assessing how easily users understand the task at hand once it is represented by designers.

Assessment Test A second type of usability test is conducted early or midway into the development of an application after the organization and general design are already determined (Rubin 2008). This kind of test can also be economical in terms of time and resources, depending upon the complexity of the design and targeted users. An assessment test assesses lower-level operations of the application, stressing the efficiency goals of the product (versus effectiveness) and how well the task is presented to users. Questions during this test might include:

- How well can users perform selected tasks?
- Are the terms in the system consistent across modules?
- Are operations displayed in a manner that allows quick detection of critical information?

During an assessment test, users perform common tasks with a system with a coded prototype. Some quantitative measures of the interaction, such as error rates, are captured and analyzed. Think aloud methods can also be used to elicit issues. Technology designers use iterative processes, typically three rounds of design, to eliminate major usability issues.

Advanced Usability Tests

Usability studies can be as advanced as an informaticist or researcher wants, again depending upon the desired results, resources, and the location of the design in the systems life cycle. Typical usability studies include validation and comparison tests but can be combined with any suitable research design.

Validation Test Late in the systems design cycle, a validation test can be conducted. Using a more mature product, a validation test assesses how this particular product compares to a predetermined standard, benchmark, or performance measure (Rubin 2008). A second purpose can be to assess how all the modules in a technology application work as an integrated whole. Questions for a validation test might be:

- Can 80% of the users retrieve the correct radiology test within 15 seconds of interacting with the system?
- Does the product adhere to the usability principles defined by Nielsen (1994a) or Dix, Finlay, Abowd, & Beale (1998)?
- Are there major or catastrophic usability issues with an electronic medication administration record?

Validation tests are typically more structured and preclude extensive interactions with informaticists or developers. An informaticist determines the specific benchmarks or standards before the test begins. Methods for a validation test can be similar rigor to those in an experimental study. A validation test could also be useful in a system selection process as decision makers could use it to decide how a new vendor supports critical tasks such as medication barcoding or decision support within CPOE.

Comparison Test Informaticists can conduct comparison studies anywhere in the systems lifecycle. Comparison tests can be used to assess different technologies, or comparing the elegance of designs from two vendors for chemotherapy protocols. Comparison tests can consume time and other resources. The major objective of this usability test is to determine which application or technology is more efficient or which design is more effective (Rubin 2008). The study design can be an informal side-by-side comparison or a classic experimental study. Designs are more easily compared if the designs are substantially different from one another.

Health informaticists can use a combination of types of usability studies and usability methods discussed in the next section.

USABILITY METHODS

Health informaticists may choose from discount usability methods mentioned earlier or others discussed here. A taxonomy of usability elements is presented in Table 9–2. Before choosing particular methods and measures, informaticists will want to determine the focus of a study and available resources, and match these to feasible measures. As may be seen, the taxonomy includes measures from three perspectives: users, experts, and organizations. Informaticists can choose more than one measure to give depth to a study and its results; however, one indicator may be adequate for some usability assessments, for example, the fit of a new physiological monitoring design with job design or workflow among staff in a same day surgery unit. A sampling of other common usability methods is presented here with examples of their use in health informatics.

Task Analysis

This method is one of the most well-known collections of techniques in HCI and usability. The generic term *task analysis* can mean a focus on cognitive processes, observable user actions, or the interaction of a user(s) with a system. Task analysis is a systematic method to understand what users are doing or required to do with technology. It focuses on tasks and behavioral actions between users and computers (Sweeney et al. 1993). Conceptually, task analysis is the process of learning about and documenting how ordinary users complete actions in a specific context (Hackos & Redish 1998; Nielsen 1993). It involves interviewing and observing users at

TABLE 9–2 Sample of Data Output From Task Analyses	
Type of Task Analysis Output	**Description**
Profiles of users	Short narrative, visual descriptions, and/or summaries about the characteristics of users
Workflow diagrams	A flow diagram of tasks or cognitive processes performed by users
Task sequences or hierarchies	Lists of tasks order by sequence or arranged to show interrelationships
Task scenarios	Detailed descriptions of events or incidents including how users handle situations
Affinity diagrams	Bottom-up groupings of facts and issues about users, tasks, and environments to generate design ideas
Video and audiotape highlights	Clips that illustrate particular observations about users and tasks in a context

Adapted from Staggers, N. (2001). Human-computer interaction in health care organizations. In S. Englebardt & R. Nelson (Eds.), *Health care informatics: An interdisciplinary approach* (pp. 321–345). St. Louis: Mosby.

their actual work sites. Task analysis is particularly useful for determining the goals users have when they interact with technology.

After observations and interviews, informaticists record user actions in flowcharts that include task descriptions. Detailed references are available for performing task analyses (Hackos & Redish 1998). Sample output from task analyses is listed in Table 9–3. For example, informaticists can videotape users as they interact with a system using Morae software, asking users to perform specific tasks and talk aloud about what they are doing.

Task analyses are helpful in identifying task completeness, the correct or existing incorrect sequencing of tasks, accuracy of actions, error recovery, and task allocation between humans and computers. Task analysis can be used throughout the systems life cycle to determine user requirements for design, redesign or to identify usability issues for complex events such as determining who in an ambulatory clinic is responsible to attend to alerts that go to various providers, to assess the match of a prototype to users' methods of work, or to determine the impact of a system on workflow.

Often task analysis is used early in the systems life cycle. For example, Staggers and Kobus videotaped nurses as they interacted with an existing inpatient clinical information system electronic medication administration records. Then, they observed nurses' actual medication management tasks as they performed them in a variety of acute care units (Staggers, Kobus, & Brown 2007). The researchers created a taskflow diagram of medication tasks and also delineated deficiencies with the current application. A novel electronic medical administration record was created using the task analysis and evaluated for user satisfaction.

Think Aloud Protocols

A third common method in usability and HCI is a think aloud protocol. In this technique, users talk aloud as they interact with an application. An informaticist determines a specific set of tasks for users to complete. An evaluator observes and records actions using one of the following: videotaping, audiotaping, paper notes, automatic capture of keystrokes, and/or user and evaluator paper and pencil diaries or logs (Dix et al. 2004). The result is a record of actions or a protocol which is then analyzed.

This method is commonly used in the design, redesign, development, or evaluation of applications at any time in the systems life cycle. It allows a detailed examination of the specified tasks, in particular to uncover major effectiveness issues. Analyzing the products from this method can be very time-consuming. Time estimates can be as much as a 10:1 ratio, analysis time to observation time, respectively. Think aloud methods may be used in conjunction with other usability methods as was seen earlier.

TABLE 9–3 Nielsen-Shneiderman Heuristics and Severity Rating Scheme

Heuristic Category	Definition
Consistency and standards	Consistency across all aspects of the technology—methods of navigation, messages and actions, meaning of buttons, terms, and icons. Congruence with known screen design principles for color, screen layout. Consistency with International Standards Organization usability guidelines
Visibility of system state	Users understand what the system is doing and what they can do with the technology by messages, information, displays
Match between system and world	The technology matches the way users think using appropriate information flow, typical options users need, expected actions by the system
Minimalist	No superfluous information. System and screen design targeted to primary information users need. Use of progressive disclosure to display details of a category of information only when needed. The exception can be designs for expert users where screen density is preferred (Staggers 1993)
Minimize memory load	Minimizing the amount of information, tasks users have to memorize to adequately use the technology. Use of sample formats for data input
Informative feedback	The technology provides prompt and useful feedback about users' interactions and actions
Flexibility and efficiency	The ability to tailor and customize to suit individuals' needs. Includes novice and expert capabilities, for example, type-ahead, hot-links
Good error messages	Tell users what error occurred and how users can recover from the error. Not abstract or general such as "Action not allowed." Need to be precise and polite and not blame the user
Prevent errors	Catastrophic errors must to be prevented, for example, medication orders well above the usual range, inadvertently deleting an order set, delivering a radiation dose with the device leaves wide open
Clear closure	Users should know when a task is completed and all information is accepted. Displays should include progress toward the completion versus multiple bars showing progress toward "100%"
Reversible actions	Whenever possible, actions and interactions should be able to be undone (within legal limits in electronic health records)
Use the users' language	The technology uses language and terms the targeted users can comprehend and expect. Health terms are used appropriately
Users in control	Users initiate actions versus having the perception that the technology is in control. Avoid surprising actions, ending up in unexpected places, loud sounds with errors
Help and documentation	Provide help for users within the context the actions occur (context-sensitive). Embed help functions throughout the application.

Severity Scale Rating Element	Definition
0—No usability problem	No need to correct the issue
1—Cosmetic problem	Correct the issue only if extra time and fiscal resources allow, lowest priority
2—Minor problem	Annoying issue with minor impact. Low priority to fix
3—Major usability problem	Issue with major impact to use or training or both. Important to fix. Considerations are the numbers and kinds of users impacted by a persistent problem. Example: Orders on a patient summary are truncated when printed
4 – Usability catastrophe	Severe issue that must be corrected before product release. Example: An IV pump button turns off the whole pump versus just one intended channel

Adapted from Zhang, J., Johnson, T. R., Patel, V. L., Paige, D. L., & Kubose, T. (2003, February–April). Using usability heuristics to evaluate patient safety of medical devices. *Journal of Biomedical Informatics*, 36(1–2), 23–30.

Usability Questionnaires

Informaticists can have users interact with technology and then completed a questionnaire that addresses the system's perceived usability. At least three examples of this type of questionnaire are available: the QUIS or Questionnaire for User Interaction Satisfaction (Norman, Shneiderman, Harper, & Slaughter 1998), the Purdue Usability Testing Questionnaire (Lin, Choong, & Salvendy 1997), and the SUMI (Software Usability Measurement Inventory) (Kirakowski & Corbett 1993). The QUIS addresses users' perceptions of the system for areas such as overall reaction, terminology, screen layout, learning, system capabilities, and other subscales such as multimedia applications. The instrument demonstrates adequate psychometric evaluations for reliability and constructs validity. QUIS subscales can be mixed and matched to fit the application at hand. In several studies, nurses completed the QUIS in 5–10 minutes (Staggers et al. 2007; Staggers & Kobus 2007).

The Purdue Usability Questionnaire also can evaluate usability of a system. Targeted to usability experts, the questionnaire has 100 open-ended questions about how features adhere to accepted guidelines, for example, how the data display is or is not consistent with user conventions. Informaticists would need to be very familiar with existing design guidelines before use. Reliability and validity assessments of the questionnaire are not reported.

Little information is published about the SUMI, including its assessed reliability and validity. The instrument has three components: an overall assessment, a usability profile, and an item consensus analysis. The usability profile examines areas such as efficiency, helpfulness, control, and learnability. The consensus component addresses adherence to well-known design alternatives such as categorical ordering of data in a simple search task.

Focused Ethnographies

Ethnography is a method from anthropology and sociology that includes fieldwork and analysis of people in cultural, social settings. Researchers describe the person of interest's point of view focusing on experience and interactions in social settings rather than the actions themselves (Dourish & Button 1998). A researcher is an observer and not a participant in the society. Detailed descriptions are generated with an emphasis on social relationships and their impact on work. In HCI and elsewhere, ethnographies can be extensive descriptions of users' experiences, from their point of view, in their settings.

Ethnographies have become important in HCI to describe the impact of new, complex applications (Dix et al. 2004). Joan Ash and colleagues have used this method extensively in their work about the impacts of CPOE in acute care facilities in the United States (Ash et al. 2009; Ash, Sittig, Dykstra, Campbell, et al. 2007; Ash, Sittig, Dykstra, Guappone, Carpenter, & Seshadri 2007; Ash, Sittig, Poon, et al. 2007). The authors used qualitative research techniques such as interviews, focus groups, and observation. They found numerous unintended consequences of CPOE to include new work/more work, workflow issues, system demands, communication, emotions, and dependence on the technology. By being immersed in the setting, Ash and colleagues could inductively derive findings and impacts on key persons and their relationships.

STEPS IN CONDUCTING USABILITY ASSESSMENTS

As a health informaticist, you will likely be expected to conduct usability tests. Step-by-step guides are available for informaticists (HIMSS 2009; Rubin 2008a). By applying material from the HCI framework(s), usability goals, types of usability tests indicators, and methods, health informaticists can conduct worthwhile usability tests. The process may be divided into five steps (Staggers 2001):

- **Define a Clear Purpose.** The specific purpose will guide informaticists in determining the type of study, the details, and methods required. Is the purpose to define user requirements for clinical documentation for a team of rehabilitation members in a busy rehabilitation hospital? Select a vendor's system to support provider activities in an ambulatory setting? Evaluate the effectiveness of a newly designed telehealth system? Each of these purposes is distinct and will point to selecting differing designs and methods for completion. For example, if the purpose relates to an assessment of a redesign of a CPOE module for the emergency department providers, an exploratory test may be indicated.

- **Assess Constraints.** Informaticists are always faced with study constraints—time, resources, availability of the software to be evaluated, availability of other equipments such as video cameras, testing labs, or users themselves, especially if the users are physicians or other specialists. These kinds of constraints may drive a section or even the whole usability test. For example, if the informaticist's goal is to evaluate an application to support transplant surgeons, these busy surgeons may not be willing to spend time in a usability test lasting more than 30 minutes.

- **Use an HCI Framework to Refine Each Component.** Assess each component of the HCI framework and match to the purpose of the study. Which users are most appropriate? What are representative, common tasks? What element of the tasks is of interest? What information needs to be exchanged, for example, between physicians and nurses during a phone call about a patient issue? What technology characteristics are needed and which actions? What setting or context? Will a naturalistic setting help determine exactly how an application will be used or will a laboratory be used to control typical interruptions? What is a representative time in the developmental trajectory or is there more than one? If the informaticists are doing a comparison study using a new and old version, how will equivalent practice be assured? The latter is a typical mistake for new usability testers. Be sure to examine this component carefully to ensure a valid comparison. The most important point is to remember that multiple tests are needed for each product being designed or redesigned.

- **Emphasize Components of Interest.** Informaticists will want to control some framework components and emphasize others for testing. With experimental or other more rigorous tests, informaticists will want to ensure that you are measuring only what you want to know in a particular test. For example, if the purpose is to compare the efficiency (speed) of user interface for robotic-assisted surgeries, informaticists will want to control for equivalency consistency in computer processors, type of users, and context. In other usability studies, informaticists may wish to test a whole team of users in the complexity of their real environments, for instance, to determine the time constraints for clinical documentation during and after a code in an acute care unit.

- **Match Methods to the Purpose, Constraints, and Framework Assessment.** Selecting methods occurs after the previous steps. Early in the systems life cycle or when little is understood about why users declined to use a module design for perioperative care, a method that produces rich results should be selected—a think aloud protocol, naturalistic observation with clarifying questions, or a cognitive walkthrough, for example. On the other hand, if the purpose of the usability study is to validate a near-final design for a personal health record, then completing a validation test using interaction task times and errors with patients may be more appropriate. Once the method is selected, you are ready to put all these pieces into action and conduct your study. The following examples show usability studies for a heuristic evaluation, requirements determination, and a comparison usability test.

Example of a Heuristic Evaluation

The purpose of this usability study was to determine whether a CPOE module for the emergency room conformed to the Nielsen-Shneiderman guidelines. The constraints for this study were the lack of funding and a short timeframe. The informaticist chose the heuristic evaluation method because of the constraints and because this descriptive study would add to the literature as no published evaluations were available for this vendor's system. Three informaticists trained in this usability inspection method completed common tasks as they spoke with emergency department physicians. The informaticists completed their assessments separately and met to resolve any differences. The usability violations were rated in severity and a lengthy list of usability issues was created.

Example of a Requirements Determination Usability Study

Staggers and Jennings completed a study to begin determining requirements to support nurses during change of shift report, a highly complex and cognitively intensive period where nurses going off-shift synthesize information about patients and communicate it to nurses coming on shift (Staggers, Guo, & Blaz 2009; Staggers & Jennings 2009). Constraints included having a small amount of research funding. Nurses used no technology, save a tape recorder, as part of shift report. More important, little research was done on shift report and none since EHRs, so little was known about modern shift report. Thus, the authors chose the type of study (requirements determination) and methods (qualitative) to obtain rich details about the process. The HCI framework guided the authors to think about requirements for different nurses—experts and novices, types of units, types of nurse such as per diem. The task component guided thoughts about different methods of giving report such as taped, face-to-face, and bedside reports. The authors sampled widely to assure various nurses were included in the study and that methods of report were varied. The researchers completed a focused ethnography on seven medical surgical units in three different acute care facilities (the context). The authors observed change of shift report, audiotaped 38 nurses, and took field notes including whether nurses interacted with the existing EHR in the facilities. The audiotapes were transcribed to determine the content and context of shift report. Four themes of information content emerged, numerous observations were made about the organization and flow of information, and the researchers were able to derive detailed information about requirements for computerized support for change of shift activities.

Example of a Comparison Study

The purpose of this study was to determine whether a new user interface for orders management was different from an older interface for performance times, errors, and user satisfaction (Staggers & Kobus 2000). The major constraint in this study was the availability of nurses at the tertiary care center. The tasks and interactions were planned to minimize the amount of time, 45 minutes, that nurses would be away from their patient care units. All data collection had to be scheduled, coordinated, and completed during a 2-week period before summer vacations began.

The informaticists used a HCI framework, similar to the HCI Health framework, to guide elements in the study. Identical computers were used to test both interfaces. The computers were disconnected from the local area network to assure that system network loads did not affect processing times. Tasks were "real-world" nursing orders that any nurse could understand, and the tasks were the same across designs. Only clinical nurses were included in the study. The environment was a computer training room, a quiet room away from patient care units and distractions. The developmental trajectory was considered in this study to assure that results were not impacted by practice time. Therefore, 40 tasks for each interface allowed nurses to become practiced with each user interface. The number of tasks was determined in pilot work.

Tasks, keystrokes, and errors were captured by computer. The QUIS was administered after each interface. Each nurse interacted with both interfaces, but the order they were presented was randomized. The results showed a significant difference for all three variables—performance speed, errors, and user satisfaction.

FUTURE DIRECTIONS

The recent interest in usability will provide interesting work for health informaticists in the future. Several trends are discussed: expanding interest in usability, increased complexity of systems, ubiquitous computing, and computer-supported cooperative work. Clearly, the current interest in usability will expand. Vendors' products can benefit from structured usability testing, redesign, and public usability ratings. The current funding toward EHR fielding is unprecedented. Usability issues will either be forced to the surface by health IT users or be designed/redesigned into submission in the future. Usability is now deemed critical enough that its expansion in the future is imperative.

Informaticists will be faced with even more complexity in systems design and concomitant usability issues. New users, such as increasing numbers of health consumers and patients and groups of users, will need to be accommodated. New types of information—in particular genetic, nanomaterials—will create layers of complexity beyond current sociotechnical system issues.

As technology disappears into everyday objects, ubiquitous computing may become a reality. Then, perhaps HCI will become just "HI" because the computer and its display will effectively be invisible. Usability issues will still likely exist and health informaticists will be challenged to work with less visible user interfaces.

Computer-supported cooperative work deserves more attention in the future. This area focuses on people as they act in their normal lives, including work lives. Support of tasks becomes intertwined with patterns of group behaviors as reflected by social or situational contexts. Examples here include the growth of groups of people as they act in virtual worlds, create blogs, and work in virtual work teams. Designing for usability is being considered only now; the reality is in the future.

CASE STUDY EXERCISE

Your facility has a history of adopting technology and information systems that are not well received or used by the staff. It was recently determined that a major effort would be made to acquire a new clinical information system. In your role as informatics nurse what actions would you take to improve user acceptance of this new system?

SUMMARY

- Current usability issues in health information technology (IT) applications include new errors in health care, uneven adoption of clinical applications, high costs associated with unusable systems, reduced provider productivity, and unintended consequences.
- The term *usability* is often used interchangeably with *human–computer interaction (HCI)*. More formally, usability is the extent to which a product can be used by specific users in a specific context to achieve predefined goals with effectiveness, efficiency, and satisfaction.
- Usability and HCI goals include the creation of advanced technology to improve decision making and the making of technology more useful, safe, satisfying, and efficient to use.
- Three axioms of usability are an early and central focus on users in the design and development of systems, iterative design of applications, and systematic usability measures.
- HCI frameworks include the major elements of patients, providers, technology, context, tasks, information, interactions, and a developmental trajectory.
- Usability tests are systematic and structured examinations of the effectiveness, efficiency, or satisfaction of any component or interactions in the HCI framework(s).
- Usability studies can be done at any point, although experts recommend they be done early and often. Informaticists can match the type of study to the constraints of available resources.

- Any informaticist can learn and conduct discount usability tests using usability inspection techniques, small-scale prototypes, and reduced numbers of users.
- Usability tests vary from scaled-down studies and methods that offer economies of time, effort, and cost to more detailed heuristic evaluations which compare applications against accepted guidelines or published usability principles.
- Common usability methods include task analysis, think aloud protocols, cognitive walkthroughs, focused ethnographies, and usability questionnaires.
- Five steps for planning and conducting usability tests include:
  - Definition of purpose
  - Assessment of constraints
  - Use of an HCI framework to refine each component
  - Emphasis on components of interest
  - Matching methods to the purpose, constraints, and framework assessment
- Expanding interest in usability, increased complexity of systems, ubiquitous computing, and computer-supported cooperative work ensure a role for informaticists in this area.

REFERENCES

Ammenwerth, E., Iller, C., & Mahler, C. (2006). IT-adoption and the interaction of task, technology and individuals: A FIT framework and a case study. *Biomed Central, 3,* 1–13.

Armijo, D., McDonnell, C., & Werner, K. (2009). *Electronic health record usability: Interface design considerations.* Rockville, MD: Agency for Healthcare Research and Quality.

Ash, J. S., Sittig, D. F., Dykstra, R., Campbell, E., & Guappone, K. (2007). Exploring the unintended consequences of computerized physician order entry. *Studies in Health Technology and Informatics, 129*(Pt. 1), 198–202.

Ash, J. S., Sittig, D. F., Dykstra, R., Campbell, E., & Guappone, K. (2009, April). The unintended consequences of computerized provider order entry: Findings from a mixed methods exploration. *International Journal of Medical Informatics, 78*(Suppl. 1), S69–S76.

Ash, J. S., Sittig, D. F., Dykstra, R. H., Guappone, K., Carpenter, J. D., & Seshadri, V. (2007, June). Categorizing the unintended sociotechnical consequences of computerized provider order entry. *International Journal of Medical Informatics, 76*(Suppl. 1), S21–S27.

Ash, J. S., Sittig, D. F., Poon, E. G., Guappone, K., Campbell, E., & Dykstra, R. H. (2007, July–August). The extent and importance of unintended consequences related to computerized provider order entry. *Journal of the American Medical Informatics Association, 14*(4), 415–423.

Beuscart-Zephir, M., Brender, J., Beuscart, R., & Menager-Depreiester, I. (1997). Cognitive evaluation: How to assess the usability of information technology in healthcare. *Computer Methods and Programs in Biomedicine, 54*(1–2), 19–38.

Cockton, G., Woolrych, A., & Lavery, D. (2008). Inspection-based evaluations. In A. Sears & J. Jacko (Eds.), *The human-computer interaction handbook: Fundamentals, evolving technologies and emerging application* (2nd ed., pp. 1172–1188). New York: Lawrence Erlbaum.

Despont-Gros, C., Mueller, H., & Lovis, C. (2005, June). Evaluating user interactions with clinical information systems: A model based on human-computer interaction models. *Journal of Biomedical Informatics, 38*(3), 244–255.

Dix, A., Finlay, J., Abowd, G., & Beale, R. (1998). *Human-computer interaction.* London: Prentice Hall Europe.

Dix, A., Finlay, J. E., Abowd, G. D., & Beale, R. (2004). *Human-computer interaction* (3rd ed.). Essex, England: Prentice Hall.

Dourish, P., & Button, G. (1998). On "technomethodology": Foundational relationships between ethnomethodology and system design. *Human-Computer Interaction, 13*(4), 395–432.

Dumas, J. S., & Fox, J. E. (2008). Usability testing: Current practice and future directions. In A. Sears & J. Jacko (Eds.), *The human-computer interaction handbook: Fundamentals, evolving technologies and emerging applications* (2nd ed.). New York: Lawrence Erlbaum.

Gould, J. D., & Lewis, C. (1985). Designing for usability: Key principles and what designers think. *Communications of the ACM, 28*(3), 300–311.

Graham, T. A., Kushniruk, A. W., Bullard, M. J., Holroyd, B. R., Meurer, D. P., & Rowe, B. H. (2008). How usability of a web-based clinical decision support system has the potential to contribute to adverse medical events. *AMIA Annual Symposium Proceedings,* 2008, 257–261.

Hackos, J. T., & Redish, J. C. (1998). *User and task analysis for interface design.* New York: John Wiley & Sons.

HIMSS. (2009). *Defining and testing EMR usability: Principles and proposed methods of EMR usability evaluation and rating.* Retrieved from http://www.himss.org/content/files/HIMSS_DefiningandTestingEMRUsability.pdf

Hollnagel, E., & Woods, D. (2005). *Joint cognitive systems: Foundations of cognitive systems engineering.* Boca Raton, FL: Taylor & Francis Group.

Jha, A. K., DesRoches, C. M., Campbell, E. G., Donelan, K., Rao, S. R., Ferris, T. G., . . . Blumenthal, D. (2009). Use of electronic health records in U.S. Hospitals. *New England Journal of Medicine, 360*(16), 1628–1638.

Johnson, C. M., Johnson, T. R., & Zhang, J. (2005). A user-centered framework for redesigning health care interfaces. *Journal of Biomedical Informatics, 38*(1), 75–87.

Karat, C. (1990). *Cost-benefit analysis of usability engineering techniques.* Paper presented at the *Proceedings of the Human Factors Society 34th Annual Meeting,* Orlando, FL.

Kirakowski, J., & Corbett, M. (1993). SUMI: The software measurement inventory. *British Journal of Educational Technology, 24*(3), 210–212.

Kuehn, B. M. (2009, March 4). IT vulnerabilities highlighted by errors, malfunctions at veterans' medical centers. *JAMA, 301*(9), 919–920.

Kushniruk, A., & Patel, V. (1995). *Cognitive computer-based video analysis: Its application in assessing the usability of medical systems.* Paper presented at the MEDINFO 95, Vancouver, Canada.

Kushniruk, A., Patel, V., & Cimino, J. (1997). Usability testing in medical informatics: Cognitive approaches to evaluation of information and user interfaces. *Conference Proceedings from the American Medical Informatics Association Annual Symposium,* pp. 218–222.

Langendoen, D., & Costa, D. (1994). *The home office computer handbook.* New York: Windcrest/McGraw-Hill.

Lin, H., Choong, Y., & Salvendy, G. (1997). A proposed index of usability: A method for comparing the relative usability of different software systems. *Behaviour and Information Technology, 16*(4/5), 267–278.

Lindgaard, G. (1992). Evaluating user interfaces in context: The ecological value of time-and-motion studies. *Applied Ergonomics, 23*(2), 105–114.

Mantovani, G. (1996). Social context in HUCI: A new framework for mental models, cooperation, and communication. *Cognitive Science, 20*(2), 237–269.

Nielsen, J. (1993). *Usability engineering.* Cambridge, MA: AP Professional.

Nielsen, J. (1994a). Heuristic evaluation. In J. Nielsen & R. L. Mack (Eds.), *Usability inspection methods* (pp. 25–64). New York: John Wiley & Sons.

Nielsen, J. (1994b). *Severity ratings for usability problems.* Retrieved from http://www.useit.com/papers/heuristic/severityrating.html

Nielsen, J. (2008). *Usability ROI declining, but still strong.* Retrieved from http://www.useit.com/alertbox/roi.html

Norman, D. (1988). *The psychology of everyday things.* New York: Basic Books.

Norman, K., Shneiderman, B., Harper, B., & Slaughter, L. (1998). *Questionnaire for user interaction satisfaction, version 7.0.* Retrieved from http://lap.umd.edu/quis/

Philpott, T. (2006, April 7). Military access drops. *Today in the Military.* Retrieved from http://www.military.com/features/0,15240,93457,00.html

Philpott, T. (2009, March 28). Doctors see bigger role in electronic health record reform. *Stars and Stripes.* Retrieved from http://www.stripes.com/news/military-update-doctors-see-bigger-role-in-electronic-health-record-reform-1.89653

Rubin, J. (2008). *Handbook of usability testing*. New York: John Wiley & Sons.

Rubin, J., & Chisnell, D. (2008). *Handbook of usability testing: How to plan, design and conduct effective tests* (2nd ed.). New York: John Wiley & Sons.

Shneiderman, B., & Plaisant, K. (2005). *Designing the user interface: Strategies for effective human-computer interaction* (4th ed.). Boston, MA: Pearson/Addison-Wesley.

Staggers, N. (1993). The impact of screen density on clinical nurses' computer task performance and subjective screen satisfaction. *International Journal of Man-Machine Studies, 39*, 775–792.

Staggers, N. (2001). Human-computer interaction in health care organizations. In S. Englebardt & R. Nelson (Eds.), *Health care informatics: An interdisciplinary approach* (pp. 321–345). St. Louis: Mosby.

Staggers, N. (2003, August). Human factors: Imperative concepts for information systems in critical care. *AACN Clinical Issues, 14*(3), 310–319, quiz 397–318.

Staggers, N., Guo, J.-W., & Blaz, J. (2009). *Clinical system design considerations for critical handoffs.* Paper presented at HCI International 2009, San Diego, CA.

Staggers, N., & Jennings, B. M. (2009, September). The content and context of change of shift report on medical and surgical units. *Journal of Nursing Administration, 39*(9), 393–398.

Staggers, N., & Kobus, D. (2000, March–April). Comparing response time, errors, and satisfaction between text-based and graphical user interfaces during nursing order tasks. *Journal of the American Medical Informatics Association, 7*(2), 164–176.

Staggers, N., Kobus, D., & Brown, C. (2007, March–April). Nurses' evaluations of a novel design for an electronic medication administration record. *Computers, Informatics, Nursing, 25*(2), 67–75.

Staggers, N., & Parks, P. L. (1992). Collaboration between unlikely disciplines in the creation of a conceptual framework for nurse-computer interactions. *Proceedings of the Annual Symposium on Computer Application in Medical Care,* 661–665.

Staggers, N., & Parks, P. L. (1993, November–December). Description and initial applications of the staggers & parks nurse-computer interaction framework. *Computers in Nursing, 11*(6), 282–290.

Stead, W., & Linn, H. S. (2009). *Computational technology for effective health care: Immediate steps and strategic directions.* Washington, DC: National Academies Press.

Sweeney, M., Maguire, M., & Shackel, B. (1993). Evaluating user-computer interaction: A framework. *International Journal of Man-Machine Studies, 38*(4), 689–711.

Thompson, C. B., Snyder-Halpern, R., & Staggers, N. (1999, September–October). Analysis, processes, and techniques. Case study. *Computers in Nursing, 17*(5), 203–206.

Yusof, M. M., Kuljis, J., Papazafeiropoulou, A., & Stergioulas, L. K. (2008, June). An evaluation framework for health information systems: Human, organization and technology-fit factors (HOT-fit). *International Journal of Medical Informatics, 77*(6), 386–398.

Yusof, M. M., Stergioulas, L., & Zugic, J. (2007). Health information systems adoption: Findings from a systematic review. *Studies in Health Technology and Informatics, 129*(Pt. 1), 262–266.

Zafar, N., Gibson, B., Chiang, Y., & Staggers, N. (2010). *A usability evaluation of Cerner FirstNet at the University of Utah Hospital.* A paper presented at the NLM Informatics Training Conference 2010 University of Colorado Anschutz Medical Campus, June 15–16, 2010.

Zhang, J., & Butler, K. A. (2007). *UFuRT: A work-centered framework and process for design and evaluation of information systems.* Paper presented at the Proceedings of HCI International 2007, Beijing, China.

Zhang, J., Johnson, T. R., Patel, V. L., Paige, D. L., & Kubose, T. (2003, February–April). Using usability heuristics to evaluate patient safety of medical devices. *Journal of Biomedical Informatics, 36*(1–2), 23–30.

CHAPTER 10

System Implementation and Maintenance

After completing this chapter, you should be able to:

1. Discuss the significance of change in a culture.

2. Understand the barriers to implementation.

3. Describe how implementation committee members are selected.

4. Discuss the importance of establishing a project timeline or schedule.

5. Explain the differences between the test, training, and production environments.

6. List the decisions that must be addressed when performing an analysis of hardware requirements.

7. Review the issues that must be addressed when developing procedures and documentation for users.

8. Discuss the factors that contribute to effective training.

9. Discuss the "go-live" process and identify the components involved in planning for it.

10. Recognize several common implementation pitfalls.

11. Name several common forms of user feedback and support.

12. Explain the significance of providing ongoing system and technical maintenance.

13. Recognize that the life cycle of an information system is an ongoing cyclical process.

Chapter 8 discussed the first two phases of the life cycle of an information system. This chapter explores system implementation and maintenance, which make up the third and fourth phases.

SYSTEM IMPLEMENTATION

Changing a Culture

> If change does not produce a notable resistance, then the change is probably not big enough.
> (Morjikian, Kimball, & Joynt 2007, 403)

Having said that, the only thing we can be certain of is that change is constant. There is an aspect of change that we can talk about and that is the Kotter Model of change. Kotter (1995) was the guru of leadership and change management, and along with Cohen gathered information from 100 interviews from employees in organizations that were undergoing internal change. They found that the key to helping people change their behavior is to help them feel differently; in other words, appeal to their emotions. When discussing implementation strategies, it is important to remember not only do training guidelines need to be developed, but training that includes some emotional emphasis relating to patient care to really drive home the reason for a whole new process of care delivery. To begin this process of change it is important to realize that there will be obstacles that may impede the progress of the strategies. Clinical operation disruption is minimized via the identification of the processes and their changes which are then included in user training and implemented by the management team. The implementation plan should include a strategy to support people and process changes (Wolf, Greenhouse, Diamond, Fera, & McCormick 2006).

Form an Implementation Committee

The implementation phase is planned prior to the purchase of the system. Once the organization has purchased the information system, the implementation phase continues. A project leader is identified and a team of hospital staff is selected to support the project as a working committee. An important factor to consider is choosing a registered nurse to serve as the project leader. As a nurse overseeing the implementation, aspects relevant to all disciplines can be addressed. Often it is the nurse leader who has the clear vision necessary to make changes relevant to patient care and provide insight into the nursing process and coordinate the plan into a feasible process. This leader must have the ability to maintain a strong relationship with all members of the implementation team. If it is not possible to utilize a nurse in this position, the chief information officer, strategy officer, an informatics specialist, project manager, or a consultant experienced in this area may serve in this capacity. It is important, however, that this person be involved in the entire selection and implementation process and possess strong leadership and communication skills. This ensures that the project leader has a firm understanding of the vision, goals, and expectations for the system. The leader needs to be someone who is trained, skilled, and experienced in managing complex information technology (IT) projects with overlapping timelines and multiple stakeholders. He or she will be the engineer who keeps the train on track and anticipates the stops ahead (Adler 2007). One of the keys to ensuring the product meets the needs of the end users is to utilize not only nurse leaders, but bedside staff who actually do the day-to-day patient care and documentation. Only after reviewing their needs can a system be fully implemented efficiently. Recruiting efforts should focus on people who display the characteristics that support effective group dynamics and represent all key stakeholders. In addition, the project leader should facilitate the development of effective group dynamics. Any effort that involves the implementation of a system for nurses or that will be used by nurses should include an informatics nurse specialist or informatics nurse, as these individuals are uniquely qualified to communicate the needs of clinical staff to information services personnel and have a working knowledge of

---

BOX 10–1   Characteristics of a Successful Implementation Committee

Characteristics of Individual Members

- Communicates openly
- Uses time and talents efficiently
- Performs effectively and produces results
- Welcomes challenges
- Cooperates rather than competes
- Is able to work independently with minimal guidance
- Provides suggestions and feedback from peers on current process
- Has the respect of peers and co-workers
- Buys into the need for the new process
- Possesses high degree of critical thinking skills and able to "think outside the box"

Group Characteristics

- Works toward a common goal
- Encourages members to teach and learn from one another
- Develops its members' skills
- Builds morale internally
- Resolves conflicts effectively
- Shows pride in its accomplishments
- Enhances diversity of its members
- Represents all disciplines in the decision-making process

---

regulatory and system requirements, strategic plans, and budgetary constraints. The informatics nurse specialist and informatics nurses are qualified to identify current problems or issues and help to choose or develop a solution. Organizations that have nursing informatics professionals are more likely to include a representative from the nursing team in decisions involving information technology selection and implementation (CDW Healthcare 2007). The committee members and organizational issues are every bit as important as the technology itself when implementing a new system. Despite the qualifications of the committee members, the group may not select the best system or create the best implementation plan (Summers & Jerard 2006). Box 10–1 lists some of the characteristics of a successful implementation committee.

Plan the Installation

The initial work of the implementation committee is to develop a comprehensive project plan or timeline, scheduling all of the critical elements for implementation. This plan should address what tasks are necessary, the scope of each task, who is responsible for accomplishing each element, start and completion dates, necessary resources, and constraints. At this point in the project, it is necessary for the project leader to set goals and realistic expectations for both individuals and the group. An excellent way to keep everyone up to date on the current state of the project is to utilize a large wall to put up a "paper timeline." A visual plan helps keep everyone on track and understanding where others are in the project. This also allows the project leader accessibility to the progress at a quick glance. Figure 10–1 shows a sample template for a system implementation.

Milestone	Person Responsible	Estimated Start Date	Completion Date
PHASE 5: **SYSTEM IMPLEMENTATION**			
Develop implementation committee			
Analyze customization requirements			
Perform system modifications and customizations			
Analyze hardware requirements			
Develop procedures and user guides			
System and integrated testing			
Provide user training			
Go-live conversion preparation and backloading			
Go-live event			

FIGURE 10–1 • Sample template for a system implementation timeline

Questions asked at this stage focus on the background of the project, its goals and sponsor, key stakeholders, benefits, and budget. Clear definition of this phase of the project requires time, energy, and lots of good communication. Failure to adequately address this phase jeopardizes successful implementation. Project planning software may be helpful in developing the project timeline or schedule and a hierarchical arrangement of all specific tasks. This type of plan is referred to as a **work breakdown structure (WBS)**. After the project is defined, it is imperative to work on team building, control and execution, and review and exit planning. Inadequate attention to these phases can also jeopardize implementation success.

The committee members should first become familiar with the information system they will be implementing. This can be accomplished in several ways. The vendor can provide on-site training, hospital staff can receive training at the vendor's corporate centers, or third-party consultants may be hired. Vendor training should provide the opportunity to continue to update the skills of employees and to subsequently use them as a resource throughout the implementation process. Once committee members have acquired an understanding of how the system functions, they will have the knowledge needed to analyze the base system as delivered from the vendor. Ideally the following issues are addressed during system selection but should be considered by the implementation committee before the system is installed in the event that clarification or changes are necessary:

- *The technology.* It is important to consider whether the technology that is used is current and can be upgraded easily or is already obsolete. It is also necessary to have a good match between the system and the needs of the area.
- *Vendor standing.* Committee members need to consider vendor history of similar projects as well as financial solvency of the vendor for long-term service and dialog with other customers to determine their implementation issues and resolution.

- *Vendor compliance with regulatory requirements.* System customization for regulatory compliance can be expensive. It is essential to determine vendor responsibility for federal and state regulatory compliance.
- *Integration with other systems.* It is important to establish how easily the selected system exchanges information with other major systems such as medical records and financial systems. One important detail to keep in mind is improved technology and increased user knowledge. As one system is implemented, the needs of the end user become more pronounced and the users are constantly challenging the system to do more. This increased desire for new and improved functionality makes it paramount to choose a system that can be easily integrated with other systems.
- *Use for different types of patient accounts.* Does the system work equally well for inpatient, outpatient, and emergency care encounters? An important aspect to consider when planning the implementation is the ease with which a product can be used in various departments throughout the hospital. This is why it is extremely important to include all disciplines in the decision-making process during implementation planning. Often a group focuses on the needs most closely resembling their care delivery and frequently forgets that the system must be functional for all patient care areas, not just inpatient areas.
- *Electronic medical record support.* Does the system support the electronic medical record?
- *Remote access.* Does the product permit secure access to patient data from all locations, particularly remote sites?
- *Clinician support.* Does the product support patient care?

The next step is to decide whether this system should be used as is or customized to meet the specific needs of the organization. This decision will act as the implementation strategy that will guide the committee through the implementation process. Regardless of which implementation strategy is followed, the committee must next gather information about the data that must be collected and processed. Consideration must be given to the data that is pertinent to each function and available to the user for entry into the system. A **function** refers to a task that may be performed manually or automated; some examples include order entry, results reporting, and documentation. The responsibility of identifying the present workflow processes used throughout all clinical areas falls to what is termed *workflow optimization.* This workflow optimization team will utilize the gap analysis to identify changes in workflow that will require changes to the present process. It is the responsibility of this part of the team to validate the future design with a prototype application which will increase user acceptance of or decrease resistance to the new system. The output of the system should also be examined. For example, the format and content of printed requisitions, result reports, worklists, and managerial reports must be evaluated. Once decisions have been made regarding system design and modification, the appropriate department head should approve these specifications before the actual changes are made. At this stage of the implementation, it is important to include not only director-level personnel, but staff as well (Mustain, Lowry, & Wilhoit 2008). The staff will have a clear vision as to what will work and challenge the proposed conversions if they do not see them as positive changes or changes that will result in major workflow interruptions. If groups meet to review new system requirements and adjustments made prior to implementation, delays can be avoided. Numerous changes delay implementation of the system and drive up costs.

At this point, the identified changes should be made to the system in the test environment. The **test environment** is one copy of the software where programming changes are initially made. After any changes are made, the software must be tested to ensure that the changed elements display and process data accurately. Before this can be accomplished, the implementation team and all responsible managers must agree on a test plan. This includes determining long-term goals and what must be tested. Testing is best accomplished by following a transaction through the system for all associated functions. In some cases vendors provide a significant cost reduction in product purchases if the buyer is willing to beta test the product. Beta testing occurs on-site under everyday working conditions. Software problems are identified, corrected, and then retested. This follows alpha testing which is an intensive examination of new software features. An example of this testing procedure might be to enter a physician's order for an x-ray into the system for a particular client. The correct printing of the requisition should be verified. Next, the results of the x-ray should be entered for this client. Both online results' retrieval and printed report content should be verified. Finally, the system should be checked to make certain that the appropriate charges have been generated and passed on to the financial system. It is important to realize that the test environment is not exactly the same as the live environment, because the live environment is much larger and more complex. As a result, the findings of the system test may not always indicate how well the system will perform in the live environment. To help ensure that testing is valid, it is essential to involve more than a handful of persons from information services, the implementation committee, or a quality assurance group. It is strongly recommended that staff level personnel be involved in script testing. These individuals are able to question the reality of a situation and determine the validity of the proposed test. They can often recognize issues during the testing that may not be evident to IT personnel.

Analyze Hardware Requirements

A separate group of tasks related to the analysis of hardware requirements must also be addressed during the implementation phase. These tasks should be initiated early in the implementation phase and continue simultaneously while system design and modifications are being completed. Some of these items include the following:

- *Network infrastructure.* The determination of network requirements, cable installation, wiring and access points, and technical standards should be initiated early in the implementation phase. The processing power, memory capacity of network components, and anticipated future needs must be addressed by the technical members of the implementation committee or other information services staff. This is particularly important because the majority of current network outages and downtime now result from cabling issues and are costly in terms of lost productivity and customer dissatisfaction (Mouton & McNees 2003). Extensive changes to network configuration are expensive and should be avoided whenever possible. Wireless technology may not be an alternative in some cases. Some functions that place a heavy demand on the network include digital imaging and archival, and telemedicine.
- *Type of workstation or mobile device.* The system may be accessed via a number of different devices. These may include a networked personal computer (PC), thin client, wireless or hand-held device such as a personal digital assistant, or mobile laptop PC that uses radiofrequency technology. The committee must investigate the advantages of each option and make recommendations regarding the type of hardware for purchase and installation. Once a decision has been made regarding the type of workstation, the appropriate number of devices per area or department must be determined. An essential step in this process of device investigation is to plan a device fair where staff can actually work with several devices being considered. They can evaluate the ease of the device and its functionality, and provide significant feedback to the committee regarding recommendation for use. This not only yields important information, but also allows the staff to become engaged and promotes staff buy in.
- *Workstation location strategy.* A related workstation decision is the strategy for locating and using the hardware. Several options are available. **Point-of-care** devices are located at the site of client care, which is often at the client's bedside in the emergency department, delivery room, operating room, and radiology. Another strategy involves a centralized approach, where workstations are located at the unit station. A third option is to use handheld or mobile devices that may be accessed wherever the staff finds it most convenient.

- *Hardware location requirements.* The area where the equipment is to be placed or used must be evaluated as to whether there are adequate electrical receptacles, cabling constraints, and/or reception and transmission capabilities. In addition, the work area may require modifications to accommodate the selected hardware. Another major consideration is the need to protect health information from casual view.
- *Printer decisions.* The various printer options should be examined although the need to print documents has decreased. The defacto standard is laser printer technology although some label printers use dot matrix. Ink jet printers appear occasionally in low traffic locations. Other decisions focus on features such as the number of paper trays and fonts. Printed output requires the same consideration for privacy of information.

Develop Procedures and Documentation

Comprehensive procedures for how the system will be used to support client care and associated administrative activities should be developed before the training process is begun. In this way, training may include procedures as well as hands-on use of the system. One approach is to examine the current nursing policy and procedure manuals and to incorporate new policies and procedures related to automation. Policies that are controlled by regulatory bodies must be rewritten to reflect the new technology and care delivery systems. There must be a clear understanding of who will take on this enormous task of categorizing the policies and making the necessary changes prior to go-live. System updates provide an opportunity to introduce new, more stringent policies that may not have been supported with the old system (Amatayakul 2007). Information should be included on backup procedures to be used in the event that the system is not running either for reasons of scheduled maintenance or unforeseen circumstances, so that staff is aware of what to do in the case of planned or unexpected system downtime. Scheduled downtime allows for the implementation of changes in the system. Unscheduled downtime may occur with server, application, network, or electrical problems. It may be beneficial to develop separate documentation that includes the downtime procedures and manual requisition forms and to have this located in an easily identifiable and accessible location. It is crucial that support staff maintain these downtime forms since system upgrades may necessitate the use of new forms to coincide with electronic versions of documentation. A process must be in place to ensure these are up to date at all times.

System user guides should also be developed at this point. These documents explain how to use the system and the printouts that the system produces (Saba & McCormick 1996). It is important that the educational team develop an end-user guide that can be used as a quick reference guide. Job aids should also be developed to help the end user determine the new role in the "electronic world." Another good reference to develop is the frequently asked question lists that can be utilized by all staff for future reference. These tools reassure the end user and can also alleviate some calls to the help desk during the initial stages. Another important aspect of documentation is the development of a dictionary of terms and mapping terms from one system to another. This ensures that everyone has a clear definition of terms and uses them in the same way. Data dictionaries do not contain actual data but list and define all terms used and provide bookkeeping information for managing data. Data dictionaries help to ensure that data are of high quality.

Testing

The process of testing includes the development of a test plan, the creation of test scripts, system testing, and integrated testing. An effective test plan cannot be created until screens and pathways have been finalized and policies and procedures determined. Otherwise, the plan must be revised one or more times. The test plan prescribes what will be examined within the new system as well as all systems with which it shares data. Successful testing requires the involvement of staff who perform day-to-day work because they are aware of the current process and expected outcomes. The test plan should include patient types and functions seen in the facility. A review is then done to identify whether functions are completed without error. Problem areas should be tested again before the person responsible for that area indicates approval and signoff. After system testing, integrated testing can start. Integrated testing looks at the exchange of data between the test system and other systems to ensure its accuracy and completeness.

Provide Training

Once all modifications have been completed in the test environment, a training environment should be established. A **training environment** is a separate copy of the software that mimics the actual system that will be used. Many organizations populate the training database with fictitious clients and make this database available for formal training classes during the implementation process and for ongoing education.

One key factor to consider prior to the actual classroom instruction for the electronic health record (EHR) is the determination of end user's computer competency. An assessment of computer knowledge is crucial to the overall success of training. It is vital to provide basic entry-level education on computer skills and realize the various levels of expertise to expect during training.

Classroom instruction requires dedicated instructors as well as sufficient proctors to assist with technical difficulties encountered so not to interfere with the flow of the class.

Training is most effective if the training session is a scheduled time independent from the learners' other work responsibilities and at a site separate from the work environment. This allows the learner to concentrate on comprehending the system without interruptions. Although this is the best scenario for learning, it presents a logistical nightmare for directors related to scheduling, but with very careful planning the obstacles can be overcome to allow training to take place for all personnel in a timely manner.

An essential part of the training plan is the designation of an educational champion. The selection of this individual should occur early in the design phase to allow time to develop the educational plan for the project. This champion should work closely with all directors as well as maintain contact with the implementation team, which will ensure that the timeline is maintained. Any difficulties in the training plan need to be communicated to the team to allow adjustments to be made to avoid a delay in the go-live. It is extremely important to insist that training be mandatory for all staff. The emphasis on training is essential if training is to be effective and ultimately the implementation successful. Planning for the training must include the following resources:

- Classrooms
- Instructors
- Computers
- Training scripts to teach the classes
- Time

Once resources have been identified and allocated, a training plan should be developed to include the class schedule and content. When planning the class schedule, it is imperative to remember that training needs to occur 24/7. An aspect that often gets overlooked is that nurses and other hospital personnel do not all work daylight; therefore not all classes should be Monday through Friday during daylight hours. The allocation of computers in the training room is vital, as it is essential that students learn hands-on, thus requiring the availability of a computer for every student.

Another important aspect of training is the timing of the classes. It is important to allow training time for not only end users, but super users as well. Super users are very important to the implementation process in the departments and must be relied upon heavily for their expertise. Because of this increased responsibility, super users need to have additional training to become proficient in this new system. In addition, learners should have a place to practice after the formal classroom instruction. If at all possible, a training domain should be made available in all departments to allow staff to "play" in a safe environment. Learning is enhanced when students have the opportunity to utilize the new skills they have learned, and the testing domain provides this opportunity. The use of a training domain has implications that impact training. IT personnel need to maintain this site and plan for possible errors arising from student error. Even though such errors impact training and increase the demands of the implementation team, this is an extremely important part of training.

One of the most important aspects of training is to be able to provide feedback to the students on concerns or questions raised during the classroom training. It is important to allow students to feel they are in a safe environment and understand that their input and opinions about this new system are valued. Students lose trust in the instructor if they feel threatened or not valued.

During the training phase of implementation, it is vital to stress to the end user the importance of confidentiality, security, and patient privacy. The EHR provides easy access to patient data and can create unsafe and unethical situations. The student must understand the implications of accessing data that should not be accessed. They do need to understand that if they have a need to access a patient chart to provide care, that is acceptable; however, it is also imperative they understand how their access can be tracked and time stamped. This understanding is extremely important to emphasize at the beginning of training.

Go-Live Planning

The committee should determine the **go-live** date, which is when the system will be operational and used to collect and process actual client data. At this point, the production environment is in effect. The **production environment** is another term that refers to the time when the new system is in operation. Some of the necessary planning surrounding this event includes the following:

- *Implementation strategy.* It must be determined whether implementation will be staggered, modular, or occur all at once. An example of a staggered implementation strategy may be to go-live in a limited number of client units but in all ancillary departments. The remaining client units would be scheduled to go-live in groups staggered over a specified time frame. The term **roll out** is sometimes used to refer to a staggered, or rolling, implementation. It may also be used in a broader context to refer to both the marketing blitz leading up to implementation and the implementation itself.

  The decision to stagger or roll out the conversion all at once is a decision that needs to be made at the beginning of the planning process. This decision drives the plan and provides a mind-set for the organization to begin to promote its decision. A factor to keep in mind while making this decision is to ensure the organization has a fully committed senior management staff as well as a strong physician champion. The implementation process will be received in a more positive light if the drive comes from the top down as well as from the bottom up. All parties need to be clear on the vision and promote the positive aspects of the project as well as maintain a grasp on reality and understand the push back that is going to happen because of the change in process.

- *Conversion to the new system.* Decisions must be made regarding what information will be **backloaded,** or preloaded into the system before the go-live date. This includes identification of who will perform this task and the methodology used to accomplish it. Plans for how orders will be backloaded must be developed. For example, a "daily × 4 days" order for a complete blood cell count should be analyzed to determine how many days will be remaining on the go-live date. This number should be entered when the backload is performed. Backloading may be needed to create accurate worklists, charges, or medication administration sheets. Plans for verification of the accuracy of preloaded data should be considered.

- *Developing the support schedule.* It often is necessary to provide on-site support around the clock during the initial go-live or conversion phase. Support personnel may include vendor representatives, information system staff, and other members of the implementation committee. It is imperative staff be involved in this support aspect and therefore staffing allowances are very important at this implementation stage. This is again where senior management needs to show their presence especially at the physician level. A clear understanding of exactly what is expected of the staff during the go-live needs to be communicated effectively and consistently to avoid major conflicts, which could interrupt patient care.
- *Developing evaluation procedures.* Satisfaction questionnaires and a method for communicating and answering questions during the go-live conversion should be provided.
- *Developing a procedure to request post go-live changes.* Priority must be given to changes required to make the system work as it should. Additional changes should go before the implementation committee or hospital steering committee to determine necessity. This process helps to keep costs manageable.

SYSTEM INSTALLATION

Once the production system is turned on, users are expected to switch from manual procedures or their prior information system. Generally it takes users longer to perform tasks during this transition period until they become acclimatized to changes in workflow and the new system. This can cause stress, frustration, and treatment delays. Adequate support staff must be available 24/7 at the point of care to help users through this process for the first few weeks until they become adept at its use. Typically this is a time that unforeseen problems will surface that might include users who did not receive training, access issues, system errors, and failure of the system to perform as designed in all cases.

Part of the planning should include what type of on-the-job training will be available once the system is turned on. The expectation should be clear that if training has not occurred, staff should not work. This expectation needs to be supported so others will not have their work impacted as they learn simply because their peers did not receive proper training. Support staff at the point of care can resolve issues quickly on-site or refer them to appropriate information services staff for follow-up.

Common Implementation Pitfalls

There are several common pitfalls with system implementation. Perhaps the most common is an inadequate understanding of how much work is required to implement the system, resulting in underestimation of necessary time and resources. While figures differ slightly, a typical system implementation generally requires 14–18 months (Lee 2007; Winsten 2005). If the initial timeline is not based on a realistic estimate of the required activities and their scope, the implementation process may fall behind schedule. Therefore, it is necessary to fully investigate the impact of the system and control the scope of the project in the early stages of planning.

A major consideration when planning the implementation is the number of hours needed to devote to the development of the project. Team members must be relieved of current jobs and duties to be able to fully commit to the venture.

Another serious problem that may occur during implementation is that of numerous revisions during design activities, creating a constantly moving target. This is sometimes known as "scope creep" or "feature creep." **Scope creep** is the unexpected and uncontrolled growth of user expectations as the project progresses. **Feature creep** is the uncontrolled addition of features or functions without regard to timelines or budget. As needed customizations and modifications are identified, it is imperative that the appropriate department heads approve and sign off on them before programming changes are made. Frequent changes can become very frustrating for the technical staff and result in missed deadlines. Ultimately, this can be very expensive and emotionally draining for the implementation team.

The amount and type of customization that is done to the information systems can also result in problems. To guide the implementation team, the implementation strategy must address the degree of customization that will be done. One strategy is using the system as delivered by the vendor, with minimal changes. The advantage of this strategy, which is often called the "vanilla system," is an easier and quicker implementation. In addition, future software upgrades may be implemented with greater ease and speed. The disadvantage of using this system is that user workflow may not match the system design.

The opposite implementation strategy is to fully customize the information system so that it reflects the current workflow. Although this may seem appealing, the disadvantages include a complicated, lengthy, and expensive implementation process. A further disadvantage is seen when system software upgrades are attempted. Many of the customizations may prohibit the upgrades from being installed without extensive programming effort. As a result, the present trend in the hospital information systems industry is to recommend use of the vanilla systems as delivered by the vendors.

Other common pitfalls include failure to consider annual maintenance contracts and related costs, providing insufficient dedicated resources to the implementation committee, and a hostile culture. The vendor's purchase price for a system is only a portion of overall costs. Vendors charge additional fees for annual technical support, customization, and license fees. These charges are levied on the size of the institution or the number of users, which may or may not be concurrent. Additional costs may include hardware; operating or report software needed to support the system; site preparation; uninterrupted power systems; installation; and ongoing operating costs such as maintenance, supplies, personnel, and upgrades. Project success is impeded by a hostile culture, resistance to change, and refusal to see the benefits of technology.

There may also be problems with testing. These can include poorly developed test scripts, inadequate time to retest problem areas, and the inability to get other systems to exchange data with the test system. Inadequate testing can lead to unpleasant surprises at the time of roll-out or go-live. The development of the test scripts needs to be a work in progress. Although the basic learning concepts must be consistent, it is important to be able to adapt the material to varied class makeups. Not all students in the class will grasp the material quickly and therefore adjustments to the class are necessary. It is also vital to make changes when concepts may not be clear to the students and suggestions are made as to how to improve the content.

All too often, training suffers from inadequate allocation of time and resources. The training environment should mirror the testing environment and later the production environment. Design may not be completed when training starts. This creates a negative impression of the system as well as confusion among end users.

Finally, it is important to continually reinforce the concept that the implementation and the information systems are owned by the users. If the users feel no ownership of the system, they may not accept the system or use it appropriately, nor will they provide feedback regarding potential system improvements. In the event that the implementation does not proceed as planned, it is important to determine the problem (Alexander, Rantz, Flesner, Diekemper, & Siem 2007; Rodriquez 2005). Common problems include a lack of communication, insufficient support, inadequate training for users and information technology staff. All stakeholders should receive frequent communication via newsletters, posters, banners, buttons, and informational meetings. Staff seem to become more engaged in the process if they are part of the process from the beginning. They will view this new change with much anticipation and often fear, but given the opportunity, they will embrace the challenge. Input from all stakeholders must be solicited and evaluated. It is important to work with the vendor to resolve issues rather than assign blame. Consider whether the scope of the project was clearly defined, responsibilities assigned, parties empowered to perform their jobs, and whether project milestones have been defined and tracked.

MAINTENANCE

After implementation of the system, ongoing maintenance must be provided.

User Feedback and Support

One important aspect of maintenance is communication. Soon after the go-live event, feedback from the implementation evaluation should be acted on in a timely manner. This is usually the first aspect of system maintenance to be addressed. The results should be compiled, analyzed, and communicated to the users and information services staff. Any suggested changes that are appropriate may then be implemented. An important avenue for staff to convey concerns or question process is through suggestion boxes that are reviewed daily to ascertain user adoption and competency at this stage of implementation.

Continued communication is imperative for sharing information and informing users of changes. Communication can be accomplished in a variety of ways. For example, a newsletter or printed announcement can be sent to the users, on either a regular or an as-needed basis. System messages can be displayed on the screen or printed at the user location. Focus groups or in-house user groups can be formed for discussion and problem solving.

Another form of user support is the help desk. The **help desk** provides round-the-clock support that is usually available by telephone. Most organizations designate one telephone number as the access point for all users who need help or support related to information systems. The help desk is usually staffed by personnel from the information systems area who have had special training and are familiar with all of the systems in use. Often they are able to help the user during the initial telephone call. If this is not possible, the help desk may refer more complex problems or questions to other staff who have specialized knowledge. The help desk should follow up with the user and provide information as soon as it is available. It is expected that end users will become very frustrated if they feel no one is there to support them during the time of "crisis." Often they just want the reassurance someone will be able to walk them through a problem. The biggest problems during go-live occur with sign-on and passwords. Users may have missed training or may not remember how to sign on to the system.

Visibility of the support staff in the user areas is another important form of support. By making regular visits to all areas, the support staff is able to gather information related to how the system is performing and impacting the work of the users. In addition, users have the opportunity to ask questions and describe problems without having to call the help desk.

System Maintenance

Ongoing system maintenance must be provided in all three environments: test, training, and production. This enables programming and development to continue in the test region without adverse effect on the training or production systems. Therefore, training can continue without interruption and the training environment can be upgraded to reflect programming changes at the appropriate time. Actual client data and workflow will not be affected in the production system until the scheduled upgrade has been thoroughly tested in the test environment.

Requests submitted by users can provide input for upgrading or making necessary changes to the system. For example, a user might request changes to standard physician orders, such as a request to delete some lab tests to contain costs, or nursing documentation related to regulatory issues or the Joint Commission recommendations, such as adding advanced directives documentation. Advanced directives are used to convey whether the client wishes to be intubated, ventilated, or receive CPR or other life-saving or life-sustaining measures in the event of a medical emergency. The requesters must provide a thorough explanation of the desired changes, as well as the reason for the request. One method of facilitating this communication is to develop a request form, to be completed by the requesting users and submitted to the

INFORMATION SERVICES REQUEST FOR SERVICES

Requested by: _____ Date: _____

Department: _____

Department Head (print) _____ Telephone #: _____

Department Head (signature) _____

Priority: _____ Routine _____ Urgent Date Request Needed: _____

Requirement: _____

_____

_____

_____

_____

Reason for Request: _____ Cost Reduction   _____ Service Improvement

_____ Client Care Improvement   _____ Organizational Requirement

_____ Regulatory Requirement   _____ Other (explain) _____

Please provide other supporting details related to the reason for the request:

FIGURE 10–2 • Request for information services form

information services department. On receiving this form, the information services staff should determine if the change is feasible and should consider whether any alternative solutions exist. Figure 10–2 provides an example of a request for services form.

Technical Maintenance

A large portion of ongoing maintenance is related to technical and equipment issues. This maintenance is the responsibility of the information services department. Some examples of technical maintenance include:

- Performing problem solving and debugging
- Maintaining a backup supply of hardware such as monitors, printers, cables, trackballs, and mice for replacement of faulty equipment in user areas
- Performing file backup procedures
- Monitoring the system for adequate file space
- Building and maintaining interfaces with other systems
- Configuring, testing, and installing system upgrades
- Maintaining and updating the disaster recovery plan

FUTURE DIRECTIONS

As users and technical support staff work with the system, they may come to identify problems and deficiencies. Eventually, these faults may become significant enough that the need to upgrade or replace the system becomes evident, illustrating the cyclical nature of the information system's life cycle. Phase 1, the needs assessment phase, is initiated again, and the life cycle continues. In other words, the life cycle is an ongoing process that never ends. Some specific considerations that point to the need for a new system include poor performance, frequent down times, dated programming languages, no vendor support, a difficult user interface, out-moded technology, and inadequate growth capability (Winsten 2005). On the other hand if the system still meets business needs, is reliable, has little unscheduled downtime, is supported by vendors, can sustain growth, presents a high risk of operational disruption with replacement, and available replacements offer no substantial benefits, then it should be retained until these conditions change. One other major consideration for the implementation of a new system is the return on investment that it can provide (Arthour 2007; Kaplin 2007; Kywi 2007; Rushnell & Slate 2007). These can include decreased costs for labor and nonlabor expenses such as maintenance, outsourcing of forms, alignment with business strategy, and increased revenue. Increasingly ROI is also measured in less tangible measures such as increased patient safety and satisfaction, improved quality of service, system usage and compliance with regulations, streamlined workflow with improved provider satisfaction which helps to attract and retain caregivers. Patient and family acceptance are also key to the successful introduction of all health information technology (Wolf, Hartman, Larue, & Arndt 2007). Acceptance is tempered by perception. As staff adjust to new tools, they must be reminded to maintain their focus on customer service and care to prevent their actions from being misconstrued as being inattentive. ROI can also be measured via increased gross revenue due to a shortened revenue cycle and better documentation and tracking (Rushnell & Slate 2007). It may take 2 or more years to realize ROI for IT investments.

The Role of Informatics Nurse Specialists

A growing number of nurses are drawn to informatics, often as a result of their involvement working on an IT project or deployment (Health Information Management Systems Society 2007; Rollins 2007). While not every clinical system is used by nurses directly, most impact nurses and the systems they use in some way. Systems development and implementation have been identified as the top responsibilities for nurse informaticists followed by liaison, quality initiatives, strategic planning, and education and vendor communication, respectively. Nurse informaticists provide credibility for IT projects. The ability to fulfill these responsibilities is largely dependent upon a supportive environment created at the executive level. Implementation of information technology is a very political process, particularly in the cost-controlled healthcare delivery systems of today. The realization of a successful system for nursing requires a strong nurse leader who is politically savvy and technologically competent (Simpson 2007). The chief nursing officer must work with the chief information officer and other key players to develop strategies to transform care, prioritizing system design to maximize the value and benefits of a clinical information system providing abundant point-of-care access and reallocating time saved in documentation and other efficiencies to improve patient care services (Ambrosini 2006; Nagle 2006; Summers & Jerard 2006). This requires executive leadership for change management, involvement of clinicians throughout every phase of the project, and commitment to extensive training of staff to ensure that everyone develops competencies in the use of the system.

CASE STUDY EXERCISE

You are the project director responsible for creating an implementation timeline that addresses the training and go-live activities for a nursing documentation system that will be implemented on 20 units and involve 350 users. Determine whether the implementation will be staggered or occur simultaneously on all units, and provide your rationale.

SUMMARY

- Change is the only constant. It is important to consider the impact of change on the organization.
- One important aspect of system implementation is the development of an effective implementation committee comprising the informatics specialists, and clinical and technical representatives.
- The first task for the committee is the development of a timeline for system implementation activities; the second task is staying with it.
- The implementation strategy must be determined by the committee. This strategy may call for using the system as it is delivered by the vendor or significantly customizing the system to match the current work needs.
- Identified modifications are made to the software in the test environment, so that actual client data and workflow are not affected.
- The following hardware considerations must be addressed during the implementation phase: server, type of workstation device, hardware location, printer options, and network requirements.
- User procedures and documentation are developed during the implementation phase, and provide support to personnel during training and actual use of the system.
- Training is a key element for a successful system implementation.
- Careful consideration must be given to planning the go-live conversion activities to minimize disruptions to client care.
- The implementation committee must be aware of the common pitfalls and problems that may negatively affect the implementation process.
- Maintenance, an ongoing part of the implementation process, includes user support and system maintenance.
- The information systems life cycle is a continuous cyclical process.

REFERENCES

Adler, K. G. (2007). How to successfully navigate your EHR implementation. *Family Practice Management, 14*(2), 1–9.

Alexander, G. L., Rantz, M., Flesner, M., Diekemper, M., & Siem, C. (2007). Clinical information systems in nursing homes. *Computers, Informatics, Nursing, 25*(4), 189–197.

Amatayakul, M. (2007). Updating policies & procedures. *ADVANCE for Health Information Executives, 11*(2), 12.

Ambrosini, R. (2006). Chief nursing officer's role in IT and the delivery of care. In C. A. Weaer, C. W. Delaney, P. Weber, & R. L. Carr (Eds.), *Nursing and informatics for the 21st century* (pp. 75–79). Chicago: Healthcare Information and Management Systems Society.

Arthour, T. (2007). True value of IT. *ADVANCE for Health Information Executives, 11*(6), 35–38.

CDW Healthcare. (2007). *Nurses talk tech 2007: The catch-22 of nursing and information technology.* Retrieved from http://webobjects.cdw.com/webobjects/docs/pdfs/healthcare/Nurses-Talk-Tech-2007.pdf

Health Information Management Systems Society (HIMSS). (2007). *HIMSS nursing informatics survey.* Retrieved from http://www.himss.org/content/files/surveyresults/2007NursingInformatics.pdf

Kaplin, J. (2007). Predicting health. *Healthcare Informatics, 24*(7), 55–56.

Kotter, J. (1995). *Leading change.* Boston, MA: Harvard Business School Press.

Kywi, A. (2007). Connecting care. *ADVANCE for Health Information Executives, 11*(6), 10–11.

Lee, T. (2007). Nurses' experiences using a nursing information system. *Computers, Informatics, Nursing, 25*(5), 294–300.

Morjikian, R. L., Kimball, B., & Joynt, J. (2007). Leading change: The nurse executive's role in implementing new care delivery models. *Journal of Nursing Administration, 37*(9), 399–404.

Mouton, A., & McNees, R. (2003, July). Does cabling need intelligent monitoring? *Communications News, 40*(7), 24.

Mustain, J., Lowry, L., & Wilhoit, K. (2008). Change readiness assessment for conversion to electronic medical records. *Journal of Nursing Administration, 38*(9), 381.

Nagle, L. N. (2006). Nurses in chief information officer positions. In C. A. Weaver, C. W. Delaney, P. Weber, & R. L. Carr (Eds.), *Nursing and informatics for the 21st century* (pp. 87–93). Chicago: Healthcare Information and Management Systems Society.

Rodriquez, V. (2005). The second time around. *ADVANCE for Health Information Executives, 9*(2), 18.

Rollins, G. (2007, April). Nurses find new calling in information technology. *Hospitals & Health Networks, 81*(4), 16–18.

Rushnell, C., & Slate, J. (2007). Improved revenue cycle. *ADVANCE for Health Information Executives, 11*(6), 26–29.

Saba, V. K., & McCormick, K. A. (1996). *Essentials of computers for nurses.* New York: McGraw-Hill.

Simpson, R. (2007, October). The politics of information technology. *Nursing Administration Quarterly, 31*(4), 354–358.

Summers, M., & Jerard, M. (2006). 12 simple rules for implementing clinical systems. *ADVANCE for Health Information Professionals, 10*(6), 47–49.

Winsten, D. (2005). Extending the life of an aging LIS. *ADVANCE for Health Information Executives, 9*(2), 50, 52, 54.

Wolf, D. M., Greenhouse, P. K., Diamond, J. N., Fera, W., & McCormick, D. L. (2006). Community hospital successfully implements eRecord and CPOE. *Computers, Informatics, Nursing, 24*(6), 307–316.

Wolf, D. M., Hartman, L. M., Larue, E. M., & Arndt, I. (2007). Patient first. *Computers, Informatics Nursing, 25*(2), 112–117.

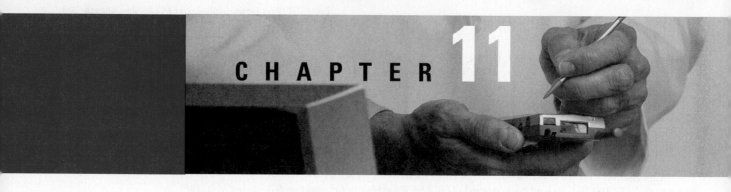

CHAPTER 11

Information Systems Training

After completing this chapter, you should be able to:

1. Describe how learning needs and objectives are determined for end users.

2. List content areas required for information system training.

3. Identify human factors related to information systems.

4. Understand training strategies and blended learning as an instructional approach.

5. Recognize factors that affect learning and knowledge retention.

6. Select training resources that match organizational requirements.

7. Compare training evaluation methods.

8. Discuss issues associated with training, including scheduling, confidentiality, cost, technology, and training environments.

9. Explain how user training can be viewed as a return on investment.

Information systems (IS) are prevalent in today's healthcare setting and provide software applications that assist clinical staff in the management of computerized client information. Healthcare settings have various needs for information systems (Hillestand et al. 2006). Smaller settings may need only basic support, such as a client database, appointment scheduling software, and the ability to process charges and perform billing functions. Larger institutions require complex financial and comprehensive clinical information systems that are able to support the **electronic health record (EHR)**. There is an increased interest in the EHR since President Barack Obama signed the American Recovery and Reinvestment Act (ARRA) into law in February 2009. Even though technology is readily available, there are many who do not understand the role that technology plays in today's healthcare environment (Leo 2009). The availability of both desktop and laptop computers, as well as other smaller computing devices connected to an information system, is an inevitable and integral part of the clinical environment. The value of technology is being evaluated in the healthcare environment for patient safety and nurse retention (Shedenhelm, Hernke, Gusa, & Twedell 2008).

Workplace training activities designed for information systems play a critical role in the adoption and integration of computer technology by healthcare workers. Nurses, physicians, allied healthcare professionals, and support staff must master computer skills in order to access client medical information and document the delivery of care (Duggan 2005). For most workers, information systems are a welcome change and the transition from paper to automation is a smooth one. Some are anxious about learning new skills and what they perceive as the forced use of computers to carry out their job duties. The emotional reaction to the infusion of workplace technology is not unfounded in some situations. As computer applications evolve and manual processes become automated, healthcare workers potentially face job loss or significant changes to work duties in order to meet client and institutional needs (Harvard Business School 2003). Organizations can minimize the perceived negative impact of information technology through a well-planned employee education program. Healthcare administrators need to recognize that education is a key to the successful use of any information system. While educational programs are costly and time consuming, the end result is a knowledgeable work force that can efficiently handle information technology and have a positive effect on the quality of healthcare (Thielst 2007).

THE TRAINING PLAN

An educational strategy aligns with the organization's strategic initiatives and defines the goals, objectives, and action plan for educating workers (Meister 1998). The educational strategy addresses work force training needs for information systems and provides the blueprint for how employees will learn new computer skills. **Training** focuses on acquiring practical knowledge and skilled behaviors and is an organized approach to providing large numbers of staff and healthcare workers with the knowledge needed to use an information system in a clinical setting. Trainers design structured lesson plans that include "learn by doing" activities and practice so that knowledge and skills that are taught can be discretely measured through class exercises and proficiency assessments. Educators associated with healthcare settings tend to view the term *training* negatively because of its association with behavioral psychology and its focus on behavior change through skill acquisition. This is in contrast to the educational approach of cognitive psychology, which concentrates on learning, thinking, and problem solving as a way to change behavior (Fleming & Levie 1993). Organizations may adopt a more inclusive definition of training and use the terms *training* and *development* to help bridge philosophical differences between trainer and educator roles. Training and development focuses on workplace learning and improving performance using both behavioral and cognitive psychology concepts (Driscoll 2000).

Information system implementation projects require a tactical strategy to deliver training (Barritt & Alderman 2004). A **training plan** is designed and developed to help ensure instructional success and address the following areas:

- *Training philosophy.* Training is most effective when instruction occurs at a dedicated time, close to the **go-live** date, is removed from the work area, and is independent of other work responsibilities. The physical environment or classroom where training takes place should be free of work-related interruptions and distractions.

- *Identification of training needs.* There is a general acknowledgment of the importance of studying a training need before deciding upon a training solution. A needs assessment is performed in response to a training request in order to gather information to make a data-driven and responsive recommendation (Rosett & Sheldon 2001). A needs assessment is commonly done early in the implementation planning timeline and leads to the development of instruction. A needs assessment will help to determine who needs to be trained, the content area to be taught, the amount of instruction time needed to master the prescribed tasks, requested equipment, and when and where training will take place. Training needs are reviewed and revised at regular intervals during implementation and when new requests are submitted by the information systems team. The need for ongoing education should be considered during this needs assessment to provide education for system upgrades and additional system functionality (Shedenhelm et al. 2008).

- *Training approach.* Once the initial needs assessment data are analyzed and the task analysis is performed, decisions need to be made about how to plan instructional interventions and deliver the training. Instructional decisions include content development and how the course will be taught. Organizations decide whether to create materials through internal resources, outsource or contract the development of content, or purchase class materials available through the software vendor. Materials purchased through the software vendor are developed for the base information system and may need to be tailored to match any customized build that the organization makes to the base system. Content development or tailoring starts once the detailed implementation plan is complete and clinical design of the system is under way and continues through implementation. Training delivery may include one or a combination of methods, for example, instructor-led, technology-based, or on-the-job training. Job aids and an **electronic performance support system (EPSS)** are integrated into the training methodology. A blended approach may prove to be effective and cost efficient because it has the capability to target different learning styles, enhance knowledge transfer, offer alternatives to classroom instruction, and deliver just in time training (Driscoll 1998).

- *Training resources.* The next step in the training plan is to identify the individuals or group who will coordinate or conduct information systems training. The selection of training resources is usually completed 6 months prior to implementation. Administrators need to evaluate the availability and skill level of internal resources or decide to contract with outside or vendor-related training professionals. Internal training resources are preferred over external trainers because of their familiarity with the organization and its operational processes and their ability to support a flexible training schedule.

- *Timetable and training schedule.* The training timetable is developed in coordination with the projected go-live date of the information system. The factors to consider include the number of users who will need training and the amount of time required to complete the training. The training schedule is designed to allow enough time for "knowledge" transfer, practice, and application of skills. The goal is to conduct training as close to implementation as possible. The timetable and schedule is a delicate balance; end user training conducted too early in the implementation process may require retraining before go-live. Individuals trained late in the implementation process may need additional support once the system is in use.

- *Budget and costs.* Training is costly and includes productivity losses during the education process (Anderson 2009). However, a well-trained workforce is a return on investment (ROI) when job satisfaction and retention is an outcome. Gartner Research reports that each hour of effective training is worth 5 hours to the organization. Well-trained users attain required skill levels in less than a quarter of the time, require less assistance from peers and fewer calls to the help desk, and spend less time correcting errors (Aldrich 2000). Although training is time consuming and labor-intensive, it should be considered an investment in enhancing work force knowledge and as a measurement in the successful implementation of an information system. The considerations for estimating the direct cost of information system training include salary for training resources, trainee coverage or replacement during training, cost of materials, educational technology and equipment, travel expenses, and space allocation.

  Implementation training requires thoughtful planning and careful allocation of resources in order to stay within budget and to minimize indirect costs, such as trainee overtime and unanticipated retraining activities. Organizations interested in determining the overall value of training can use ROI metrics. ROI utilizes industry standard financial investment indicators that compare dollar costs to the value-added benefits of an innovation. An ROI study done after the implementation of an information system may measure all direct training costs compared to reported reductions in medical errors, timeliness of charting, a decrease in staff turnover, and an increase in employee job satisfaction and productivity (Phillips & Phillips 2005).

- *Evaluation strategy.* The purpose of an information systems training evaluation strategy is to collect subjective participant feedback about the learning experience, identify pre- and post-training skill gaps, and measure knowledge and performance of the stated learning objectives. The ultimate success of training is measured by the ability of the participant to perform the targeted computer skills.

There are two popular program evaluation models for training intervention and evaluation: a traditional approach and a process evaluation approach. The Kirkpatrick Level 4 Model is an example of a simple, intervention-based approach to evaluation. Many organizations have been interested in a process-based evaluation and have adopted the targeted evaluation process (TEP) as an evaluation methodology. TEP is a process approach that allows for a full range of evaluation tools, technology, and techniques (Combs & Falletta 2000).

Some organizations require proficiency testing and provide remediation so that all employees can achieve the necessary skill level. If instruction is delivered through the use of technology, it can often be set up to provide immediate feedback and supplemental practice for employees to learn the new skills. Technology-based instruction can evaluate, measure progress, and track the acquisition of skills of each employee (Newbold 1996).

IDENTIFICATION OF TRAINING NEEDS

The training preparation process begins by identifying user needs, determining content, establishing learning objectives, and deciding upon the approach and evaluation strategy. The delivery process begins by creating the training timetable, allocating space, and defining hardware and software requirements. The training budget and all associated costs are monitored throughout the preparation and delivery process. Administrators review budget reports and may request adjustments to how training dollars are being spent at any point during implementation. Budgetary changes during the course of implementation may affect how training content is created and delivered; for example, an instructor-led approach may switch to a technology-based one, or external trainers may be replaced by internal training resources.

End User Training Needs

Healthcare workers who use an information system to view or document client information are called **end users**. End users are identified and grouped by job class responsibilities to guide what applications and level of access they will have in the information system. The training needs of each job class are determined according to what functions each will perform. Shrager (2010) also noted that in addition to training users in the functions they will need, successful training provides sufficient practice time and helps end users to understand the relationships between different screens and functions. Administrators decide what applications or modules will be automated first, and end user training is delivered respective to these decisions. The client database and registration modules for admissions, discharges, and transfers are usually implemented first, followed by clinical documentation and physician order entry.

Most end users have access to view client demographic data, allergies, diagnosis, emergency contacts, and recent medical history. Information systems are designed so that security levels can be set and access, or functionality, can be restricted for some job classes and not others. Access to sensitive client information and advanced system functionality may be given to physicians, nurses, and supervisors while restricted to administrative support personnel. Laws governing professional practice also help to determine the degree of access assigned to an end user. See Box 11–1 for a matrix of end users who may need information system training.

User class defines the level of access to an information system. A **user class** is defined and categorized as the personnel who perform similar functions. Representatives from clinical areas can help identify user classes based upon job descriptions. The user class refines the types of training classes needed for implementation. For example, provider training classes may include physicians, residents, nurse practitioners, and physician assistants as they use similar information.

BOX 11–1   Who Might Need Training?

Providers

- Physicians and residents
- Nurse practitioners
- Midwives
- Physician assistants
- Dentists

Non-providers who provide care

- Registered nurses
- Licensed practical nurses
- Pharmacists
- Nutritionists and dieticians
- Respiratory therapists
- Occupational therapists
- Speech therapists
- Physical therapists
- X-ray technicians
- Patient care and medical assistants

Students

- Students from all professional and technical healthcare programs
- Medical students

Support personnel

- Admission clerks
- Dietary personnel
- Social service staff
- Home healthcare personnel
- Pastoral care staff
- Housekeeping personnel
- Central supply staff
- Case managers
- Unit clerks and secretaries
- Infection control and quality assurance personnel
- Persons who check insurance authorization; billers and individuals who enter charges

However, physicians would have additional security access to allow them to review and co-sign orders. Non-provider training classes may include registered nurses (RNs) and ancillary department staff. RNs are provided with a higher level of security in accordance with their scope of practice to include order entry, processing of physician orders, charting medication administration, and documenting client medical information. The licensed practical nurse (LPN) is another example; an LPN needs to view and document client information but may not perform order entry functions. Higher-level user classes, such as RNs, may perform functions assigned to lower classes to allow them to carry out functions assigned to support personnel when these personnel are unavailable.

Replacement staff and students who commonly rotate through institutions also need to use the information system. The degree of automation within the institution determines what groups require computer training. For example, if physician order entry is the only automated function, then neither replacement staff nor students may need training. In healthcare settings where system access is required for the retrieval of data or to document client information, training is necessary for replacement staff to perform their job. Students may opt to attend training as an educational experience in order to learn and acquire job-related computer skills.

Training Class Content

Project scope is the information systems term used to describe the details of the system functionality that is slated for automation. Learning objectives and training class content are developed in accordance with the project scope document and when changes are made during implementation. Learning objectives reflect the information system functionality defined for the users within a user class. For example, learning objectives for the documentation of vital signs by a nursing assistant would include the ability to log in to the system, access the client record, accurately record and save the vital sign data, and retrieve the entered vital signs at the end of the training activity.

Training class content should address the following topics:

- *Computer-related policies.* The training class provides an excellent environment to discuss client confidentiality policies, ethical computing, and penalties for the inappropriate use and access to data within the information system. Most organizations require employees to sign confidentiality statements that advise against sharing user access codes and passwords. Employees may receive their user access code and password at the completion of training.

In some organizations, the application for access to the information system is completed by the employee's supervisor. An **access code** or user ID is some form of unique identifier and provides authentication of the end user's identity within the information system. The entry point or log in to the information system may require both an access code and a password. Note that some information systems have a more sophisticated mechanism to identify an end user, such as biometric fingerprint authentication, iris or retinal scans, and voice recognition technology (Woodward, Orlans, & Higgins 2002). Equipment will need to be available to support the training of these technologies.

- *Access privileges.* End users, such as students and other nonemployees, may be required to sign additional documents regarding access to an information system. Organizations need to protect client information, and any misuse of privileges should result in loss of clinical privileges and possible legal action. Two examples of misuse might include viewing the medical record of a high-profile client for no clinical reason and failure to properly handle and dispose of confidential paper reports.

- *Human factors.* The implementation of an information system presents a major disruption in the work setting, especially when an organization transitions from minimal automation to a complex computing environment (Harvard Business Review 2003). Organizations may use educational strategies to prepare the workforce for technology. Preimplementation presentations, hands-on demonstrations, bulletin board messages, tent cards, newsletter articles, administrative role modeling, and unit level champions help to ease the associated anxiety and uncertainty of change. The classroom may provide a safe place for employees to learn about change, ask questions, and realize the benefit of automating their work processes.

- *Computer literacy.* Employees may lack fundamental computer skills and knowledge. A separate needs assessment may be required in the preimplementation phase. This needs assessment may be completed through human resources so that basic job competencies can be identified and met before the introduction of an information system and its associated training. Organizations that need to provide basic computer literacy training may send employees to outside computer training classes, provide on-site sessions, or use computer-based training software.

- *Workflow.* The transition from manual work to automation is considered a cultural change in the work setting (Harvard Business Review 2003). Employees are expected to learn new ways to carry out current job duties or accept new responsibilities in a technology-enhanced work environment. Workflow diagrams that visually display new processes help end users understand what is expected of them and ease their transition into the information age.

- *Scenario and step-by-step design of instruction.* Training content can be designed in formats that enhance end user knowledge retention and target different learning styles. Scenario-based content provides medical case studies in a realistic frame of reference in which trainees work through, for example, the client admission process (Guite, Lang, & McCartan 2006). Another effective instructional technique is the use of step-by-step exercise and practice that can be used to demonstrate the electronic order entry process. For example, trainees can practice entering different types of orders and then view the expected results. The accurate completion of step-by-step exercises can serve as proof of skill acquisition.

- *Electronic help.* Reference documents, context-level help screens, and online tutorials can be beneficial provided that they are accurate, easily accessible, user friendly, and that the end user knows of their existence. Reference documents are usually a minimum of two pages in length, provide topic-specific help, and are saved in portable document format (PDF). Reference documents are most helpful if they can be accessed through a **hyperlink** within the information system, have a logical name, and are alphabetically organized on a list. **Context sensitive help** topics are available throughout the software and provide directions at the screen and field level to help end users complete a particular task. **Online tutorials** provide computer animation or written instructions for how to use the software application or one of its features. Online tutorials are available for referral at any time. Training classes should introduce online help features, demonstrate their use, and provide directions for how to access them.

- *Error messages.* **Error messages** are generated by an information system to warn of missing information or data entry errors. Error messages alert end users that they need to correct or add information. Some examples include missing data in a required field or a medication order that needs one or more of the following fields completed or corrected: drug name, dosage, route, or administration schedule. Failure to satisfy the error message may prevent the end user from proceeding or completing an order, procedure, or documentation. Error messages are a safety feature designed to reduce or prevent client documentation or clinical charting-related mistakes. Class content should address how error messages are generated, tips to prevent them, and how they can be corrected in the information system.

- *Error correction.* Data entry errors result from typographical or misspelled words within free text fields or by selecting an incorrect choice from selection boxes or drop-down menus. Corrections can be made at the time of entry and before saving or at a later date and time. For example, some clinical documentation systems provide an opportunity to review and correct information before processing the data. Data entry errors can be corrected after processing; however, the information system maintains an audit trail that records all changes made to the computer record. Quality assurance personnel may review the audit logs and track data entry errors for frequency, severity, and degree of risk to client safety. These audit trail error logs also provide information systems analysts with data. Trends in data entry errors can be studied so that changes to the information system can be made that would help to reduce these common data entry errors. Training content should include drill and practice exercises to familiarize end users with performing accurate data entry and completing electronic forms.

- *Screen and system "freezes."* **Freezing** refers to a situation where the end user is logged in to the information system but is unable to enter or process data. Possible causes include a workstation malfunction, computer network overload, order queue processing issue, or a system crash. Depending on the root cause, a freeze may be a momentary slow-down or a more serious problem resulting in downtime. Training content should include basic troubleshooting guidelines and information about how to report a problem to the information systems help desk.

- *System idiosyncrasies.* Information system developers attempt to develop software applications that are intuitive and easy to use (Thielst 2007). System design, programming, and technical platform determine what an information system can and cannot do. One goal of software development is to provide automated solutions to manual processes. Automated solutions often handle information in a way that is very different from the manual process. This change in process may initially disrupt the **comfort zone** of the end user and seem counterintuitive. Graphical user interfaces (GUI) help end users adjust to doing their work electronically. In some situations, major programming changes need to be done to accommodate complex workflows. Programming changes and customization are costly and require development time. Organizations may decide to delay or forego system enhancements. For this reason, healthcare workers need to understand the limitations of their information system.

- *Equipment maintenance and basic troubleshooting.* Some problems are easy to fix, such as a loose computer cable or unplugged electrical cord. Most printing issues stem from an empty paper tray or toner cartridge. Other problems are more complex and require some basic troubleshooting knowledge. Training content should include instructions for creating desktop shortcuts and icons and for adjusting computer settings, such as mouse speed and screen colors. Organizations may lock down workstations in order to limit end user changes to the desktop, for example, to prohibit changes to the display background or to the screen saver. The importance of logging out of both the workstation and the information system should be emphasized in the training session. End users who know how to troubleshoot and know who to contact for help will save time and maintain a high level of productivity (Regan & O'Connor 2002).

- *Downtime procedures.* Information systems personnel carefully plan computer downtime to perform system or code maintenance and upgrades. Planned downtime is scheduled at a time when few end users are routinely logged into the information system, usually during the early morning hours. Unplanned but scheduled downtime can happen at any time; for example, a software fix is necessary and needs to be installed immediately into the information system. Unplanned and unscheduled downtime can happen at any time when the network or computer hardware malfunctions. Downtime procedures are not implemented unless downtime is expected to last for several hours. The administrator on call usually decides when to start using downtime procedures. Paper medication administration records, clinical and lab reports, and manual requisitions are used during an information system downtime. Downtime procedures should be introduced during training and should be reviewed annually. It is also important to review downtime procedures if the system will be out of operation for an extended schedule downtime.

- *Ability to retrieve and view clinical information.* An information system changes the way nurses and healthcare workers view clinical data. Data elements can be sorted, filtered, and displayed in different ways; for example, test results can be displayed by test, by date, or graphically on a flow sheet. Training activities should include hands-on activities to practice how to retrieve data. Table 11–1 displays sample screen options that permit review of a client's laboratory results using any one of a variety of data sorting and filtering options.

TABLE 11–1   Sample Screen Options for Retrieving Lab Result and Graphical Display

Screen Option	Training Activity	Information Retrieved
For the most recent tests	Filter on a date range or sort chronologically	Provides results of the most recent results
For today	Sort by date	Lists all laboratory results for the current date
For the previous 2 days	Filter on a date range	Shows laboratory results from the previous 2 days
From the time of admission	Column sort by order	Displays all laboratory results from admission to the present time, in either chronological or reverse chronological order
Previous admissions	Retrieval by admission date	Lists laboratory findings by dates of previous admissions
Department specific, e.g., chemistry, hematology, or microbiology	Filter or sort by department	Allows practitioners to quickly find a particular result, such as a wound culture
Glucose values for a date range	Graphical display	

Class Schedules

The timing of end user training can be a challenge that requires careful planning and flexibility when scheduling class times. Factors to consider include trainee availability, class length, and location. Healthcare organizations are a 24/7 operation. Since employees may work rotating, flexible, or steady shifts, the class schedule must accommodate end user availability to attend classes. Class length depends on the amount of content that needs to be covered and can range from 1- to 8-hour sessions. It is often difficult for employees to leave their clinical area during a shift for training without disrupting patient care and ensuring adequate coverage. Conversely, scheduling classes before or after work shifts will contribute to fatigue, decreased concentration, and lack of attention to the training. Employees who are tired or distracted will not retain what they need to know regarding the use of the information system. Successful training strategies provide a plan that includes dedicated training days in which the participants are relieved of clinical duties and can focus on training activities.

Instructors need to be available to deliver training to accommodate employees working all shifts. Preparation time for each class must be factored into the training team schedule, as back-to-back classes may target different audiences. Planning and preparation in advance will make the training effort and classroom experience less stressful and more productive for both the trainers and trainees. As mentioned earlier in this chapter, the timetable for training should be developed to allow adequate days to reach all end users and should be scheduled as close to the go-live date as possible. Computer instruction is most effective when provided no more than 1 month before the actual anticipated use in the work setting (Craig 2002).

Hardware, Software, and Environment Requirements

The end user learning experience is most effective when the hardware, software, and computer training environment match what the end user will use in the clinical setting. Administrators who understand the importance of training will support these requirements. Ideally, each trainee will have a networked computer workstation that is connected to peripherals, such as printers, fax machines, scanners, hand-held devices, and any other specialized equipment. The **computer training environment** is defined as a software or application copy of the information system's production environment. The environment is stripped, which means that actual client or **live data** and employee data are removed after the copy process. This ensures that client and employee data are kept confidential. The copy of the production environment for the training environment is done close to the start of implementation training in order to capture as much of the customized application build as possible. Any additional changes made to the production environment must be replicated for training. The trainers are responsible for creating training data that will be uploaded into the training environment. Training data includes simulated client and employee databases, log in and access codes, orders and procedures, medications, alerts, admission history, and test results. Trainers design instruction and the training environment to meet the learning needs of the various user classes and disciplines employed within the organization. Since no training should occur on the actual system, the training and information system teams work together to coordinate and plan the creation, support, and maintenance of the training environment. The training team needs to be included in the information systems project team status meetings to keep up to date with application build and production environment changes, such as code and software updates that may impact the training environment.

Training Costs

The largest line item in a training initiative budget is salary for trainers, administrative support, replacement staff, and for end users and their replacement while attending training sessions. Training is considered expensive primarily because of the personnel hours required to support a training function (Filipczak 1996). For this reason, salary costs for the following staff must be considered:

- *Trainers.* Trainers are accountable for the development of training to support an information system implementation. Trainer time is spent assessing, developing, delivering, evaluating, and supporting training activities. External, contract, or vendor-supplied trainers may prove to be costly in the long run. Organizations may choose to hire trainers or recruit current employees for information system training.
- *Administrative support staff.* Staff is needed to support the trainers and training function through clerical support, typing, copying, collating materials, and registering and tracking attendees. Administrative support staff may also help with preparing class materials, such as using specialized software to prepare job aids, create presentations, and convert files for electronic and Web applications.
- *Employee training.* End users can be either salaried or hourly employees. Compensation for time spent in training may be considered a "work" day for exempt employees and documented at the regular hourly rate for nonexempt staff. Employee overtime can be kept to a minimum if the training schedule is flexible and can accommodate the various shift and work schedules. Clinical and department supervisors should have access to the training schedule in advance in order to schedule employee training and plan for coverage or replacement staff. Training classes held on the weekend may accommodate exempt and weekday employees, who can use compensation time at a later date.
- *Replacement staff.* Implementation training is mandatory in most organizations. Unit and department supervisors must arrange coverage for employees attending training. Replacement staff may be needed during times when regular staff is not available to cover the clinical areas.

Some other line items in the training budget to consider include the purchase of training materials from the vendor and desktop software applications to support training and development, such as file conversion software, authoring packages, and Web development tools. Training materials, if purchased from the vendor, usually need to be edited due to information system customization. Some organizations may decide to develop training materials and not purchase them. In either scenario, trainer desktop workstations may need additional memory or disk space to support the training software applications.

Training Center

The training center or classroom space planning starts in the early phase of the implementation plan. As emphasized in this chapter, learning and knowledge transfer is most effective when instruction is conducted away from the work area and free of work-related interruptions and distractions. A dedicated training space allows for trainees to focus on what is being taught and encourages retention of information. Training conducted in the work areas should be limited to short in-services and just-in-time sessions to address critical issues. Classroom space located within the organization is recommended in terms of convenience, travel, and parking, and closeness to technical support. In multisite facilities, temporary classrooms can be strategically set up for implementation training. When classroom space is not available within the organization, convenience of location, travel time, parking or shuttle service, and technical connectivity are considerations for the selection of an off-site facility. Box 11–2 lists some factors to consider when selecting a training site. The physical and learning environment of the classroom or facility should be a comfortable and calm learning space. The use of ambient lighting, a comfortable temperature and ventilation, and workstation ergonomics that allow chair, desk, and workstation adjustments minimize fatigue and prevent repetitive stress injuries. Once the implementation training is complete, the classroom space may serve other purposes, for example, as the implementation system go-live command center, for one-on-one training and support, computer-based learning, and end user requests for space to practice and review the information system. The workstations can be set up to access either the training environment or the production system.

Training Approaches

The overall training approach should be consistent with the organization's philosophy and should consider the various disciplines that make up the workforce (Abla 1995; Fender & Jennerich 1997; Glydura, Michelman, & Wilson 1995). A blended approach to training may prove to be effective to target different learning styles and promote knowledge transfer (Horton 2001). A blended approach includes one or a combination of methods, for example, instructor-led, technology-based, or on-the-job training (Troha 2002). Job aids and an EPSS are considered adjuncts to training and are integrated into the approach (Driscoll 1998). Classroom technology and teaching tools are welcome and necessary elements for supporting the training approach. The minimum equipment includes a separate instructor workstation connected to a printer, ceiling mounted data projector, wireless mouse, white boards, and laser pens. Classroom techniques that engage the participants, such as active participation, group activities, hands-on exercises, and other various instructional approaches enhance attention and learning. The use of an **advanced organizer** is a way to guide the instruction, manage time, and allow for logical breaks in the classroom instruction (Fleming & Levie 1993). A sample scenario describing a blended approach is described as follows:

> The instructor welcomes the class, reviews housekeeping details, and introduces participants to each other through an icebreaker. A slideshow follows that explains the class content. A copy of the agenda is distributed in the advanced organizer format. The instructor demonstrates system access and log in through the trainer workstation and data projector. The participants practice logging

with a training access code and password, following step-by-step instructions listed in their training manual. The instructor uses a slideshow and lecture to review confidentiality policies. There is a short break. The instructor proceeds with the training session using a combination of lecture, scenario-based demonstrations, and hands-on practice. A case study is presented and the participants work as a group to complete the assignment. After lunch, the participants log in to the workstation and access a **computer-based training (CBT)** module located on the organization's intranet to learn about Order Entry. The CBT is completed at the learner's own pace. The learner completes an online evaluation of the CBT, which automatically provides feedback to the instructor and creates a computer generated report and proficiency assessment score of the participant's progress for Order Entry. After the afternoon break, the session continues with instructor-led lecture, drill and practice exercises, and step-by-step assignments that are reviewed one on one with the instructor. Another group exercise follows.

At the end of the training session, the participants complete an online proficiency test, which is automatically scored. Participants return for remediation, as needed. The instructor records attendance and test scores, then prepares for the next class. This use of blended delivery includes a combination of approaches to maximize retention, target learning styles, and allow the participant to actively participate in learning activities. See Box 11–3 for factors to consider when choosing training methods.

Many types of training delivery method options exist, including instructor-led classroom instruction, computer-based training, online multimedia or Web-based training, online tutorials, on-the-job training, peer training, videotaped sessions, job aids, and self-directed text-based exercises. Other options include threaded discussions, video conferencing, and simulation (Simonson, Smaldino, Albright, & Zvacek 2003). Instructor-led instruction continues to be the most popular approach even though it is resource intensive (Zielstorff 1996). Box 11–3 provides specific factors to consider when selecting a training method, and Table 11–2 outlines advantages, disadvantages, and organizational tips for each instructional approach.

Blended learning has grown in popularity; however, adopting this approach for information systems training requires that it is appropriate for the content that needs to be taught (Rosett & Sheldon 2001) and that the organization's network infrastructure can support electronic training delivery. Web-based training may prove appropriate for information systems training. **Webcasts** are a popular push technology in which Web-based information is sent to participants. Webcasts can be live or recorded instruction. This format allows multiple learners to access a Web site to attend a scheduled class. The learners are able to view a slideshow or multimedia presentation online. Data and audio transmission is usually

---

BOX 11–3 Selecting a Training Method: Factors to Consider

- **Time.** The time required to develop and present material using each instructional approach varies; for example, lectures can be written and revised quickly and content can be delivered to a large number of participants at one time.

- **Cost.** Initial content development time and subsequent revisions can be lengthy for computer-based training. CBT may be cost prohibitive in terms of the number of personnel hours needed to develop, support, and revise this approach.

- **Learning styles.** Blended delivery includes a combination of approaches that target learning styles and allow learners to actively participate in training activities.

- **Learning retention.** Active participation through scenarios, case studies, practice exercises, and repetition provide opportunities for learning, applying job skills, and retaining knowledge.

TABLE 11–2 Advantages, Disadvantages, and Tips Associated with Various Training Approaches

Training Approach	Advantages	Disadvantages	Tips for Effective Organizational Use
Instructor-led class	Flexible Easy to update Can include demonstration Allows for individual help Can test proficiency	Often relies on lecture ↑ Class size ↓ effectiveness of demonstrations Consistency varies with trainer Difficult to maintain pace good for all	For each user group: • Keep a file with objectives and exercises • Use the same presentation order • Use generic examples unlikely to change overtime Never rely on just one trainer—leaves no paper trail for others to follow
Computer-based training (CBT)	Self-paced Interactive ↑ Retention—uses technology to teach technology 24-hour availability Can be offered online or offline Can be done in increments Facilitates mastery learning Emulates "real" system without threat of harm	Time and labor intensive to develop and revise Requires great attention to accompanying materials Limited usefulness of vendor supplied materials that are not specific to customization Lacks the flexibility of access to an actual information system—only programmed options can be tried	Trainer serves as a facilitator Needs specific, well-prepared learning aids
Online multimedia	Interactive Stimulates multiple senses for ↑ retention May allow user to bookmark and return to the same spot Can test proficiency	Requires intense planning, resources for design, and revision Less flexible to revise	Use and revise carefully
Online tutorials	24-hour availability Allows immediate application of learning Can test proficiency May allow user to bookmark and return to the same spot	Design and revision more involved than instructor-led training	Must have access from all locations and availability must be known
E-mail	Provides individual feedback on entry errors Provides a mechanism for all users to ask questions	Too slow for actual training	Effective for announcements and updates
Video	24-hour availability Easily revised/updated Extends resources	Not interactive Appropriateness limited to select content such as ethical issues—not actual training	Use on a limited basis

(*continued*)

TABLE 11–2 (continued)			
Training Approach	**Advantages**	**Disadvantages**	**Tips for Effective Organizational Use**
Web-based	Can be accessed from any networked PC	Requires knowledgeable Webmaster	Include online learner assessment
	Provides 24-hour availability	Requires an existing intranet that can be accessed by all employees	
	Easily updated and revised		
	May allow user to bookmark and return to the same spot		
	Can test proficiency		
On-the-job training	Individualized	Trainer often does not know educational principles	Trainer must know basic adult education principles
	Permits immediate application	May lose productivity of two workers	May work well for unit clerks, working in pairs
	Can test proficiency	Seasoned employees may pass on poor habits	
		Difficult to achieve with many interruptions	
Peer training	Training specific to function	Trainer often does not know educational principles	Trainer must know basic adult education principles
	Can test proficiency	Seasoned employees may pass on poor habits	May work well for unit clerks, working in pairs or to learn PC applications
Super User	Acquainted with clinical area and the information system	Spends time away from clinical responsibilities for additional information system training and meetings	May serve as resource persons particularly during off-shifts
	May come from any user class		May assist with training other users
	Serves as communication link between end users and information system personnel to help resolve issues		
Job aids	↓ Need to memorize	Not effective if access is limited	Make accessible and user friendly
	↓ Training time		
	↓ Help requests		
	Can be created quickly and inexpensively		
Self-directed text-based courses	Self-paced	Requires high level of motivation	Need highly structured materials
	Can test proficiency		
	Lacks interaction with training hospital/system		

one-way unless a dial-up communication bridge is used for two-way audio communication between the instructor and the participants. Webcasts generally provide some means for electronic interaction, including online question and answer forums. **Video conferencing** is a media-rich, synchronous training approach and has the capability of linking the instructor with participants from various remote sites. Video conferencing is an appropriate delivery approach but requires the organization to purchase and maintain video equipment at various locations and stream compressed video over the computer network (Simonson et al. 2003).

Training Materials

Well-designed instructional materials are critical to successful information system training (Abla 1995; Filipczak 1996; Henry & Swartz 1995). **Learning aids** are materials intended to supplement or reinforce lecture- or computer-based training. Learning aids may include outlines, diagrams, charts, or conceptual maps. **Job aids** are written instructions designed to be used as a reference in both the training and work settings. Materials supplied by the software vendor needs to be evaluated for quality and consistency and usually require edits due to information system customization. Some organizations may decide to develop training materials and not purchase them. The development can start once the detailed implementation plan is complete and clinical design of the system is under way. The development and revision of training materials may continue throughout implementation. Operational owners should review training materials and content for ease of use, accuracy, and clarity and to ensure that materials reflect workflow processes.

Proficiency Assessments

Some organizations require proficiency assessments. Instruction that is technology based and testing that is done online can be monitored electronically and provide immediate feedback and test scores that measure the acquisition of skills (Vaillancourt 2000). Proficiency assessments are designed to measure learner knowledge retention and ensure that learners can perform the required new job skills. Any instructional approach can accommodate proficiency testing (Sittig et al. 1995). Proficiency assessments can be a criterion-referenced measure to evaluate predetermined competencies, or norm-referenced tools can be used to assess performance relative to peers or other participants. Norm-referenced testing is useful in competitive hiring situations where there are more applicants than positions available. However, this type of testing is not typically used for information system training. If proficiency assessments are administered, procedures need to be in place to score and store paper-based tests, analyze training needs and prescribe remediation from the results, and report findings to administration, as required. Human resources may participate in developing policies and procedures for storing the tests and results.

Whenever possible, proficiency assessments should be administered electronically to facilitate scoring, storing, and retrieving individual examination results (White & Weight 2000).

Information System Trainers Administrators decide who will conduct the information system training. Decisions are made based upon available resources, cost factors, recommendations from the information systems project team, stakeholders, and the system selection committee. Training resources may include internal training staff, employees selected who will learn how to deliver training, external and vendor-supplied trainers, and consultants. Organizations must weigh the advantages and disadvantages of each group. Internal training staff are familiar with the culture, operation, and procedures of the organization but may know little about the information system. The choice to use internal trainers can be a positive decision and seen as a reward, an incentive, or promotion. External, vendor-supplied trainers, and consultants are knowledgeable about the information system but know little about the organization and may not be able to support a flexible training schedule, ongoing content changes, and long-term training evaluation. External, vendor-supplied trainers, and consultants may leave after the initial implementation training is complete, allowing the organization to select internal staff to take over the responsibility

---

BOX 11–4   Selecting a Trainer: Factors to Consider

- **Teaching skills and experience**. Previous training and content development experience is helpful, as well as experience using an information system.
- **Ability to interact with groups and individuals.** Most information system training occurs in a classroom with several trainees. The ability to communicate clearly and manage the training needs of the group requires patience and skill. Experienced trainers are adept at keeping the group focused and on schedule. One-on-one communication and occasional individualized training may be needed during implementation.
- **Understanding end users and their responsibilities.** Trainers must have an understanding of the various user classes and their job needs and information system requirements.
- **Training approach.** Trainers should be knowledgeable and comfortable with the selected approach. For example, if computer-based training is used, instructors must be familiar with access, content, and navigational features of the software.
- **Centralized versus departmental training.** Centralized training provides the general principles and overall functionality of the information system. Departmental training is workflow oriented, customized, and focused on individual user class responsibilities in a given area.

---

of training new employees and new system functionality. Box 11–4 lists factors to consider when selecting trainers.

Organizations frequently develop a core set of instructors chosen from their own personnel ranks. These individuals receive their initial system training from the vendor and are then responsible for teaching the system to employees. Instructors often come from the following areas:

- *Hospital-wide or staff development educators.* Educators may know the basic principles of adult education but may lack familiarity with specific day-to-day unit routines and workflows.
- *Clinicians.* Clinicians have expertise within their clinical practice areas.
- *Department supervisors.* Supervisors are knowledgeable about their clinical area and workflow but may be unable to leave their supervisory responsibilities.
- *Information system personnel.* These individuals may include systems analysts who understand the software application and functionality, but lack a clinical perspective and have no teaching or instructional design experience.

An ideal training team would consist of a combination of clinical and information technology staff who have good communication skills and who have knowledge and experience with classroom instruction, educational technology, and curriculum development. A dedicated core group of trainers helps to provide consistent delivery of instruction. The need for training does not end once the information system has been implemented and in use. There are ongoing demands and requests to train newly hired employees, communicate new functionality, and provide post-go training support to end users.

Super User Another training resource to consider is the **super user**. Super users are employees who are proficient in the use of the information system and can serve as mentors to other end users in their department. Super users may be from any user class and have specialized knowledge in both the information system and the clinical area. This knowledge and skill set enables super users to assist with implementation training and to support and troubleshoot issues after go-live. Super users may be available on all shifts to answer questions and provide assistance. Some organizations have incentive programs that encourage staff to serve as super users.

Another popular option is virtual training. Box 11–5 provides information about virtual training.

BOX 11–5 Virtual Training

Virtual training is a term that has been used somewhat loosely to refer to activities that can include almost any form of Web-based learning, virtual reality, and more recently the use of Web 2.0 and simulation in virtual worlds such as Second Life. Virtual training has been widely used by the military and Department of Defense, aviation, many industries, and for the acquisition of surgical skills.

Virtual training continues to gain popularity as a means to provide necessary skills in an environment free of risks to employees and customers. More than one-half U.S. companies use virtual training to some degree, relying primarily on Web conferencing or course management software. Significant advances in the gaming industry and Department of Defense applications helped to make virtual training feasible. Virtual training can also be run on a variety of hardware platforms. The advantages of virtual training for the provider include:

- Ease of control and editing
- Effective use of scarce resources such as trainers, space, dedicated equipment, and shrinking budgets
- The ability to provide large-scale training to employees without regard to their location
- Just-in-time training
- A realistic environment
- Economy of scale
- 24/7 access
- Consistency in approach
- The ability to match training to user needs and to provide learning experiences that while important may not occur frequently

The benefits of virtual training for learners include control over pace of learning, ability to repeat content, the ability to access training at times and from places convenient to them without a commute. The interactive learning environment also appeals to digital natives.

There are several factors to weigh when considering virtual training for your setting. These include the cost to create versus the overall benefits, the realism of the environment, learning goals, and any risks to its use. As with any instructional activity, virtual training requires detailed planning. The use of storyboards is recommended. Authoring tools facilitate the rapid creation of animation, interactive activities, and simulations for virtual environments, minimizing time-intensive, laborious coding. Unlike the limited capacity of traditional training environments, virtual training potentially has no limits to the numbers of users that it can accommodate, driving down costs per user. Virtual training allows trainers to be used more effectively as they monitor the training environment and provide answers to questions rather than repeat content.

Given that the purpose of training is to help users acquire skills that they need in real situations, it is important to create a realistic training environment. Using computers to access information system training is logical given that users are accustomed to standard keyboards and displays. Visual, auditory, and haptic feedback can be added to enhance the realism of the experience. Virtual training is particularly attractive for large healthcare delivery systems that employ thousands of employees in multiple sites over a large geographic area.

ADDITIONAL TRAINING CONSIDERATIONS

Organizations support an information systems training function in order to provide employees with the knowledge required to understand and utilize workplace technology. There are several issues related to training that should be addressed in every setting. These include but are not limited to the following:

- *Responsibility for training costs.* Institutions handle training costs differently. Some organizations may charge back training fees to each department or clinical unit. This requires an attendance tracking mechanism and a standard process for monitoring departmental training budgets. Other organizations absorb the cost of training through the information systems departmental budget.

- *Responsibility for trainers.* Internal trainers are frequently recruited from several departments and training assignments may run a course of several months. Organizations need to consider transferring these employees temporarily to the information systems department. This alleviates confusion about reporting structures and relieves the trainer of clinical duties.
- *Workflow training.* Most end users benefit from training that simulates their own workflow. Training is effective when the approach incorporates realistic, job-related scenarios and examples that are seen in day-to-day practice.
- *Confidentiality.* A well-planned and designed computer training environment complies with the confidentiality policies of the organization. The training client database must not contain the names of actual clients or cases, nor should they be discussed in the training session.
- *System updates.* System updates and enhancements are an integral part of an information system. A communication and in-service strategy must be in place so that end users are informed of new functionality, such as new forms and documentation, changes to the electronic medication administration record, nursing care plans, or critical pathway management. Any regulatory changes related to the use of the electronic medical record must be reviewed against current system functionality and relayed to the end users who are affected by the change.
- *The employee who fails to demonstrate system competence.* Some employees need extra training time, practice, and remediation regarding the acquisition of computer skills. Learning styles should be respected and difficult situations should be handled on a case-by-case basis. It is appropriate to seek the advice of human resources when an employee cannot or will not develop new job skills.
- *Training personnel from other institutions.* As hospitals and organizations merge and computer applications expand, information systems trainers may be asked to teach end users from other hospitals who are in various stages of an implementation. A review of the acquired hospital's initial needs assessment data, training strategy, and project scope and plan may help identify the information system training needs of the newly acquired hospital.
- *Training students.* Disciplines within the organization need to take responsibility for ensuring that students have a quality clinical experience. Training plans and content for students should be developed in conjunction with coordinators from each discipline; examples include medical, nursing, physical therapy, and pharmacy students.

Training Students

Training plans for students are reevaluated periodically to ensure that the needs of the student and the quality of the clinical experience are met. The training of students takes the same amount of time and resources as employee training, since students need to be able to review a client chart, view test results, complete assessments, and document findings in the information system. Organizations do not benefit from training students unless they seek employment with them after graduation. Organizations may consider a few options regarding student training. One option is to include students in existing end user classes, thus eliminating the need to create a separate curriculum track and instructional materials. For example, nursing students may benefit from the experience of attending a class with registered nurses, and medical students may learn from an opportunity to attend class with providers and medical staff.

Other options include the use of technology-based learning, utilizing faculty to instruct students, and integrating an informatics course into the curriculum. Any information system educational opportunity will enhance the student's clinical experience and his or her marketability upon graduation. Students should receive some degree of training so that they have the experience and responsibility of using an information system. Faculty can then act as mentors in the learning process instead of entering all documentation for their students during clinical rotations.

FUTURE DIRECTIONS

Skilled use of information systems is an expectation of today's healthcare workforce. That expectation makes effective information system training critical. As the realization of that criticality grows, additional attention will be accorded to the development and implementation of a training strategy that includes the use of proven training methods and measures of competency.

Movement in this direction will accord training the respect, and subsequently the resources, that it deserves. Until that time, millions of dollars will be spent on the purchase and implementation of systems without realizing many of the benefits that they can provide because employees, and providers, do not use systems according to design.

Visit nursing.pearsonhighered.com for additional cases, information, and weblinks.

CASE STUDY EXERCISE

Kevin Gallagher, RN, has access to all client records on his medical-surgical unit. Consider each of the following situations:

- Kevin's mother is admitted to the unit. Is it appropriate for him to view his mother's electronic medical record? Why or why not?
- Kevin's unit clerk also has access to Mrs. Gallagher's record. Is it appropriate for her to view Mrs. Gallagher's record? Why or why not?
- Kevin's co-worker, Kaneesha, is a client on the unit assigned to another staff nurse's care. Is it appropriate for Kevin to review her chart or laboratory results? Why or why not?

SUMMARY

- Education is key to the successful use of an information system. Education should be guided by a training strategy and plan that identifies end user needs and includes a teaching philosophy, learning objectives, and training approach. A timetable and training schedule are essential to meeting the implementation plan time line.
- Once users are identified, a needs assessment is completed so that training content can be developed according to user class and job responsibilities. The examples of user classes include physicians, nurses, and administrative support staff. User classes are assigned different levels of access privileges needed to perform their job duties within the information system.
- The transition from manual work to automation is considered a cultural change in the work setting. End users who experience difficulty with change, use of technology, or training may affect the learning experience for both the trainer and other participants in the classroom.
- The training needs of students and replacement staff need to be evaluated to determine if these individuals are required to retrieve and document client information.

- Ideally, training sessions are conducted in classroom settings and not in the clinical areas. Classrooms provide a setting free of work-related distractions. In-services and one-on-one support sessions may be held in client areas on an as-needed basis. Information systems trainers need to ensure client confidentiality. A training environment is created that is a close parallel to the production system and simulates the features and functionality that the end users will be using once the information system is in use.
- Training is time consuming and labor-intensive and should be considered an investment in enhancing workforce knowledge and as a measurement in the successful implementation of an information system.
- Information systems training may be delivered by internal resources, such as staff development educators, clinicians, information systems analysts, the software vendor, or external consultants. Internal training resources are preferable because of their familiarity with the organization and ability to maintain a flexible training schedule.
- Super users are clinical and departmental employees with additional information system training who have an above-average mastery of the software applications. They serve as resources in their departments and are capable of providing support, troubleshooting assistance, and collaborating with others to solve problems. Super users may come from any user class and should be able to help most end users.
- Proficiency assessments and review of classroom exercises and assignments may be included in the training activity to ensure that learners can demonstrate the expected job skills and demonstrate knowledge transfer.
- End users of an information system require technical, operational, and training support. Some training considerations include system upgrades to the computer training environment, training responsibility for updates regarding regulatory changes, training budget and costs, trainer selection and supervision, realism in training, confidentiality, end user competency, and meeting the training needs of all end users.

REFERENCES

Abla, S. (1995). The who, what, where, when, and how of computer education. *Computers in Nursing, 13*(3), 114–117.

Aldrich, C. (2000). The justification of IT training. *Gartner Research*, Note DF-11–3614.

Anderson, H. (2009). Kaiser's long and winding road. *Health Data Management, 17*(8), 34–40.

Barritt, C., & Alderman, F. L. (2004). *Creating a learning objects strategy. Leveraging information in a knowledge economy.* San Francisco, CA: Pfeiffer.

Combs, W. L., & Falletta, S. V. (2000). *The targeted evaluation process. A performance consultant's guide to asking the right questions and getting the results you trust.* Alexandria, VA: American Society for Training and Development.

Craig, J. (2002). The life cycle of a health care information system. In S. Englebardt & R. Nelson (Eds.), *Health care informatics* (pp. 181–208). St. Louis, MO: Mosby.

Driscoll, M. (1998). *Web-based training. Using technology to design adult learning experiences.* San Francisco, CA: Jossey-Bass Pfeiffer.

Driscoll, M. P. (2000). *Psychology of learning for instruction* (2nd ed.). Needham Heights, MA: Allyn & Bacon.

Duggan, C. M. (2005). Designing effective training. *Journal of American Health Information Management Association, 76*(6), 28–32.

Fender, M., & Jennerich, B. (1997). The real key to success with new technology: Understanding people. *Enterprise Systems Journal, 12*(4), 38, 40, 42, 44, 46.

Filipczak, B. (1996). Training on the cheap. *Training, 33*(5), 28–34.

Fleming, M., & Levie, W. H. (1993). *Instructional message design principles from the behavioral and cognitive sciences* (2nd ed.). Englewood Cliffs, NJ: Educational Technology Publications.

Glydura, A. J., Michelman, J. E., & Wilson, C. N. (1995). Multimedia training in nursing education. *Computers in Nursing, 13*(4), 169–175.

Guite, J., Lang, M., & McCartan, P. (2006). Nursing admissions process redesigned to leverage EHR. *Journal of Healthcare Information Management, 20*(2), 55–64.

Harvard Business School. (2003). *Guide to managing change and transition.* Boston, MA: Harvard Business School Publishing Company.

Henry, S. A., & Swartz, R. G. (1995). Enhancing healthcare education with accelerated learning techniques. *Journal of Nursing Staff Development, 11*(1), 21–24.

Hillestand, R., Bigelow, J., Bower, A., Girosi, F., Meilli, R., Scoville, R. & Taylor, R. (2006). Can electronic medical record systems transform health care? Potential health benefits, savings, and costs. *Health Affairs, 24*(5), 1103–1117.

Horton, W. (2001). *Leading e-learning.* Alexandria, VA: American Society for Training and Development.

Leo, J. (2009). EMR: One hospital that got it right. *Health Management Technology, 30*(8), 14–17.

Meister, J. C. (1998). *Corporate universities: Lessons in building a world-class workforce.* New York: McGraw-Hill.

Newbold, S. K. (1996). Maximizing technology for cost-effective staff education and training. In M. C. Mills, C. A. Romano, & B. R. Heller (Eds.), *Information management in nursing and health care* (pp. 216–221). Springhouse, PA: Springhouse Corporation.

Phillips, P. P., & Phillips, J. J. (2005). *Return on investment (ROI) basics.* Alexandria, VA: American Society for Training and Development.

Regan, E. A., & O'Connor, B. N. (2002). *End-user information systems: Implementing individual and work group technologies* (2nd ed.). Upper Saddle River, NJ: Prentice Hall.

Rossett, A., & Sheldon, K. (2001). *Beyond the podium, delivering training and performance in the digital world.* San Francisco, CA: Jossey-Bass Pfeiffer.

Shedenhelm, H. J., Hernke, D. A., Gusa, D. A., & Twedell, D. M. (2008). EMR implementation and ongoing education. *Nursing Management, 39*(7), 51–53.

Shrager, F. E. (2010, January/February). Revamping end-user training. *Computers, Informatics, Nursing,* 5–7.

Simonson, M., Smaldino, S., Albright, M., & Zvacek, S. (2003). *Teaching and learning at a distance: Foundations of distance education* (2nd ed.). Upper Saddle River, NJ: Merrill Prentice Hall.

Sittig, D. F., Jiang, Z., Manfre, S., Sinkfeld, K., Ginn, R., Smith, L., . . . Borden, R. (1995). Evaluating a computer-based experiential learning simulation: A case study using criterion-referenced testing. *Computers in Nursing, 13*(1), 17–24.

Thielst, C. B. (2007). Effective management of technology implementation. *Journal of Healthcare Management, 52*(4), 216–219.

Troha, F. J. (2002). The right mix: A bullet proof mode for designing blended learning. *E-learning, 3*(6), 34–37.

Vaillancourt, S. (2000, May 4). *Technology delivered learning.* Presented at Tri-State Nursing Computer Network, Pittsburgh, PA.

White, K. W., & Weight, B. H. (2000). *The online teaching guide: A handbook of attitudes, strategies, and techniques for the virtual classroom.* Needham Heights, MA: Allyn & Bacon.

Woodward, J. D., Orlans, N. M., & Higgins, P. T. (2002). *Biometrics: Identity assurance in the information age.* Berkeley, CA: McGraw-Hill Osborne.

Zielstorff, R. (1996). Training issues in system implementation. In M. C. Mills, C. A. Romano, & B. R. Heller (Eds.), *Information management in nursing and health care* (pp. 128–138). Springhouse, PA: Springhouse Corporation.

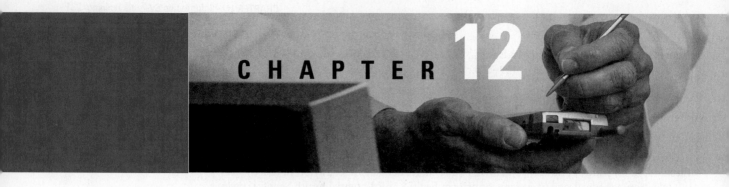

Information Security and Confidentiality

After completing this chapter, you should be able to:

1. Understand the differences between privacy, confidentiality, information privacy, and information security and the relationships among them.

2. Discuss how information system security affects privacy, confidentiality, and security.

3. Understand the significance of security for information integrity.

4. Recognize potential threats to system security and information.

5. Identify several security measures designed to protect information and discuss how they function.

6. Compare and contrast available methods of authentication in terms of levels of security, costs, and ease of use.

7. Distinguish between appropriate and inappropriate password selection and processing.

8. Provide common examples of confidential forms and communication seen in healthcare settings and identify proper disposal techniques for each.

9. Discuss the impact that Internet technology has on the security of health-related information.

10. Discuss the implications of the HIPAA privacy and security rules as they relate to the protection of medical information.

The need for increased levels of security management in organizations continues to grow. With increasing globalization and the increased use of the Internet, information technology (IT)–related risks have multiplied, including identity theft, fraudulent transactions, privacy violations, lack of authentication, redirection, phishing and spoofing, data sniffing and interception, false identities, and fraud attempts. Information system security, integrity, privacy, accessibility, and the confidentiality of personal information are major concerns in today's society as reports of stolen and compromised financial information and medical records continue to grow at an increasing rate. The fast-growing and increasingly widespread use of information technology and electronic business conducted through the Internet, along with numerous occurrences of information system penetrations and national and international terrorism, have created a need for better methods of protecting computer systems and the information they store, process, and transmit.

Healthcare information systems are required to provide rapid access to accurate and complete client information for legitimate users, while at the same time safeguarding client privacy and confidentiality. Electronic healthcare applications and databases facilitate efficient and effective sharing of information, but the ease with which healthcare applications and associated systems can be accessed creates concerns over the security of the information that they store and transmit (Sax, Kohane, & Mandl 2005). As a result, healthcare administrators must implement policies and procedures that protect information in order to comply with the Health Insurance Portability and Accountability Act (HIPAA) requirements and also meet accreditation criteria set forth by the Joint Commission (1996). These criteria continue to evolve as technology evolves and intrusion techniques become more sophisticated. The HIPAA security rule does not specify the utilization of particular technologies; instead it requires organizations to determine threats and appropriate protective measures for information, not only in electronic formats, but in all formats. Protection of client privacy and confidentiality requires an understanding of privacy, confidentiality, information privacy, and system security, as well as potential threats to these issues within an organization. Although there have been numerous improvements in information technology security capabilities as well as legal and regulatory standards, breaches of security continue to occur. This fact highlights the need for constant vigilance on the part of an organization's administrators, and all employees, to determine threats and implement protective measures for information in all formats. Continuing reports of intrusion and violations of privacy events are clear indications that electronic records are particularly susceptible to compromise on a large scale via loss, theft, or penetration of system safeguards. In the absence of a single, large-scale national authentication infrastructure, information must be protected through a combination of electronic and manual methods.

PRIVACY, CONFIDENTIALITY, AND SECURITY

While the terms *privacy* and *confidentiality* are often used interchangeably, they are not the same.

Privacy is a state of mind, a specific place, freedom from intrusion, or control over the exposure of self or of personal information (Blair 2003; Kelly & McKenzie 2002; Kmentt 1987; Reagan 2003; Windslade 1982). Privacy includes the right to determine what information is collected about an individual, how it is used, and the ability to access collected personal information to review its security and accuracy. Anonymity may be requested by an individual because he or she holds public office or is a celebrity. HIPAA regulations require that clients be given clearly written explanations of how facilities and providers may use and disclose their health information (Calloway & Venegas 2002). The content and limits of what is considered private differs among cultures and even among individuals, but they do share some basic common themes (Wikipedia.org 2009a). The efforts to protect privacy have become an international trend. The European Union established the European Network and Information Security Agency (ENISA) to address potential risks associated with the widespread use of information technology

(Mitrakas 2006). Canada established its Office of the Privacy Commissioner, and Australia and South Africa also have passed privacy legislation (Australia's privacy legislation 2002; Olinger, Britz, & Olivier 2007). Ethiopia's work to establish an e-health program and related legislation to address access, privacy, and liability issues represents a focus on health information. Privacy is typically related to personal information. Personal information is information that identifies a person or could identify a person. Obvious examples of identifying personal information include name, address, phone number, or e-mail address but could also be photos, videos, workplace name, as well as opinions and preferences. Such identifying information can potentially allow unauthorized access to medical records, financial records, birth records, educational records, credit records, work records, and so on. There is a trend toward integrating privacy commissions or agencies with information technology agencies to be in a better position to coordinate laws and regulations with information technology developments and intrusion prevention measures (Australian Government, Office of the Australian Information Commission 2010).

Confidentiality refers to a situation in which a relationship has been established and private information is shared (Romano 1987). In a healthcare environment, it is the ethical principle or legal obligation that a healthcare professional will not disclose information relating to a patient unless the patient gives consent permitting the disclosure. Confidentiality is essential for the accurate assessment, diagnosis, and treatment of health-related problems. Once a client discloses confidential information, control over the release of this information lies with the persons who access it. Confidentiality is one of the core tenets of medical practice. Yet every day, healthcare professionals face challenges to this long-standing obligation to keep all information between them and patients private (Edwards 2008). Private information should be shared only with parties who require it for client treatment (Hill 2003). The ethical duty of confidentiality entails keeping information shared during the course of a professional relationship secure and secret from others. This obligation involves making appropriate security arrangements for the storage and transmission of private information, and ensuring that the hardware, software, and networks used for storage and transmission of information is secure and that measures are implemented to prevent the interception of e-mail, instant messages (IMs), faxes, and other types of correspondence that contain private information. Nurses are obligated by the American Nurses' Association Code of Ethics and state practice laws to protect patient privacy (Blair 2003). Inappropriate redisclosure can be extremely damaging. For example, insurance companies may deny coverage based on information revealed to them without the client's knowledge or consent. Inappropriate disclosure can also damage reputations and personal relationships or result in loss of employment.

Most breeches of confidentiality often occur as a result of carelessness and can be avoided through rigorous control over client records and by not discussing clients in public areas or with persons who do not have a "need-to-know." The obligation of confidentiality prohibits healthcare professionals from disclosing information about a patient's case to other interested parties and encourages them to take precautions with the information to ensure that only authorized access occurs. But the context of medical practice makes it difficult to constrain the healthcare professional's obligation to protect patient confidentiality. In the course of caring for patients, a healthcare professional will find himself or herself exchanging information about patients with other healthcare professionals. These discussions are often critical for patient care and are an integral part of the learning experience in a teaching hospital. As such, they are justifiable so long as precautions are taken to limit the ability of others to hear or see confidential information. Computerized patient records pose new and unique challenges to confidentiality, and healthcare professionals should follow prescribed procedures for computer access and security as an added measure to protect patient information (Edwards 2008).

Information/data privacy is the relationship between data collection, information technology, an individual's expectation of privacy, and the legal, ethical, and political issues related to these relationships. It is the right to choose the conditions and extent to which information and beliefs are shared (Murdock 1980). Informed consent for the release of specific information illustrates information privacy in practice. Information privacy also includes the right to ensure the accuracy of information collected by an organization (Murdock 1980). Information privacy concerns exist wherever personally identifiable information is collected and stored in digital form or any other format. Improper or nonexistent disclosure control can be the root cause for privacy issues. Data privacy issues can arise in response to information from a wide range of sources, such as:

- Healthcare records
- Criminal justice investigations and proceedings
- Financial institutions and transactions
- Biological traits, such as genetic material
- Residence and geographic records
- Ethnicity
- Social networking

The challenge for information/data privacy is to share data while protecting personally identifiable information. The areas of information/data security utilize software, hardware, and human resources to address this issue (Wikipedia.org 2009b).

Information security is the protection of information against threats to its integrity, inadvertent disclosure, or availability (Griffiths 2003). Information systems can improve protection for client information in some ways and endanger it in others. Unlike the paper record that can be read by anyone, the automated record cannot easily be viewed without an access code and privileges. Poorly secured information systems can threaten record confidentiality because records may be accessed from multiple sites with immediate dissemination of information, making clients vulnerable to the redisclosure of sensitive information. The HIPAA Privacy Rule was crafted to protect the privacy of people who seek healthcare (Blair 2003). Effective information security systems incorporate a range of policies, security products, technologies, and procedures. Software applications that provide firewall information security and virus scanners are not enough on their own to protect the security of information. A set of policies, procedures, and security systems needs to be applied to effectively deter access to information (Crystal 2010).

Consent is the process by which an individual authorizes healthcare personnel to process his or her information based on an informed understanding of how this information will be used (Kelly & McKenzie 2002). Obtaining consent should include making the individual aware of any risks that may exist to privacy as well as measures implemented to protect privacy. HIPAA has adopted a consent form for the release of health-related information that is intended to protect a patient's privacy. The HIPAA consent form is based on rules and restrictions on who may see or be notified of a patient's protected health information (PHI). These restrictions do not include the normal interchange of information necessary to provide a patient with office services but attempt to balance these needs with the goal of providing a patient with quality professional service and care (Wulf 2007).

INFORMATION SYSTEM SECURITY

Information system security is the continuous protection of both information housed on a computer system and the system itself from threats or disruption (Ramanathan 2006; Vidalis & Kazmi 2007). The primary goals of healthcare information system security are the protection of client confidentiality and information integrity and the timely availability of information when it is needed. Availability is necessary in today's information-driven world, yet it is constantly challenged as emerging technologies expand traditional security perimeters. Availability is dependent upon **survivability.**

Survivability is "the capability of a system as a whole to fulfill its mission, in a timely manner, in the presence of attacks, failures, or accidents" (Ramanathan 2006, p. 50). The goals of healthcare information system security are best accomplished when security is planned rather than applied to an existing system after problems occur. Planning for security saves time and money and should be regarded as a form of insurance against downtime, breaches in confidentiality, loss of consumer confidence, cybercrime, liability, and lost productivity. Good security practices are necessary to ensure compliance with HIPAA legislation. Effective security starts with a thorough assessment of assets and risks, as well as necessary resources, a well-crafted security plan and policy, and a supportive organizational culture and structure. Administrative support is essential to this effort. In addition to being secure, systems must still be easily accessible for legitimate users.

Risks

Risk is a function of the likelihood of a given **threat-source** exercising a particular potential vulnerability, and the resulting impact of that adverse event on an organization (NIST 2002).

Every component in a network is constantly under attack to some degree at any one time (Ramanathan 2006). Potential threats to information and system security come from a variety of sources. These can include thieves, hackers, crackers, denial of service attacks, terrorists, viruses, snatched Web sites, flooding sites with fictitious data, power fluctuations that damage systems or data, revenge attacks, fires and natural disasters, and human error.

Espion, an advisory practice specializing in information security, ranked the top security threats for 2010 as (Espion 2010):

1. *Social networking.* Sites such as Facebook, Bebo, and MySpace offer cybercriminals a vast new world in which to target unsuspecting users.
2. *Malware attacks.* Cyber criminals are using more creative means to package and deliver malware (viruses, worms, Trojan horses, etc.), especially in e-mails.
3. *Scareware.* Attackers and fraudsters use online pop-ups designed to look like messages from the operating system, warning of a problem or virus infection to coerce users to download a program to "correct" the problem.
4. *Microsoft.* Windows 7 is expected to be widely adopted by Microsoft users worldwide. This massive user base is a prime target for the opportunistic hacker looking to attack a new, unfamiliar operating system.
5. *The insider threat.* Information is stored in files and folders, accessible remotely by large numbers of users.
6. *Localized attacks.* Often attempts to deceive victims fail because they are clearly fraudulent, text used is grammatically incorrect, spelling errors raise red flags, and graphics are poor replicas.
7. *Smartphones.* The convergence of telecommunications and computing is creating a new target for hackers.
8. *Mac OS X.* There is a widespread misconception that relative to personal computers (PCs), Macs are resistant to attack.
9. *Embedded computing.* As society relies increasingly on information and communications technology (ICT) across all aspects of life, national critical information infrastructures—such as energy, transport, and telecommunications—will become more and more connected to and reliant on the Internet.
10. *Virtualization and cloud computing.* Lower budgets and improvements in distributed computing and high-speed Internet access make cloud computing and virtualization appealing alternatives to costly and complex conventional computing methods but open alternative paths for intrusion (Espion 2010).
11. *Wireless networks (WLANs)*—The increase in the use of WiFi networks in healthcare facilities can make patient information and associated information system vulnerable if not properly secured.

These threats may result in jammed networks, violations to confidentiality, identity theft, information integrity violations, disruption in the delivery of services, monetary losses, and violation of privacy regulations. Confidential client information may also be exposed through file-sharing applications running on employee workstations as well as unauthorized access via e-mail, instant messaging, file transfers, and Internet chat sites. For this reason, it is essential to have a real-time threat management system in place at all times. A threat management system includes automatic intrusion detection and audit software, as well as security training for all employees. One aspect of security training is the identification of risks and methods to minimize these risks. Professionals can be hired to test a system for vulnerabilities.

Vulnerability is a flaw or weakness in system security procedures, design, implementation, or internal controls that could be accidentally triggered or intentionally utilized that result in a security breach or a violation of the system's security policy. Vulnerability can be a weak point in any part of the system. Vulnerabilities are not merely weaknesses in the technical protections provided by a system because vulnerabilities can be embedded in activities such as the standard operating procedures that system administrators perform, the process that the help desk personnel use to reset passwords, or inadequate log reviews. Vulnerabilities may also be identified at the policy level. For example, the lack of a clearly defined risk management or security testing policy may be responsible for the lack of vulnerability scanning.

Viruses, **worms**, and **malicious software** are programs that someone writes with the intent to steal information, cause annoyance and mayhem, or conceal what he or she is doing. Viruses, worms, Trojan horses, spyware, and root kits are all forms of malicious software. In general, malicious software may:

- Attempt to reproduce itself automatically and secretly
- Try to conceal itself from routine forms of detection (e.g., using random file names) and elimination (e.g., turning off your antivirus software)
- Spread itself to other computers via the network, such as by e-mail, unsecured file shares, password guessing, or exploiting security problems on other computers
- Modify the operating system or other legitimate software
- Make copies of itself to floppy disks, USB storage devices, CD-RW discs, or other writable media
- Send personal information gleaned from your computer back to the maker of the malicious software, or his or her criminal associates, for purposes of identity theft or to collect market data
- Display unwanted advertising banners on Web sites or in pop-up windows
- Allow malicious individuals to monitor your computer remotely over the network
- Delete, damage, or modify your documents and data files

Viruses attach themselves to other computer programs. They may, or may not, damage data or disrupt system operation. Some viruses are likened to electronic graffiti in that the writer leaves his or her mark by displaying a message. Infected e-mail and IM attachments are common means to spread malware. Executing, or opening, an attached file spreads the virus to the host computer, which then infects the hard drive. Unfortunately, viruses are frequently already widespread at the time of detection. Viruses can also be spread by downloading files from the Internet, visiting certain Web pages, and transferring data from infected CDs, DVDs, and flash drives from one computer or network to another. The personal use of the Internet and e-mail when a virus is involved can end up compromising a single computer or the entire network to which it is connected. The infectious period for viruses varies and it may occur any time that an infected program is run, or the virus may remain active in the computer memory until the computer is turned off. Viruses are not the only program types that can damage data or disrupt computing. Other malicious programs include worms, Trojan horses, logic bombs, root kits, and bacteria. See Table 12–1 for definitions and characteristics associated with each program type.

TABLE 12–1	Characteristics of Malicious Programs
Program Type	**Characteristics**
Viruses	Require normal computer operations to spread
	May or may not disrupt operations or damage data
Worms	Named for pattern of damage left behind
	Often use local area and wide area network communication practices as a means to spread and reproduce
	Usually affect memory and/or hard disk space
Trojan horses	Appear to do (or actually do) one function while performing another undesired action
	One common example resembles a regular system log-in but records user names and passwords for another program for illicit use
	Do not self-replicate
	Are easily confined once discovered
Logic bombs	Are triggered by a specific piece of data such as a date, user name, account name, or identification or another event
	May be part of a regular program or contained in a separate program
	May not activate on the first run of the program
	May be included in virus-infected programs and with Trojan horses
Root kits	Modify the operating system to hide themselves
	Use worm-like methods to propagate to other computers
Spyware	Sends information about the computer, your personal information, or your Internet browsing activities to a third party
Bacteria	Are a class of viral programs
	Do not affix themselves to existing programs

Although antivirus software can locate and eradicate viruses and other destructive programs, the best defense against malicious programs is knowledge obtained from talking with computer users and experts about problems experienced. Some people are experts in viral detection and eradication. Box 12–1 provides tips for how to avoid malicious programs. If a virus is contained on one machine, it must be isolated and disinfected with antivirus software. Suspect files should be deleted.

All backup materials should be considered suspect. It should not be necessary to reformat the hard drive to eliminate the virus(es).—Viruses, worms, and other malicious viruses are detrimental to the economy because of the loss of productivity and resources required to restore functionality.

Phishing is the criminally fraudulent process of attempting to acquire sensitive information, such as usernames, passwords, and credit card details, by masquerading as a trustworthy entity in an electronic communication (Ollmann 2005). Phishing attempts to get consumers to divulge personal information such as financial data and credit card and bank account numbers through social engineering and technical subterfuge (McMillan 2007). Phishing is typically carried out by e-mail or IM, and it often directs users to enter details at a fake Web site whose look and feel are almost identical to the legitimate one. Social engineering schemes use fraudulent e-mails to lead consumers to counterfeit Web sites, which then ask them to supply private information. Technical subterfuge schemes plant software onto computers that steals credentials directly, often by recording keystrokes. The number of phishing sites continues to increase. The Anti-Phishing Working Group is an industry association focused on eliminating the identity theft and fraud that result from the growing problem of phishing; the group provides information on attacks, resources, and consumer advice.

BOX 12–1 How to Avoid Malicious Programs

- Do not permit overprivileged users or overprivileged programs.
- Use only licensed software.
- Run the latest version of virus detection software routinely. Upload updates on a regular basis.
- Use an Internet firewall
- Never open any file attachment from an unfamiliar source.
- Use designated machines to check portable drives, storage media, and software for viruses before use.
- Maintain a list of all program files, their size, and date of creation, and review them periodically for changes.
- Retain backup copies of original software, work files, and directory structure for each PC. Backup can quickly restore system setup and work.
- Keep a record of all CD product keys and the number on the package to facilitate reinstallation.
- Keep a list of vendors, purchase dates, and serial numbers for all hardware and software items to facilitate virus tracking.
- If a virus is found, send a copy to an expert for tracking purposes.
- Watch for and download software patches that eliminate security problems.
- Ensure that system safeguards have been put into place by information technology staff. Safeguards may include programming e-mail servers to reject e-mail containing viruses, setting up policies related to e-mail and IM use, and educating the workforce.
- Stay informed of potential threats.

Spam is the use of electronic messaging systems to send unsolicited bulk messages indiscriminately. While the most widely recognized form of spam is e-mail, the term *spam* can be applied to similar actions in other media such as IM spam, Usenet newsgroup spam, Web search engine spam, spam in blogs, wiki spam, online classified ads spam, mobile phone messaging spam, Internet forum spam, junk fax transmissions, social networking spam, television advertising, and file-sharing network spam. Because the barriers to entry are low, spammers are numerous, and the volume of unsolicited mail has become extremely high. The costs, such as lost productivity and fraud, are borne by the public and by Internet service providers, which have been forced to add extra capacity to cope with the volume of spam. Spamming has been the subject of legislation in many jurisdictions (Spamhaus Project Ltd 2010). Spam is considered unwanted or "junk" e-mail, but it threatens security when it serves as a vehicle for the introduction of malware and when it threatens ready access to information by overloading networks and consuming valuable resources.

System Penetration

Even the most secure systems can be penetrated. This could result from poor or improper system configuration, both known and unknown hardware or software flaws, and operational weaknesses in processes or technical countermeasures. The best that can be hoped for is that security strategies will minimize instances of system penetration and minimize damages. One way to reduce attacks is called a penetration test, occasionally called a pentest, which is a method of evaluating the security of a computer system or network by simulating an attack from a malicious source, known as a Black Hat Hacker, or Cracker. The process involves an active analysis of the system for any potential vulnerability. A 2003 survey (Tuesday 2003) found that retail, financial services, healthcare, and federal and local governments were among the top industry sectors targeted by attackers. Significant financial losses occur annually as a result of compromised systems. A 2006 Computer Security Institute survey, conducted in conjunction with the FBI, found the average cost of a computer attack was \$203,606 (Gordon, Loeb, Lucyshyn, & Richardson 2006). Barriers to effective security include inadequate resources, money, time, and attention from management; the complexity of training; and the increasing sophistication of users.

- **Cybercrime** is now a larger threat than other physical security problems. Cybercrime commonly refers to the ability to steal personal information, such as Social Security numbers stored on computers. Cyberattackers use widely available hacker tools to find network weaknesses and gain undetected access. Netcrime refers, more precisely, to criminal exploitation of the Internet. Issues surrounding this type of crime have become high profile, particularly those surrounding hacking, copyright infringement, child pornography, and child luring. There are also problems of privacy when confidential information is lost or intercepted, lawfully or otherwise. Inconsistent and inadequate approaches to security risks allow entry. The May 2010 monthly antifraud report from RSA (2010), a trade publication from the security division of a corporation that provides information infrastructure solutions, claims that cybercriminals are focusing their criminal efforts on exploiting the healthcare industry and, more specifically, patient data. The following types of individuals may become involved in system penetration and computer crime:
- *Opportunists.* Opportunists take advantage of a situation and their access to information for uses not associated with their jobs.
- *Hackers.* Hackers are individuals who have an average, or above-average, knowledge of computer technology and who dislike rules and restrictions. Hackers penetrate systems as a challenge, and many do not regard their acts as criminal. Other hackers, however, break into systems with the intent of obtaining information, creating confusion, destroying files, or gaining a financial benefit. Members of this group are referred to as *crackers* or *black hats.*
- *Computer or information specialists.* These individuals are knowledgeable about how networks and computers work and are in an ideal position to commit computer crime and disable systems while avoiding detection.
- *Unauthorized users and over privileged users.* Although the most common fear is that a system will be penetrated from outside, the greatest threat actually comes from inside sources, namely employees, contractors, consultants, outsourced services, and vendors who view information inappropriately, disrupt information availability, or corrupt data integrity (Steele & Wargo 2007). Such access constitutes unauthorized use and may occur at any level within an organization. Consideration must be given to the access rights accorded to all employees, including system administrators.

Even though healthcare professionals have codes of ethics to maintain client confidentiality, not all professionals act ethically. System safeguards for all users are needed for this reason. As healthcare alliances grow and client records become more accessible, the likelihood of unauthorized system access increases. For an individual client, legal protection was limited in the United States until HIPAA compliance became mandatory. The Data Protection Act provides protection for confidentiality in the United Kingdom (Kelly & McKenzie 2002). Australia has taken action to protect health information as well. The right to data privacy is heavily regulated and rigidly enforced in Europe based on Article 8 of the European Convention on Human Rights (ECHR). Other nations are working on this issue. Consumer groups and healthcare professionals need to serve as advocates for healthcare consumers in the protection of privacy and confidentiality.

Concern for client confidentiality is not limited to the period in which a client is receiving active treatment. Access to client records may occur after treatment through loopholes that exist in automated systems (Hebda, Sakerka, & Czar 1994). These loopholes can be found by curious users and must be corrected as soon as information system (IS) personnel and administrators become aware of them. One example may be illustrated by the automated system that restricts access to client records during treatment but allows retrieval of any record or laboratory value after a client is discharged. Healthcare alliance physicians and office staff often need to see test results after the client's admission but should be able to view only the results for their clients. This type of problem represents an oversight in the system design process that must be corrected. Commercial software vendors are now under greater pressure to improve the security of their products as customers use their purchasing power to exert better security demands. The U.S. government has started to stipulate security provisions that vendors must meet to win contracts with the government.

Sabotage

The destruction of computer equipment or data or the disruption of normal system operation is known as **sabotage**. IS staff typically have system privileges that would permit this type of destruction, but in fact any worker may commit sabotage. Employees who are satisfied, well informed, and feel a vested interest in maintaining information and system security are less likely to perform destructive acts on a system. A positive work environment, a well-defined institutional ethics policy, and intact security mechanisms help to deter intentional information or system misuse or destruction. Consideration should be given to having background checks performed on employees and all other persons who manage and maintain computer systems or are in a position to misuse information, as a means to avert this type of threat. Insider threat management is an emerging focus area in information security and operational risk management (Steele & Wargo 2007).

Errors and Other Disasters

Errors may result from poor design, system changes that permit users more access than they require, failure to follow policies and procedures, poorly trained personnel, the absence of policies and procedures, or poorly written policies and procedures. One example of poor design is when information restricted during inpatient treatment is available to all users after the patient is discharged whether the users have a need to know or not.

Errors may also arise from incorrect user entries such as inadvertent selection of the wrong client for data retrieval or documentation. A 2006 Computing Technology Industry Association survey found that nearly 60% of the surveyed organizations reported that their last security breach was due to human error (McCarthy 2006a, 2006b). This same survey found that only about one-third of respondents' IT staffs and users received security training. Lack of adherence to established policies has resulted in several high-profile data losses when laptops and portable drives were lost or stolen. During disasters, manual backup procedures may compromise information because the primary focus is on maintaining services. One example of this is when paper reports of laboratory findings are not enclosed in envelopes for delivery to client care units.

Poor Password Management

Additional threats to information and system security come from poor password management, sharing passwords, posting log-on IDs and passwords on workstations, leaving logged-on devices unattended, and compromised handheld devices. Poor password management is likely to occur when users have multiple passwords to manage and it becomes difficult to remember them all. Password management best practices should be utilized (Hitachi ID Systems 2010).

Compromised Devices

As more and more people use personal digital assistants (PDAs) and smartphones for job-related tasks and functions, security breaches are quickly moving from the realm of theory to corporate reality. The damages are no longer just personal inconvenience but can include data theft, private information broadcasts on the Web, significant personal expense, and corporate network vulnerability. Indeed, as the "office" is defined less by a physical space and more by the location of its employees at any given time, the security of data held on PDAs, cell phones, and mobile devices has become a top concern for chief information officers and IT managers in businesses and organizations of all sizes.

Handheld devices can transmit viruses and worms to a hospital network, threatening applications, devices, and network security. Given the increased risk factor associated with these devices, experts recommend that handheld devices connect to the rest of the network through a firewall to optimize security (Malin 2007). Another security-related concern is that handheld devices can easily be stolen because of their size and portability. Theft of information may occur once the devices are in the hands of an unauthorized user or when wireless transmissions are heard or intercepted by unauthorized users.

SECURITY MECHANISMS

The security of information and computer systems should receive top priority. Typically, security mechanisms use a combination of logical and physical restrictions to provide a greater level of protection than is possible with either approach alone. This includes measures such as firewalls and the installation of antivirus and spyware detection software. These measures should also be reevaluated periodically to determine what modifications need to be made. A simple example of a logical restriction is automatic sign-off after a period of no activity.

Automatic sign-off is a mechanism that logs a user off the system after a specified period of inactivity on his or her computer. This procedure is recommended in all client care areas, as well as any other area in which sensitive data exist. The level of security provided should reflect the value of the information. Some levels of information may have no particular value and do not need protection from theft, only from unauthorized change.

Physical Security

The top 10 best practices for physical security are:

1. Lock up the server room
2. Set up surveillance
3. Make sure the most vulnerable devices are in that locked room
4. Use rack mount servers
5. Safeguard the workstations
6. Keep intruders from opening the case
7. Protect the portables
8. Pack up the backups
9. Disable the drives
10. Protect your printers

Physical security measures include the placement of computers, file servers, routers, switches, and computers in restricted areas. The server room is the heart of the physical network, and someone with physical access to the servers, switches, routers, cables, and other devices in the server room can do enormous damage. When this is not possible, equipment should be removed or locked. Physical security is a challenge for remote access. **Remote access** is the ability to use the health enterprise's information system from outside locations, such as a physician's office or home. Secure modems and encryption are particularly useful in conjunction with remote access.

Physical security is challenged by the growing use of mobile wireless devices such as notebooks; tablet PCs, and PDAs, as well as portable storage devices such as thumb drives. These items may fall into the hands of unauthorized individuals. Security cables, motion detectors, or alarms used with these devices help prevent theft. Secure, lockable briefcases should be considered for the storage of devices not in use. In the event that mobile devices are stolen, some measure of protection can be provided by making the boot-up process password protected; setting passwords on individual files; storing files in zipped, password-protected folders; and/or encrypting the hard drive. These actions are not foolproof because hard drives can be removed, decrypted, and copied. Daily backups and portable storage devices such as an external drive help to prevent data loss. It is essential to include wireless devices as part of organizational standards, policies, and procedures to ensure that risk management and preventive measures are taken.

Another facet of physical security is introduced when healthcare enterprises provide Internet access within the facility for visitors and patients. Increasingly this is an expected amenity as it is available in hotels, public areas, and coffeehouses (Stern 2007). Individuals who opt to use free wireless connections in public places should employ the following precautions:

- *Look for posted signs that provide the exact name of the hotspot.* This will help to avoid fake networks that are designed to collect passwords, credit card information, and other personal data.
- *Change settings so that permission is required before connecting to a new network.* This measure helps to avoid fake networks.
- *Avoid networks that are computer-to-computer.* Free wireless networks should be noted as such. Computer-to-computer networks are generally fake networks set up for spurious purposes.
- *Turn off file sharing.* This will keep passersby from accessing stored data.
- *Refrain from online banking or shopping.* These activities should be avoided unless network security can be guaranteed.
- *Do not store passwords on your computer or other mobile devices.* These may be accessed through suspect connections or compromised when the physical device is stolen.
- *Verify that a PC's software firewall is turned on.*

Public Internet access should not be provided on the same network that is used to transmit secure health data unless extensive measures are used to maintain the security of that data.

Authentication

Authentication is the process of determining whether someone is who he or she professes to be. This usually involves a username and a password, but can include other methods of proving identity, such as a smart card, retina scan, voice recognition, or fingerprints. Authentication is equivalent to showing your driver's license or passport at the ticket counter at the airport. Several methods of authentication exist, ranging from log-on passwords to digital certificates to public or private keys used for encryption and biometric measures. Authentication is one component of identity management (ID management).

ID management is a broad administrative area that deals with identifying individuals in a system and controlling their access to resources within that system by associating user rights and restrictions with an established identity. ID management provides managers a unique view of the IT environment for each user, determined primarily by job function and security concerns. ID management software is available, but it requires more work for what is typically an already overworked IT office. Organizations have to develop a central database to maintain identities, manage the access rights for every user on the network, and enforce a strict policy for how that database will be managed.

Passwords are simply secret words or phrases. They can be compromised in many ways:

- Users may write them down or share them, so that they are no longer really secret.
- Passwords can be guessed, either by a person or by a program designed to try numerous possible combinations in rapid succession.

- Passwords may be transmitted over a network either in plain text or encoded in a way that can be readily converted back to plaintext.
- Passwords may be stored on a workstation, server, or backup media in plain text or encoded in a way that can be readily converted back to plaintext.

Each of these vulnerabilities makes it easier for someone to acquire the password value and consequently pose as the user whose identity the password protects. Conversely, if passwords are managed securely by users and if password systems are constructed so as to prevent brute-force attacks and inspection or decryption of passwords in transit and in storage, then passwords can actually be quite secure.

Access codes and passwords are a common means to authenticate access to automated records, mainly because they represent a familiar, available, and inexpensive technology (Campbell, Kleeman, & Ma 2007; Lemos 2006). A password is a collection of alphanumeric characters that the user enters into the computer. This may be required after the entry and acceptance of an access code, sometimes referred to as the *user name.* IS administrators sometimes need this information to problem-solve or reissue passwords. The password does not appear on the screen when it is entered and it should not be known to anyone but the user and IS administrators.

The keys to password strength are length and complexity. An ideal password is long and has letters, punctuation marks, symbols, and numbers. The greater the variety of characters in a password, the greater is its strength. Recommendations for password selection and use are given in Box 12–2. Obvious passwords such as the user's name, house number, or dictionary words are easily compromised. Strong passwords use combinations of letters, numbers, and symbols that are not easily guessed. Software is available to test and eliminate easily compromised passwords before use.

Individuals should not share passwords or leave computers logged on and unattended. System administrators must keep files that contain password lists safe from view or copying by unauthorized individuals. One compromised password can jeopardize information and the system that contains it. For this reason, users should not use the same password for access to more than one site or system. Using the same password at various sites reduces security. System administrators need to allow legitimate users the opportunity to access the system while refusing entry to others. One means to accomplish this is to shut down a workstation after a random number of unsuccessful access attempts and send security personnel to check that area. Although passwords provide considerable system protection, other defenses are still necessary.

BOX 12–2   Recommendations for Password Selection and Use

- Choose passwords that are at least 12, preferably 14, characters long.
- Select stronger passwords for higher levels of security.
- Avoid using the same password for more than one application.
- Do not use the browser "password save" feature.
- Use combinations of uppercase and lowercase letters, numbers, punctuation marks, and symbols.
- Do not use proper names, initials, words taken from the dictionary, or account names.
- Do not use words that are spelled backwards or with reversed syllables.
- Do not use dates or telephone number, license plate, or Social Security numbers.
- Do not store or automate passwords in the computer.
- Avoid repeated numbers or letters.
- Keep passwords private.
- Change passwords frequently, with no reuse of passwords for a specified period.
- Use the entire keyboard, not just the letters and characters you use or see most often.

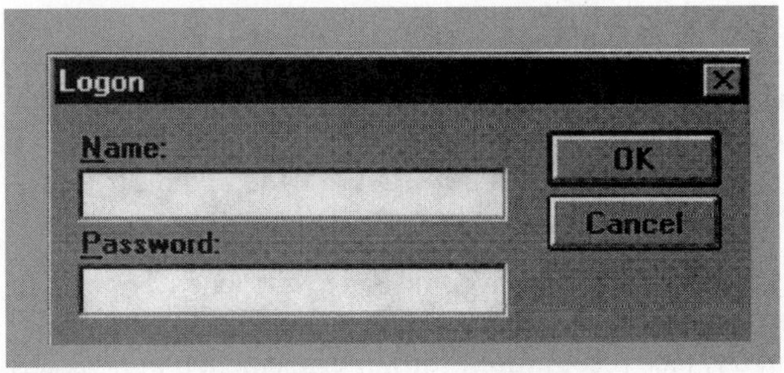

FIGURE 12–1 • Screenshot of a log-on screen

These include measures to verify user identity. Figure 12–1 shows a screen shot of a typical log-on screen.

Sign-on/log-on access codes and passwords are generally assigned on successful completion of system training. Passwords may be difficult for a user to recall. This leads some people to write passwords down and post them in conspicuous places. This practice should be prohibited. Users who find it necessary to record the dozens of passwords used to access various sites and systems must store them in an area away from the computer and out of casual view. Storing passwords in a file on the computer is a problem if the device is shared by others or if the hard drive crashes or is replaced. A file-cleaning utility should be used to permanently erase the drive so that password files cannot be restored. When a file is used to store passwords, it should be encrypted and password protected. Passwords should be regarded as an electronic signature. There is software available to check the strength of a password and it would be useful to test your password with a password checker. A password checker evaluates a password's strength automatically.

Frequent and random password change is recommended as a routine security mechanism. This can be a time-consuming and unpleasant task because it is difficult for users to remember new passwords. There are, however, situations that mandate immediate change or deletion of access codes and passwords, including suspicion of unauthorized access and termination of employees. Codes and passwords should also be deleted with status changes such as resignations; leaves of absence; and the completion of rotations for students, faculty, and residents. Because IS staff can view any information in the system, all members of the department should receive new passwords when IS personnel leave. In the event that an IS employee is terminated, department door locks or combinations should be changed as well.

Disadvantages associated with the use of passwords include the following:

- They are typically poorly managed, are frequently forgotten, and often need to be reset by help desk staff.
- They can be shared or stolen.
- Users often choose very guessable passwords.
- The complex rules for password generation are largely unenforceable.
- The purpose of passwords is defeated when the user sets the browser to remember them.

Public key infrastructure (PKI) is a set of hardware, software, people, policies, and procedures used to create, manage, distribute, use, store, and revoke digital certificates (Toorani and Shirazi 2008). Encrypted key-based authentication is a more secure technology than simply using passwords. **PKI** is an arrangement that binds public keys with respective user identities by means of a **certificate authority (CA).** The term **trusted third party (TTP)** may also be used for *certificate authority.* PKI uses an encrypted passkey that can be provided to the user in various formats, including a smartcard, token, or wireless transmitter. The passkey provides a secret value that is verified against a registered digital certificate. The user submits the passkey information during the sign-on/log-on process, and the PKI system compares it against the registered digital certificate ID to verify a match. Digital certificates include information about the owner, such as systems that he or she may access, level of access, and biometric measures. Digital certificates provide assurance of the identity, rights, and privileges of the user. Security tokens that resemble key chain fobs are an example of this technology. Tokens strengthen authentication because the user must use both the token and a special PIN code to gain access. PKI can provide a common infrastructure that allows access to multiple delivery systems across an organization or organizations.

Biometrics Scanned employee identification may include a name badge but generally refers to biometric authentication, which is based on a unique biological trait, such as a fingerprint, voice or iris pattern, retinal scan, hand geometry, face recognition, ear pattern, smell, blood vessels in the palm, gait recognition, or keystroke cadence (Sturdevant 2007). Biometric technology is feasible and can be very accurate. Unlike passwords or devices that can be forgotten or stolen, biometric measures are always with the individual, barring major injury, and cannot be lost, stolen, or used without user consent.

The quality of biometric authentication varies by device and software used. Finger print scanning is a popular biometric employee identification technique but may result in a high rate of failure of first print readings as the number of users increases. This situation may require a second or third reading. Individuals must learn the proper method of placing their fingers into scanners. Skin moisture and temperature also affect the quality of the scan. Very moist or dry skin and cold fingers negatively affect reading. Some readers can be fooled by using tape, gelatin, or other measures. Infection control is a related concern when biometric authentication requires contact. No contact is required to scan the voice or iris pattern, retina, hand geometry, face, ear pattern, smell, blood vessels in the palm, or for gait recognition. Biometric authentication helps organizations to better comply with regulations and reduces the amount of time that help staff spend resetting passwords. The use of biometric measures for authentication is expected to replace password use in the near future.

Other authentication devices include proximity radio systems that detect user badges within a specified distance, picture authentication packages that use pictures instead of passwords, and digital certificates. Users should have different authentication requirements, depending upon the sensitivity or value of the resources that they access. Authentication can be strengthened by requiring multifactor authentication. Authentication policies should outline acceptable forms of authentication, depending on multiple factors, including class of user, type of resources, location, and time of day. The policy must also protect authentication systems from attack and sabotage. Building an authentication policy is one thing but implementing, managing, and enforcing it is another.

Firewalls and Other Network Devices

A **firewall** is a component of a computer system or network that is designed to block unauthorized access while permitting authorized communications. It is a device or set of devices that are configured to permit or deny network transmissions based upon a set of rules and other criteria. Firewalls can be implemented in either hardware or software, or a combination of both. A typical firewall is a combination of hardware and software that forms a barrier between systems, or different parts of a single system, to protect those systems from unauthorized access. Firewalls screen traffic, allow only approved transactions to pass through them, and restrict access to other systems or sensitive areas such as client information, payroll, or personnel data. There are several types of firewall techniques:

1. *Packet filter.* Packet filtering inspects each packet passing through the network and accepts or rejects it based on user-defined rules. Although difficult to configure, it is fairly effective and mostly transparent to its users. It is susceptible to IP spoofing, a situation in which IP addresses are forged in order to conceal the identity of the sender.
2. *Application gateway.* Applies security mechanisms to specific applications, such as FTP and Telnet servers. This is very effective, but can impose performance degradation.

3. *Circuit-level gateway.* Applies security mechanisms when a Transmission Control Protocol (TCP) or User Datagram Protocol (UDP) connection to the Internet is established. Once the connection has been made, packets can flow between the hosts without further checking.

4. *Proxy server.* Intercepts all messages entering and leaving the network. The proxy server effectively hides the true network addresses (Wikipedia.org 2008).

Firewalls, or a separate device behind them, may be able to inspect transmissions for anomalies that help to identify malware (Britt 2005). Multiple firewalls can increase protection. Strong security policies and practices strengthen firewall protection. Once a user has passed through the firewall, controlling access to individual applications takes place elsewhere. Firewalls are not foolproof. Specialists periodically create "patches" to counter flaws in security software. It is imperative to apply security patches as soon as they become available. Security protocols on network switches and routers also help. Another means to safeguard information is to segment a network into different levels of security each with its own level of priorities and set of policies (Malin 2007). It is also essential to train and remind employees about their role in security.

Wireless Network Security

After assessing the risks associated with an installed wireless network, the following steps may be taken to secure a wireless network (McCullough 2004):

1. Change the default service set identifier (SSID), the unique identifier attached to the packets of information sent a wireless network.
2. Disable the SSID broadcast.
3. Change the default IP address.
4. Consider disabling the dynamic host configuration protocol (DHCP) that assigns IP addresses to devices as they join a network.
5. Enable MAC address filtering, a security access control methodology that assigns unique address to network cards and permits or denies access via the use of a list.
6. Change the default administrative passwords.
7. Change default user names.
8. Enable wired equivalent privacy (WEP) or WiFi–protected access (WPA) encryption to protect data from inadvertent access.
9. Adjust broadcast power to limit access.
10. Set minimum connection speeds required for access.
11. Set access times to limit access.

Application Security

Another area of concern is application security, which encompasses measures taken throughout an application program's lifecycle to prevent exceptions in the security policy of an application or the underlying system (vulnerabilities) through flaws in the design, development, deployment, upgrade, or maintenance of an application. Application security measures should be used with the client information system and other systems such as payroll records. Security testing techniques look for vulnerabilities or security holes in applications. These vulnerabilities leave applications open to exploitation. Ideally, security testing is implemented throughout the entire software development life cycle (SDLC) so that vulnerabilities may be addressed in a timely and thorough manner. Unfortunately, testing is often conducted as an afterthought at the end of the development cycle. Likewise, it is important for employees to sign off when they leave a workstation or computer or are finished using a particular software application, because failure to do so may allow others to use their code to access information. Automatic sign-off has been designed as a security measure when employees fail to properly exit a program or step away from a computer.

Antivirus Software

Antivirus software is a set of computer programs that can locate and eradicate malware, including computer viruses, worms, and Trojan horses. Such programs may also prevent and remove adware, spyware, and other forms of malware from scanned memory sticks, storage devices, individual computers, and networks. The continuous creation of new viruses makes it necessary to update antivirus software frequently. Antivirus software may come preloaded on new computers or be obtained in computer stores or over the Internet. The user must then frequently download updated virus definitions from the vendor's Web site. Some vendors automatically notify users as new virus definitions become available. Users can set up antivirus software to automatically run a virus check on the PC or server on a scheduled basis in addition to performing random checks. Networked computers are generally set by the administrator to include a virus scan at routine start-up, automatically scan new files, and update antivirus files. Network administrators can also set privileges to prohibit unauthorized file downloads.

Spyware Detection Software

Spyware is a data collection mechanism that installs itself without the user's permission. This often happens when a user is browsing the Web or downloading software. Spyware can include cookies that track Web use as well as applications that capture credit card, bank, and PIN numbers or other personal health information (PHI) stored on that computer for illicit purposes by an unauthorized person. This is a concern for all healthcare providers because it threatens PHI. No computer that is attached to the Internet is immune.

Clues that spyware has infected a computer include the presence of pop-up ads, keys that do not work, random error messages, and poor system performance. Because of the security threat that this represents, spyware detection software should be utilized.

ADMINISTRATIVE AND PERSONNEL ISSUES

The final responsibility for creating and managing the infrastructure to protect client privacy and confidentiality lies with healthcare administrators. This involves developing a plan, policies, designated structure for implementation, user access levels, and an adequate budget (Rainer, Marshall, Knapp, & Montgomery 2007). Upper-level management must have security awareness training and set a positive example for all stakeholders, including employees, students, consultants, and contractors, because privacy and security is a responsibility shared by everyone in the organization. Administration must also work with IS personnel to establish the following centralized security functions:

- *A comprehensive security plan.* This plan needs to be developed with input from administrators, information services personnel, and clinical staff. It should define security responsibilities for each level of personnel as well as a timeline for the development and implementation of policies, procedures, and physical infrastructure. Incorporation of computer forensics as a plan component helps to build and maintain a strong security image. **Computer forensics** refers to the collection of electronic evidence for purposes of formal litigation and simple internal investigations.
- *Accurate and complete information security policies, procedures, and standards.* These should be published online for easy access, with e-mail notification of employees as new policies are released.
- *Information asset ownership and sensitivity classifications.* Ownership in this context refers to who is responsible for the information, including its security. Sensitivity classification is a determination of how damaging an item of information might be if it were disclosed inappropriately. The level of sensitivity may be used to determine what information should be encrypted.

- *Identification of a comprehensive security program.* A well-defined security plan can avert or minimize threats. A key part of the plan is the identification of responsibility for information integrity, privacy, and confidentiality. A strong plan incorporates computer forensics.
- *Information security training and user support.* Education is an important component in fostering proper system use. Most problems with information system security are primarily related to the human factor, rather than the technical one.
- *An institution-wide information security awareness program.* Formal IS training and frequent suggestions are needed to remind users of the need to protect information.

For an information security plan to be effective, responsibility must be shared by healthcare administrators, IS and healthcare professionals, and all system users. Involving users in system security development fosters ownership of this responsibility and facilitates the ability to trace problems, limit damage, and make corrective changes. This involvement can occur on an individual level or through an institutional security committee. Security committees should consider routine maintenance, confidentiality clauses in vendor contracts, third-party payer needs, legal issues inclusive of monitoring, ongoing security needs as the institution and system evolve, and disaster planning. The IS department should address these areas when there is no security committee. Individual users are responsible for protecting their passwords, saving and backing up work files on a regular basis, securing removable storage media, and not leaving confidential information unattended on the computer screen or in paper form. They should also be responsible for reporting any observed unauthorized access. It may be necessary to outsource security if there are insufficient resources internally, but this decision needs to be carefully weighed. A set of 33 principles for securing information technology systems is provided by NIST SP 800-14 "Generally Accepted Principles and Practices for Securing Information Technology Systems." These principles can act as a basis for establishing a security plan (Whitman and Mattord 2009).

LEVELS OF ACCESS

Access should be strictly granted on a need-to-know basis. This means no personnel, including IS staff, should have routine access to confidential information unless it is required by a particular event, at which time an audit trail should be established. IS personnel must be held to the same confidentiality requirements that are applied to other personnel.

Access Limitations

Access should be determined based on who needs a medical record and under what conditions and locations. For example, direct care providers require information about their clients under a wide range of conditions and locations. Access levels should be decided by defining roles for every level of personnel. Levels of personnel can be referred to as "user classes." Each user class has a different set of privileges. Initial system access should be contingent on successful completion of system training and demonstration of competence. User training should address appropriate uses of information and the consequences of information misuse. User roles and audits must be incorporated into the design of information systems to best ensure security, privacy, accessibility, and confidentiality. Attempts to define user roles and implement audits into older hospital information systems are extremely difficult. A definition of each user role is instrumental in preventing unauthorized access to sensitive healthcare information. For example, nursing assistants are responsible for the documentation of hygiene, dietary intakes, vital signs, and fluid intake and output but this user should not be able to access diagnostic and historical information.

User Authentication

Access by authorized individuals can be verified through user authentication. User authentication can be based on (a) what you know, for example, passwords; (b) what you have, for example, smartcard; (c) what you are, for example, fingerprint; or (d) what you do, for example, voice recognition. Third-party authentication systems such as Kerberos and Sesame can be used. One common form of authentication is the appearance of the user's name on the screen. In the event that other staff members discover a discrepancy, they have the responsibility to report it immediately. It is important to develop authentication policies jointly with IT personnel, business staff, and end users. It is also critical to factor in time to install and test drivers and hardware, as well as to consider the time and resources required to enroll and update users. Support costs and training times increase as the complexity of the authentication process increases. Unwieldy authentication systems can reduce staff productivity.

Personnel Issues

Clear policies and procedures must be established and communicated to all personnel who handle information. Staff education is a key element for information and system security. Education for information handling and system use should include an orientation, system training, and a discussion of what is acceptable and unacceptable behavior. Staff should also be informed of the consequences for unauthorized access and information misuse, the use of audit trails, and ongoing measures to heighten security awareness. Staff needs to know what constitutes an incident and how it should be handled. There should be periodic reminders that client information belongs to the client as well as what constitutes professional, legal, and ethical behavior. Yearly review of the ethical computing statement is one way to emphasize the importance of ethical behavior. Figure 12–2 displays an example of such a statement. Education and monitoring activities show administrative commitment to ethical information use. Explicit written policies and procedures provide the discipline to achieve information and system security. Policies and procedures should address information ethics, training, access control, system monitoring, data entry, backup procedures, responsibilities for the use of information on mobile devices and at remote sites, and exchange of client information with other healthcare providers. Information ethics policies should do the following:

- *Plan for audit trails.* **Audit trails** are a record of IS activity. Users should know that their system access is monitored and that audit trail records will be kept for a period of years.
- *Establish acceptable computer uses.* This includes authorized access and using only authorized and legal copies of software. One example of how this might be enforced is requiring licenses for all software used within the institution.
- *Collect only required data.* Limiting the collection of information to what is needed, and no more, eliminates the danger of inappropriate disclosure of unneeded information and may lessen the workload.
- *Encourage client review of files for accuracy and error correction.* Client inspection of records ensures information integrity.
- *Establish controls for the use of information after hours and off-site.* As many employees and physicians work at home or complete projects on their own time, it is important to develop policies related to downloading files or carrying information off the premises. Both the types of information that may be carried on mobile devices and the responsibilities of the staff member to safeguard that information must be communicated to all employees.

For information security, integrity, confidentiality, accessibility, and privacy policies to be effective, they must meet the following criteria:

- Be disseminated
- Be reviewed
- Be understandable
- Be compliant
- Be enforceable and enforced

ST. FRANCIS HEALTH SYSTEM
INFORMATION SYSTEM
USER SIGN-ON CODE RECEIPT

[] St. Francis Medical Center
[] St. Francis Hospital of New Castle
[] St. Francis Central Hospital
[] _____

ST. FRANCIS HEALTH SYSTEM

Hospital Personnel or Hospital Based Physician Sign-On codes are confidential. Disclosure of your Sign-On code, attempts to discover another person's Sign-On code, or unauthorized use of a Sign-On code are grounds for immediate dismissal.

I, the undersigned, acknowledge receipt of my User Sign-On Code and understand that:

1. My User Sign-On Code is equivalent of my signature; (Please note that the electronic signature is recognized by the Health Care Finance Administration (HCFA) and the Commonwealth of Pennsylvania).

2. Accessing the system via my Sign-On Code, is recorded permanently;

3. If assigned a User Sign-On Code, I will not disclose this code to anyone;

4. I will not attempt to learn another user's User Sign-On Code;

5. I will not attempt to access information in the system by using a User Sign-On Code other than my own;

6. I will access only that information which is necessary to perform my authorized functions;

7. If I have reason to believe that the confidentiality of my User Sign-On Code has been broken, I will contact Information Services immediately so that the suspect code can be deleted and a new code assigned to me; and

I understand that if I violate any of the above statements, it will be referred to the appropriate authority.

I further understand that my User Sign-On Code will be deleted from the system when I no longer hold an appointment or am no longer employed at St. Francis or authorization is otherwise revoked.

I have read the above statements and understand the implications if confidentiality of Sign-On code is violated.

_____ Social Security #_____-_____-_____
Name (Please print)

Dept:_____ Supervisor:_____ Position:_____

System: MIS:_____ MEDIPAC:_____ G/L:_____ A/P:_____ CYBORG:_____ OTHER:_____

Signature of Code Recipient_____ Date:___/___/___

* Trainer Signature:_____ Date:___/___/___

* Dept. Head Authorization:_____ Date:___/___/___

Issuer Signature:_____ Date:___/___/___
        Information Services

Code will not be issued without proper identification and signature in presence of issuer.
* Signature **must** be present prior to issuance of code.   MIS User Class:_____

FORM H-1280 Date of Origin: 2/85
         Revised: 10/95

File: Personnel Department
Physicians: Medical Staff Office

FIGURE 12–2 • Sample ethical computing statement (reprinted by permission of St. Francis Health System, Pittsburgh, PA)

Information ethics policies are most credible when practiced by top administrators and IS personnel. After policies have been developed and implemented, a Security Education, Training, and Awareness program (SETA) must be implemented. A SETA program should consist of three elements: security education, security training, and security awareness.

System Security Management

System security involves protection against deliberate attacks, errors, omissions, and disasters. Good system management is a key component of a strong framework for security because it encompasses the following tasks:

- Monitoring
- Maintenance

- Operations
- Traffic management
- Supervision
- Risk management

Monitoring includes setting and enforcing standards, tracking changes, and observing all system activity in the operational environment. Monitoring also alerts managers to problems such as intruders or the introduction of a virus. Maintenance encompasses all activity needed for proper operation of hardware, including preventive measures such as testing, periodic applications of patches, and replacement of select components to ensure that data are available when needed. Maintenance includes documentation of all configuration settings, server protocols, and network addresses and changes to any mentioned earlier, so that records are available in the event that the system must be restored. Operations management includes all activities needed to provide, sustain, modify, or cease system and telecommunications. Traffic management permits rerouting of transmissions for better system performance. Supervision requires monitoring traffic as well as system performance and taking measures to prevent system overload and crashes.

Risk management helps to identify and curtail high-risk problem areas in a timely fashion. Although software is available to facilitate system management tasks, the lack of comprehensive commercial packages available for the management of systems across networks has forced institutions to develop in-house solutions or use outsourcing agents for customized applications. Many organizations have different staff members for network and systems management. Network staff traditionally focus on hardware such as switches, routers, and connections, whereas IS personnel track information and software use. The security officer plays a pivotal role in tracking personnel information about system use. It is the security officer who should assign access codes and passwords to authorized users and who deletes codes for staff no longer with the organization and changes access rights when personnel move from one department to another. Increased computing needs and limited budgets require greater staff efficiency. Effective use of system and network management tools will help to provide that efficiency, minimize the number of required support staff, reduce support costs, and improve information security.

AUDIT TRAILS

Audit trails maintain a record of system activity both by system and application processes and by user activity of systems and applications. In conjunction with appropriate tools and procedures, audit trails can assist in detecting security violations, performance problems, and flaws in applications. Auditing software helps to maintain security by recording unauthorized access to certain programs, screens, or records. Audits show access to records by user or by password and all access by an individual or level of employee, for example, user class. For this reason all users should sign off after each use; if they encounter an active session that belongs to another user, they should log that user off and sign in under their own access credentials. Frequent review of audit trails for unusual activity quickly identifies inappropriate use. Poorly audited systems invite fraud and abuse. The level of control in many audit systems is not sufficient for HIPAA compliance. Optimally, audits should be able to track all access, creations, updates, and edits at the data element level for each patient record. This ability will support a consumer's right to view logs of who accessed his or her data, what they saw, and when the data were accessed. Audit trail records must now be available for longer periods of time. Before HIPAA, audit logs were usually kept for limited periods. Consideration must be given now to the retention period for audit logs. Department managers must be advised when audit trails indicate that members of their staff have accessed records without a justifiable need. Audit trails are essential but may still fail to capture the full range of security issues. In the event that an audit trail identifies unauthorized access, it is important to enforce written security policy. At a minimum, this should be a verbal reprimand or possibly a notation on the employee's performance evaluation. In many institutions, however, employees are held to the statement they signed on receipt of their access code and password, acknowledging termination of employment as a possible consequence of inappropriate system use. When employees are terminated for this reason, they may be escorted off the premises by the security department to prevent any further opportunity for unauthorized access. Audit trails may also reveal unauthorized access from outside sources, although little legal recourse has been available to punish the guilty parties until recently. There is now an increased legislative activity to prevent and punish cybercrime.

HANDLING AND DISPOSAL OF CONFIDENTIAL INFORMATION

Although most people recognize the need to keep electronic medical records confidential, many pay less attention to safeguarding information printed from the record or extracted from it electronically for reporting purposes. All client record information should be treated as confidential and kept from being viewed by unauthorized persons regardless of its form or format.

Computer Printouts

In the past, the primary sources of inadvertent disclosure of information were printouts of portions of client records and faxes. All papers containing personal health information (PHI), such as prescriptions, laboratory specimen labels, identification bracelets, meal descriptions, addressograph plates, and any other items that carry a patient's name, address, Social Security number, date of birth, or age must be destroyed. This may entail using shredders or locked receptacles for shredding and incineration later. Shredding on-site may offer better control as well as cost savings. Nurses may also be responsible for erasing from a computer's hard drive files containing calendars, surgery schedules, or other daily records that include PHI. Disposal policies for records must be clear and enforced. For tracking purposes, each page of output should have a serial number or other means of identification so that an audit trail is maintained that identifies what each paper record is as well as the date and method for destruction and the identity of individuals witnessing the destruction. The person designated to oversee this destruction can vary but it may be a secretary or staff from information services. Control must be established over the materials that users print or fax. Some institutions include a header on all printouts such as lab results that display the word *confidential* in capital letters. This reminds staff to dispose of materials appropriately.

Faxes

Institutional and departmental policies must dictate the types of information that can be sent, allowable recipients, the location to which transmissions are sent, and the verification process. Information should not exceed that requested or required for immediate clinical needs. Legal counsel should review policies for consistency with federal and state law. Clients should sign a release form before faxing any client information. The following measures enhance fax security:

- *Confirm that fax numbers are correct before sending information.* This helps to ensure that information is appropriately directed.
- *The use of a cover sheet.* This is a particularly important practice when the fax machine serves a number of different users. A cover sheet eliminates the need for the recipient to read the fax transmission to determine who gets it. The cover sheet may also contain a statement to remind recipients of the presence of confidential information. Figure 12–3 displays an example of a fax cover sheet.
- *Authentication at both ends of the transmission before data transmission.* This action verifies that the source and destination are correct. This is done through the use of a fax cover sheet

ST. FRANCIS MEDICAL CENTER
FAX TRANSMITTAL FORM

ST. FRANCIS HEALTH SYSTEM

DATE: _____   NO. OF PAGES: _____
(including cover sheet)

FROM: _____

FACILITY: _____

DEPARTMENT: _____

TELEPHONE: _____   FAX: _____

TO: _____

FACILITY: _____

DEPARTMENT: _____

TELEPHONE: _____   FAX: _____

COMMENTS: _____

_____

_____

_____

_____

_____

This fax contains privileged and confidential information intended only for the use of the recipient named above. If you are not the intended recipient of this fax or the employee or agent responsible for delivering it to the intended recipient, you are hereby notified that any dissemination or copying of this fax is strictly prohibited. If you have received this fax in error, please notify sender listed above; and return the original to the above address via U.S. mail.

This information has been disclosed to you from records whose confidentiality is protected by state and federal law. Any further disclosure of this information without the prior written consent of the person to whom it pertains may be prohibited.

FIGURE 12–3 • Sample fax cover sheet (reprinted by permission of St. Francis Health System, Pittsburgh, PA)

listing intended recipient, the sender, both phone and fax numbers, and the transmittal confirmation sheet that lists the fax number.

- *Programmed speed-dial keys.* Programmed keys eliminate the chance of dialing errors and misdirected fax transmissions.
- *Encryption.* Encoding transmissions makes it impossible to read confidential information without the encryption key. This safeguards fax transmissions that might be sent to a wrong number.
- *Sealed envelopes for delivery.* The enclosure of confidential information in sealed envelopes provides a barrier to discourage casual viewing.
- *Fax machine placement in secure areas.* Secure areas have limited traffic and few, if any, strangers.
- *Limited machine access by designated individuals.* Restricting access to a few people makes it easier to enforce accountability for actions and to identify any transgressions.

- *Inclusion of a request to return documents by mail.* Inadvertent entry of a wrong telephone number can jeopardize sensitive information. In the event that information is faxed to a wrong number, a request to return documents may limit further disclosure.
- *A log of all fax transmissions.* A roster of all faxes sent and received provides a means to keep track of what information is sent and to help ensure that only appropriate information is sent.

Electronic Files

Given that virtually all documents originate in electronic format, the destruction of paper print-outs is almost incidental. For this reason, measures must be taken to ensure that confidential information contained on storage media, computers, and hard drives that is no longer needed is also disposed of properly. This method must go beyond the dumpster to include destruction of the storage media or electronically writing over files to ensure that no information can be retrieved from them. This is particularly important as equipment is often moved from one area of an organization to another and may even be donated to outside entities.

E-Mail, Instant Messages, and the Internet

E-mail, IM, and the Internet are discussed at length in Chapter 4. Policy should dictate what types of information may be allowed. E-mail and IM are great means of disseminating information, such as announcements, to large numbers of people quickly and inexpensively. However, information that is potentially sensitive should not be sent via these routes unless it is encrypted. Nonencrypted messages can be read, and public e-mail password protection of mailboxes can be cracked. When looking at encryption, ask whether e-mail and IM software encrypts all messages between users, whether messages are encrypted both in transit and when stored in the mailbox, and whether messages remain encrypted when sent between different e-mail programs. Unauthorized, or dormant, mail accounts should be destroyed and firewalls used for additional protection. It is easy to inadvertently send out messages to the wrong party, attach the wrong document, or include persons who are not authorized to see the information. Software can be used to monitor network traffic for patterns that represent client information such as lists or Social Security numbers. This same software can detect requests for files, and monitor IM and Web-based mail to determine if requests come from appropriate parties or if there are problems with information being sent to unauthorized recipients.

HIPAA regulations affect e-mail use and routing infrastructures. Most e-mail networks allow messages to travel through any available simple mail transfer protocol (SMTP) relay until it reaches its destination. Messages are stored at each relay and then forwarded. These relays can be hacked; encryption helps to ensure that intercepted mail cannot be read but it does not keep it secure. Security lies with access and control of decryption keys. Central administration for encryption, key management, and disclosure should be addressed via policies and training. Another concern related to e-mail and information system security is spam. **Spam** is unsolicited e-mail that uses valuable server space and employee time and can serve as an entry for malicious programs. E-mail security software can filter out spam. The downside is that this process may result in the loss of a small percentage of legitimate mail. Monitoring e-mail is important to avoid legal liability and maintain network security, employee productivity, and confidentiality of information.

Web-Based Applications for Healthcare

There is a high level of concern over the security of health information transmitted via the World Wide Web. The debate over whether the Web is safe enough to use for health information is likely to continue for some time. Technology and good practices can provide adequate security but increase the cost of such application. Economic concerns may reduce implementing adequate safeguards. Internet use for healthcare information over the Web continues to grow. Protection of health information can be increased by spelling out liability for its compromise and insurance.

Electronic Storage

Increased access to information through an ever-increasing number of interconnected storage devices and networks also creates additional concerns over security. Security threats to stored information mirror those that may affect any network. Unauthorized access to information is a major threat that can be curtailed through careful management of the interfaces between systems. It is crucial to ensure that authorized users can access information when they need it but that sufficient security measures are in place to prevent unauthorized access. These measures include requirements for user identification and encrypted passwords to access the various components of the network. Confidential information may also be copied from the system in the form of electronic records. Administrators may download these records for report purposes. Once the records are no longer needed, electronic copies of sensitive data should be deleted or subjected to shredder software. **File deletion software** overwrites files with meaningless information so that sensitive information cannot be accessed.

SPECIAL CONSIDERATIONS WITH MOBILE COMPUTING

Mobile computing has the potential to improve information access, enhance workflow, and promote evidence-based practice to make informed and effective decisions at the point of care (Lu, Xiao, Sears, & Jacko 2005; Pohjonen, Ross, Blickman, & Kamman 2007). Handheld computers, PDAs, and smartphones offer portable and unobtrusive access to clinical data and relevant information at the point of care. They also prove useful in areas of documentation and medical reference. For these reasons mobile devices are used widely in healthcare providers' practice, and the level of use continues to rise. Despite these many benefits, there are also security problems. According to a survey by the *British Journal of Healthcare Computing and Information Management,* one fifth of devices used to store data in the healthcare sector had no security (Survey reveals 2006). This study was limited to 117 medical professionals and IT managers. It included laptops, PDAs, BlackBerrys, and phones, most of which were individually owned. Individual devices must be subjected to the same types of safeguards applied to healthcare information systems. No patient specific information should be placed on a device unless it is protected. For example, students can use their PDAs for reference and make notes on their patient assignments but should never input identifiable information.

Staff who use mobile devices should work with the information services department to help secure those devices from unauthorized view. Other problems identified with the adoption of mobile technology include usability and lack of technical and organizational support. Point-of-care devices and the software that they use must actually serve to facilitate, not hinder, the work of the bedside caregiver in order to realize the benefits associated with point-of-care technology. The mobility that provides an advantage can also pose problems because mobile devices may be left unattended in patient care areas subject to unauthorized view or theft. WiFi is vulnerable in a number of ways that wired networks are not. The main reason is because WiFi signals are simultaneously broadcast in all directions. Therefore, special care must be taken to secure all mobile devices used by healthcare professionals.

FUTURE DIRECTIONS

The necessity of uninterrupted access to information makes it imperative that the systems that store, process, and transmit the information are adequately secured. The goal of adopting electronic health records nationwide by 2014 has spurred the increased use of information technology for recording, processing, and transmitting confidential information. Unfortunately security has not received the attention that it deserves, as is evident from the continuing number of high-profile cases of identity theft, loss, and accidental disclosure of personal and health information. Greater awareness, sufficient resources, and an organization-wide commitment to information security are needed, particularly as development proceeds toward the realization of a lifetime electronic health record. Healthcare institutions and providers have an ethical and legal obligation to consumers to secure health information. Present methods have shown that they are not good enough. New technologies continue to emerge to meet this need, and existing measures such as biometric authentication will become more common. For example in 2010, a technique was developed to automatically generate filters to protect applications against malicious attacks until vendors develop and release patches. Likewise, increased legislation and harsher penalties for cybercriminals are likely to reduce the number of incidents that violate privacy and confidentiality.

Visit nursing.pearsonhighered.com for additional cases, information, and weblinks.

CASE STUDY EXERCISE

In the course of conversation, your nurse manager tells you that she loaded a copy of the spreadsheet program she uses on her home office PC onto one of the unit PCs so that she can work on projects at both locations. Your institution has a well-publicized policy against the use of unauthorized, unlicensed software copies. As a staff nurse, what should you do? Explain your response.

SUMMARY

- The primary goals of healthcare information system security are the protection of client confidentiality and information availability and integrity.
- Privacy and confidentiality are important terms in healthcare information management. Privacy is a choice to disclose personal information, while confidentiality assumes a relationship in which private information has been shared for the purpose of health treatment.
- Information privacy is the right to choose the conditions under which information is shared and to ensure the accuracy of collected information.
- Threats to information and system security and confidentiality come from a variety of sources, including system penetration by thieves, hackers, unauthorized use, denial of service and terrorist attacks, cybercrime, errors and disasters, sabotage, viruses, and human error.
- Planning for security saves time and money and is a form of insurance against downtime, breaches in confidentiality, and lost productivity.
- Security mechanisms combine physical and logical restrictions.
- Examples include automatic sign-off, physical restriction of computer equipment, strong password protection, and firewalls.
- Ultimately, healthcare administrators are responsible for protecting client privacy and confidentiality through education, policy, and creating an ongoing awareness of security.
- One aspect of system security management includes monitoring the system for unusual record access patterns, as might be seen when a celebrity receives treatment.
- Health information on the Internet requires the same types of safeguards provided for information found in private offices and information systems.

- All chart printouts, forms, and computer files containing client information should be given the same consideration as the client record itself to safeguard confidentiality.
- More secure methods of authentication are needed as even the best passwords can be compromised.

REFERENCES

Australian Government. (2010). Office of the Australian Information Commission. Retrieved from http://www.privacy.gov.au/law/apply

Australia's privacy legislation: A guide for nurses. (2002). *Australian Nursing Journal, 10*(2), 24.

Blair, P. D. (2003). Make room for patient privacy. *Nursing Management, 34*(6), 28.

Britt, P. (2005). Protecting private information. *Information Today, 22*(5), 1–38.

Calloway, S. D., & Venegas, L. M. (2002). The new HIPAA law on privacy and confidentiality. *Nursing Administration Quarterly, 26*(4), 40.

Campbell, J., Kleeman, D., & Ma, W. (2007). The good and not so good of enforcing password composition rules. *Information Systems Security, 16*(1), 2–8.

Crystal, G. (2010, October 24). *What is information security?* Retrieved from http://www.wisegeek.com/what-is-information-security.htm

Edwards, K. A. (2008). *Confidentiality.* Retrieved from http://depts.washington.edu/bioethx/topics/confiden.html

Espion. (2010). *Espion's top 10 information security risks for 2010.* Retrieved from http://practicepr.wordpress.com/2010/01/05/espions-top-10-information-security-risks-for-2010/

Gordon, L. A., Loeb, M. P., Lucyshyn, W., & Richardson, R. (2006). *2006 CSI/FBI computer crime and security survey. Computer Security Institute.* Retrieved from http://i.cmpnet.com/gocsi/db_area/pdfs/fbi/FBI2006.pdf

Griffiths, D. (2003, April 22). Treat IT security as if the law required it. *Computer Weekly,* p. 44.

Hebda, T., Sakerka, L., & Czar, P. (1994). Educating nurses to maintain patient confidentiality on automated information systems. In S. J. Grobe & E. S. P. Pluyter-Wenting (Eds.), *Nursing informatics: An international overview for nursing in a technological era.* Proceedings of the Fifth IMIA International Conference on Nursing Use of Computers and Information Science. New York: Elsevier Science.

Hill, J. (2003, March 29). Speak no evil. *Lancet, 361*(9363), 1140.

Hitachi ID Systems. (2010). *Password management best practices.* Retrieved from http://www.psynch.com/docs/password-management-best-practices.html

Joint Commission on Accreditation of Healthcare Organizations. (1996). *Medical records process.* Chicago, IL: Accreditation Manual for Hospitals.

Kelly, G., & McKenzie, B. (2002). Security, privacy, and confidentiality issues on the Internet. *Journal of Medical Internet Research, 4*(2), e12. Retrieved from http://www.jmir.org/2002/2/e12/

Kmentt, K. A. (1987, Winter). Private medical records: Are they public property? *Medical Trial Technique Quarterly, 33,* 274–307.

Lemos, R. (2006, May 9). Password policies. *PC Magazine, 25*(9), 116.

Lu, Y. C., Xiao, Y., Sears, A., & Jacko, J. A. (2005). A review and a framework of handheld computer adoption in healthcare. *International Journal of Medical Informatics, 74*(5), 409–422.

Malin, A. (2007). Designing networks that enforce information security policies. *Information Systems Security, 16*(1), 47–53.

McCarthy, B. (2006a). Close the security disconnect between awareness and practice. *Electronic Design, 54*(19), 20.

McCarthy, B. (2006b). Security efforts still falling short. *eWeek, 23*(46), E4.

McCullough, J. (2004). *185 wireless secrets.* Indianapolis, IN: Wiley Publishing, p. 281.

McMillan, R. (2007). Phishing sites explode on the web. *PC World, 25*(4), 22.

Mitrakas, A. (2006, March). Information security and law in Europe: Risks checked? *Information & Communications Technology Law, 15*(1), 33–53.

Murdock, L. E. (1980). The use and abuse of computerized information: Striking a balance between personal privacy interests and organizational information needs. *Albany Law Review, 44*(3), 589–619.

Murphy, C. (2010, January 5). *Espion's top 10 information security risks for 2010*. Retrieved from http://www.iia.ie/news/item/1453/espions-top-10-information-security-risks-for-2010/

National Institute of Standards and Technology (NIST). (2002, July). *Risk management guide for information technology systems*. National Institute of Standards and Technology Special Publication 800-30, p. 8. Retrieved from http://csrc.nist.gov/publications/nistpubs/800-30/sp800-30.pdf

Olinger, H. N., Britz, J. J., & Olivier, M. S. (2007). Western privacy and/or Ubuntu? Some critical comments on the influences in the forthcoming data privacy bill in South Africa. *International Information & Library Review, 39*(1), 31–43.

Ollmann, G. (2005). *The phishing guide: Understanding and preventing phishing attacks. Technical Info*. Retrieved from http://www.technicalinfo.net/papers/Phishing.html

Pohjonen, H., Ross, P., Blickman, J. G., & Kamman, R. (2007). Pervasive access to images and data—The use of computing grids and mobile/wireless devices across healthcare enterprises. *IEEE Transactions on Information Technology in Biomedicine, 11*(1), 81–86.

Rainer, R. K., Marshall, T. E., Knapp, K. J., & Montgomery, G. H. (2007). Do information security professionals and business managers view information security issues differently? *Information Systems Security, 16*(2), 100–108.

Ramanathan, R. (2006). Thinking beyond security. *Security Management, 15*(2), 49–54.

Reagan, M. (2003). *Electronic eye can protect your health information*. Retrieved from http://health-information.advanceweb.com/Article/An-Electronic-Eye-Can-Help-Protect-Your-Private-Health-Information.aspx

Romano, C. (1987). Confidentiality and security of computerized systems: The nursing responsibility. *Computers in Nursing, 5*(3), 99–104.

RSA. (2010, May). *RSA online fraud report*. Retrieved from http://www.rsa.com/solutions/consumer_authentication/intelreport/10947_Online_Fraud_report_0510.pdf

Sax, U., Kohane, I., & Mandl, K. D. (2005). Wireless technology infrastructures for authentication of patients: PKI that rings. *Journal of the American Medical Informatics Association, 12*(3), 263–268.

Spamhaus Project Ltd. (2010). *The definition of spam*. Retrieved from http://www.spamhaus.org/definition.html

Steele, S., & Wargo, C. (2007). An introduction to insider threat management. *Information Systems Security, 16*(1), 23–33.

Stern, L. (2007, October 29). When to be wary of "free wi-fi." *Newsweek*, pp. 62–63.

Sturdevant, C. (2007, May 7). Keystrokes are us. *eWeek*, p. 32.

Survey reveals NHS failing to secure data on mobile devices. (2006, June 27). Retrieved from http://www.bjhc.co.uk/news/1/2006/n606012.htm

Toorani, M., & Shirazi, A. A. B. (2008, November). *LPKI: A lightweight public key infrastructure for the mobile environments*. Proceedings of the 11th IEEE International Conference on Communication Systems (IEEE ICCS'08) (pp. 162–166), Guangzhou, China.

Tuesday, V. (2003, April 21). Security log. *Computerworld, 37*(16), 35.

Vidalis, S., & Kazmi, Z. (2007). Security through deception. *Information Systems Security, 16*(1), 34–41.

Whitman, M. E., & Mattord, H. (2009). *Principles of information security* (3rd ed.). Boston, MA: Course Technology.

Wikipedia.org. (2008, February 10). *Firewall*. Retrieved November 1, 2010, from http://en.wikipedia.org/wiki/Firewall_(computing)

Wikipedia.org. (2009a, January 4). *Privacy*. Retrieved November 1, 2010, from http://en.wikipedia.org/wiki/Privacy

Wikipedia.org. (2009b, November). *Privacy*. Retrieved November 1, 2010, from http://en.wikipedia.org/wiki/Information_privacy

Windslade, W. J. (1982). Confidentiality of medical records: An overview of concepts and legal policies. *Journal of Legal Medicine, 3*(4), 497–533.

Wulf, G. (2007). *HIPAA information and consent form*. Retrieved from http://www.wulfclinic.com/document/hipaaform.pdf

CHAPTER 13

System Integration and Interoperability

After completing this chapter, you should be able to:

1. Recognize the importance of system integration and interoperability for healthcare delivery.

2. Explain what an interface engine is and how it works.

3. Identify several integration issues, including factors that impede the process.

4. Discuss the relevance to system integration efforts of the data dictionary, master patient index, uniform language efforts, and clinical data repository.

5. Consider how standards for the exchange of clinical data affect integration efforts.

6. Review the benefits of successful information system integration for healthcare providers and healthcare professionals.

7. Define the role of the nurse in system integration efforts.

8. Understand how Web-based tools can provide an alternative method for obtaining patient information from diverse information systems.

The need to exchange data and information electronically is a mandate in today's society. The healthcare delivery system lags behind finance and business in the ability to exchange data although progress has been made. Scholtzer and Madsen (2010, p. 161) noted that interoperability between "systems using different database designs, different terminologies, and different structures is difficult but not impossible." Achieving interoperability, and the subsequent exchange of meaningful information, requires a combination of technical and political approaches. This chapter addresses the mechanisms that allow the exchange of data and information.

It is a rare hospital or healthcare provider that does not have computer information systems in place in some, if not all, of their major departments. Historically, financial systems were computerized first, followed by registration, laboratory, order entry, pharmacy, radiology, and monitoring systems (not necessarily in that order). Some of these computer information systems were first implemented as stand-alone systems. Most departments select the information system that best meets their needs or that hospital administrators approve because of cost reasons, promises to vendors, or the preexistence of other products by the same vendor in the institution. It is rare for all departments in a given healthcare institution to agree that one vendor's product meets their information system needs. As a consequence, most institutions have several different systems that do not readily communicate or share data. Some level of customization of information systems to meet individual department and institutional specifications is common. This customization, however, complicates integration. Integration needs have increased dramatically as single institutions and providers use more systems internally and as they join with other institutions to form enterprises, alliances, and networks. In addition, integration must be achieved before the electronic health record (EHR) can be realized.

Integration is the process by which different information systems are able to exchange data in a fashion that is seamless to the end user. The physical aspects of joining networks together are not nearly as complicated as getting unlike systems to exchange information in a seamless manner. Traditionally, communication between and among most disparate systems has been the result of costly, time-consuming efforts to build interfaces. In other words, interface programs are the tools used to achieve integration. An **interface** is a computer program that tells two different systems how to exchange data.

Without integration, providers cannot realize the full advantages of automation, since sharing data across multiple systems is limited and redundant data entry by various personnel takes place. When this occurs, the likelihood of errors is increased. This situation is unacceptable in a time when institutions need to realize the benefits of automation to compete in today's healthcare delivery system. Box 13–1 lists some benefits associated with integration.

INTERFACES

Interfaces between different information systems should be invisible to the user. Many vendors claim their products are based on open systems technology, which is the ability to communicate with other systems. The reality is that there has been little financial incentive for vendors to

---

BOX 13–1   The Benefits of Integration

- Allows instant access to applications and data
- Improves data integrity with single entry of data
- Decreases labor costs with single entry of data
- Facilitates the formulation of a more accurate, complete client record
- Facilitates information tracking for accurate cost determinations

market products that readily work with their competitors' products. Another problem is that the customization of vendor products by individual providers precludes off-the-shelf interface solutions, necessitating costly and time-consuming design of custom interfaces. This is one reason why there has been a movement away from customization. Another problem with customized interfaces is pinpointing the responsibility for any problems that occur. Each vendor responsible for developing an interface tends to blame the other for any difficulties encountered. Without a determination of responsibility, problem resolution is delayed and no one can be held accountable for the cost of solving the problem. All too often the institution must absorb the costs for this process; yet competition in a managed care environment does not permit this luxury. In addition, the timely flow of information is critical to cost-cutting measures and institutional survival.

There are two general types of interfaces: **point-to-point** and those using integration engine software. A point-to-point interface is an interface that directly connects two information systems. Communication and transfer of data take place only between these systems. Historically these were the first types of interfaces used in healthcare. This type of interface is achieved through customized programming and for this reason is expensive and labor-intensive to build and maintain.

More recent technology uses **interface engine** software to create and manage interfaces. This provides the ability to transfer information from the sending system to one or many receiving systems and allows users of different information systems to access and exchange information both in real-time and batch processing. **Real-time processing** occurs immediately, or with only a slight delay, whereas **batch processing** typically occurs once daily. In this situation, data are often not processed until the end of the day and therefore are not available to users until that time. Although batch processing was very common in the past, current use is primarily limited to transactions that are less time critical, such as processing charges for procedures, supplies, and special equipment.

The interface engine provides seamless integration and presentation of information results. Interface engines work in the background and are not seen by the user. This technology allows applications to interact with hardware and other applications. Interface engines allow different systems that use unlike terminology to exchange information without the need to build expensive point-to-point interfaces (Freedman 2007). This is done through the use of translation tables to move data from each system to the **clinical data repository**, a database where collective data from all information systems are stored and managed. The clinical data repository provides data definition consistency through mapping. The clinical data repository may also be referred to as the clinical data warehouse (CDW). Over time the CDW has evolved to support financial as well as clinical applications. The CDW was once developed within individual facilities but may be managed through vendors. **Mapping** is the process in which terms defined in one system are associated with comparable terms in another system. The major impact of using interface engines is that mappings for multiple receiving systems can be built for each sending system. For example, a client registration system can send registration transactions to the interface engine, which then forwards them on to any number of ancillary systems such as laboratory, radiology, and pharmacy. Each of these systems is able to receive updated client healthcare and demographic information, eliminating the need to manually register the client in the ancillary system. Box 13–2 discusses some of the benefits associated with the use of interface engines.

Interfacing of laboratory orders and results provides another example of how the interface engine is used in a hospital setting. On a client's admission, the client's demographic information is entered in the hospital registration system, and portions of these data are transmitted to the clinical data repository via the interface engine. When a laboratory order is entered into the order entry system, the appropriate client demographic information is retrieved from the clinical data repository and used by the order entry system. After the order is entered, the order information may be transmitted via the interface engine to the clinical data repository and the

> **BOX 13–2 Interface Engine Benefits**
>
> - Improves timeliness and availability of critical administrative and clinical data
> - Decreases integration costs by providing an alternative to customized point-to-point interface application programming
> - Improves data quality because of data mapping and consistent use of terms
> - Allows clients to select the best system for their needs
> - Preserves institutional investment in existing systems
> - Simplifies the administration of healthcare data processing
> - Simplifies systems integration efforts
> - Shortens the time required for integration
> - Improves management of care, the financial tracking of care rendered, and efficacy of treatment

laboratory system. When testing is complete, the results are transferred via the interface engine from the laboratory system to the clinical data repository. At this point, they are available for retrieval using the order entry system or another clinical information system.

Interface engine management requires an analyst who can identify initial and ongoing interface specifications, coordinate any changes that will impact interfaces, maintain a database for translation tables, and ascertain that data integrity is intact for all data to be sent through the interface engine.

Most discussions that involve the large-scale electronic exchange of healthcare information across enterprises for the purpose of accessing and maintaining longitudinal health records speak of interoperability. Definitions for interoperability vary but a common definition for **interoperability** is the ability of two entities, whether those are human or machine, to exchange and predictably use data or information while retaining the original meaning of that data (Freedman 2007; Mead 2006; Schwend 2007).While the terms *interface* and *interoperability* are sometimes used interchangeably, the interface engine routes information from one system to another but stops short of enabling the second system to understand and use that information. Benson (2010) noted that The HL7 EHR Interoperability Work Group framework included three types of interoperability: technical, semantic, and process. **Technical interoperability** is the ability to exchange the data from one point to another. *Syntactic* and *functional interoperability* are additional terms that refer to the movement of data that does not necessarily ensure the meaning of the data. **Semantic interoperability** guarantees that the meaning of the exchanged data remains the same on both ends of the transaction. This is critical for clinical data. **Process interoperability** coordinates processes to enable business processes at the organization(s), housing the systems to work together. There have been several standardization efforts to achieve interoperability for EHRs. These include the Health Level Seven (HL7) Clinical Document Architecture (CDA); the European Committee for Standardization (CEN) EN 13606-1, also known as EHRcom; and the openEHR. All provide specifications for how information should be exchanged (Kilic & Dogac 2007). HL7 relies upon XML markup language for the storage and movement of clinical documents between systems. The International Organization for Standardization (2007) considers EN 13606-1 to be a communications standard in development. The primary focus of EN 13606-1 is to support direct care given to individuals, or to support population monitoring systems such as disease registries and public health surveillance, although EN 13606-1 may also allow the use of health records for secondary purposes such as disease registries, teaching, audits, reports, and anonymous aggregation of individual records for epidemiology or research.

The openEHR initiative is an international effort to provide semantic interoperability through the creation of specifications, open source software, and tools (Kalra 2007; Kilic & Dogac 2007; openEHR Foundation 2007). It builds upon more than 15 years of international research on the EHR. In the clinical arena, it strives to create high-quality, reusable clinical models of content and process that are defined by clinicians and are known as **archetypes**, as well as formal interfaces to terminology. Each archetype contains a header, definition, and ontology section. The header has a unique code identifying the clinical concept defined as well as descriptive information such as author, version, and status. The definition includes restrictions obtained from the information model. The ontology section contains codes representing the meanings of nodes and constraints on text or terms, as well as linkages to terminologies such as SNOMED or LOINC. The Archetype Definition Language (ADL) is a formal language for the expression of archetypes.

On a second level the openEHR initiative supports the use of archetypes to model and share knowledge (Garde, Knaup, & Hovenga 2005). The development and maintenance of archetypes must be coordinated at an international level with input from health professionals for success (Garde, Knaup, Hovenga, & Heard 2007). Archetypes must be consistent, link to terminology systems in an appropriate way, and meet quality standards for the capture, processing, and communication of clinical data (Kalra 2007). The EuroRec Institute has partnered with the openEHR Foundation to address quality criteria. The openEHR Foundation (2011) announced the first release of openEHR.NET with the aim to help all developers share the same core classes and collaborate on a single library, rather than each working independently. Despite these and other efforts, there is no single standard in place at present that enjoys widespread acceptance or provides complete interoperability for EHRs. Integrating Healthcare Enterprise (IHE) is a global initiative dedicated to improving patient care by promoting the way that computer systems in healthcare share information by promoting the adoption of standards such as DICOM and HL7 and interoperability (HIMSS 2007). IHE was conceived in the late 1990s. There have been other projects for interoperability in the United States, Canada, and the European Union over the years.

Another proposed solution to interoperability is **service-oriented architecture (SOA)** (Choi, Nazareth, & Jain 2010; Lewis, Morris, Simanta, & Wrage 2008; Rajini & Bhuvaneswari 2010). SOA calls for placing key functions into modules that, along with new capabilities, may be reused, similar to object-oriented programming. SOA defines a service as a self-contained unit of work that has well defined and understood capabilities. A service may be an entire process, a function supporting a process, or a step of a business process. Services may be built into a library that can be used to address enterprise needs. SOA does not require reengineering of existing systems. SOA goes beyond other technologies in that it is vendor and technology neutral and does not require specific equipment or standards for operation. SOA can support information exchange among systems that use different programming languages. Its other characteristics hold promise for streamlining health information exchange. These include the ability to maintain a registry of services at the enterprise level that can be invoked after lookup, and the ability to provide quality service that includes security requirements such as authentication, authorization, and reliable messaging and policies.

INTEGRATION AND INTEROPERABILITY ISSUES

Integration is a massive project within institutions and enterprises. It generally requires more time and effort than originally projected. Several factors contribute to this situation. First, vendors frequently make promises about their products that they may not be able to meet to make a sale. Second, merged institutions may keep their own systems rather than accept a uniform standard that would be easier to manage which ultimately requires further negotiation and additional programming. Third, as each department and institution tries to retain its own identity and political

> **BOX 13–3 Factors That Slow Integration**
>
> - **Unrealistic vendor promises.** Vendors often promise that their information systems are interoperable with other systems. Many customers find, however, they face difficult, lengthy, and costly integration efforts after they have already purchased a system.
> - **Unrealistic institutional timetable.** This is often based on a lack of understanding of the complexity of the integration process.
> - **Changing user specifications.** As the integration process proceeds, users frequently request additional capabilities or change their minds regarding initial specifications.
> - **Lack of vendor support.** Vendors may not provide enough support and assistance to facilitate integration efforts.
> - **Insufficient documentation.** Information regarding existing systems and related programming is imperative for achieving successful integration.
> - **Lack of agreement among merged institutions.** Individual facilities within a merged enterprise may wish to continue use of their existing systems. This means there are more systems to integrate.
> - **All components of a vendor's products may not work together.** Although difficulties are expected in attempts to integrate competing vendors' products, there may also be problems in integrating products developed by the same vendor.

power, it is difficult to come to an agreement on a common data dictionary, data mapping, and clinical data repository issues. Another issue is that integration brings a number of concerns for individuals, including changes in job description, learning new skills, the fear of job loss, and the general fear of change. Box 13–3 identifies several factors that may impede the integration process.

Freedman (2007) noted that progress toward attaining true large-scale interoperability has been impeded by a lack of consensus as to how it should be achieved. Some experts feel that perfect harmonization of standards between technology systems must occur first, while others oversimplify the issue by stating that interoperability can be attained merely by mapping codes from one system to another. Rather than waiting until the issue is fully resolved, Freedman advocated using extant technology that can provide some level of semantic interoperability, and then building upon that foundation. SOA allows enterprises to shift their efforts from maintaining a complex interface strategy to creating service-oriented applications that support interoperability while focusing more closely on the business of healthcare delivery. With the additional adoption and use of SOA within the healthcare industry, collections of services will be available for purchase or subscription serving with the end result that providers can focus on their primary business rather than duplicating the efforts of those who went before them. Other interoperability issues include:

- The need to select interoperability solutions that work with present and evolving standards
- Need for consensus on archetypes for broad clinical application
- Safe use of processes such as decision support across sites, which requires a consistent approach for naming and organizing EHR entries so that all needed information can be obtained (Kalra 2007)

NATIONAL HEALTHCARE INFORMATION NETWORK

Several developments led to the creation of the National Healthcare Information Network (NHIN). These included the Institute of Medicine's 2001 report *Crossing the Quality Chasm: A New Health System for the 21st Century,* which called for the development of a national health information network as a means to advance healthcare information technology and realize the benefits that a health information exchange (HIE) could offer. Interoperability provides many benefits, including improved physician workflow, productivity and patient care, improved safety, fully standardized healthcare information exchange, and an estimated annual savings equivalent to approximately 5% of annual U.S. healthcare expenditures (Kaushal et al. 2005; Schwend 2007). Interoperability also enables large-scale data exchange that is needed to support comparative effectiveness research (CER) (McKinney 2010) and the intent of Meaningful Use requirements to improve patient care (Martin, Monsen, & Bowles 2011). The Markle Foundation started the Connecting for Health project in 2001 to promote the interconnection of healthcare information systems, then announced a contribution of $1.9 million to launch a Regional Health Information Organization interconnectivity project in 2005. The Robert Wood Johnson Foundation also provided financial support to this effort. In 2004 President Bush issued a directive for interoperable EHRs by 2014. In late 2007 Mike Leavitt, secretary of the Department of Health and Human Services, announced the award of contracts totaling $22.5 million to nine HIEs to begin trial implementations of the NHIN (DHHS 2007). President Obama also supported an interoperable EHR, signing the American Recovery and Reinvestment Act in law in 2009 along with the Health Information Technology for Economic and Clinical Health Act (ARRA 2009), which provided economic incentives for the adoption of certified EHR software. These efforts represent a start but the road to the NHIN will be an expensive one. In 2005 a study published by Kaushal et al. (2005) estimated the cost to implement the NHIN at $103 billion in total capital with another $27 billion annually for operating costs. Enrado (2007) and Larsen (2005) suggested the focus should instead be the incentives for establishing the NHIN, namely the benefits such as improved quality of care, safety, and decreased costs related to redundant services. Larsen also noted the need to establish a roadmap to establishing the NHIN, one that will allow the cost to be broken down into steps as well as a reexamination of what is meant by interoperability. In the interim, work continues on developing the framework to support NHIN. In late 2007 the Healthcare Information Technology Standards Panel, a multistakeholder group working with the U.S. DHHS to assure the interoperability of EHRs in the United States, approved recommendations designed to facilitate the secure exchange of information. These recommendations were sent to the American Health Information Community, which made further recommendations to Secretary Leavitt (ANSI 2007). Other organizations involved in this effort included:

- The Office of Interoperability and Standards for the Office of the National Coordinator for Health Information Technology, or ONCHIT
- The Certification Commission on Healthcare Information Technology
- Commission on Systemic Interoperability
- National Committee on Vital and Health Statistics
- The Center for Information Technology Leadership

THE NEED FOR INTEGRATION STANDARDS

The need to exchange health data continues to grow in response to the demands placed by managed care, consumers seeking improved levels of healthcare, Meaningful Use requirements, and the mandate for comparative effectiveness research. To derive the utmost benefit from data, it must have a consistent or standard meaning across institution, enterprise, and alliance boundaries, facilitating the exchange of client data. This is the basis for developing a data dictionary within an enterprise and a uniform language for use on a national and global scale. It is becoming increasingly important for hospitals and information system vendors to adopt and use uniform standards for the electronic exchange of clinical information. The use of uniform standards will provide safer and more efficient healthcare delivery systems and also play a critical role in compliance with government healthcare regulations.

So many standards exist now that it adds to the difficulty of standardization. Multinational vendors are reluctant to commit to the adoption of standards that are not universal (Nusbaum

2007). In some cases only local interoperability is available. Recent initiatives such as IHE and national harmonization initiatives in the United States and abroad may help to solve that problem as they strive to create a "plug and play" solution by eliminating the optional features individual vendors supply with their version of standards such as DICOM and HL7.

Data Dictionary

The **data dictionary** defines terminology to ensure consistent understanding and use across the enterprise. Terms defined in the data dictionary should include synonyms found in the various systems used within the enterprise. This may be achieved, in some cases, through the use of the interface engine. For example, a term or data element may be a diagnosis or a laboratory test, such as "potassium." Potassium may be known in the nursing order entry system as "potassium" but be called "K" in the laboratory system. The use of the data dictionary and interface engine facilitates integration and allows for the collection of aggregate data.

Master Patient Index

The integration process may require enhancements to the data dictionary, the clinical data repository, and the master patient index. The **master patient index (MPI)** is a database that lists all identifiers assigned to one client in all the information systems used within an enterprise. It assigns a global identification number for each client and allows clients to be identified by demographic information provided at the point of care. The MPI may use first and last names, birthdates, Social Security numbers, and driver's license numbers. It cannot rely on a single type of number such as the Social Security number, because of duplicates and the fact that some people, such as noncitizens, may not have one. When the MPI cannot match records based on demographic data, all possible matches are provided for the user to view and select. The MPI is a critical component in supporting successful integration. Not all healthcare enterprises have a data dictionary, a clinical data repository, or an MPI, or these components may be in various stages of development. The move toward creating a lifetime patient record creates the need to access client encounters across time. This is particularly important in a multi-institutional enterprise. The MPI, data dictionary, and clinical data repository are tools that support this effort.

The MPI saves work because vital information can be obtained from the database rather than rekeyed with each client visit. This decreases the possibility of making a mistake and eliminates the inadvertent creation of duplicate records. As a result, the registration clerk now plays a greater role in the maintenance of data integrity.

Some of the key features of an effective MPI include the following:

- It locates records in real time for timely retrieval of information.
- It is flexible enough to allow inclusion of additional identification.
- It is easily reconfigured to accommodate network changes.
- It can grow to fit an organization of any size.

It is possible to exchange information without first creating an MPI (Getting started 2007). A research group of the American Health Information Management Association recommended starting with clinical messaging for the exchange of clinical information, such as lab results, and then adding additional information and services such as medication history, clinical summaries, quality measurement, reporting services, and administrative data.

Uniform Language

One major step in the integration process is the development of a uniform definition of terms, or language. This is essential for the easy location and manipulation of data. Uniform languages are essential to ensure semantic interoperability within EHRs. There have been many efforts to develop uniform languages in the healthcare arena. The discussion of the role of standardized terminologies in EHRs is covered in depth in Chapter 15. The Systematized Nomenclature of Medicine-Clinical Terms (SNOMED-CT) is globally recognized as a common language for electronic health applications (IHTSDO n.d). The American Nurses Association (ANA) recognizes SNOMED-CT as a standardized terminology for nursing, and ANA-recognized terminologies are integrated within SNOMED. The American Nurses Association's Committee for Nursing Practice Information Infrastructure (CNPII) recognizes nursing terminologies (Warren & Bakken 2002). The National Library of Medicine developed the Unified Medical Language System (UMLS), which "integrates and distributes key terminology, classification and coding standards" in an effort to foster more effective and interoperable systems (NLM 2011). The adoption and use of nursing terminologies provides visibility for the contributions made by nursing because they facilitate the collection of data related to nursing care, making it possible to cost out care, demonstrate contributions to patient outcomes, and support research and data mining.

In addition to SNOMED and nursing nomenclatures, coding systems are used in other areas of healthcare to communicate information about medical diagnoses and procedures performed. One common application is the use of the International Classification of Diseases (ICD) classification system and Current Procedural Terminology (CPT) codes to collect information used for billing and third-party payment reimbursement.

Data Exchange Standards

In addition to the uniform definition of terms, integration standards facilitate the exchange of client data by providing a set of rules and structure for formatting the data.

HL7 A major standard for the exchange of clinical data for integration is Health Level 7 (HL7). HL7 refers to both an organization and its standards for the exchange of clinical data. The mission statement of Health Level 7 International states that its purpose is to provide standards for interoperability "that improve care delivery, optimize workflow, reduce ambiguity and enhance knowledge transfer among all of our stakeholders" (Health Level 7 2011). In particular, these standards address definitions of data to be exchanged, the timing of the exchanges, and communication of certain errors between applications. HL7 provides a structure that defines data and elements and specifies how the data are coded. The structure of the data element must follow HL7 rules, such as those specifying the length of the fields and the code nomenclature. The use of HL7 standards in individual applications improves the integration of these applications with other applications or systems using an interface engine. Benefits include easier and less costly integration within an organization and more accurate and useful data integration nationally and globally. Integration efforts and the development and use of integration standards, including HL7, are taking place at many levels. For example, integration is seen beyond the hospital setting in the form of integrated delivery systems. Although efforts are under way to develop both national and international health data networks, competition has not yet facilitated this type of information sharing. Sometimes HL7 standards have been modified by information system vendors to support various applications, creating integration issues. HL7 Version 3 was developed in response to a growing awareness that Version 2 did not guarantee meaningful exchange of data across enterprise boundaries in a cost-effective manner (Mead 2006).

HL7 standards are not the only standards that have been evolving to fit the changing healthcare model. Other organizations instrumental in supporting the development of standards and in helping to define data exchange include the Institute of Medicine, National Institute of Standards and Technology, the National Science Foundation, the National Library of Medicine, the National Committee for Health Statistics, the Centers for Medicare and Medicare Services, the National Coordinator for Health Information Technology, the American Health Information Management Association, the American Medical Informatics Association, and the Healthcare Information and Management Systems Society.

DICOM DICOM (Digital Imaging and Communications in Medicine) refers to both an organization and a standard. The DICOM standard was first developed for the transmission of medical images and their associated information. It is now used in nearly all hospitals worldwide for the production, display, storage, retrieval, and printing of medical images and derived structured documents, as well as to manage related workflow (DICOM 2011). DICOM's goals are to achieve compatibility and improve workflow efficiency between imaging systems and other information systems. DICOM also addresses the integration of information produced by specialty imaging applications into the electronic health system, defining the network and media interchange services that allow storage and access to these DICOM objects for EHR systems.

THE BENEFITS OF INTEGRATION AND INTEROPERABILITY

It is integration that allows data from many disparate information systems to be accessed from one point by the user, but it is interoperability that allows for the meaningful exchange of information that retains its meaning as it crosses from one system to another, ultimately providing a complete record for each client. When information system professionals speak of integration, interoperability is the implied outcome. At this point the clinical data repository remains a key element of the EHR. It provides a storage facility for clinical data over time. The data in the clinical data repository may be generated from various systems and locations. For example, laboratory data is generated by a laboratory system and collected in an acute, ambulatory, or long-term care setting. Other data may be included from clinical systems such as radiology, pharmacy, and order entry. Decision-support applications that use clinical repository data benefit other facilities if data from all facilities can be mapped to the data dictionary. Poor documentation regarding term definitions in the individual systems collecting the data has been a stumbling block to the creation and maintenance of the clinical data repository. Figure 13–1 depicts an example of mapping with laboratory test terms. The adoption of standardized terminology helps to eliminate ambiguity in how terms are defined.

Hospitals, healthcare enterprises, providers, and patients all benefit from integration and interoperability because it eliminates redundant data entry and interventions, provides access to more complete data along the care continuum and through additional information systems and sites, improves the quality of documentation, and permits improved tracking of patients and patient outcomes. Integration of related systems such as radiology information system, picture archiving communication system (PACS), and the EHR provides clinicians with a more comprehensive view of the patient that can be accessed from many points within the hospital, or remotely. This provides the ability to view an electronic text report related to a radiology examination from the EHR and then seamlessly view the associated electronic images from the PACS

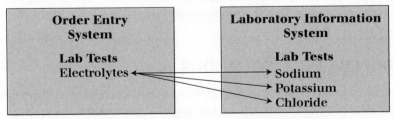

The order entry system lists a test called Electrolytes. The laboratory information system does not list a test called Electrolytes but lists its individual component tests. Before the interface engine can allow exchange of data, the relationships between the tests listed in both systems must be established by mapping.

FIGURE 13–1 • Mapping of laboratory test terms

systems. A standard client identifier used by all the organizations' information systems is key to creating this type of integration.

The lack of interoperability has long been a barrier to effective data reporting and analysis. For example, executive information needs may require data regarding all aspects of an obstetric client's care, including prenatal care, risk factors, complications before admission, length of hospital stay, and cost of the entire episode of care. Some of this information may be stored in an independent information system in the physician's office. Other data may be found in the hospital clinical information system and in the financial system. The inability to exchange this clinical, financial, and administrative data makes it difficult to impossible for administrators to make good decision to integrate decision support tools.

Interoperability also facilitates data collection for accreditation processes. For example, the Joint Commission requirements call for the ability to provide aggregate data. These requirements include the following:

- Uniform definition of data
- Uniform methods for data capture
- Ability to provide client-specific as well as aggregate data

These information standards allow the Joint Commission to compare data within and among healthcare enterprises.

IMPLICATIONS FOR NURSING

The nursing profession needs to take an active role in the design of interfaces and interoperability solutions (While & Thomas 2007). Nurses must be involved in identifying and defining data elements that an interface may be able to supply. One way to ensure this is to recruit staff nurses to provide input during the interface design.

Another concern is ensuring that data will be collected in only one system and shared via the interface engine and clinical data repository with all other systems requiring it. This eliminates redundant effort while ensuring data integrity. For example, a client's allergies should be identified and documented by a nurse and entered into a clinical information system. These data are then transmitted to the clinical data repository via the interface engine, where they are available for retrieval by other systems that may require them, such as a pharmacy system.

The nursing profession must also be involved in determining measures to assure the quality of the data that are exchanged among individual information systems and in the formation and maintenance of the EHR. If data quality cannot be assured, then clinical decision support and other important features will be suspect. One means to ensure the collection of quality information is the adoption and use of standardized languages, especially nursing terminologies, because terms have a common meaning. Also the structure of standardized terminologies facilitate the collection of aggregate data that can demonstrate the value of nursing contributions, cost out nursing services, support research and the development of new nursing knowledge, and facilitate tracking of outcomes.

EMERGING INTEROPERABILITY SOLUTIONS

Several years ago Web-based tools and Internet technology were seen as a means to provide access to data from disparate information systems. This was largely a local solution that improved access to clinical information for the providers at a single hospital or healthcare system, but did nothing to advance exchange of data on a larger scale or ensure that data could be used in the same manner in both sending and receiving systems. Since that time data exchange standards have been refined, national priorities set, and work has started on building the framework needed to make interoperability of electronic health data a reality. Interoperability will become increasingly vital for the optimal management of patient care and financial success of individual institutions. What remains unclear is the exact means by which this will be accomplished, or whether it will build on one of several existing models or architectures. Much work lies ahead. The road will not be easy, quick, or cheap but the promised benefits will be immeasurable.

FUTURE DIRECTIONS

At this point in time many facilities are still working toward implementing information systems and getting those systems to exchange data with other systems within their working environment. For example, many physician offices are in the process of installing systems now largely because of financial incentives offered via reimbursement for services for providers using EHR systems certified to meet Meaningful Use requirements for the purpose of improving patient outcomes (Blumenthal 2010, p. 501). Other settings such as clinics that offer care to poor and transient populations remain paper based. The type of data exchange required by the lifetime EHR proposed by presidents Bush and Obama largely remains a work in process since out-of-the box "plug and play" interoperability between different information systems does not now exist.

The importance of interoperability will continue to grow. One driver will be the 2010 Affordable Care Act Medicare Shared Savings Program calls for the operation of **Accountable Care Organizations (ACOs)** for Medicare in 2012 (Harris, Grauman, & Hemnani 2010; Taylor 2010). An ACO is a provider organization that assumes the responsibility of providing for the health needs of a defined population which includes the total cost of care and quality and effectiveness of services (Accountable care 2011). While an ACO may be a single hospital and affiliating physicians, it may be comprised of larger entities. The concept behind the ACO is to shift the paradigm away from payment per service rendered instead to a model that focuses upon wellness. ACOs will require high levels of interoperability among participants to facilitate the care of assigned populations and track outcomes. A high level of integration and interoperability will be required to enhance clinical and administrative aspects of care (Gooch 2010; Terry 2011).

CASE STUDY EXERCISE

You have been selected as a member of the Integration Project Team, which is charged with identifying ways that system integration could improve information flow. You work on an inpatient unit that uses a stand-alone nursing documentation system that is not interfaced or integrated with any other hospital information system. Identify the implications of this situation, and suggest integration options that could improve information flow.

SUMMARY

- An interface is a computer program that tells two different systems how to exchange data.
- Most healthcare providers have a variety of automated information systems that do not readily share data unless major efforts are made to build interfaces.
- Integration is the process by which different information systems are able to exchange data without any special effort on the part of the end user.
- The creation of networks to exchange data between systems and the process of integration are essential in today's healthcare information world, where an institution or enterprise may have multiple disparate clinical information systems.

- The interface engine is a software application designed to allow users of different information systems to exchange information without the need to build direct customized interfaces between systems.
- Other processes that facilitate the move toward and the exchange of health information include the clinical data repository, mapping, the data dictionary, the master patient index, uniform language efforts, and data exchange standards.
- The clinical data repository is a database that collects and stores data from all information systems.
- Mapping of terms establishes the relationship between terms defined in one system and those used in another.
- The data dictionary defines terms used within an enterprise to ensure consistent use.
- The master patient index lists all identifiers assigned to one client in all information systems and assigns a global identification code as a means to locate all records for a given client.
- Standardization of clinical terms through a uniform language is one means to facilitate the exchange of information across healthcare enterprises.
- Health Level 7 and DICOM are standards for the exchange of clinical data that provide rules and structure for how data are formatted.
- Integration improves data integrity and access for caregivers, eliminates redundant data collection, and improves data collection for staffing, for finding financial trends and client outcome trends, and for meeting requirements of regulatory and accrediting organizations.
- Integration is a necessary component for the development of the electronic health record and for integrated delivery systems.
- Interoperability is the ability of two entities, whether those are human or machine, to exchange and predictably use data or information while retaining the original meaning of that data.
- Technical interoperability, also known as syntactic and functional interoperability, is the ability to exchange the data from one point to another.
- Semantic interoperability guarantees that the meaning of the exchanged data remains the same on both ends of the transaction which is critical for clinical data.
- Process interoperability coordinates processes to enable business processes at the organization(s), housing the systems to work together.
- The National Healthcare Information Network (NHIN) is a proposed structure for the exchange of electronic data among individual healthcare enterprises for the purpose of supporting a longitudinal birth-to-death health record, with all of its attendant benefits, for all individuals.
- The nursing profession needs to take an active role in the design of interfaces and interoperability solutions.
- One driver for information system interoperability will be Accountable Care Organizations (ACOs).

REFERENCES

Accountable care organizations in "very early stages" of growth [Cover story]. (2011). *Healthcare Benchmarks & Quality Improvement, 18*(1), 1–4.

American National Standards Institute (ANSI). (2007, December 18). HITSP delivers next round of interoperability specifications to support U.S. nationwide health information network. *Earthtimes.org*. Retrieved from http://www.earthtimes.org/articles/show/news_press_release,244569.shtml

The American Reinvestment and Recovery Act (ARRA) H.R.1. (2009, January 6). Retrieved from http://frwebgate.access.gpo.gov/cgi-bin/getdoc.cgi?dbname=111_cong_bills&docid=f:h1enr.pdffrwebgate.access.gpo

Benson, T. (2010). *Principles of health interoperability HL7 and SNOMED.* London: Springer. doi:10.1007/978-1-84882-803-2

Blumenthal, D. (2010). The "meaningful use" regulation for electronic health records. *New England Journal of Medicine, 363*(6), 501–504. doi:10.1056/NEJMp1006114

Choi, J., Nazareth, D. L., & Jain, H. K. (2010). Implementing service-oriented architecture in organizations. *Journal of Management Information Systems, 26*(4), 253–286. doi:10.2753/M1S0742-1222260409

DICOM. (2011, March 31). *Strategic document V11.1.* Retrieved from http://medical.nema.org/dicom/geninfo/Strategy.pdf

Enrado, P. (2007, December 12). NHIN forum: Value of HIEs needs attention. *Healthcare IT News.* Retrieved from http://www.healthcareitnews.com/story.cms?d=8293&page=1

Freedman, I. (2007). What does "interoperability really mean"? *Health Management Technology, 28*(10), 50–51.

Garde, S., Knaup, P., & Hovenga, E. (2005). *OpenEHR archetypes in electronic health records: The path to semantic interoperability?* Retrieved from http://healthinformatics.cqu.edu.au/downloads/garde_gmds_2005.pdf

Garde, S., Knaup, P., Hovenga, E., & Heard, S. (2007). Towards semantic interoperability for electronic health records. *Methods of Information in Medicine, 46*(3), 332–343.

Getting started. (2007). *Hospitals & Health Networks, 81*(5), 14. Retrieved from Health Source: Nursing/Academic Edition database.

Gooch, J. J. (2010). Pilots key to ACO implementation. *Managed Healthcare Executive, 20*(8), 6–7.

Harris, J., Grauman, D., & Hemnani, R. (2010). Solving the ACO conundrum. *Healthcare Financial Management, 64*(11), 67.

Health Level Seven. (2011). *Mission statement.* Retrieved from http://www.hl7.org/about/index.cfm?ef=nav

Healthcare Information and Management Systems Society (HIMSS). (2007). *IHE.* Retrieved from http://www.himss.org/ASP/topics_ihe.asp

Institute of Medicine. (2001). *Crossing the quality chasm: A new health system for the 21st century.* Washington, DC: National Academies Press.

International Health Terminology Standards Development Organisation (IHTSDO). (n.d.). *About SNOMED CT.* Retrieved from http://www.ihtsdo.org/snomed-ct/snomed-ct0/

International Organization for Standardization (ISO). (2007). *ISO/FDIS 13606–1.* Retrieved from http://www.iso.org/iso/iso_catalogue/catalogue_tc/catalogue_detail.htm?csnumber=40784

Kalra, D. (2007). *Trustworthy decision support: Is the electronic health record dependable?* Retrieved from http://www.haifa.il.ibm.com/Workshops/hcls2007/papers/trustworthy_decision_support.pdf

Kaushal, R., Blumenthal, D., Poon, E. G., Jha, A. K., Franz, C., Middleton, B., . . . Bates D. W. (2005). The costs of a national health information network. *Annals of Internal Medicine, 143*(3), 165–173.

Kilic, O., & Dogac, A. (2009). Achieving clinical statement interoperability using R-MIM and archetype-based semantic transformations. *IEEE Transactions on Information Technology in Biomedicine, 13*(4), 467–477. Retrieved from http://www.srdc.metu.edu.tr/webpage/projects/ride/publications/KilicDogac.pdf

Larsen, E. (2005, October). *Estimating the costs of NHIN functions and interoperability. HIMSS standards insight summary.* Retrieved from http://www.himss.org/content/files/standardsinsight/summaries/2005-10.pdf

Lewis, G. A., Morris, E., Simanta, S., & Wrage, L. (2008). Effects of service-oriented architecture on software development lifecycle activities. *Software Process Improvement and Practice, 13,* 135–144. doi:10.1002/splp.372

Martin, K. S., Monsen, K. A., & Bowles, K. H. (2011). The Omaha system and meaningful use: Applications for practice, education, and research. *Computers, Informatics, Nursing, 29*(1), 52–58. doi:10.1097/NCN.0b013e3181f9ddc6

McKinney, M. (2010). "Huge potential" for EHRs and comparative effectiveness. *Hospitals & Health Networks/AHA, 84*(4), 41–42.

Mead, C. N. (2006). Data interchange standards in healthcare IT—Computable semantic interoperability: Now possible but still difficult, do we really need a better mousetrap? *Journal of Healthcare Information Management, 20*(1), 71–78.

National Library of Medicine. (2011, April 6). *United medical language system (UMLS)*. Retrieved from http://www.nlm.nih.gov/research/umls/

Nusbaum, M. H. (2007, December). Global interoperability now within reach. *Healthcare IT News,* p. 9.

OpenEHR Foundation. (2007). *Welcome to open EHR*. Retrieved from http://www.openehr.org/home.html

OpenEHR Foundation. (2011, April 3). *News: First open source release of openEHR.NET available on codeplex*. Retrieved from http://www.openehr.org/news_events/news.html

Rajini, S. N. S., & Bhuvaneswari, T. (2010). SOS in business organization. *The IUP Journal of Computer Sciences, IV*(4), 22–27.

Schlotzer, A., & Madsen, M. (2010). Health information systems: Requirements and characteristics. *Studies in Health Technology and Informatics, 151,* 156–166. doi:10.3233/978-1-60750-476-4-156

Schwend, G. T. (2007). Searching for Oz. *ADVANCE for Health Information Executives, 11*(2), 79.

Taylor, M. (2010). The ABCs of ACOs [Cover story]. *Hospitals & Health Networks, 84*(5), 26–38.

Terry, K. (2011). You'll need the right IT tools to build an ACO. *Hospitals & Health Networks, 85*(1), 23.

U.S. Department of Health and Human Services (DHHS). (2007, October 5). *News release: HHS awards contracts for trial implementations of the nationwide health information network*. Retrieved from http://www.hhs.gov/news/press/2007pres/10/pr20071005a.html

Warren, J. J., & Bakken, S. (2002). Update on standardized nursing data sets and terminologies. *Journal of the American Health Information Management Association, 73*(7), 78–83, quiz: 85–76.

While, A., & Thomas, P. (2007). Should nurses be leaders of integrated health care? *Journal of Nursing Management, 15*(6), 643–648.

CHAPTER 14

The Electronic Health Record

After completing this chapter, you should be able to:

1. Define the term *electronic health record* (*EHR*).

2. Define the term *electronic medical record* (*EMR*).

3. Define the term *computer-based patient record* (*CPR*).

4. Discuss the similarities and differences between the EHR, EMR, and the CPR.

5. Understand the significance of the 12 characteristics of the CPR defined by the Institute of Medicine for today's EHR.

6. Discuss the benefits associated with the EHR.

7. Review the current status of the EHR, including impediments.

8. List several concerns that must be resolved before implementation of the EHR.

9. Recognize the relationship between Meaningful Use and the adoption and use of the EHR in hospitals, physician offices, and other settings.

Requirements for the management of healthcare information are evolving—transforming the ways that healthcare providers store, access, and use information. The traditional paper medical record that reports client status and test results no longer meets the needs of today's healthcare industry. Paper records are episode-oriented with a separate record for each client visit. Key information, such as allergies, may be lost from one episode to the next, jeopardizing patient safety. Another drawback to paper records is that only one person can access the record at any given time, leading to wasted time spent looking for paper records and treatment delays. Different versions of the same information may be stored in several places. Paper records cannot incorporate diagnostic studies that include images and sound, nor do they make use of decision-support systems. Paper records impede the collection of data for tracking patient outcomes and comparative effectiveness research. The electronic health record (EHR) has the potential to integrate all pertinent patient information into one lifetime record, which will help to improve the quality of health information, improve care coordination, patient safety, and productivity; contain costs; support research; decrease wait time for treatment; and contribute to the body of healthcare knowledge (Hagens & Krose 2009; IOM 2003; Persell & Bufalino 2008). The Bush administration called for the adoption of the EHR by 2014 as a means to help transform U.S. healthcare, and provide a life-long EHR for every citizen. Following this directive the American Recovery and Reimbursement Act of 2009 mandated the implementation of "meaningful use benchmarks" (Bell & Thornton 2011; Hogan & Kissam 2010; Montandon 2009; Sullivan 2010). These benchmarks require healthcare providers to report certain data. Compliance with mandated reporting requirements is contingent upon the adoption and use of certified EHR systems capable of collecting and sharing the specified data which is linked to financial incentives for the adoption of EHR technology. The intent of Meaningful Use is to encourage the implementation and use of the EHR for the improvement of the overall quality of care.

DEFINITIONS

Numerous terms have been used over the years to describe the concept of an EHR, leading to confusion about the definitions. *EHR* has been used as a generic term for all electronic healthcare systems and recently became the favored term for the lifetime computerized record. Some other frequently used terms include *electronic medical record (EMR), electronic patient record (EPR), computer-based patient record (CPR), CPR system, and Shared Electronic Health Record (SEHR).* HIMSS Analytics, a not-for-profit subsidiary of the Healthcare Information and Management Systems Society (HIMSS) outlined the differences between the terms *electronic medical record* and *electronic health record,* defining the **electronic medical record (EMR)** as the "legal record created in hospitals and ambulatory environments that is the source of data for the EHR (Garets & Davis 2006)." The EMR typically referred to a single encounter with no, or very limited, ability to carry information from one visit to another within a care delivery system. That situation has changed so that it is possible to bring information forward from prior visits within the organization or delivery system. Basic EMR components include:

- Clinical messaging and e-mail
- Results reporting
- Data repository
- Decision support
- Clinical documentation
- Order entry

EMR result reporting and data repository components include unstructured data, which are data that do not follow any particular format and often are provided as a text report. Examples are reports produced by transcription services, including history and physical assessments, consultation findings, operative reports, and discharge summaries. The EMR also includes structured data, which are data that follow a predefined format and are often presented as discrete data elements. Structured data are often obtained from automated ancillary reporting systems; a primary example is laboratory results from an automated laboratory information system. Another type of data that may be included in the EMR is electronic imaging produced by diagnostic studies, including tomography, ultrasonography, and magnetic resonance imaging. The data in the EMR is the legal record of patient care during an encounter at the healthcare delivery system and is owned by that system.

While most hospitals have some level of automation, few have attained a fully electronic environment. At present approximately one-half of physician offices have implemented an electronic record (Lewis 2010). Ambulatory care and long-term care settings are in the process of implementing electronic records. In 2008 the National Alliance for Health Information Technology (p. 17) sought to eliminate the confusion in terms when it defined the **electronic health record (EHR)** as "an electronic record of health-related information on an individual that conforms to nationally recognized interoperability standards and that can be created, managed, and consulted by authorized clinicians and staff across more than one health care organization." The Alliance also noted that the primary distinction between the EMR and EHR was the ability to exchange information outside of a single healthcare delivery system.

Given that the EMR is considered a building block in the creation of the EHR, it is important to note the status of healthcare delivery systems in the attainment of EMR capabilities. The HIMSS Analytics EMR Adoption Model was developed in 2005 and was recently revised to show how individual hospitals and integrated healthcare systems in the United States and Canada fared in their levels of EMR capabilities (Hoyt n.d.). The stages of the model range from minimal automation at stage 0 to full automation at stage 7. Each subsequent stage presumes the existence of the functionalities listed for the preceding stage. HIMSS added European hospitals to the EMR adoption survey in 2010. Data from the HIMSS Analytics U.S. Adoption Model indicated that 10% of the more than 5,000 organizations that participated in the survey had progressed to stage 4 with approximately one-half having achieved stage 3 (HIMSS Analytics 2011). The criteria associated with each stage are listed here.

Stage 0: Some clinical automation exists but the laboratory, pharmacy, and radiology systems are not all operational.

Stage 1: The major ancillary clinical systems—the laboratory, pharmacy, and radiology systems—are all installed.

Stage 2: Major ancillary clinical systems send data to a clinical data repository (CDR) that allows physicians to retrieve and review results. The CDR also contains a controlled medical vocabulary and clinical decision rules engine that checks for conflict. Document imaging systems may also be linked to the CDR.

Stage 3: Basic clinical documentation (vital signs, flow sheets) is required. Nurses' notes, care plans, and/or electronic medical administration records may be present and are integrated with the CDR for at least one hospital service. Basic clinical decision support is available for error checking with order entry. Some availability is present for the retrieval and storage of diagnostic imaging. Typically this refers to the picture archiving communications systems (PACS) used for x-rays and other diagnostic images.

Stage 4: Computerized provider order entry (CPOE) and a second level of clinical decision support for evidence-based practice are added to the previous stages.

Stage 5: At least one service area has the closed loop medication administration process where barcode medication administration (BCMA), radio frequency identification (RFID), or other identification technology is in place and integrated with CPOE and the pharmacy to maximize patient safety.

Stage 6: At least one service area has full physician documentation, third-level clinical decision support for all clinicians for protocols and outcomes with variance and compliance alerts, and a full PACS system.

Stage 7: This is a paperless environment where all information is shared electronically and the EHR can produce a continuity of care document (CCD).

The **electronic patient record (EPR)** is an electronic client record, but not necessarily a lifetime record, that focuses on relevant information for the current episode of care.

The computerized patient record (CPR) is a comprehensive lifetime record that includes all information from all specialties (Andrew, Bruegel, & Gasch 2007). The classic definition and attributes of the CPR, as identified by the Institute of Medicine (IOM), provide the basis for today's understanding of the EHR.

The U.S. Department of Health and Human Services (DHHS) said that the EHR is a "digital collection of patient's medical history and could include items like diagnosed medical conditions, prescribed medications, vital signs, immunizations, lab results, and personnel characteristics like age and weight" (DHHS news release 2005). HIMSS (2011a) defines the EHR as

> . . . a longitudinal electronic record of patient health information generated by one or more encounters in any care delivery setting. Included in this information are patient demographics, progress notes, problems, medications, vital signs, past medical history, immunizations, laboratory data and radiology reports. The EHR automates and streamlines the clinician's workflow. The EHR has the ability to generate a complete record of a clinical patient encounter—as well as supporting other care-related activities directly or indirectly via interface—including evidence-based decision support, quality management, and outcomes reporting.

Information in the EHR may be owned by the patient or stakeholder although recent developments favor a more consumer-centric approach. Unlike the EMR, the EHR provides interactive patient access as well as the ability for the patient to append information. The Department of Defense (DOD) added dental records to the list of EHR components (Anderson 2007). The development of the EHR relies upon the presence of fully operational EMRs, interoperability (National Alliance for Health Information Technology 2008), and a national health information network (NHIN). In 2003, HIMSS identified the following attributes of the EHR:

1. Provides secure, reliable real-time access to client health record information where and when it is needed to support care

2. Records and manages episodic and longitudinal EHR information

3. Functions as clinicians' primary information resources during the provision of client care

4. Assists with the work of planning and delivery of evidence-based care to individual and groups of clients

5. Captures data used for continuous quality improvement, utilization review, risk management, resource planning, and performance management

6. Captures the patient health-related information needed for medical record and reimbursement

7. Provides longitudinal, appropriately masked information to support clinical research, public health reporting, and population health initiatives

8. Supports clinical trials and evidence-based research

The EHR must provide secure, real-time, point-of-care (POC), patient-centric information for clinicians at the time and place that clinicians need it. The EHR must also provide evidence-based decision support, automate and streamline the clinician's workflow, and support the collection of data for uses other than direct client care. These indirect uses include billing, quality management, outcomes reporting, resource planning, and public health disease surveillance and reporting (HIMSS 2003, p. 2).

In July 2003, the DHHS announced the formation of the EHR Collaborative. This group of founding stakeholder organizations was charged with the task of facilitating rapid input from the healthcare community to support the adoption of standards for the EHR. Member organizations included the following:

- American Health Information Management Association
- American Medical Association
- American Medical Informatics Association
- American Nurses Association
- College of Healthcare Information Management Executives (CHIME)
- eHealth Initiative (eHI)
- Healthcare Information and Management Systems Society (HIMSS)
- National Alliance for Health Information Technology (NAHIT)

The EHR Collaborative sponsored a series of open forum meetings to solicit input, which were published as the *Final Report: Public Response to HL7EHR Ballot 1.* In 2005, the American Health Information Community (AHIC) was chartered as a federal advisory body to make recommendations to the secretary of the DHHS on how to accelerate the development and adoption of health information technology. AHIC concluded operations in 2008. President Bush recognized the need to support ongoing efforts to adopt and use health information technology when he established the position of National Coordinator for Health Information Technology in 2004. The Office of the National Coordinator (ONC) was later mandated legislatively in the Health Information Technology for Economic and Clinical Health Act (HITECH Act) of 2009 (DHHS 2006, 2009). During the intervening years work continued to develop a functional model and agreed-on standards because the EHR requires both technical and clinical standards. The adoption of nationally agreed-on standards for the EHR will impact all sectors of the healthcare community including:

- Hospitals
- Physicians
- Payers
- Researchers
- Pharmacies
- Public health agencies
- Long-term facilities
- Consumers

The International Organization for Standards' (ISO) Technical Committee 215 recommended definitions of electronic medical and health records that are used throughout most of the world but these were not adopted by the United States (Walton 2007). The United States instead became a charter member of the International Health Terminology Standards Development Organization (IHTSDO), which acquired the Systemized Nomenclature of Medicine Clinical Terms (SNOMED-CT) as a means to foster the rapid development and adoption of standard clinical terminology for EHRs (DHHS 2007). SNOMED-CT has subsequently been chosen as the common language required by 2015 for certified EHRs (Manos 2009). SNOMED-CT and other standardized nomenclatures and languages are discussed in greater detail in Chapter 15.

Another concept with electronic records is the **continuity of care document (CCD).** This record is intended to improve continuity of care when clients move between various points of care. The CCD is comprised of contributions from many types of caregivers, including physicians, nurses, physical therapists, and social workers with each providing a summary of care provided (Conn 2007). The record supports the patient's safety and has a positive impact on the quality and continuity of care. The Health Level 7 (HL7) and ASTM International standards groups created the CCD based upon work done by earlier groups. The CCD is a snapshot of patient status, rather than a comprehensive record. The CCD has been named in U.S. Meaningful Use regulations for the exchange of clinical information (HL7 2010).

HISTORICAL DEVELOPMENTS

The IOM identified the following 12 major components of the CPR, which it considered the "gold standard" attributes (Andrew & Bruegel 2003):

1. Provides a problem list that indicates current clinical problems for each encounter, the number of occurrences associated with all past and current problems, and the current status of the problem

2. Evaluates and records health status and functional levels using accepted measures

3. Documents the clinical reasoning/rationale for diagnoses and conclusions. Allows sharing of clinical reasoning with other caregivers and automates and tracks decision making.

4. Provides a longitudinal or lifetime client record by linking all client data from previous encounters

5. Supports confidentiality, privacy, and audit trails

6. Provides continuous access to authorized users at any time

7. Allows simultaneous and customized views of the client data

8. Supports links to local or remote information resources, such as various databases using the Internet or organization-based intranet resources

9. Supports decision analysis tools

10. Supports direct entry of client data by physicians

11. Includes mechanisms for measuring the cost and quality of care

12. Supports existing and evolving clinical needs by being flexible and expandable

Most of the data included in the CPR are structured data. Other data formats may also be linked to the CPR, including dictation and transcription, images, video, and text. These data, and collective data from all systems, are stored and managed in the clinical data repository. This database allows retrieval of multiple elements of client data regardless of their system of origin. For example, the user may retrieve a lab result from the clinical data repository that was originally produced by the laboratory information system, along with a radiology report that was generated in the radiology information system from a transcribed dictation. Collectively, these various systems and the clinical data repository make up the CPR. Data exchange standards would permit the uniform capture of data required to build a longitudinal record comprised of integrated information systems from multiple vendors.

MEANINGFUL USE

The framework for Meaningful Use of the EHR evolved from a set of national priorities to help focus performance improvement efforts identified in the *National Priorities & Goals* report released by the National Priorities Partnership (2008), which was convened by the National Quality Forum. These priorities included (Meaningful Use Workgroup 2009):

- Patient engagement
- Reducing racial disparities
- Improved efficiency

- Increased safety
- Coordination of care
- Measures to improve population health

The HITECH, part of the 2009 American Recovery and Reinvestment Act, authorized CMS to reimburse providers who succeed at becoming "Meaningful Users" of the EHR starting in 2011. Incentives will decrease gradually with penalties imposed for failure to achieve Meaningful Use by 2015. The Meaningful Use requirement is a major driver in the adoption and use of EHR systems across U.S. healthcare delivery systems and physician practices today (Bell & Thornton 2011; Hewlett Packard 2010). CMS estimates for incentives paid to eligible providers and hospitals range between $9.78 and $27.4 billion (Harris 2010). The Office of the National Coordinator created the criteria for what the EHR should be able to do while CMS created the clinical quality measures that must be met by hospitals and providers to quality for financial incentives (Klepacki, Lamer, & Sattler n.d.). The clinical quality measures identified by CMS differ from those established for the Medicare pay-for-reporting program and the MIPPA E-Prescribing Incentive Program (CMS 2011a; Jarousse 2010). Box 14–1 lists the 14 core requirements for hospitals. The Meaningful Use requirement is being implemented in stages. Stage 1 measures focus on patient movement through the emergency department, stroke care, and treatment of blood clots. CMS has identified the degree of expected compliance to meet each measure. Additionally hospitals must meet 5 of the 10 requirements that are depicted in Box 14–2 although they have the latitude to choose which measures they will adopt from this second list. Stage I emphasizes the electronic capture and sharing of health information in coded format, and the use of that information to track conditions and coordinate care. Physicians must meet the core requirements for inpatient facilities plus the additional requirements of (Bigalke & Morris 2010; Classen, Newcomb, & Drazen 2009):

- E-prescribing
- Generating lists of patients with specific conditions
- Progress notes

BOX 14–1 Stage I Meaningful Use Core Requirements for Hospitals

1. Record demographic information (preferred language, gender, race ethnic background, date of birth, date/cause of death (inpatient setting only)).
2. Computerized provider order entry.
3. Clinical decision support and the ability to track compliance with rule(s).
4. Automatic, real-time drug-drug and drug-allergy interaction checks based on the medication list, allergy list.
5. Maintain an active medication list.
6. Maintain an active medication allergy list.
7. Record and retrieve vital signs (height, weight, blood pressure, BMI, growth charts for ages 2–20 years).
8. Record smoking status for patients 13 years old and older.
9. Mechanisms to protect information created or maintained by the certified EHR technology that include access control.
10. Electronically exchange key clinical information among providers and patient-authorized entities.
11. Supply patients with an electronic copy of their health information upon request.
12. Supply patients with an electronic copy of their discharge instructions upon request.
13. Report required clinical quality measures to CMS.
14. Maintain up-to-date problem lists of current and active patient diagnoses.

Source: U.S. Department of Health and Human Services, Centers for Medicare & Medicaid Services Medicare and Medicaid Programs. (July 28, 2010). Electronic Health Record Incentive Program Final Rule. *Federal Register, 75* (144), 44313–44588. Retrieved from http://edocket.access.gpo.gov/2010/pdf/2010-17207.pdf

---

BOX 14–2   Menu Set of 10 Optional Stage I Meaningful Use Core Measures

1. Incorporate clinical lab test results as structured data.
2. Generate patient lists by specific conditions to use for quality improvement, reduction of disparities, research or outreach.
3. Submit electronic data to immunization registries.
4. Submit syndromic public health surveillance data electronically in accordance with applicable law.
5. Identify and provide patient-specific education resources.
6. Drug-formulary checks.
7. Support medication reconciliation.
8. Generate summary care records for transition of care/referral.
9. Electronic submission of reportable lab results.
10. Advance directives for patients 65 years old and older.

Source: U.S. Department of Health and Human Services, Centers for Medicare & Medicaid Services Medicare and Medicaid Programs. (July 28, 2010). Electronic Health Record Incentive Program Final Rule. *Federal Register, 75*(144), 44313–44588. Retrieved from http://edocket.access.gpo.gov/2010/pdf/2010-17207.pdf

---

The rules for Stages 2 and 3 have not been finalized as yet, but Stage 2 focuses on HIT use at the point of care for continuous quality improvement and exchange of information in a structured format (Jarousse 2010; Markle Connecting for Health 2009). Financial incentives for Stage 2 compliance will be available in 2013. Stage 3 focuses on improved outcomes and population health via improvements in safety, quality, efficiency, and expanded EHR functionality. Financial incentives for Stage 3 will be available in 2015. Bigalke and Morris (2010) noted that providers need to make meeting Meaningful Use requirements a priority that is guided by goals and expected outcomes with established timelines and designation of resources.

Eligibility for Meaningful Use incentives also requires the adoption and use of EHRs that have been certified although certification alone does not guarantee incentives—only the demonstrated use of certified EHRs in meaningful ways will qualify providers for incentives. Certified technology provides the assurance that an EHR system has the technical capacity, functionality, and security to meet the Meaningful Use criteria for a given stage (CMS 2011b). The final rule for permanent certification of EHRs was established in January 2011 by the Office of the National Coordinator (ONC 2011a).

BENEFITS OF THE EHR

Thompson, Velasco, Classen, and Raddemann (2010) stated that most of the benefits resulting from EHR implementation are enabled by the EHR rather than produced solely through its implementation. They also noted that the potential financial benefits far exceed those netted from government financial incentives for meeting Meaningful Use requirements. Some of the benefits are general, but others relate to nurses, physicians, and other care providers, as well as the healthcare enterprise.

General Benefits

- *Improved data integrity.* Information is more readable, better organized, and more accurate and complete.
- *Increased productivity.* Caregivers are able to access client information whenever it is needed and at multiple convenient locations. This can result in improved client care due to their ability to make timely decisions based on appropriate data.

- *Improved quality of care.* The EHR supports clinical decision-making processes for physicians and nurses. For example, the clinician can tailor a view of patient information that shows the most recent labs, vital signs, and current medications on one screen or select another view that graphs lab values and vital signs over time. This capability could be used to show renal response to ordered medications or for any number of other scenarios.
- *Increased satisfaction for caregivers.* Caregivers are able to take advantage of easy access to client data as well as other services, including drug information sources, rules-based decision support, and literature searches.

Nursing Benefits

- Facilitates comparisons of current data and data from previous events
- Supports an ongoing record of the client's education and learning response across encounters or visits
- Eliminates the need to repeat collection of baseline demographic data with each encounter, saving nursing time
- Provides universal data access to all who have access to the EHR
- Improves data access and quality for research
- Provides prompts to ensure administration and documentation of medications and treatments
- Improves documentation and quality of care (Nelson 2007)
- Facilitates automation of critical and clinical pathways
- Supports the development of a database that facilitates research, provides information useful to administrators and clinicians, and allows recognition of nursing work in measurable units when used with a common unified structure for nursing language

Benefits for Healthcare Providers

- Improved eligibility for reimbursement
- Simultaneous record access by multiple users
- Previous encounters may be accessed easily
- Faster chart access waiting for old paper records to be located and delivered from the medical records department
- More comprehensive information is available
- Fewer lost records than with paper systems
- Improved efficiency of billing inclusive of automated charge capture
- Better reporting tools. Trends and clinical graphics are available on demand.
- Reduced liability through better decision making and documentation
- Improved reimbursement rates
- Enhanced compliance through system-generated prompts with preventive care protocols (Martin 2007; Mitchell 2007)
- Enhanced ability to meet regulatory requirements such as the physician quality reporting initiative (Bell & Thornton 2011)
- Supports pay-for-performance bonuses
- Early warnings of changes in patient status
- Supports benchmarking for how well physicians manage patients with chronic disease conditions (Novogoratz 2007)
- Improved population health
- Increased efficiencies in workflow

Healthcare Enterprise Benefits

- Improved client record security
- Instant notice of authorization for procedures with integration with payer-based health records
- Strengthened communications
- Fewer lost records
- Decreased need for record storage
- Reduced medical record department costs because pulling, filing, and copying of charts are decreased
- Improved verification of client eligibility for healthcare coverage
- Faster turnaround for outstanding accounts with electronic coding and claim submission
- Decreased need for x-ray film and physical filing, storage, and transport of films
- Improved cost evaluation based on clinical outcomes and resource utilization data
- Decreased length of stay (Thompson et al. 2010)
- Enhanced compliance with regulatory requirements

Consumer Benefits

- Decreased wait time for treatment
- Improved access and control over health information.
- Increased use of best practices with incorporation of decision support
- Improved ability to ask informed questions
- Greater responsibility for one's own care
- Increased medication safety
- Quicker turnaround time for ordered treatments (Thompson et al. 2010)
- Alerts and reminders for upcoming appointments and scheduled tests
- Increased use of preventive care
- Increased satisfaction
- Greater clarity to discharge instructions
- Improved understanding of treatment choices (Martin 2007; Mitchell 2007)

Payer Benefits

- Supports pay for performance as quality measures are gathered (Martin 2007)
- Supports disease management, lowering costs for expensive diagnoses

Despite this lengthy list of potential benefits, limited research in past years made it difficult for healthcare executives to adequately evaluate the costs, benefits, and risks of a commercial EMR purchase. HIMSS created a Clinical Information Systems (CIS) Benefits Task Force to create a database of actual provider experiences and thereby lead to better purchase decisions and the implementation of necessary organizational changes to realize EHR benefits (Thompson, Osheroff, Classen, & Sittig 2007). Puffer et al. (2007) cautioned that the mere implementation of an EMR does not guarantee that benefits will be achieved. A major concern associated with the rush to implement EHR systems for Meaningful Use compliance is that hasty decisions will lead to poor purchase decisions and inadequate planning for change, which, in turn, will lead to the failure to fully realize EHR benefits (Hewlett Packard 2010).

CURRENT STATUS OF THE EHR

While no country has yet implemented an operational national EHR, the HITECH Act has sparked new interest and brings focus and consistency to U.S. EHR adoption efforts, making clear what needs to be done even if the time that it will take remains unclear (Sullivan 2010).

The HITECH Act also helps move U.S. efforts toward the adoption of specific standards to ensure the interoperability that will allow the data collection and exchange required to comply with Meaningful Use requirements. Meaningful Use rules provide direction as to the technical and content standards for the EHR. For example, the content standard for a patient summary will be the CCD or continuity of care record. SNOMED-CT, NCPDP Script, RxNorm, HL7, and LOINC are standardized terminologies that have been identified as a means to enable the interoperability required to realize Meaningful Use of EHRs. The ONC has provided leadership for the development and implementation of an interoperable health information technology infrastructure to improve quality and efficiency of care.

The DOD and the Department of Veterans Affairs (VA) lead the United States in EHR adoption. Together they operate two of the nation's largest healthcare systems using EHRs to manage patient information. Both are involved in an initiative to modernize their systems and work collaboratively to establish the virtual lifetime electronic record (Electronic Health Records 2011).

Many other organizations and entities have also been active in shaping the EHR. The Healthcare Information Technology Standards Panel (HITSP), a partnership between the public and private sectors, was formed for the purpose of harmonizing and integrating standards for information sharing. HITSP recently completed a contract with the DHHS (HITSP n.d.). The Markle Foundation is a U.S. organization that focuses upon harnessing the potential of information and information technology to advance the quality of healthcare. Informatics and professional organizations have long voiced their views on the adoption of technology in healthcare. The ONC also encourages the public to comment on HIT.

While many organizations struggle with the slow piecemeal conversion to electronic medical records, unintended negative outcomes may be seen. These include increased workloads and delayed information retrieval as clinicians are forced to search multiple data sources for client information. For example the clinician may need to find or document key information which now requires several steps instead of one.

CONSIDERATIONS WHEN IMPLEMENTING THE EHR

Information system vendors as well as healthcare providers are aware of the pressing need to develop and deploy the EHR. Compliance with regulatory and reimbursement issues, particularly Meaningful Use, is a major driver. This requires the use of certified EHRs or strategies to update existing EHR systems. Development of an electronic infrastructure and cost have been two of the biggest impediments to the creation of a fully functioning EHR. The principal requirement is that the major participants in the healthcare arena, including healthcare facilities, payers, and physicians, must be linked electronically. This is a costly undertaking. Other issues have included the lack of a common vocabulary, privacy, security, and confidentiality issues; resistance among caregivers; failure to adequately consider organizational change; determining a realistic timeline; a lack of IT staff to create and support the necessary infrastructure; and legal issues surrounding the discovery of medical information (Maynard 2010).

ONC-Authorized Testing and Certification

The ONC established a temporary certification program for health information technology (health IT) as a means to facilitate the adoption of interoperable EHRs capable of meeting Meaningful Use core requirements. The purpose of the testing and certification program is to provide a way for organizations to become authorized by the National Coordinator to test and certify EHR technology. Certification in turn provides the assurance that EHR technology adopted is capable of helping organizations meet Meaningful Use criteria. According to the ONC (2011b) the recent adoption of the final rule for certification "represents the first step in an incremental approach to adopting standards, implementation specifications, and certification criteria to enhance the interoperability, functionality, utility, and security of health IT and to support its meaningful use."

Initially only two entities were authorized as ONC-Authorized Testing and Certification Bodies (ONC-ATCBs), The Certification Commission for Health Information Technology and the Drummond Group Inc. (DHHS 2010). The list of ONC-ATCBs has since been expanded and is available on the ONC Web site (ONC 2010). ONC issued the final rule to establish the permanent health information technology certification program in January 2011. Box 14–3 lists functionality required for EHR certification although required functions may be added at future dates.

BOX 14–3 Functionality Required for Certified EHRs		
Function	**Inpatient Settings/ Hospitals**	**Outpatient Settings/ Physician Offices**
Record demographic information	X	X
• Preferred language		
• Gender		
• Race		
• Ethnic background		
• Date of birth		
Date/cause of death (inpatient setting only)		
Computerized provider order entry	X	X
Clinical decision support and the ability to track compliance with rule(s)	X	X
Automatic, real-time drug-drug and drug-allergy interaction checks based on the medication list and allergy list	X	X
Maintain an active medication list	X	X
Maintain an active medication allergy list	X	X
Record and retrieve vital signs	X	X
• Height		
• Weight		
• Blood pressure		
• BMI		
• Growth charts and BMI ages 2–20 years		
Record smoking status for patients 13 years old and older	X	X
Mechanisms to protect information created or maintained by the certified EHR technology that include access control	X	X
Electronically exchange key clinical information among providers and patient-authorized entities	X	X
Supply patients with an electronic copy of their health information upon request	X	X
Supply patients with an electronic copy of their discharge instructions upon request	X	N/A
Report required clinical quality measures to CMS	X	X
Maintain up-to-date problem lists of current and active patient diagnoses	X	X

BOX 14–3 (*continued*)

Function	Inpatient Settings/ Hospitals	Outpatient Settings/ Physician Offices
Incorporate clinical lab-test results as structured data	X	X
Generate patient lists by specific conditions to use for quality improvement, reduction of disparities, research or outreach	X	X
Submit electronic data to immunization registries	X	X
Submit syndromic public health surveillance data electronically in accordance with applicable law	X	X
Identify and provide patient-specific education resources		
Drug-formulary checks	X	X
Support medication reconciliation	X	X
Generate summary care records for transition of care/referral	X	X
Electronic submission of reportable lab results	X	N/A
Advance directives	X	
Patient reminders for preventive and/or follow-up care	N/A	X
Provide patients with timely electronic access to their information	N/A	X
Check insurance eligibility electronically	X	X
Submit claims electronically	X	X
Support electronic prescriptions	N/A	X

Source: U.S. Department of Health and Human Services, Centers for Medicare & Medicaid Services Medicare and Medicaid Programs. (July 28, 2010). Electronic Health Record Incentive Program Final Rule. *Federal Register, 75* (144), 44313–44588. Retrieved from http://edocket.access.gpo.gov/2010/pdf/2010-17207.pdf

Electronic Infrastructure

The healthcare facilities, payers, physicians, and nurses all need the ability to access and update the client's longitudinal record. This ability requires linkage of the various information systems that support these stakeholders via a network infrastructure. Agreement must be reached regarding the nature and format of client data to be stored, as well as the mechanisms for data exchange, storage, and retrieval. This means that all participants use common data communication standards. The lack of standards has been a key barrier to establishing this type of electronic connectivity. First and most important is the decision regarding the recognition of a universal client identifier or MPI (master patient index) number, so that all client data can be associated with the correct client. The Social Security number has been widely used for this purpose, but it is unreliable because it may be stolen or inaccurately provided; in addition, some individuals have used more than one number, while others do not have one. Improvements in connectivity alone are not enough to support the EHR. It is also important to include components such as interoperability, comparability, decision support, and POC data capture to achieve a longitudinal electronic record.

Cost

Another impediment to the EHR is cost. Initial and ongoing costs for deploying and maintaining IT systems were cited as the greatest barrier to IT. According to recent CMS estimates, eligible providers will spend an average of $54,000 to purchase and implement a certified EHR for their offices and eligible hospitals will spend an average of $5,000,000 for the purchase and installation; those figures do not include annual maintenance costs (Harris 2010). Furthermore the development of the electronic links forming the infrastructure is costly, and the allocation of fiscal responsibilities is difficult. Until the introduction of Meaningful Use incentives most of the expense for EHR development has been underwritten by each individual provider, hospital, or healthcare enterprise. Links to other facilities and agencies are rare and for the most part limited to provider–payer arrangements.

Vocabulary Standardization

Standardization in clinical terms used in patient records facilitates interoperability as it ensures a common understanding of terms. Standardized languages make it possible to generalize research findings across settings, countries, and cultures; compare patient outcomes; facilitate communication with other disciplines and delivery systems; and showcase nursing's contributions to healthcare. Despite these clear advantages, adoption of standard nomenclature has been slow. The increased acceleration of EHR adoption can be used as an opportunity to realize the benefits associated with standardized nomenclature for the entire healthcare sector as well as for nurses who could use the power of standardized nursing nomenclatures to demonstrate contributions made by nurses. In-depth discussion of standardized nomenclature takes place in Chapter 15.

Setting a Realistic Timeline

While the intent of ARRA was to escalate the adoption of HIT, the unwanted side effect is an overly rushed implementation process that can negate many of the potential benefits associated with EHRs and potentially sacrifice patient safety (Ames, Ciotti, & Mathis 2011). The enormity of switching from a paper process to a new EHR system must be fully considered (Raths 2009). Knowledge management challenges include bringing forward information from old legacy systems and how to combine paper and electronic records. Maximizing realization of EHR benefits requires careful planning as well as culture changes and work redesign.

Security and Confidentiality

Security and confidentiality concerns are critical considerations in EHR development and use. Even as EHR adoption increases, patients remain concerned that the electronic storage of personal health information will make inappropriate access to that information easier (Lewis 2010). The EHR system must be configured to allow access only to those who have been identified as authorized users. The system must authenticate the user's identity with user IDs and passwords and possibly biometrics. HIPAA considerations include the need to be able to provide the client, upon request, with a log of caregivers who have accessed his or her chart. In addition, client information should not be available to anyone without the client's approval. Data that are communicated via the Internet must be encrypted. Firewalls must be in place when data are sent and received via the Internet to safeguard data integrity. Meaningful Use requirements also include measures to protect patient information that strengthen HIPAA requirements.

Caregiver Resistance

Resistance by caregivers such as physicians and nurses can delay the development and use of the EHR. This resistance is, in part, attributed to the fact that many EHRs lack essential features or are perceived as awkward or inconvenient to use. A study conducted by Ford, Menachemi, Peterson, and Huerta (2009) that compared EHR adoption rates before and after 2004 found that resistance to adoption increased after 2004, but this work was submitted prior to the enactment of ARRA. Likewise Simon et al. (2009) noted that despite an increased use of EHRs in physician practices, many physicians still do not use the full functionality of available EHRs. The fully developed EHR necessitates that all caregivers use the EHR during the course of their daily routine. Some individuals have been unable or unwilling to use computers for various factors such as the complexity of software, the need to learn multiple systems, the availability of workstations, and resistance to change in the work patterns. Some physicians believe that data entry is demeaning and a waste of time and interferes with their ability to provide client care on a timely basis. In addition, they may resist perceived changes to the way they practice medicine that will be required by the EHR system. As a result some physicians are choosing to ignore the incentives, indicating the penalties will be less costly than implementing a new office EHR. The implications of this "inaction" may lead physicians to decrease or refuse to accept patients on Medicare/Medicaid since this is the focus of this incentive. However, reimbursement issues are forcing the adoption of EHRs in most sectors of the healthcare delivery systems. Financial incentives provided through ARRA are expected to decrease resistance to EHR adoption.

Data Integrity

Data integrity can be compromised in three ways: incorrect entry, data tampering, and system failure. In general, data integrity can be improved by implementing security measures, including the use of audit trails, as well as the development of detailed procedures and policies.

Incorrect Data Entry The client data found in the EHR are only as accurate as the person who enters them and the systems that transfer them. Therefore, critical information, such as allergies and code status, should be verified for accuracy at each encounter. This will allow the correction of data entry errors and screen for changes that have occurred in client status. This is especially crucial because data may be entered or modified from many different encounters in the healthcare arena, such as hospitals, clinics, and home care visits. Data integrity is also compromised if an interface is not receiving or sending data correctly. When corrections to the data in the electronic record must be made, data must be corrected in multiple areas. The data in the initial system must be corrected, as well as any receiving systems. For example, if information is incorrect in the hospital information system, it must be corrected there. Any other systems that derive information from this, such as physician office systems and ancillary systems, must also be updated. This may involve correction using interface transactions or manual intervention. Some systems may not allow automated correction, which means that a person must make changes.

Data Correction An effective audit trail procedure permits the tracking of who entered or modified each data element, allowing appropriate follow-up measures. Policies need to be in place for the correction and updating of data, particularly when erroneous data is discovered.

Master File Maintenance

The development and maintenance of master files and data dictionaries is critical to preserving data integrity. Careful attention to initial development of the files, including documentation, will ensure that data are accurate and communicate valid information. Periodic review and validation of master files, at least annually, is necessary to maintain current and accurate data.

System Updates and Maintenance The robust nature of today's technology requires frequent system updates and maintenance in order to comply with new regulations and/or organizational needs. In the clinical setting this can be disruptive and lead to issues with data integrity. Scheduled system maintenance is a common occurrence with most EHRs and may require the clinician to revert to paper forms and alternate communication methods if the downtime is lengthy. Major system updates can change the database structure and cause loss of important information unless version control is carefully monitored. Downtime policies and procedures need to be developed and communicated to ensure appropriate steps are taken to enter lost data due to system updates or maintenance.

System Failure Hardware and software malfunctions, such as a system crash, may result in incomplete or lost data. Once the problem has been resolved, it may be necessary to verify the client data that could have been affected. It may then be necessary to append paper records or manually enter data once the system is restored. Downtime procedures and disaster recovery plans should be developed during the initial EHR implementation process and updated on an ongoing basis in preparation for potential system failure. These documents should outline the roles, responsibilities, policies, and procedures necessary to continue business as usual while recovering a failed system.

Ownership of the Patient Record

Currently, paper medical records are the property of the institution at which they are created. This institution is responsible for ensuring the accuracy and completeness of the record. With the development of the EHR, however, ownership issues become more complex. Because many providers use the same data, it is unclear who actually owns them and is responsible for maintaining their accuracy. Because the data are shared and updated from many sites, decisions must be made regarding who can access the data and how the data will be used. In addition, it must be determined where the data will actually be stored. With Meaningful Use requirements mechanisms must be in place to allow patients timely access to their data as well as provide electronic copies of their records, which helps to ensure that patients "own" information and can take steps to correct errors or omissions.

Privacy and Confidentiality

Preservation of the client's privacy is one of the most basic and important duties of the healthcare provider. Because one of the key attributes of the EHR is the ease of data sharing, the client's privacy rights may not be guarded by all who have access to the record. Legislation such as HIPAA has been initiated that addresses electronic access to client records. In addition, healthcare providers must address client privacy rights when developing the electronic record. In a recent survey consumers indicated that they were ready to accept electronic records if they could be assured that their health information would be kept private and secure (Chhanabhai & Holt 2007).

Electronic Signature

The healthcare provider has always been required to authenticate entries into the paper medical record with a handwritten signature. This cannot be done with the EHR because all entries are electronic. An electronic signature must be used to authenticate electronic data entries. A user's computer access code and/or password recognizes that individual by name and credentials and allows access to the system. The user should be required to sign a confidentiality statement before obtaining an access code, stating that no other person will be permitted to use the code. Other technologies, such as private encryption keys and biometric authentication, should also be used when developing an electronic signature mechanism to guarantee the source of the document.

Systems typically affix a date and time log to each entry, as well as the identity of the user in the form of an audit trail. The electronic signature is automatically and permanently attached to the document when it is created. This electronic signature cannot be forged or transferred to any other transaction and provides authentication of the healthcare provider. In the United States the Food and Drug Administration and the e-sign bill address the importance of digital signatures. The European Union has its own set of guidelines (Aharoni & Schlerf 2007).

Legal Aspects Related to Online Documentation

The move toward the EHR brings forth new legal issues and highlights old ones. Maynard (2010) noted that the rules of discovery for lawsuits are rapidly changing as healthcare moves to the EHR. Federal law has been amended to address the discovery of electronically stored information. Many states have also updated their laws in this area. In a study conducted by Saleem et al. (2009) in a Veterans Affairs Medical Center with a fully implemented EHR, persistent use of paper work-arounds was found which were categorized into 11 different types. Saleem et al. concluded that that there were occasions when paper was an important tool that assisted healthcare personnel to perform their work but in other cases paper work-arounds circumvented the intended use of the EHR resulting in potential gaps in documentation as well as possible errors. Another documentation issue with the EHR comes into play when there are multiple data entry sites—such as hospitals, clinics, physician offices—and who is ultimately responsible for updating key information as it becomes known. For example, if a patient exhibits or reports an allergic reaction when visiting a physician, who should enter that change into the EHR? Also, how will the mix of unstructured data from physician offices that do not have EHRs be integrated into the EHR? And what might the implications of important unstructured data present in an era of increased automation? Many of the issues related to discoverable information have not been fully addressed as yet and will require new areas of expertise.

Smart Cards

One of the technologies associated with the EHR is the smart card. The smart card is used to store client information such as demographics, allergies, blood type, current medications, current health problems, payer or insurance provider, and possibly a photograph. The smart card resembles a plastic credit card. It contains a microprocessor chip, which can store thousand more bits than a magnetic strip card. Smart cards permit quick access to client information through an electronic card reader, which may be important during an emergency. In nonemergency situations, the smart card allows the client to provide his or her history easily and accurately. The Smart Card Alliance, a consortium of companies and government entities, provides extensive information on all issues related to smart card use. The mission for the Alliance is to promote widespread adoption and use throughout North America (Smart Card Alliance 2011).

FUTURE DIRECTIONS

There are many questions as to whether or not a fully operational EHR for every American is attainable by 2014 despite presidential goals and financial incentives tied to compliance with Meaningful Use requirements. At the time of this writing approximately one-half of U.S. hospitals have attained stage 3 of 7 for EMR adoption, which is a building block for the EHR. Another

13% of participating hospitals reported reaching stage 4 of 7, 7% reported reaching stage 5 of 7, and just over 4% reported that they had attained stage 6 of 7 (HIMSS Analytics 2011). This *HIMSS Analytics* report indicated that more than one-half of U.S. hospitals are well positioned to meet Meaningful Use requirements (HIMSS 2011a, 2011b). Davis (2009) indicated that that hospitals that survive the transformation in healthcare delivery will be the organizations that understand how to leverage technology to collect data and manage information in a manner that will continually improve care delivery processes using evidence-based practice. Additional guidance may be needed to help hospitals plan their EHR strategies. A government survey conducted between 2009 and 2010 showed that the number of physicians using electronic health or medical records has passed the 50% mark although another survey report published by the President's Council of Advisors on Science and Technology (PCAST) found that nearly 80% of physicians, primarily those in small, independent practices, did not have digital records (Lewis 2010). This latter report was corroborated by Rao et al. (2011) in a national survey that found an alarmingly low rate of adoption in solo and two-physician practices. According to Hogan and Kissam (2010) the majority of physicians who have EHRs already use functions that meet some of the proposed Meaningful Use criteria although gaps remain that must be addressed by researchers and policy makers. Collins and Wise (2010) caution that physicians and ambulatory settings about to embark on the Meaningful Use journey lack the knowledge and skills required to successfully implement EHRs and should actively learn more about EHRs, proceed with caution, and take full advantage of potential EHR benefits.

Obviously much work lies ahead before the benefits associated with the EHR can be realized. The U.S. DHHS Agency for Healthcare Research and Quality (AHRQ) announced its intention to seek approval for a two-year project to look at barriers to achieving Meaningful Use for providers so that AHRQ can develop appropriate support services (McKinney 2011). However, not all changes will occur quickly or easily. Rowe (2011) expressed concerns by the College of Healthcare Information Management Executives (CHIME) that ONC should consider slowing down the Meaningful Use implementation schedule to allow greater success in attaining each stage. Meaningful Use will provide invaluable information that will improve patient outcomes and population health, changing many current practices as the United States transforms its healthcare delivery system. The increased emphasis upon patient engagement and empowerment will change the way healthcare consumers and practitioners interact. This transformation may not occur as quickly as desired; it will take longer for some consumers and practitioners to make the transition since changes must also be seen in attitudes. Individual consumers will have greater responsibility for managing their own health with tracking and benchmarking information at their fingertips.

In conclusion, the EHR has tremendous potential to support nurses and advance nursing knowledge in the following ways (Watkins et al. 2009; Westra et al. 2010):

- Elimination of redundant efforts
- Redesigning the workflow
- Demonstrating the contributions that nurses make to patient care and outcomes
- Contributing to the body of nursing knowledge through the incorporation of standardized nursing languages

Visit nursing.pearsonhighered.com for additional cases, information, and weblinks.

CASE STUDY EXERCISE

As a new student gathering information about your assigned patients via an EHR, what advantages can this approach provide you over traditional paper records?

SUMMARY

- The electronic medical record (EMR) is the legal record created in hospitals and ambulatory environments and often is restricted to a single episode of care.
- The electronic health record (EHR) is a longitudinal record that includes client data, demographics, clinician notes, medications, diagnostic findings, and other essential healthcare information.
- The EMR serves as a building block for the electronic health record EHR.
- Few hospitals or physician practices have attained the advanced stages of the EMR.
- The Institute of Medicine identified 12 major components or characteristics of the CPR, which continue to provide the standard for current EHR systems with only slight refinement.
- A major driver for U.S. adoption of the EHR at this time are the "Meaningful Use" financial incentives legislated by the Health Information Technology for Economic and Clinical Health Act (HITECH) of the 2009 American Recovery and Reinvestment Act.
- The EHR offers benefits to nurses, physicians, and other healthcare providers, the healthcare enterprise, and, most importantly, the consumer.
- The HITECH has sparked new interest in EHRs and brings focus and consistency to U.S. EHR adoption efforts.
- One of the major considerations in the implementation of an EHR system at this time is the selection of a system certified as capable of supporting Meaningful Use requirements to enable eligible providers to receive financial incentives.
- Other considerations in the adoption of EHR systems include creating the perquisite infrastructure, costs associated with system purchase and support, and the integration of standardized nomenclatures to support interoperability and research. Despite its many benefits, setting realistic expectations, planning for culture change, instituting safeguards to protect patient information, and caregiver resistance are the major impediments to the development of an EHR.
- Issues that must be considered when developing the EHR include data integrity, ownership of the patient record, privacy, and electronic signature.

REFERENCES

Aharoni, G., & Schlerf, R. (2007, June). The value of digital signatures in e-clinical applications. *Applied Clinical Trials*. Retrieved from http://www.actmagazine.com/appliedclinicaltrials/article/articleDetail.jsp?id=43192

Ames, E., Ciotti, V., & Mathis, B. (2011). Meaningful abuse: The rush toward EHR implementation. *Healthcare Financial Management, 65*(2), 70–73.

Anderson, H. J. (2007). EHR pioneers try to stay out front. *Health Data Management, 15*(5), 26–34.

Andrew, W., & Bruegel, R. (2003). 2003 CPR systems. *ADVANCE for Health Information Executives, 7*(9), 59–64.

Andrew, W. F., Bruegel, R. B., & Gasch, A. E. (2007). 2K6 EHR systems market summary. *ADVANCE for Health Information Executives, 11*(1), 41–44, 46, 56.

Bell, B., & Thornton, K. (2011). From promise to reality achieving the value of an EHR (cover story). *Healthcare Financial Management, 65*(2), 50–56.

Bigalke, J. T., & Morris, M. (2010). Meaningful use update. *Healthcare Financial Management, 64*(11), 114–188.

Centers for Medicare & Medicaid Services (CMS). (2011a, April 12). *Eligibility: Participating in the EHR incentive program and other current CMS incentive programs*. Retrieved from https://www.cms.gov/EHRIncentivePrograms/15_Eligibility.asp#TopOfPage

Centers for Medicare & Medicaid Services (CMS). (2011b, January 11). *Electronic health record (EHR) or electronic medical record (EMR)*. Retrieved from http://www.cms.gov/EHRIncentivePrograms/

Chhanabhai, P., & Holt, A. (2007). Consumers are ready to accept the transition to online and electronic records if they can be assured of the security measures. *Medscape General Medicine, 9*(1), 8. Retrieved from http://www.pubmedcentral.nih.gov/articlerender.fcgi?ool=pubmed&pubmedid=17435617

Classen, D., Newcomb, P., & Drazen, E. (2009). *Update on meaningful use.* Retrieved from http://www.federalnewsradio.com/pdfs/CSC_Update_on_Meaningful_Use.pdf

Collins, D. A., & Wise, P. B. (2010). Meaningful use: Lessons learned on the path to excellence in ambulatory care. Prepared for California HealthCare Foundation. Retrieved from http://www.himss.org/davies/docs/MeaningfulUseLessonsLearnedPathEHRExcellenceAmbCare.pdf

Conn, J. (2007). Agreement could put EHRs on fast track. *Modern Healthcare, 37*(9), 22.

Davis, M. W. (2009). *The state of U.S. hospitals relative to achieving meaningful use requirements.* HIMSS Analytics. Retrieved from http://www.himssanalytics.org/docs/HA_ARRA_100509.pdf

Electronic health records: DOD and VA should remove barriers and improve efforts to meet their common system needs. (2011, February 2). *GAO Reports,* 1–74.

Ford, E. W., Menachemi, N., Peterson, L. T., & Huerta, T. R. (2009). Resistance is futile: But it is slowing the pace of EHR adoption nonetheless. *Journal of the American Medical Informatics Association, 16*(3), 274–281. doi:10.1197/jamia.M3042

Garets, D., & Davis, M. (2006). *Electronic medical records vs. electronic health records: Yes, there is a difference.* A HIMSS AnalyticsTM White Paper. Retrieved from http://www.himssanalytics.org/docs/WP_EMR_EHR.pdf

Hagens, S., & Krose, A. (2009). Evolution of a national approach to evaluating the benefits of the electronic health record. *Studies in Health Technology and Informatics,* 143389–143394.

Harris, C. M. (2010). *An overview of the meaningful use final rule.* Retrieved from http://www.himss.org/content/files/MU_Final_Rule_Overview_PPT.pdf

Healthcare Information and Management Systems Society (HIMSS). (2003). *Electronic health record definitional model,* version 1.1. Retrieved from http://www.himss.org/content/files/ehrattributes070703.pdf

Healthcare Information and Management Systems Society (HIMSS). (2011a). *EHR: Electronic health record.* Retrieved from http://www.himss.org/ASP/topics_ehr.asp

Healthcare Information and Management Systems Society (HIMSS). (2011b). *HIMSS news: HIMSS Analytics report confirms increase in hospitals expected to achieve meaningful use.* Retrieved from http://www.himss.org/ASP/ContentRedirector.asp?type=HIMSSNewsItem&ContentId=78732

The Healthcare Information Technology Standards Panel (HITSP). (n.d.). Retrieved from http://www.hitsp.org/

Hewlett Packard Development Company, L. P. (2010). *Four EHR change management mistakes and how your medical practice can avoid them. White paper.* Available at http://www.hp.com/sbso/solutions/healthcare/expertise/whitepaper/index.html

HIMSS Analytics. (2011). *US EMR adoption model SM.* Retrieved from http://www.himssanalytics.org/stagesGraph.asp

HL7. (2010, last modified May 3). *Product CCD.* Retrieved from http://wiki.hl7.org/index.php?itle=Product_CCD

Hogan, S. O., & Kissam, S. M. (2010). Measuring meaningful use. *Health Affairs, 29*(4), 601–606. doi:10.1377/hlthaff.2009.1023

Hoyt, J. P. (n.d.). *HIMSS news: State of the industry: Informatics perspectives on the EMR adoption model.* Retrieved from http://www.himss.org/ASP/ContentRedirector.asp?ContentId=75059&type=HIMSSNewsItem&src=cii20101108

Institute of Medicine (IOM). (2003). *Key capabilities of an electronic health record system.* A letter report Committee on Data Standards for Patient Safety and Board on Health Care Services. Washington, DC: National Academies Press. Retrieved from http://books.nap.edu/catalog/10781.html

Jarousse, L. A. (2010). What you need to know about meaningful use. *Hospitals & Health Networks, 84*(10), 32.

Klepacki, S., Lamer, S., & Sattler, J. (n.d.). *What you need to know about meaningful use.* Retrieved from http://www.ihs.gov/recovery/documents/OverviewofMU020110.pdf

Lewis, N. (2010, December 13). EHR adoption crosses 50% threshold. *InformationWeek*. Retrieved from http://www.informationweek.com/news/healthcare/EMR/ showArticle.jhtml?rticleID=228800286

Manos, D. (2009, August 30). SNOMED CT will be required by 2015 for bonuses under economic recovery law. *Healthcare IT News*. Retrieved from http://www.healthcareitnews.com/news/ snomed-ct-will-be-required-2015-bonuses-under-economic-recovery-law

Markle Connecting for Health. (2009, April 30). *Achieving the health IT objectives of the American Recovery and Reinvestment Act*. Retrieved from http://www.markle.org/ publications/403-achieving-health-it-objectives-american-recovery-and-reinvestment-act

Martin, A. (2007). Payers get personal with online records. *Health Data Management, 15*(2), 88, 90, 92, 94, 96.

Maynard, K. G. (2010, Jan–Feb). Trends and issues with electronic discovery of medical information. *Physician Executive*. Retrieved from http://findarticles.com/p/articles/mi_m0843/is_1_36/ ai_n48840395/

Meaningful Use Workgroup. (2009, June 16). *Meaningful use: A definition. Recommendations from the meaningful use workgroup to the Health IT Policy Committee*. Retrieved from http:// healthit.hhs.gov/portal/server.pt?CommunityID=1206&spaceID=399&parentname=&control= SetCommunity&parentid=&PageID=0&space=CommunityPage&in_hi_totalgroups=1&in_hi_ req_ddfolder=6652&in_ra_topoperator=or&in_hi_depth_1=0&in_hi_req_page=20&control= advancedstart&in_hi_req_objtype=18&in_hi_req_objtype=512&in_hi_req_objtype=514&in_ hi_req_apps=1&in_hi_revealed_1=0&in_hi_userid=8969&in_hi_groupoperator_1=or&in_hi_ model_mode=browse&cached=false&in_ra_groupoperator_1=or&in_tx_fulltext=%22meaning ful+use%3A+a+definition%22%2B2009

McKinney, M. (2011, January 18). AHRQ seeks to identify EHR barriers. *Modern Healthcare*. Retrieved from http://www.modernhealthcare.com/article/20110118/NEWS/301189989

Mitchell, R. N. (2007). News monitor. *ADVANCE for Health Information Executives, 11*(4), 12.

Montandon, E. (2009). Health IT: Stimulus creates challenges. *Government Technology, 22*(5), 48.

National Alliance for Health Information Technology (Alliance). (2008, April 28). *Report to the office of the national coordinator for health information technology on defining key health information technology terms*. Retrieved from http://www.himss.org/content/files/ HITTermsFinalReport.pdf

National Priorities Partnership. (2008, November). *National priorities & goals*. Retrieved from http:// www.nationalprioritiespartnership.org/uploadedFiles/NPP/About_NPP/ExecSum_no_ticks.pdf

Nelson, R. (2007). Electronic health records: Useful tools or high-tech headache? *American Journal of Nursing, 107*(3), 25–26.

Novogoratz, S. (2007). Using EMRs to improve quality of care. *ADVANCE for Health Information Executives, 11*(1), 51–55.

Office of the National Coordinator for Health Information Technology (ONC). (2010, December 28). *ONC-authorized testing and certification bodies*. Retrieved from http://healthit.hhs.gov/ portal/server.pt?pen=512&mode=2&objID=3120

Office of the National Coordinator for Health Information Technology (ONC). (2011a). *Certification programs*. Retrieved from http://healthit.hhs.gov/portal/server.pt/community/ healthit_hhs_gov__certification_program/2884

Office of the National Coordinator for Health Information Technology (ONC). (2011b). *Standards & certification criteria final rule*. Retrieved from http://healthit.hhs.gov/portal/server.pt/ community/healthit_hhs_gov__standards_ifr/1195

Persell, S., & Bufalino, V. (2008). So, how are electronic health records working out for office practices? *Journal of Family Practice, 57,* S14–S16.

Puffer, M. J., Ferguson, J. A., Wright, B. C., Osborn, J., Anshus, A. L., Cahill, P., . . . Ryan, M. J. (2007). Partnering with clinical providers to enhance the efficiency of an EMR. *Journal of Healthcare Information Management, 21*(1), 24–32.

Rao, S. R., DesRoches, C. M., Donelan, K., Campbell, E. G., Miralles, P. D., & Jha, A. K. (2011). Electronic health records in small physician practices: Availability, use, and perceived benefits. *Journal of the American Medical Informatics Association, 18*(3), 271–275. doi:10.1136/amiajnl-2010-000010

Raths, D. (2009). A healthy dose of content management. *KM World, 18*(9), 14–15.

Rizk, E. (2007). Data hub. *ADVANCE for Health Information Executives, 11*(5), 43.

Romano, M. (2006). Moving IT forward. Government advances plans for electronic records. *Modern Healthcare, 36*(6), 7.

Rowe, J. (2011, April 21). *CHIME pitches balance and caution to ONC. HITECHWatch.* Retrieved from http://hitechwatch.com/blog/chime-pitches-balance-and-caution-onc

Rowland, C. (2007, May 14). Hospitals' move to e-files spurs a labor shortage. *The Boston Globe.* Retrieved from http://www.boston.com/business/technology/articles/2007/05/14/hospitals_move_to_e_files_spurs_a_labor_shortage/

Saleem, J. J., Russ, A. L., Justice, C. F., Hagg, H., Ebright, P. R., Woodbridge, P. A., & Doebbeling, B. N. (2009). Exploring the persistence of paper with the electronic health record. *International Journal of Medical Informatics, 78*(9), 618–628. doi:10.1016/j.ijmedinf.2009.04001

Simon, S. R., Soran, C. S., Kaushal, R., Jenter, C. A., Volk, L. A., Burdick, E., . . . Bates, D. W. (2009). Physicians' use of key functions in electronic health records from 2005 to 2007: A statewide survey. *Journal of the American Medical Informatics Association, 16*(4), 465–470.

Simpson, R. (2007). Easing the way for the electronic health record. *American Nurse Today, 2*(2), 48–50.

Smart Card Alliance. (2011). Homepage. Retrieved from http://www.smartcardalliance.org/

Standards for Health IT: Meaningful Use and Beyond. Testimony before the Subcommittee on Technology and Innovation Committee on Science and Technology, U.S. House of Representatives [Testimony of Richard Gibson]. (2010, September 30).

Sullivan, M. (2010). Playing catch-up in health care technology. *Journal of Health Care Compliance, 12*(3), 25–30.

Thompson, D., Velasco, F., Classen, D., & Raddemann, R. J. (2010). Reducing clinical costs with an EHR. *Healthcare Financial Management, 64*(10), 106–114.

Thompson, D. I., Osheroff, J., Classen, D., & Sittig, D. F. (2007). A review of methods to estimate the benefits of electronic medical records in hospitals and the need for a national benefits database. *Journal of Healthcare Information Management, 21*(1), 62–68.

U.S. Department of Health and Human Services (DHHS). (2005, June 6). *HHS news release "Secretary Leavitt takes new steps to advance health IT national collaboration and RFPs will pave the way for interoperability."* Retrieved from http://www.hhs.gov/news/press/2005pres/20050606.html

U.S. Department of Health and Human Services (DHHS). (2006, October 8). *Office of the national coordinator for health information technology (ONC) executive summary.* Retrieved from http://www.himss.org/handouts/executiveSummary.pdf

U.S. Department of Health and Human Services (DHHS). (2007, April 26). *HHS news release "HHS joins international partners to promote electronic health records standards."* Retrieved from http://www.hhs.gov/news/press/2007pres/04/pr20070426a.html

U.S. Department of Health and Human Services (DHHS). (2009, October 30). *American health information community (AHIC).* Retrieved from http://healthit.hhs.gov/portal/server.pt/community/american_health_information_community_(ahic)/1199/home/15512

U.S. Department of Health and Human Services (DHHS). (2010, August 30). *Initial EHR certification bodies named.* Retrieved from http://www.hhs.gov/news/press/2010pres/08/20100830d.html

Walton, G. (2007). The status of acute care EMRs. *ADVANCE for Health Information Executives, 11*(5), 59.

Watkins, T. J., Haskell, R. E., Lundberg, C. B., Brokel, J. M., Wilson, M. L., & Hardiker, N. (2009). Terminology use in electronic health records: Basic principles. *Urologic Nursing, 29*(5), 321–326. Retrieved from http://www.suna.org/cgi-bin/WebObjects/SUNAMain.woa/1/wa/viewSection?_id=1073743840&ss_id=536872962&wosid=KEgD1YLkWvyW2qGLud6kd6K74ko

Westra, B. L., Subramanian, A., Hart, C., Matney, S., Wilson, P., Huff, S., . . . & Delaney, C. (2010). Achieving "meaningful use" of electronic health records through the integration of the nursing management minimum data set. *Journal of Nursing Administration, 40*(7/8), 336–343. doi: 10.1097/NNA.0b013e3181e93994

CHAPTER 15

The Role of Standardized Terminology and Language in Informatics

After completing this chapter, you should be able to:

1. Understand what standardized healthcare terminology is and why it is important to nursing.

2. Describe the American Nurses Association (ANA) recognition criteria established for recognizing standardized terminologies.

3. Describe each of the ANA-recognized terminologies and the benefits of use when implemented within an electronic healthcare record.

4. Discuss standardized terminologies used for the different parts of the nursing process and their similarities and differences.

5. Define the different types of terminology structures, such as a classification system (e.g., NANDA, NIC, NOC) versus a reference terminology (ICNP, SNOMED-CT).

6. Demonstrate how standard terminologies facilitate the use of evidence-based practice and decision-support rules.

7. Illustrate how using standardized healthcare terminologies correlates to the U.S. Meaningful Use criteria.

8. Identify the benefits of using structured terminologies within electronic healthcare records.

INTRODUCTION TO TERMINOLOGY

Treating patients in a variety of settings across the entire healthcare continuum requires the ability to share the most accurate and up-to-date information among a multitude of providers and care settings (C. B. Lundberg 2009). The current state of information use in the healthcare community is evolving from paper-based to computerized records. The introduction of computerized information systems and their increasing use has amplified the need for structured and controlled vocabularies that can be used to represent patient care.

Standardized Terminology

Standardized terminologies have been developed for use within the electronic health record (EHR). **Standardized terminologies** are structured and controlled languages that have been developed according to terminology development guidelines and have been approved by an authoritative body (HIMSS 2006). These terminologies are often referred to as *controlled terminologies.*

Healthcare terminology standards are designed to enable and support widespread interoperability among healthcare software applications for the purpose of sharing information. The use of standardized terminology is a means of ensuring that the data collection is accurate and valid (The Joint Commission 2010; Westra, Delaney, Konicek, & Keenan 2008). The requirement for standardized terminology development has increased tremendously to support the use of national and international health information standards.

Standardized terminology is essential for successful development and implementation of an EHR. Terminology is required to represent, communicate, exchange, manage, and report data, information, and knowledge. It enables safe, patient-centric, high-quality healthcare that optimizes data collection for the measurement of patient outcomes. EHRs can no longer be developed or implemented without standardized terminologies. Data exchange between EHR application systems must take place without loss of meaning. "The adoption of EHRs implemented with standardized terminology is proving to be a positive effect on the improvement of healthcare quality, efficiency, and patient safety" (U.S. Department of Health and Human Services [HHS] 2009).

The implementation of standardized terminology within the EHR is essential for healthcare organizations to meet the criteria of Meaningful Use. The American Recovery and Reinvestment Act of 2009 defines **Meaningful Use** as a certified EHR technology used in a meaningful way. Meaningful Use is one piece of a broader health information technology (HIT) infrastructure needed to reform the healthcare system and improve healthcare quality and efficiency and patient safety (HHS, 2009). One of the primary criteria identified for Meaningful Use is the use of standardized terminologies. The goal of Meaningful Use is to exchange clinical structured data in a manner that it is accurate and complete to improve patient care in a cost-efficient way.

Terminology Definitions Before we discuss the specific terminologies, some basic elements need to be explained: concepts, codes, and the different types of terminologies. A **concept** is defined as an expression with a single unambiguous meaning (ISO/IEC 17115 2007). A concept can have one or more representations called *synonyms* or *terms.* Clinical concepts are used to document ideas or express orders, assessment, and outcomes within an EHR. Concepts have unique identifiers known as codes. **Codes** are made up of letters, numbers, or a combination of both, used to designate concepts in a computer system (de Keizer, Abu-Hanna, & Zwetslook-Schonk 2000). A concept with an assigned code is considered **codified.** Concept codes facilitate the development of evidence-based practice and decision-support rules, reporting of administrative and financial healthcare standards for diagnoses, procedures, and drugs, and the core quality measures. Codified data is used to track key clinical data such as disorders, nursing problems, allergies, procedures, and signs and symptoms. Providers use the data collected for care coordination purposes, data retrieval, initiating the reporting of clinical quality measures, and public health information. Although many individuals working within the healthcare industry recognize coded data only as the source for determining reimbursement, Health Information Management professionals have always understood the immeasurable uses of coded data.

Clinical terminology enables the capture of data at the level of detail necessary for patient care documentation and is used to describe health conditions and healthcare activities (ISO/IEC 17115 2007). Clinical terminologies consist of concepts that support diagnostic studies, history and physical examinations, visit notes, ancillary department information, nursing notes, assessments, flow sheets, vital signs, and outcome measures. A clinical terminology can be mapped to a broader classification system for administrative, regulatory, and fiscal reporting requirements (Giannangelo 2010, p. 3).

Types of Terminologies   Different types of clinical terminological systems are used in healthcare (de Keizer et al. 2000). Table 15–1 outlines the terminology types.

A **classification system** is used to categorize the details of the clinical encounter. It does not capture the level of detail necessary to document specific items at the point of care. Classifications consist of mutually exclusive categories that can be used for specific purposes. An example would be to group data to determine costs and outcomes of treatment. A classification system provides data to consumers on costs and outcomes of treatment options. It is used in the collection and reporting of health statistics. The International Classification of Diseases (ICD), which is a classification system, does not consist of definitions or definitional relationships between terms.

The term **ontology** is frequently used within the healthcare information technology world. Ontologies help to facilitate interoperability in that concepts are organized by their concept meaning that describes the definitional structure-relationship, for example, concept of *finger* is a part of the concept of *hand*. Ontologies also organize concepts for storage and retrieval of semantically accurate data. The concepts in the ontologies have unique codes.

Reference Versus Point-of-Care Terminology

Terminologies are used two different ways within EHR systems: first, as a reference terminology and second, as a point-of-care terminology. A **reference terminology** consists of a set of concepts with definitional relationships. A reference terminology is frequently an ontology and can therefore be used to support data aggregation, disaggregation, and retrieval. A reference terminology is necessary to analyze data, develop evidence-based practice, and improve the quality of care. A reference terminology is used to retrieve data across healthcare settings, domains, and specialties, in a standardized manner. A **point-of-care terminology,** frequently referred to as an *interface terminology,* is what the clinicians see on the screen and consists of terms of which clinicians are familiar with (Rosenbloom, Miller, Johnson, Elkin, & Brown 2006). It is usually made

TABLE 15–1 Types of Healthcare Terminologies		
Types of Terminology	**Description**	**Example**
Nomenclature	A set of terms composed according to pre-established rules	LOINC, NANDA-I
Terminology	A set of terms representing concepts in a particular field or domain, for example, problems, observations	
Vocabulary	A terminology accompanied by definitions or descriptions	
Classification	An arrangement of concepts based on essential characteristics. Arranged in a single hierarchy	ICD, CPT, NIC, NOC
Ontology	A set of concepts formally organized by meaning	SNOMED-CT, ICNP

up of synonyms from the reference terminology and supports entry of patient-related information into computer programs.

Terminology Development Guidelines Standard terminologies are developed according to terminology development guidelines. These guidelines, or rules, were clearly articulated by Cimino (1998) and have been adopted as a gold standard in the healthcare industry by which terminologies are evaluated. Table 15–2 depicts these guidelines.

Terminology and Nursing For years, nurses have expressed nursing care using different terms to say the same thing. A straightforward definition of standardized nursing language is a "common language, readily understood by all nurses, to describe care" (Keenan 1999, p. 12). A uniform representation of nursing care supports a complete and unambiguous description of how nursing problems, interventions, and outcomes are documented. The use of coded standardized terminology for nurses is vital to bedside nursing and to the nursing profession. It is essential because it enables consistent use of terminologies across clinical settings and specialists. The use of standardized nursing terminology will result in better communication to the interdisciplinary team, increase the visibility of nursing interventions, enhance data collection used to evaluate and analyze patient care outcomes, and support greater adherence to standards of care. Further, the use of standardized nursing terminology can be used to assess nursing competency. Healthcare facilities are required to demonstrate the competency of staff for the Joint Commission. The nursing interventions delineated in standardized terminologies can be used as a means to assess nurse competency in the performance of these interventions (Rutherford 2008).

TABLE 15–2   Cimino's 12 Terminology Development Guidelines

Guideline	Explanation
1. Content	Medical terminologies should be rich in content.
2. Concept orientation	Medical terminologies should be based on concepts, rather than on terms. Terms must correspond to at least one meaning (nonvagueness) with no more than one meaning (nonambiguity). The meanings correspond to no more than one term (nonredundancy).
3. Concept permanence	Once a concept enters a terminology, it should not be deleted or reused.
4. Nonsemantic concept identifier	Concept identifiers are the codes that identify concepts in a terminology. The code must have no meaning, and each concept must have a unique identifier.
5. Polyhierarchy	A strict hierarchy consists of a root concept used for traversing the hierarchies.
6. Formal definition	Formal definitions add semantic exactness to a terminology by making the relationship between concepts explicit.
7. Reject "not elsewhere classified"	The problem with such terms is that they can never have formal definition other than one of exclusion.
8. Multiple granularities	Terminologies should not restrict users or applications to terms at some particular level of granularity.
9. Multiple consistent views	It should be possible to view the concept hierarchies in multiple consistent ways.
10. Beyond medical concepts representing context	Terminologies should not specify how different pieces on clinical information are related.
11. Evolve gracefully	The terminology should allow for long-term growth.
12. Recognize redundancy	Redundancy is the condition in which the same information can be stated in two different ways.

The need for standardization in nursing documentation is critical to support interoperability, the ability to share comparable data with other healthcare organizations. The collection of standardized nursing care documentation can enable a comparison of different terminologies that can be used to research patient care outcomes nationally and worldwide. Given that the healthcare requirements involve the implementation of EHRs, there is a need to establish standards for the implementation within the EHR. Healthcare terminology needs to be universally understood across all healthcare providers and organizations in order for healthcare systems to be interoperable and to uniformly exchange data. To accomplish interoperability, standardized clinical terminologies must be implemented within the EHR (Foley & Garrett 2006).

LANGUAGES AND CLASSIFICATION

Billing Codes

Healthcare encounters are coded for billing by code sets mandated by the **Health Insurance Portability and Accountability Act (HIPAA)**. HIPAA mandates that all electronic transactions include only HIPAA-compliant codes (Giannangelo 2010). The code sets described here are the International Classification of Disease (ICD), Common Procedural Terminology codes, and the Alternative Billing Codes (ABC). These codes are used to classify and catalog diseases and procedures. These code sets are reviewed and subject to modification annually. Use of billing codes at the point of care is discouraged, but some systems use them to build problem and procedure lists. This chapter will give only a brief overview of the code sets and is not intended for training of Health Information Management professionals.

International Classification of Disease The **International Classification of Disease (ICD-9/ICD-10),** developed by the World Health Organization (WHO), is the international standard diagnostic classification for all general epidemiological, many health management purposes, and clinical use. The ICD diagnoses are used to classify mortality and morbidity data from inpatient and outpatient records. They are used to classify diseases and other health problems recorded on many types of health and vital records, including death certificates and health records. In addition to enabling the storage and retrieval of diagnostic information for clinical, epidemiological, and quality purposes, these records also provide the basis for the compilation of national mortality and morbidity statistics used throughout the world.

The original intent of ICD was diagnostic and procedural coding for statistics and research. Since 1983, ICD has also been used for reimbursement. ICD-9-CM is currently used in the United States for diagnosis reimbursement. Two departments within the Department of Health and Human Services (HHS), the Centers for Medicare & Medicaid Services (CMS) and the National Center for Health Statistics (NCHS), develop and maintain the ICD-9-CM official Guidelines for Coding and Reporting. The guidelines should be used as a companion document to the official version of ICD-9-CM. ICD-10 is used by the rest of the world, and ICD-10-CM and ICD-10-PCS will be used for billing in the United States in October 2013. WHO requires that mortality data be submitted as ICD-10. Some facilities have mapped their problem list to ICD-9-CM to support their diagnosis reimbursement, but diagnosis may also be mapped to SNOMED-CT so that the problem list data collected can be used for Meaningful Use. ICD has many uses that include morbidity and mortality classification, indexing hospital records by disease, analyzing payments, monitoring resource utilization, and tracking public health risks.

The official ICD-9-CM is currently comprised of the following three volumes:

Volume 1, Diseases: Tabular List

Volume 2, Diseases: Alphabetical Index

Volume 3, Procedures: Tabular List and Alphabetical Index

TABLE 15–3	Examples of ICD-9-CM Codes
ICD-9-CM	**Diagnosis**
760–763.99	Maternal causes of perinatal morbidity and mortality
762	Fetus or newborn affected by complications of placenta, cord, and membranes
762.7	Chorioamnionitis affecting fetus or newborn
240–279.99	Endocrine, nutritional and metabolic diseases, and immunity disorders
249–259.99	Diseases of other endocrine glands
250	Diabetes mellitus
250.2	Diabetes mellitus with hyperosmolarity
250.21	Diabetes mellitus, type I [insulin dependent type] [IDDM] [juvenile type] with hyperosmolarity, not stated as uncontrolled
ICD-9-CM	**Procedure**
42–54.99	Operations on the digestive system
43	Incision and excision of stomach
43.1	Gastrostomy
43.11	Percutaneous [endoscopic] gastrostomy [PEG]

The ICD classification system consists of a monohierarchy, which means that the concepts are classified by a disease header with the disease variations underneath. The monohierarchy provides a means of data collection against one point of view. The collection of the ICD data does not support the specificity necessary for clinical description of patients, research quality analysis, and health policy development. The ICD-9-CM codes are from three to five characters. Table 15–3 provides some examples of ICD-9-CM codes.

Common Procedural Terminology Codes The American Medical Association (AMA) **Current Procedural Terminology (CPT)** is a classification system used for billing and reimbursement of outpatient procedures and interventions. CPT is the most widely accepted medical nomenclature used to report medical procedures and services under public and private health insurance programs. CPT codes are used to code all medical procedures performed in healthcare except for alternative medicine. CPT code sets are copyrighted by the AMA and are released once each year.

The CPT listings have divisions including: Evaluation and Management, Anesthesia, Surgery, Radiology, Pathology, and Laboratory and Medicine. Within these divisions are subsections that include Section Headings, Subsections, Categories, and Subcategories; Guidelines, Symbols, Colons, and Semicolons; Modifiers, Appendices, Indices, and Examples. For example, CPT codes that fall under Pathology and Laboratory range from 80048 to 89356. If a urinalysis was done under this category, the code would range from 81000 to 81099 and is classified according to its specific type of urinalysis performed, for example, urinalysis microscopic. The range's specific details or procedures would dictate the precise number. When trying to locate a surgery code (10000 to 69999), locate that section's heading and then find the corresponding subheading to classify what type of procedure was conducted and where on the body it was performed. For example, if it took place within the patient's intergumentary system (10040 to 19499) and an excision was done on a benign lesion (11400 to 11471), detail should be coded regarding where the incision was made and how big it was. Table 15–4 displays some examples of CPT codes.

Clinical Terminologies

Clinical terminologies are those used for documenting patient care within the EHR. This section will give a brief overview of two categories of clinical terminologies, multidisciplinary and nursing specific.

TABLE 15–4 Examples of CPT Codes	
CPT Code	**Description**
Level 1: 80000–89398	Pathology and laboratory tests
Level 2: 81000–81099	Urinalysis procedures
81015	Urinalysis; microscopic only
81005	Urinalysis; qualitative or semiquantitative, except immunoassays
Level 2: 80100–80103	Drug testing
80100	Drug screen, qualitative; multiple drug classes chromatographic method, each procedure

Most of the terminologies discussed here are listed as source vocabularies within the **Unified Medical Language System (UMLS)** developed by the National Library of Medicine (NLM). The UMLS is a large metathesaurus that contains more than a hundred source vocabularies (NLM 2009). The NLM provides a Web-based application to the UMLS in which users can do multiple types of searches such as finding synonymous terms from two or more sources and the association between concepts (Humphreys, McCray, & Cheh 1997; NLM 2010b).

The American Nurses Association (ANA), through the Committee for Nursing Practice Information Infrastructure (CNPII), recognizes terminologies appropriate for use by nursing (Warren & Bakken 2002). Terminologies must meet defined criteria for approval. The criteria specify that terminologies must be used to support nursing practice reflecting the nursing process. The nursing process data elements include assessment, diagnosis, outcome identification (goal), planning, implementation (interventions), and evaluation. The terminologies have to contain concepts that are clear and unambiguous with a unique identifier. The terminology developer should have an outlined maintenance and submission process. The Nursing Management Minimum Data Set, Nursing Minimum Data Set, and ABC are data sets approved by the ANA but will not be discussed in this chapter. All of the approved terminologies are outlined in Table 15–5.

Multidisciplinary Terminologies

Systematized Nomenclature of Human and Veterinary Medicine Clinical Terms

Systematized Nomenclature of Human and Veterinary Medicine Clinical Terms (SNOMED-CT) is a globally recognized controlled healthcare vocabulary that provides a common language for electronic health applications. SNOMED-CT enables a consistent way of capturing, sharing, and aggregating health data across specialties and sites of care. The use of SNOMED-CT within EHRs provides interoperable data collection that can be analyzed and used in the implementation of evidence-based practice, decision-support rules, reporting of quality measures, and administrative billing.

SNOMED-CT is in conformance with national industry regulatory standards and the Consolidated Health Initiative (NLM 2010b). The National Committee on Vital and Health Statistics in 2003 rated SNOMED-CT highest among all terminologies evaluated for EHR as it met the essential criteria defined according to sound medical informatics practices (DHHS 2003).

In 2007, the College of American Pathologists transferred the SNOMED-CT intellectual property to the International Health Terminology Standards Development Organization (IHTSDO) to support the development of an international effort to produce and enhance a global clinical terminology standard (IHTSDO 2010). The IHTSDO has developed a set of principles that guide decision making of SNOMED-CT. The IHTSDO consisted of

TABLE 15–5   ANA-Recognized Nursing Languages

Terminology	Web site	Diagnosis/ Problem	Intervention	Outcome	Other
Alternative Billing Concepts (ABC Codes)	http://www.abccodes.com				Billing Codes
Clinical Care Classification (CCC)	http://www.sabacare.com	X	X	X	
International Classification of Nursing Practice (ICNP)	http://www.icn.ch/icnp.htm	X	X	X	Assessment
Logical Identifiers Names and Codes (LOINC)	http://loinc.org/			X	Assessment
North American Nursing Diagnosis International (NANDA-I)	http://www.nanda.org	X			
Nursing Intervention Classification (NIC)	http://www.nursing.uiowa.edu/cnc/		X		
Nursing Outcomes Classification (NOC)	http://www.nursing.uiowa.edu/cnc/			X	
Nursing Management Minimum Data Set	http://www.nursing.umn.edu/ICNP/ USANMMDS/home.html				Nursing Management Codes
Nursing Minimum Data Set	http://www.nursing.umn.edu/ICNP/				
Omaha System	http://www.con.ufl.edu/omaha	X	X	X	
Perioperative Nursing Data Set (PNDS)	http://www.aorn.org	X	X	X	
SNOMED-CT	http://www.ihtsdo.org/snomed-ct	X	X	X	

9 founding country members, which recently increased to 15 member countries. Each member country has a SNOMED-CT release center responsible for managing concept requests and distributing SNOMED-CT. SNOMED-CT is continually updated to meet the needs of users around the world. Revisions to the international version of SNOMED-CT are released twice a year, once at the end of January and again at the end of July. Each release includes the core of the terminology (concepts, descriptions, and relationships), together with works to support the implementation of SNOMED-CT.

SNOMED-CT updates are driven by users of the terminology, who can request new concepts and submit them through the IHTSDO. Examples include refinements to descriptions, remodeling of new concepts to place them into the correct hierarchy, or the addition of new concepts. Prior to the release, SNOMED-CT undergoes a clinical quality review process to ensure that concepts have been defined accurately.

SNOMED-CT is recognized by the ANA as one of the standardized terminologies for nursing. The College of American Pathologists and SNOMED Editorial Board collaborated with the ANA-recognized nursing developers listed in Table 15–6 to integrate the content of their terminologies within SNOMED Reference Terminology (SNOMED RT). The relationship began in 1998 by collaborating with each of the nursing terminology developers to discuss the need of integrating the nursing classifications within SNOMED RT. Once the ANA-recognized terminologies were integrated within SNOMED RT, and before they were released within SNOMED core, the terminology developers validated the mappings to ensure accurate representation of the nursing concepts and that the concepts were defined equivalently as represented within the classification system. In March 2010, a collaboration agreement was signed between the International Council of Nurses (ICN) and IHTSDO (eHealthNews 2010) to establish a Harmonization Board with the objective of future integration between ICNP and SNOMED-CT. Table 15–6 displays ANA-recognized terminologies integrated within SNOMED-CT.

TABLE 15–6	ANA-Recognized Terminologies Integrated within SNOMED-CT	
ANA-Recognized Terminology	**Data Elements in SNOMED-CT**	**Domain in SNOMED-CT**
Clinical Care Classification (CCC)	Diagnoses and Intervention	Diagnoses—Clinical findings
		Interventions—Procedures
NANDA International (NANDA-I)	Nursing diagnoses	Diagnoses—Clinical findings
Nursing Intervention Classification (NIC)	Intervention Labels	Interventions—Procedures
Nursing Outcomes Classification (NOC)	Outcome labels	Outcome labels—Observable entity
Omaha System	Problem Classification Scheme	Problem classification scheme
		Signs and symptoms—Clinical findings
		Intervention scheme interventions—Procedures
Perioperative Nursing Data Set (PNDS)	Diagnoses, Intervention, and Outcome	Diagnoses—Clinical findings
		Interventions—Procedures
		Outcomes—Clinical findings

Source: Lundberg, C., Warren, J., Brokel, J. M., Bulechek, G., Butcher, H., McCloskey Dochterman, J., et al. (2008). Selecting a Standardized Terminology for the Electronic Health Record that Reveals the Impact of Nursing on Patient Care. *Online Journal of Nursing Informatics, 12*(2). Retrieved from http:ojni.org/12_2/lundberg.pdf.

SNOMED-CT is a clinical terminology comprised of codes, concepts, and relationships used in recording and representing clinical information across the scope of healthcare. SNOMED-CT is concept-based, meaning that each concept has a distinct definition with a unique code identifier. SNOMED-CT consists of 19 top-level hierarchies: procedures (medical and surgical procedures, laboratory and radiology procedures, interventions, education, and management procedures), clinical findings (nursing diagnoses, disorders, diseases that are necessarily abnormal, and signs and symptoms [also known as assessments]), body structures, observable entity (questions being asked during an assessment), devices, substances, and medications.

SNOMED-CT hierarchies are created through defining relationships linking one concept to another concept for the purpose of defining each concept down to its specific meaning. Defining concepts by using parent-child relationship begins to build vertical hierarchies within SNOMED-CT. Concepts lower in the hierarchy are more specific in meaning than those higher up in the hierarchy, creating multiple levels of granularity. Defining relationship attributes further defines the concept's meaning by relating all necessary and sufficient to fully represent the concept's definition. An example of how the NANDA-I concept of *ineffective breathing* is mapped within SNOMED-CT is illustrated in Table 15–7.

SNOMED-CT is used to document care by clinicians, specialists, and domains using an interdisciplinary approach. It is used to document patient care across all sites of care and healthcare facilities (acute care, home care, hospice care, spiritual health, long-term care, and healthcare clinic visits, as well as community and public health). The documentation of assessments, flow sheets, care plans, task lists, order sets, education plans, problem lists, allergies and allergic reactions, task lists, and medication administration records can be encoded to SNOMED-CT.

Logical Observation Identifiers Names and Codes

The Logical Observation Identifiers, Names, and Codes (LOINC) is a terminology that includes laboratory and clinical observations. The laboratory portion of the LOINC database contains the usual laboratory categories such as chemistry, hematology, and microbiology. The domain and scope of clinical LOINC is extremely broad. Some of the sections of terms include vital signs, obstetric measurements, clinical assessment scales, outcomes from standardized

---

TABLE 15–7 SNOMED-CT Example: Ineffective Breathing

SNOMED CT: Ineffective breathing pattern (finding)

SNOMED Concept ID: 20573003

Is_A Clinical finding

Is_A Finding related to ability to perform breathing functions (finding)

IsA Respiration alteration (finding)

Finding Site: Structure of respiratory system (body structure)

Interprets: Ability to perform breathing functions (observable entity)

---

nursing terminologies, and research instruments (Scichilone 2008). LOINC is also used for document and section names (Hyun 2006).

Nursing content is one of the domains with a special focus on clinical LOINC (Matney 2003). In 2002, LOINC was recognized by the ANA. The ANA determined that both laboratory and clinical LOINC are appropriate for use by nursing. Because of their breadth and the early focus on laboratory testing, nursing assessment observations are not yet well represented.

LOINC provides identifiers and names for observations, not values. Each LOINC record corresponds to a single observation, measurement, or test result. The record includes the axis fields specified in Table 15–8.

Nursing Terminologies

Clinical Care Classification The **Clinical Care Classification (CCC) System** is a nursing classification designed to document the six steps of the nursing process across the care continuum (Saba 2007). It facilitates patient care documentation at the point of care. CCC was developed in 1991 and revised in 2005. The CCC consists of two interconnected terminologies, the CCC of nursing diagnosis and outcomes and the CCC of nursing interventions. The two taxonomies are tools that support the documentation of nursing care. Both terminologies are classified by 21 care components that represent the functional, health, behavioral, physiological, and psychological patterns of a patient.

TABLE 15–8 LOINC Axes With Examples

Axis	Description of the Axis	Sample Values
Component (analyte)	The substance or entity measured, evaluated, or observed	Systolic blood pressure, pain onset, and sodium
Kind of property	The characteristic or attribute of the component measured, evaluated, or observed	Length, volume, time stamp, mass, ratio, number, and temperature
Time aspect	The interval of time over which the observation or measurement was made	"Point in time" and "over an 8-hour period"
System	The system (context) or specimen type with which the observation was made	Urine, serum, fetus, patient (person), and family
Type of scale	The scale of measure	Quantitative (a true measurement), ordinal (a ranked set of options), nominal, or narrative
Type of method	The procedure used to make the measurement or observation. Method is the only axis that is optional and is only included when different methodologies would significantly change the interpretation of the result	Patient reported, measured

CCC nursing diagnosis consists of 182 diagnostic concepts classified into 59 major categories and 123 subcategories. Outcomes are assigned by expanding the nursing diagnosis concepts with one of three qualifiers: "improved," "stabilized," or "deteriorated."

CCC uses a five-character code to codify the terminology. Each code can be decomposed to determine the meaning. The syntax of the code categorization is as follows:

Code 1 = care component

Codes 2 and 3 = major category (followed by a decimal point)

Code 4 = one digit code for a subcategory (followed by a decimal point)

Code 5 = one of three expected outcomes *or* one of four nursing intervention types

CCC nursing interventions consist of 198 categories classified into 72 major categories and 126 subcategories that represent interventions, procedures, treatments, and activities. The interventions can be modified by one of four intervention types: (1) assess or monitor, (2) care or direct or perform, (3) teach or instruct, or (4) manage or refer.

CCC is an open source terminology with no license fees. The terminology tables can be freely downloaded from http://www.sabacare.com. CCC is copyrighted and, its use within an EHR requires written permission.

CCC is integrated within SNOMED-CT. CCC codes are stored in cross map tables that can be obtained from the College of American Pathologists—SNOMED Terminology Solutions or the UMLS. CCC outcomes are also mapped to LOINC.

International Classification of Nursing Practice The **International Classification of Nursing Practice (ICNP)** is a unified nursing language system developed by the ICN) in Geneva, Switzerland (J. Warren & Coenen 1998). ICN is responsible for ensuring that the content reflects the domain of nursing. ICNP Version 2.0 was released in 2009. ICNP is a compositional terminology for nursing practice that facilitates the development of and the cross-mapping among local terms and existing terminologies. ICNP has been implemented as both a point-of-care (ICNP Catalogues) and reference terminology.

ICNP contains nursing phenomena (diagnoses), nursing actions, and nursing outcomes (ICN 2010). ICNP is represented using a seven-axis model. The seven axes are defined in Table 15–9 (ICN 2005):

The ICNP has developed specific guidelines for using the seven-axis model to develop nursing diagnosis, outcome, and intervention statements.

TABLE 15–9 ICNP Axes With Examples

Axis	Description of the Axis	Sample Values
Focus	The area of attention	Mobility, pain, parenting, knowledge
Judgment	Critical opinion or determination related to the focus of nursing practice	Actual, risk, high
Means	A manner or method of accomplishing an intervention	Bandage, walker, video
Action	An intentional process applied to or performed by a client	Educate, assess, monitor
Time	The point, period, instance, interval, or duration of an occurrence	Admission, child birth, chronic
Location	Anatomical and spatial orientation of a diagnosis or intervention	Abdomen, head, healthcare department
Client	Subject to which a diagnosis refers and who is the recipient of an intervention	Newborn, caregiver, family, community

ICNP diagnosis:

A term from the focus axis is required.

A term from the judgment axis is required.

Additional terms from the focus, judgment, and other axes are included as needed.

ICNP intervention:

A term from the action axis is required.

At least one target term is required. Target terms come from all of the other seven axes except for judgment.

ICN recognized early that the terminology would need to be organized so it could be used at the point of care (Coenen & Bartz 2010). The ICNP Catalogues are being developed to fulfill this need. ICNP catalogues are designed to support clinical documentation in an EHR. The first two catalogues published by ICN are "Partnering with Individuals and Families to Promote Adherence to Treatment" and "Palliative Care for Dignified Dying." More catalogues are in development and testing. This will generate more content that nurses can use to document care.

North American Nursing Diagnosis International North American Nursing Diagnosis International (**NANDA-I**) dates back to 1970 and was the first terminology to be recognized by the ANA (Gordon 1994). A nursing diagnosis is a clinical judgment about individual, family, or community experiences and responses to actual or potential health problems and life processes.

NANDA-I diagnoses are used to identify human responses to health promotion, risk, and disease (C. Lundberg et al. 2008). Each nursing diagnosis has a description, a definition, and defining characteristics. The defining characteristics are manifestations, signs, and symptoms that assist the nurse in determining the correct diagnosis to assign (Scroggins 2008).

NANDA-I is classified into 13 domains. Within each domain are two or more classes. The domains and classes have formal definitions. Below is a list of the domains with examples of the classes below them:

Domain 1: Health Promotion—Classes Health Awareness and Health Management

Domain 2: Nutrition

Domain 3: Elimination/Exchange

Domain 4: Activity/Rest

Domain 5: Perception/Cognition

Domain 6: Self-Perception

Domain 7: Role Relationship

Domain 8: Sexuality

Domain 9: Coping/Stress Tolerance

Domain 10: Life Principles

Domain 11: Safety/Protection

Domain 12: Comfort

Domain 13: Growth/Development

The first NANDA-I taxonomy was an alphabetical listing of the nursing diagnosis. In 2001 NANDA-I released NANDA-I Taxonomy II in which the nursing diagnoses are formatted using a multiaxial structure. The seven axes of the taxonomy are dimensions of the human response (Scroggins 2008). Table 15–10 depicts the NANDA-I axes with examples.

NANDA-I is used to document nursing diagnoses within all settings and across the care continuum. The coding system can be used within the EHR. NANDA-I has been linked to the

TABLE 15–10 NANDA-I Axes With Examples

Axis	Description of the Axis	Sample Values
Axis 1: The diagnostic concept	The principle element or root of the diagnostic statement. May consist of one or more nouns.	Activity intolerance Fatigue Fear Pain Sorrow
Axis 2: Time	Duration of a period or interval.	Acute, chronic, short-term, long-term
Axis 3: Unit of care	Person or population for which the nursing diagnosis is determined.	Individual, family, community
Axis 4: Age	Physical development stage.	Fetus, adolescent, young adult, old, old adult
Axis 5: Health status		Wellness, actual, risk for
Axis 6: Descriptor	A modifier that limits or defines the nursing diagnosis meaning.	Ability, decrease, delayed, excessive, impaired
Axis 7: Topology	Parts or regions of the body.	Auditory, bowel, urinary, skin

NIC interventions and NOC outcomes. The NANDA-I coding system can be used within the EHR either by mapping the nursing problems that nurses document directly or by mapping to the NANDA-I, NIC, and NOC linkages. The linkages can be loaded into an EHR and can be used together to document the elements of the nursing process within the care plan.

Nursing Interventions Classification The **Nursing Interventions Classification (NIC)** is a standardized classification of interventions that describes the activities that nurses perform. NIC is used in all care settings. An intervention is described as "any treatment, based upon clinical judgment and knowledge, that a nurse performs to enhance patient/client outcomes" (The University of Iowa 2010a). The current NIC edition (2008) has 542 interventions (Bulechek, Butcher, & Dochterman 2008). The interventions are grouped together by 30 classes and 7 domains. Each intervention includes a label name, a definition, a unique code, and associated nursing activities. There are more than 1,200 activities. Below is a list of the NIC domains:

Domain 1: Physiological: Basic

Domain 2: Physiological: Complex

Domain 3: Behavioral

Domain 4: Safety

Domain 5: Family

Domain 6: Health System

Domain 7: Community

The NIC coding system can be used within the EHR either by mapping the nursing interventions and activities that nurses perform directly or by mapping to the NANDA-I, NIC, and NOC linkages. The linkages can be loaded into an EHR. They were developed to be used together to document the elements of the nursing process within the care plan.

Nursing Outcomes Classification The **Nursing Outcomes Classification (NOC)** is a classification system that describes patient outcomes sensitive to nursing interventions. The NOC is a system to evaluate the effects of nursing care as a part of healthcare. NOC consists of outcomes for individual patients, families, and communities. An outcome is "a measurable individual, family, or community state, behavior, or perception that is measured along a continuum and is responsive to nursing interventions" (The University of Iowa 2010b). NOC can be used across all clinical settings and specialties. The NOC classification is structured using three levels: domains, classes, and outcomes. The outcomes are organized into 31 classes and 7 domains (Moorhead, Johnson, Maas, & Swanson 2008). Each outcome concept consists of a definition, a measurement scale, a list of associated indicators, and supporting references. Below is a list of the NOC domains:

Domain 1: Functional Health

Domain 2: Physiological Health

Domain 3: Psychosocial Health

Domain 4: Health Knowledge and Behavior

Domain 5: Perceived Health

Domain 6: Family Health

Domain 7: Community Health

Each outcome, associated indicators, and measurement scale(s) are coded for use in EHRs.

The NOC coding system can be used within the EHR either by mapping the nursing outcomes directly or by mapping to the NANDA-I, NIC, and NOC linkages. The linkages can be loaded into an EHR. They were developed to be used together to document the elements of the nursing process within the care plan.

The Omaha System The **Omaha System** is a research-based taxonomy that provides a framework for integrating and sharing clinical data. It is widely used in settings such as home care, hospice, public health, school health, and prisons (Martin 2005). ANA initially recognized the Omaha System in 1992 as a standardized terminology to support nursing practice.

The Omaha System consists of three relational components: an assessment component (Problem Classification Scheme), an intervention component (Intervention Scheme), and an outcomes component (Problem Rating Scale for Outcomes) ("The Omaha System: Solving the Clinical Data-Information Puzzle" 2009). The three components are designed to be used together and create a comprehensive problem-solving model for practice, education, and research. Concepts from the components can be assigned to an individual, family or group, or community (Correll & Martin 2009). Table 15–11 provides an overview of the Omaha System.

Perioperative Nursing Data Set The **Perioperative Nursing Data Set (PNDS),** developed by the Association of periOperative Registered Nurses (AORN), is a standardized perioperative nursing vocabulary that provides nurses a clear, precise, and universal language for clinical problems and surgical treatments. The AORN's initial goal was to develop a unified language for nursing care that could be systematically quantified, coded, and easily captured in a computerized format in the perioperative setting (AORN Inc. 2002, p. 13). It provides a clinical approach to describe patient care outcomes. The PNDS provides a systematic approach to define and recognize the contributions of the perioperative nurse in healthcare.

PNDS provides wording and definitions for nursing diagnoses, interventions, and outcomes, thus furnishing clinicians with the same terms to describe patient care for the perioperative settings. This consistency of terms supports documentation using the same terms across clinical situations and settings. This allows data to be collected in a uniform way and subsequently be analyzed. For example, nurses within an institution consistently document "skin remains smooth, intact, non-reddened, non-irritated, and free from bruising other than surgical incision" after surgery. If this statement is recorded in a consistent manner, characteristics can be collected

TABLE 15–11 Omaha System Overview		
Component	**Terms**	**Purpose**
Problem Classification Scheme	• Four domains • Forty-two problems • Two sets of modifiers • Clusters of problem-specific signs or symptoms	Organize assessment (needs and strengths) for individuals, families, and communities
Intervention Scheme	• Four categories • Seventy-five targets and one "other" • Client-specific information	Organize multidisciplinary practitioners' care plans and the services they deliver
Problem Rating Scale for Outcomes	• Three concepts • Five-point Likert-type scale	Individual, family, community

A full description of the components is available online at http://www.omahasystem.org.

Source: Garvin, J. H., Martin, K. S., Stassen, D. L., & Bowles, K. H. (2008). Omaha System: Coded data that describe patient care. *Journal of the American Health Information Management Association, 79*(3), 44–49.

about the patients who acquire a skin injury as well as the percentage of cases and the staff mix for those cases. In addition, if nursing interventions are recorded in a consistent manner, the most effective interventions can be determined. If other institutions document outcomes using the same vocabulary, benchmarking on an outcome can be meaningful.

In addition to the development of the PNDS, AORN has created a theoretical model and framework for perioperative nursing practice. The Perioperative Patient-Focused Model in combination with the PNDS was the beginning point to help registered nurses document and describe perioperative patient care. The patient and their family are at the core of the model that provides the focus of perioperative nursing care. Within the model, circles expand beyond the patient and family representing the perioperative nursing domains and elements. The model illustrates the relationship between the patient, family, and care provided by the perioperative nurse. The model is divided into four quadrants, three representing patient-centric domains: safety of the patient, patient physiological responses to surgery, and patient and family behavioral responses to surgery. The fourth quadrant represents the health system in which the perioperative care is delivered. The health system domain designates administrative concerns and structural elements, for example, staff, equipment, environmental factors, and supplies that are essential to successful surgical intervention (AORN Inc. 2002).

The PNDS consists of four components: patient problems that nurses identify, interventions that nurses perform, the intensity of care, and the outcomes that are achieved. The second version of the PNDS consists of 75 nursing diagnoses, 135 nursing interventions, and 27 nurse-sensitive patient care outcomes. The PNDS also includes activities that are related to the 135 interventions that are not coded. Table 15–12 provides an example of the PNDS.

The PNDS supports the nursing process by providing the foundation for determining the patient's needs and establishing the plan of care for the perioperative clinical setting. Subjective and objective assessment data support the identification of potential nursing diagnoses. Assessment data is used in the identification of signs and symptoms of a nursing diagnosis. The etiology of a clinical problem and the desired outcome determine the appropriate nursing interventions. Assessment data collected regarding the patient's health status and response to the interventions performed in the intraoperative setting contribute to the evaluation process (AORN Inc. 2002).

The PNDS provides the framework and terminology for identifying clinical problems, nursing interventions, and clinical outcomes that are used in standards of care, standard care plans or clinical pathways, generic documentation forms, and individualized care plans. For example, a

TABLE 15-12	Perioperative Nursing Data Set Example
Outcome	Patient is free from signs and symptoms of infection.
Outcome definition	The patient is free from signs and symptoms of nosocomial surgical site infection such as pain, induration, foul odor, purulent drainage, and/or fever through 30 days following the perioperative procedure.
Outcome indicators	Immune status Skin condition (surgical wound) Medication regimen Clinical documentation
Nursing diagnoses	Risk for infection Risk for impaired skin integrity Impaired skin integrity Delayed surgical recovery
Nursing interventions	Implements aseptic technique Assesses susceptibility for infection Classifies surgical wound Performs skin preparations Monitors for signs and symptoms of infection Protects from cross contamination Minimizes the length of invasive procedure by planning care

Source: AORN Inc. (2002). *Perioperative nursing data set: The perioperative nursing vocabulary.* Denver, CO: AORN Inc.

perioperative clinical pathway can begin in the physician's office and continue to the preoperative department for presurgical testing, then onto ambulatory care, holding, the operating room, and through the PACU if interoperable standardized terminology is implemented. The development of perioperative clinical pathways assist in the identification of specific patient problems that name specific outcomes defined in the PNDS for the patient population addressed in the pathway. The identified outcomes delineate the specific interventions that need to be performed. When all data fields that are linked to the interventions are completely filled in, the outcome is flagged as achieved.

In summary, this section has described the terminologies used within an EHR. The ANA-recognized nursing classifications codify data used during the nursing process such as assessments, nurse-sensitive problems, interventions, and outcomes. One or more terminologies can be used for nursing documentation. The next section will illustrate a use case showing how the nursing terminologies can be used for documenting nursing care.

Storyboard Illustrating Terminology Use

The following storyboard is an example that illustrates the use of SNOMED-CT, LOINC, CCC, ICNP, NANDA, NIC, and NOC. Examples show encoding concepts used in the nursing process and not for everything that can be encoded within the storyboard (e.g., gender = male):

> Joe is a 24-year-old male paraplegic admitted to an inpatient unit from his home with right lower lobe pneumonia. During his admission assessment, the nurse notes that he has no sensation from the shoulders down. He is confined to a wheelchair and requires two-person assistance with movement. He could move himself with his upper body before this illness. His oxygen saturation is 85% on room air by pulse oxymetry. Evaluation of his vitals shows a temperature of 101°F. His skin is moist and clammy.

Assessment The process of nursing assessment includes items such as vital signs, physiological signs, and patient symptoms within the realm of the nursing practice (Matney,

Bakken, & Huff 2003). Assessments are observations documented as a name-value, or question-and-answer, pair. Assessment name-value pairs depicted in the storyboard are oxygen saturation = 85%, temperature = 101°F, skin type = moist and clammy, and skin temperature = cold. SNOMED-CT and LOINC both include content that supports the encoding of point-of-care assessments. Table 15–13 illustrates how the assessments can be encoded.

Nursing Diagnosis/Problem and ICD-9 Coding After the patient has been assessed, a nursing diagnosis or problem is determined. Even though Joe is a paraplegic, he has impaired mobility because he could move himself with his upper body before his pneumonia. Other nursing diagnoses for Joe include impaired gas exchange and hypothermia. Table 15–14 illustrates NANDA, ICNP, and CCC coding examples. It should also be noted that Omaha System, PNDS, and SNOMED-CT contain nursing diagnoses.

Joe will be assigned an ICD-9-CM billing code for his pneumonia by the medical coders of the hospital after discharge. The ICD-9-CM code for "Pneumonia, organism unspecified" is "486."

TABLE 15–13 Nursing Assessment Coding Examples

Assessment Measure	SNOMED-CT	LOINC	Assessment Value
Oxygen saturation	**Fully Specified Name:** Hemoglobin saturation with oxygen (observable entity) **Concept Code:** 103228002 **Defined as:** Is A: hematologic function	**Name:** Oxygen saturation in capillary blood **Code:** 2709-4 **Fully Specified Name:** Oxygen saturation:MFr:PT:BldC:QN:: Component = Oxygen Property = Mass fraction Time = Point in time System = Blood mixed venous Scale = Quantitative	**Numeric value = 85** **Units of measure = Percent**
Temperature	**Fully Specified Name:** Body temperature (observable entity) **Concept Code:** 386725007 **Defined as:** Is A: body temperature measure Is A: vital signs	**Name:** Body temperature **Code:** 8310-5 **Fully Specified Name:** Body Temperature:Temp:PT: ^Patient:QN:: Component = Body temperature Property = Temperature Time = Point in time System = Patient Scale = Quantitative	**Numeric value = 85** **Units of measure = Degrees Fahrenheit**
Skin moisture	**Fully Specified Name:** Moistness of skin (observable entity) **Concept Code:** 364532007 **Defined as:** Is A: skin observable	**Name:** Moisture of Skin **Code:** 39129-2 **Fully Specified Name:** Moisture:Type:PT:Skin:Nom:: Component = Moisture Property = Type Time = Point in time System = Skin Scale = Nominal	**Coded Value** **SNOMED-CT Code = Fully Specified Name:** Clammy skin (finding) **Concept Code:** 102598000 **Defined as:** Is A: Finding of moistness of skin

TABLE 15–14	Nursing Diagnosis/Problem Coding Examples		
Diagnosis/Problem	**NANDA-I**	**ICNP**	**CCC**
Impaired mobility	Impaired physical mobility **Axes:** **The diagnostic concept =** Physical mobility **Descriptor =** Impaired	Impaired mobility **Concept Code:** 10001219 **Axes:** **Focus** = Ability to mobilize **Judgment** = Impaired	Physical mobility impairment **Concept Code:** A01.5 **Concept Categorization:** Component 'A' = Activity Major category '01' = Alteration
Impaired gas exchange	Impaired gas exchange **Axes:** **The diagnostic concept =** Gas exchange **Descriptor** = Impaired **Defining Characteristic:** Hypoxia	Impaired gas exchange **Concept Code:** 10001177 **Axes:** **Focus** = Gaseous exchange **Judgment** = Impaired	Gas exchange Impairment **Concept Code:** L26.3 **Concept Categorization:** **Component 'L' =** Respiratory **Major Category '26'=** Alteration
Hyperthermia	Hyperthermia **Axes:** **The diagnostic concept =** **Descriptor =** **Defining Characteristic:** Body temp above normal range	Hyperthermia **Concept Code:** 10000757 **Axes:** **Focus** = Hyperthermia **Judgment** = Negative	Hyperthermia **Concept Code:** K25.2 **Concept Categorization:** Component 'K' = Physical regulation Major category '25' = Alteration

Nursing Interventions Nursing interventions are acts performed by or with the client. Nursing interventions include acts such as assess, evaluate, educate, and monitor. Using Joe's example, the interventions on his care plan include assist with transfer, oxygen therapy, and monitor temperature. Table 15–15 shows NIC, ICNP, and CCC examples. It should also be noted that the Omaha System, PNDS, and SNOMED-CT contain nursing interventions.

Goals and Potential Nursing Outcomes A goal is the desired outcome for the future. It is a scheduled observation in the future. Based on Joe's diagnoses, the nurse sets measurable goals that include improved mobility, improved gas exchange, and normothermia. The assessment data, diagnoses, and goals are written in the care plan for other care providers to access. When the goal is evaluated and given an outcome measurement value, such as improved, it is then considered an outcome. Table 15–16 shows NOC, ICNP, and CCC examples. It should also be noted that the Omaha System, PNDS, and SNOMED-CT contain nursing outcomes.

BENEFITS OF IMPLEMENTING STANDARDIZED TERMINOLOGIES

Implementing standardized terminology has many benefits to multiple beneficiaries. Beneficiaries include the patient, the provider, the organization, and the healthcare industry in general. Using standardized terminologies ensures compliance with standards coming forth for Meaningful Use, quality measures, and interoperability. Terminology facilitates the monitoring of trends and problems of the health of populations, developing clinical decision support, and expanding our knowledge of diseases and treatments and outcomes through research and clinical data mining.

TABLE 15–15	Nursing Intervention Coding Examples		
Nursing Intervention	**NIC**	**ICNP**	**CCC**
Assist with transfers	Transfer **Domain:** Physiological domain: Basic **Class:** Immobility management **Definition:** Moving a patient from one location to another	Transferring act **Concept Code:** 10020030 **Axes:** **Action:** Transferring **Description:** Positioning: Moving somebody or something from one place to another	Transfer care **Concept Code:** A03.3 **Categorization:** **Component:** 'A' = Activity **Concept:** '03.3' = Transfer care **Definition:** Actions performed to assist in moving from one place to another
Oxygen therapy	Oxygen therapy **Domain:** Physiological domain: Complex **Class:** Respiratory management **Definition:** Administration of oxygen and monitoring of its effectiveness	Oxygen therapy **Concept Code:** 10013921 **Axes:** **Action:** Therapy **Description:** Therapy	Oxygen therapy care **Concept Code:** L.35 **Categorization:** **Component:** 'L' = Respiratory **Concept:** 35 Oxygen therapy care **Definition:** Actions performed to support the administration of oxygen treatment
Monitor temperature	Temperature Regulation: Fever treatment **Domain:** Physiological domain: Complex **Class:** Thermoregulation **Definition:** Attaining and/ or maintaining body temperature within normal range	Monitoring body temperature **Concept Code:** 10012165 **Axes:** **Focus:** Body temperature **Action** = Monitoring **Description:** Monitoring	Temperature **Concept Code:** K33.2 **Categorization:** **Component:** 'K' = Physical regulation **Concept:** '33.2' = Temperature **Definition:** Actions performed to measure body temperature

Patient-Specific Benefits

Patient care benefits include decreased costs, increased quality across the continuum of care, improved outcomes, and improved safety. Standard terminologies provide a means of sharing chart data electronically between other departments, facilities, and settings. The use of collected interoperable data can be analyzed to identify ways to reduce errors of omission via reminders and alerts (clinical decision support) that are developed within an EHR. Costs can be reduced by eliminating redundant testing and diagnostic investigation. Value is derived by maintaining continuity of care. With standardized clinical terminology, patient data will be available across the full spectrum of healthcare settings: Family history, medications, allergies, diseases, treatments, and interventions can be coded and shared among clinicians, sites of care, and even across national and international geographic boundaries that improves communication, resulting in improved patient safety and outcomes. The ability to track a patient's health maintenance, follow-up activity, compliance, and progress will provide important information regarding quality-of-care outcomes.

TABLE 15–16 Nursing Goal/Potential Outcome Coding Examples

Nursing Goal/Outcome	NOC	ICNP	CCC
Improved mobility	Immobility consequences: Physiological **Domain:** Functional health **Class:** Mobility **Definition:** Severity of compromise in physiological functioning due to impaired physical mobility	Effective mobility **Concept Code:** 10028461 **Axes:** **Focus** = Ability to mobilize **Judgment** = Positive	Physical mobility impairment improved **Concept Code:** A01.5.1 **Concept Categorization:** Improved = Fifth digit. '1' added to the diagnosis
Improved gas exchange	Respiratory status: Gas exchange **Domain:** Physiologic health **Class:** Cardiopulmonary **Definition:** Alveolar exchange of carbon dioxide and oxygen to maintain arterial blood gas exchange	Effective gas exchange **Concept Code:** 10027993 **Axes:** **Focus** = Gaseous exchange **Judgment** = Positive	Gas exchange impairment improved **Concept Code:** L26.3.1 **Concept Categorization:** Improved = Fifth digit. '1' added to the diagnosis
Normothermia	Thermoregulation: Vital sign status **Domain:** Physiologic health **Class:** Metabolic regulation **Definition:** Balance among heat production, heat gain, and heat loss	Thermoregulation **Concept Code:** 10014973 **Axes:** **Focus** = Thermoregulation **Judgment** = Positive	Hyperthermia improved **Concept Code:** K25.2.1 **Concept Categorization:** Improved = Fifth digit. "1" added to the diagnosis

Provider and Nursing Benefits

Providers and nurses will benefit by having access to complete data along the continuum of care. Healthcare organizations around the world are working to integrate EHRs. Using structured vocabularies within and between systems will provide access to complete and accurate healthcare data. Lack of complete and accurate data is currently a frustration to providers who want to give the best patient care. This frustration occurs when important clinical information for the patient is unavailable at the point of care. These systems will provide access to medical records that will gain better control over healthcare information quickly and when the information is needed most, at the point of care.

Nurses will benefit from using a standardized nursing language by enhanced efficiency, accuracy, and effectiveness, resulting in a significant improvement in patient care. Recently, Smith and Smith (2007) described several examples in which the implementation of a standardized nursing terminology made a significant impact on patient outcomes. The study reported using standardized nursing terminology incorporated into the electronic nursing care plan supplies the necessary tools to effectively disseminate evidence-based protocols, to list pertinent nursing interventions, and to provide consistent methods to track patient outcomes. The study demonstrated that nurse-driven care supported by a standardized nursing terminology decreased the number of average ventilation days for all ventilator-associated pneumonia patients from 14 to 10 days. Furthermore, the study demonstrated a decrease in the number of ventilator-associated pneumonia from orally colonized types of pathogens (*Pseudomonas, Acinetobacter,* or *Klebsiella*) from 55 to 0.

Organizational Benefits

The organization can benefit by cost savings, decision-support rules, outcomes measurement, and the ability to use the data for data mining. Using standardized clinical terminology allows sharing of accurate health information across departments and facilities. The necessity of streamlining care processes to capture efficient gains that require fewer physician and staff hours devoted to administrative care will result in reduced hospital costs. Organizations that implement EHRs using standard terminologies will observe benefits such as the ability to measure an improvement in patient care outcomes and cost efficiency. For example, healthcare organizations will experience a reduction in transcription errors and reduce coding and billing errors, resulting in reduced healthcare claim denials. The ability to track a patient's health maintenance, follow-up activity, compliance, and a patient's progress will provide important information regarding the quality of patient care outcomes.

Standardized terminologies support the development of **decision-support software (DSS)**. Decision support is the alerts and reminders used within an EHR. The ability to collect codified data provides vital information that can be used for decision support (Huff, Rocha, Parker, & Matney 2006). Clinical decision-support software is highly dependent on clinical information to function. To be useful, the clinical information must contain sufficient detail with respect to the right variables, the right wording and codes, and the right information modeling and must thus be structured in a way that the decision-support software understands DSS is used to prevent negative outcomes and support positive outcomes of patient care.

Documentation of healthcare using a standardized terminology is vital to support **data mining**. Data mining is the process of analyzing healthcare data from different perspectives and summarizing it into useful information that can be used to improve patient safety and quality of care and cut costs. It is becoming an important tool to transform data into information. Data mining is the key component in the analysis of workflow in complex healthcare organizations. It is also used for research (Holzemer 2009). The data mining process is carried out by the collection of standardized data with their associated codes from EHRs. Analyzed results from data mining can identify patterns or trends in patient care and outcomes. The use of data mining by organizations can provide analysis for the identification of important questions that are directly related to increased errors causing a reduction in patient safety, resulting in high healthcare costs. For example, a hospital organization may want to analyze questions like how many patients are at risk for falls and actually fall, resulting in injury, while in the hospital resulting in injury. The data collected and mined for these important questions can provide important information regarding patient falls and identify an improvement in the interventions provided for patients who are at risk for falls and education that can lead to a reduction in the occurrence of falls.

NATIONAL HEALTHCARE REPORTING REQUIREMENTS

The Health Information Technology for Economic and Clinical Health (HITECH) Act seeks to improve American healthcare delivery and patient care through the adoption of interoperable EHRs. The provisions of the HITECH Act are specifically designed to work together to provide the necessary assistance and technical support to providers, enable coordination and alignment within and among states, establish connectivity to the public health community in case of emergencies, and ensure that the workforce is properly trained and equipped to be Meaningful Users of EHRs (HHS 2009, p. 1).

Medicare has various initiatives that require standardized terminologies. CMS is collaborating with public agencies and private organizations including the National Quality Forum (NQF), the Joint Commission of the Accreditation of Health Care Organizations, the National

Committee for Quality Assurance, the Agency for Health Care Research and Quality, the AMA, and many other organizations (CMS 2005). For CMS-eligible hospitals and physicians who meet the Meaningful Use requirements, the use of standardized terminology is necessary for data collection and reporting of established quality measures. For example, smoking status and venous thrombosis prophylaxis is required to be tracked and collected to report to NQF in order to be eligible for the Meaningful Use 2011 financial incentive. Also, the HIT standards committee has defined that hospitals are required to maintain an active problem list mapped to ICD-9-CM or SNOMED-CT by 2011, and by 2015 problem lists will be mapped to SNOMED-CT (HHS 2009). HL7 is an ANSI-accredited standards development organization dedicated to providing a comprehensive framework and related standards for the exchange, integration, sharing, and retrieval of electronic health information (Health Level Seven 2010). Healthcare organizations are required to send HL7 messages containing patient demographic and clinical data. Messages sent containing laboratory test names and results are required to be sent using LOINC codes. Messages sent containing allergies should use SNOMED-CT and RxNorm, a standardized nomenclature for clinical drugs and drug delivery devices, developed by the NLM (DHHS 2009). In summary, to meet the CMS Meaningful Use criteria and financial incentives, as well as provide safer patient care with improved quality, the implementation of standardized terminology is required.

ISSUES AND CONCERNS

It is not easy to use standardized terminology within systems (Rector 1999). There are many issues related to the implementation and maintenance of standardized terminologies, and we will address three high-level issues in this chapter. First, there are numerous systems in use today with locally defined concepts, which will need to map or link their local terminology to standardized terminology. Second, determining which terminology or terminologies to use is still a challenge. Third, data entry, presentation, and retrieval for clinical tasks must be considered. The mandate for the use of standardized terminologies in EHRs for Meaningful Use has increased the need for systems to use standardized terminologies. Many systems in use today, both home grown and vended, have been created without using standard terminologies. The applications will have to be rewritten to use standardized terminologies. Methods will need to be developed to convert stored data or retrieve data from the old system so that patient's data will not be lost. Developers will need to determine how terminologies will be maintained and updated when new versions are released.

Specific terminologies have been mandated for laboratory and clinical systems, but the only nursing mandate is that SNOMED-CT be used to message nursing data between systems. This causes two challenges: First, nurses need to determine which nursing terminologies they want to use to support the nursing process. Second, the terminology they choose will have to include a mapping to SNOMED-CT to send patient data to other systems such as a nursing home.

Finally, point-of-care terms and synonyms for data entry, presentation, and retrieval for clinical tasks must be locally developed. Clinicians use different terms for the same concept across specialty and even between nursing units and settings. For example, a pediatrician or advanced nurse practitioner will want to know that the newborn experienced "transient tachypnea of the newborn." The display should be spelled out for them, but providers in the NICU would rather see "TTN." Both of these are synonyms of the concept and should be created based on context of use. Synonyms are also used differently from country to country. For example, a "diaper" in the United States is a "nappy" in the United Kingdom. Operational resources will be required for the development of the synonyms.

FUTURE DIRECTIONS

In July 2009, the NLM announced the release of the first version of the Clinical Observations Recording and Encoding (CORE) Subset of SNOMED-CT. The primary purpose of this subset was to facilitate coding of problem list data in EHRs using SNOMED-CT and to enable more Meaningful Use to improve patient safety, healthcare quality, and health information exchange (NLM 2010a). The purpose of the UMLS CORE Project was to define a subset most useful for documentation and encoding of clinical information at a summary level, such as problem list, discharge diagnosis, or reason of encounter. The key feature of the CORE problem subset is the collection and analysis of datasets collected from healthcare institutions that use controlled vocabularies for data entry. These datasets contain the list of controlled terms and their frequency of use in clinical databases. The CORE Problem list also can be used to generate ICD-9-CM codes for reimbursement and other purposes in many EHRs.

HIT allows comprehensive management of clinical information and its secure exchange between healthcare providers. Broad use of HIT has the potential to improve quality, prevent medical errors, increase administrative efficiencies, decrease paperwork, expand access to affordable care, and improve population and community health. The HITECH Act of 2009 sets forth a plan for the advancement of the Meaningful Use of HIT to improve the quality of care and to establish the foundation of the U.S. health reform. The Office of the National Coordinator (ONC) for HIT is at the forefront of the administration's HIT efforts and is a source to support the adoption of HIT and the promotion of a nationwide health information exchange to improve healthcare (Health Information Technology 2010). To meet the standards defined by HITECH Act, the EHR will need to provide complete, accurate, and searchable health information, available at the point of diagnosis and care, permitting more informed decision making to enhance the quality and reliability of the healthcare delivery. Other HITECH Act requirements needed to meet the standards include the need to develop a more efficient and convenient functionality, without waiting for the exchange of records and without requiring unnecessary or repetitive tests or procedures. EHRs are required to support the reduction in adverse events through a stronger understanding of a patient's medical history and potential for drug-drug interactions providing an improvement in patient safety. Finally, systems are required to support more efficient administrative duties, allowing for more interactions with and for the transfer of information to patients, caregivers, clinical case managers, and the monitoring of patient care.

We have illustrated in this chapter that there has been significant advances in the development and adoption of clinical terminologies and terminology standards. In the last decade, and with the requirement to build EHRs that meet the 2009 Meaningful Use criteria, the use of coded data has expanded to include pay-for-performance initiatives, care coordination, patient safety monitoring, and public health surveillance. Many benefits have yet to be realized from the point of care to research and the development of evidence-based practice. There are still hurdles that need to be jumped in order for systems to fully use terminologies. We will know we have succeeded when clinical terminologies are used and reused to capture healthcare data in a standardized format that has global meaning and can be applied at both the individual and aggregate levels.

CASE STUDY EXERCISE

As the only informatics nurse at your small community hospital your chief nursing officer heavily relies upon you to translate major developments in policy and reimbursement that have direct implications for the department and facility. How would you go about explaining the relationship between standardized terminologies and financial rewards related to Meaningful Use?

Visit nursing.pearsonhighered.com for additional cases, information, and weblinks.

SUMMARY

- Standardized terminologies have been developed for use within the electronic health record (EHR) as a means to ensure accurate, consistent meaning of data that is collected and shared across the healthcare delivery system.
- The implementation of standardized terminology within the EHR is essential for healthcare organizations to meet the criteria of Meaningful Use.
- Concept codes, used to designate concepts in a computer system, facilitate the development of evidence-based practice, decision support, and reporting.
- Clinical terminology enables the capture of data at the level of detail necessary for patient care documentation. Clinical terminologies consist of concepts that support diagnostic studies, history and physical examinations, visit notes, ancillary department information, nursing notes, assessments, flow sheets, vital signs, and outcome measures.
- Standardization in nursing documentation supports research across settings on patient outcomes and interoperability.
- Healthcare encounters are coded for billing by code sets mandated by the Health Insurance Portability and Accountability Act (HIPAA). HIPAA mandates that all electronic transactions include only HIPAA-compliant codes. These include the International Classification of Disease (ICD), Common Procedural Terminology codes, and the Alternative Billing Codes (ABC).
- Reference terminology supports data aggregation, analysis, and retrieval. Point-of-care terminology represents what clinicians see on the screen.
- The American Nurses Association (ANA) Committee for Nursing Practice Information Infrastructure (CNPII) recognizes terminologies appropriate for use by nursing.
- Nursing terminologies include:
  - Clinical Care Classification (CCC)
  - International Classification of Nursing Practice (ICNP)
  - North American Nursing Diagnosis International (NANDA-I)
  - Nursing Interventions Classification (NIC)
  - Nursing Outcomes Classification (NOC)
  - The Omaha System
  - Perioperative Nursing Data Set (PNDS)
- Standardized terminology beneficiaries include the patient, the provider, the organization, and the healthcare industry. The use of standardized terminologies provides access to complete and accurate healthcare data and ensures compliance with standards coming forth for Meaningful Use, quality measures, and interoperability.
- Documentation of healthcare using a standardized terminology supports data mining, a process of analyzing healthcare data from different perspectives, and summarizing it into useful information that can be used to improve patient safety and quality of care and cut costs.
- Issues associated with the implementation of standardized terminology within systems include mapping considerations, determination of the most suitable terminologies, and retrofitting standardized terminologies into existing systems.
- Multidisciplinary terminologies include Systematized Nomenclature of Human and Veterinary Medicine Clinical Terms (SNOMED-CT), a comprehensive clinical terminology covering nursing, medicine, and allied health, and the Logical Observation Identifiers, Names, and Codes (LOINC), a terminology that includes laboratory and clinical observations.

REFERENCES

AORN Inc. (2002). *Perioperative nursing data set: The perioperative nursing vocabulary*. Denver, CO: AORN Inc.

Bulechek, G. M., Butcher, H. K., & Dochterman, J. M. (2008). *Nursing intervention classification* (5th ed.). St. Louis, MO: Mosby/Elsevier.

Centers for Medicare & Medicaid Services (CMS). (2005). *Partners healthcare. Medicare pay for performance (P4P) initiatives*. Retrieved from http://www.connected-health.org/policy/medicare-and-medicaid/external-resources/medicare-pay-for-performance-(p4p)-initiatives.aspx

Cimino, J. J. (1998). Desiderata for controlled medical vocabularies in the twenty-first century. *Methods of Information in Medicine, 37*(4–5), 394–403.

Coenen, A., & Bartz, C. (2010). ICNP: Nursing terminology to improve healthcare worldwide. In C. A. Weaver, C. Delaney, P. Weber, & R. L. Carr (Eds.), *Nursing and informatics for the 21st century: An international look at practice, education and EHR trends* (2nd ed., pp. 207–218). Chicago, IL: Healthcare Information and Management Systems Society.

Correll, P. J., & Martin, K. S. (2009). The Omaha system helps a public health nursing organization find its voice. *Computer, Informatics, Nursing, 27*(1), 12–16.

eHealthNews. (2010). *ICN and IHTSDO team-up to ensure a common health terminology*. Retrieved from http://www.ehealthnews.eu/research/1980-icn-and-ihtsdo-team-up-to-ensure-a-common-health-terminology

Foley, M., & Garrett, G. (2006). The code ahead: Key issues shaping clinical terminology and classification. *Journal of the American Health Information Management Association, 77*(7), 24–30.

Garvin, J. H., Martin, K. S., Stassen, D. L., & Bowles, K. H. (2008). Omaha system: Coded data that describe patient care. *Journal of the American Health Information Management Association, 79*(3), 44–49.

Giannangelo, K. (2010). *Healthcare code sets, clinical terminologies, and classification systems* (2nd ed.). Chicago, IL: American Health Information Management System.

Gordon, M. (1994). *Nursing diagnosis: Process and application* (3rd ed.). St. Louis, MO: Mosby.

Health and Human Services. (2009). HIT Standards Committee Joint Working Groups on Quality and Operations Meaningful Use Measure Grid. Retrieved from healthit.hhs.gov/portal/server.pt/gateway/PTARGS_0_11113_880493_0_0_18/MU Grid Data Element Standards_08202009.pdf

Health Information Technology. (2010). *The office of the national coordinator for health information technology (ONC)*. Retrieved from http://healthit.hhs.gov/portal/server.pt?open=512&objID=1200&mode=2

Health Level Seven. (2010). *About HL7*. Retrieved from http://www.hl7.org/about/index.cfm

HIMSS. (2006). *HIMSS dictionary of healthcare information technology terms, acronyms and organizations*. Chicago, IL: Author.

Holzemer, W. L. (Ed.). (2009). *Improving health through nursing research*. West Sussex, UK: Wiley-Blackwell.

Huff, S. M., Rocha, R., Parker, C. G., & Matney, S. (2006). Ontologies, vocabularies and data models. In R. A. Greenes (Ed.), *Medical decision-making: Computer based approaches to achieving healthcare quality and safety*. Burlington, MA: Elsevier.

Humphreys, B. L., McCray, A. T., & Cheh, M. L. (1997). Evaluating the coverage of controlled health data terminologies: Report on the results of the NLM/AHCPR large scale vocabulary test. *Journal of American Medical Informatics Association, 4*(6), 484–500.

Hyun, S. (2006, June). *Toward the creation of an ontology for nursing document sections: Mapping section names to the LOINC semantic model*. Paper presented at the AMIA, Washington, DC.

ICN. (2005). *International classification for nursing practice—Version 1*. Geneva, Switzerland: Author.

ICN. (2010). *International classification for nursing practice*. Retrieved from http://www.icn.ch/icnp_def.htm

IHTSDO. (2010). *International health terminology standards development organisation*. Retrieved from http://www.ihtsdo.org/

ISO/IEC 17115. (2007). *Health informatics—Vocabulary for terminological systems*. Geneva, Switzerland: Author.

The Joint Commission. (2010). *Health care staffing services standards FAQs*. Retrieved from http://www.jointcommission.org/CertificationPrograms/HealthCareStaffingServices/Standards/09_FAQs/

Keenan, G. (1999). Use of standardized nursing language will make nursing visible. *Michigan Nurse, 72*(2), 12–13. Retrieved from http://www.minurses.org/prac/snl/snlvisible.shtml

de Keizer, N. F., Abu-Hanna, A., & Zwetslook-Schonk, J. H. M. (2000). Understanding terminological systems I: Terminology and typology. *Methods of Information in Medicine, 39,* 16–21.

Lundberg, C., Warren, J., Brokel, J. M., Bulechek, G., Butcher, H., McCloskey Dochterman, J., . . . Giarrizzo-Wilson, S. (2008). Selecting a standardized terminology for the electronic health record that reveals the impact of nursing on patient care. *Online Journal of Nursing Informatics, 12*(2). Retrieved from http:ojni.org/12_2/lundberg.pdf

Lundberg, C. B. (2009). Accurate electronic patient charts—A standardized clinical language is key to success. *For The Record, 20*(20), 6. Retrieved from http://www.fortherecordmag.com/archives/ftr_092908p6.shtml

Martin, K. S. (2005). *The Omaha system: A key to practice, documentation, and information management.* (2nd ed.). St. Louis, MO: Elsevier.

Matney, S. (2003). Logical observation identifier names and codes (LOINC) ANA recognition commentary. *Online Journal of Nursing Informatics, 7*(3).

Matney, S., Bakken, S., & Huff, S. M. (2003). Representing nursing assessments in clinical information systems using the logical observation identifiers, names, and codes database. *Journal of Biomedical Informatics, 36*(4–5), 287–293.

Moorhead, S., Johnson, M., Maas, M., & Swanson, E. (2008). *Nursing outcomes classification* (4th ed.). St. Louis, MO: Mosby.

National Library of Medicine (NLM). (2009, November 3). *Unified medical language system source vocabularies—2009AB release*. Retrieved from http://www.nlm.nih.gov/research/umls/knowledge_sources/metathesaurus/release/source_vocabularies.html

National Library of Medicine (NLM). (2010a). *UMLS knowledge source server (UMLSKS)*. Retrieved from https://login.nlm.nih.gov/cas/login?service=http://umlsks.nlm.nih.gov/uPortal/Login

National Library of Medicine (NLM). (2010b). *The CORE problem list subset of SNOMED CT*. Retrieved from http://www.nlm.nih.gov/research/umls/Snomed/core_subset.html

The Omaha system: Solving the clinical data-information puzzle. (2009). Retrieved from http://www.omahasystem.org/index.html

Rector, A. L. (1999). Clinical terminology: Why is it so hard? *Methods of Information in Medicine, 38*(4–5), 239–252.

Rosenbloom, S. T., Miller, R. A., Johnson, K. B., Elkin, P. L., & Brown, S. H. (2006). Interface terminologies: Facilitating direct entry of clinical data into electronic health record systems. *Journal of American Medical Informatics Association, 13*(3), 277–288.

Rutherford, M. (2008). Standardized nursing language: What does it mean for nursing practice? *Online Journal of Issues in Nursing, 13*(1). Retrieved from http://www.nursingworld.org/MainMenuCategories/ANAMarketplace/ANAPeriodicals/OJIN/TableofContents/vol132008/No1Jan08/ArticlePreviousTopic/StandardizedNursingLanguage.aspx

Saba, V. K. (2007). *Clinical care classification (CCC) system manual*. New York: Springer.

Scichilone, R. A. (2008). The benefits of using SNOMED CT and LOINC in assessment instruments. *Journal of the American Health Information Management Association, 79*(7), 56–57.

Scroggins, L. M. (2008). The developmental processes for NANDA international nursing diagnoses. *International Journal of Nursing Terminologies and Classifications: The Official Journal of NANDA International, 19*(2), 57–64.

Smith, V., & Smith, K. (2007, March 28). *Supporting evidence-based practice through the use of standardized nursing language*. Retrieved from http://www.himss.org/content/files/NI_March28_audio_conf.pdf

The University of Iowa. (2010a). *Nursing interventions classification (NIC)*. Retrieved from http://www.nursing.uiowa.edu/excellence/nursing_knowledge/clinical_effectiveness/nocoverview.htm

The University of Iowa. (2010b). *Nursing outcomes classification (NOC)*. Retrieved from http://www.nursing.uiowa.edu/excellence/nursing_knowledge/clinical_effectiveness/nocoverview.htm

U.S. Department of Health and Human Services (DHHS). (2003). Proceedings of meeting of the Subcommittee on Standards and Security. December 9, 2003. Retrieved from http://ncvhs.hhs .gov/031209tr.htm

U.S. Department of Health and Human Services (DHHS). (2009). CMS and ONC issue regulations proposing a definition of "meaningful use" and setting standards for electronic health record incentive program. *Earth Times.* Retrieved from http://www.earthtimes.org/articles/show/ cms-and-onc-issue-regulations,1103814.shtml

U.S. Department of Health and Human Services (DHHS). (2011). *The Office of the National Coordinator for Health Information Technology.* Retrieved from http://healthit.hhs.gov/portal/ server.pt?open=512&objID=1487&mode=2

Warren, J., & Coenen, A. (1998). International classification for nursing practice (ICNP): Most-frequently asked questions. *Journal of the American Medical Informatics Association, 5*(4), 335–336.

Warren, J. J., & Bakken, S. (2002). Update on standardized nursing data sets and terminologies. *Journal of the American Health Information Management Association, 73*(7), 78–83, quiz: 85–76.

Westra, B. L., Delaney, C. W., Konicek, D., & Keenan, G. (2008). Nursing standards to support the electronic health record. *Nursing Outlook, 56*(5), 258–266, e251.

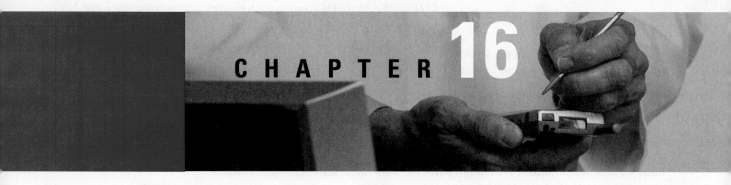

CHAPTER 16

Personal Health Records

After completing this chapter, you should be able to:

1. Define the term *personal health record (PHR)*.

2. Understand the differences between stand-alone, tethered, and integrated PHRs.

3. Discuss common functionality available in the PHR.

4. Discuss the patient-centered benefits associated with PHRs.

5. Identify at least two large health systems using PHRs.

6. List several barriers related to patient use of PHRs.

7. List several concerns related to patient self-entered data.

These are exciting and very promising times for the widespread application of information technology to improve the quality of healthcare delivery, while also reducing costs, but there is much yet to do. I want to note especially the importance of the resource most often under-utilized in our information systems: our patients.

CHARLES SAFRAN, MD, TESTIMONY TO HOUSE WAYS AND
MEANS SUBCOMMITTEE ON HEALTH, JUNE 2004

INTRODUCTION

Consumers in the United States and around the world are using technology and the Internet in ways that were inconceivable only a short time ago. From online banking to e-commerce, to digital entertainment and social networking, digital tools have transformed people's lives. Indeed, electronic tools have become so commonplace that getting through the day using any other means is rare. While a digital divide remains—particularly among those residing in rural areas, older adults, and those not completing high school—technology access gaps are narrowing ("Who's Online—Internet Demographics" 2010).

Amid the boom of the digital revolution, a quieter transformation is happening: the era of the personal health record (PHR). For consumers and caregivers the digital revolution has brought health information technology (HIT) tools that facilitate customizing care, sharing information, increasing transparency, and providing patients greater control over their own information. PHRs are accelerating this change.

Definitions of Personal Health Records

The definition of a PHR continues to evolve as technology and information exchange advances. A variety of organizations contribute to PHR's definitions, including the American Health Information Management Association and the American Association of Retired Persons. Some believe PHRs should refer only to data that is accessible to the patient and that comes from a provider or health system electronic health record (EHR), that is, data generated by clinicians or other staff. Others feel information created and *inputted by the patient* is a core PHR element. Functionality such as online medication refill and secure e-mail with providers are also seen as important, patient-centered services complementing PHR data. One definition, developed by a joint PHR Task Force of the Medical Library Association and the National Library of Medicine (Jones, Shipman, Plaut, & Selden 2010), states:

> Electronic personal health record (PHR) [is]: a private, secure application through which an individual may access, manage and share his or her health information. The PHR can include information that is entered by the consumer and/or data from other sources such as pharmacies, labs, and health care providers. The PHR may or may not include information from the electronic health record (EHR) that is maintained by the health care provider and is not synonymous with the EHR. PHR sponsors include vendors who may or may not charge a fee, health care organizations such as hospitals, health insurance companies, or employers.

We support a more comprehensive definition of the PHR that includes multiple sources of health information (including information created by the patient) and services. In their simplest concept, PHRs are electronic systems that allow people to record, access, and share health-related information in order to help them better manage their health and healthcare. The Markle Foundation, bringing together public and private stakeholders through the *Connecting for Health* Personal Health Working Group defines the PHR as: "an electronic tool that enables individuals or their authorized representatives to control personal health information, supports them in managing their health and well-being, and enhances their interactions with health care professionals" (Markle Foundation 2008).

CONNECTING FOR HEALTH COMMON FRAMEWORK, 2006 MARKLE FOUNDATION

Attributes of an Ideal Personal Health Record

1. Each person controls his or her own PHR.
2. PHRs contain information from one's entire lifetime.
3. PHRs contain information from all healthcare providers.
4. PHRs are accessible from any place at any time.
5. PHRs are private and secure.
6. PHRs are transparent. Individuals can see who entered each piece of data, where it was transferred from, and who has viewed it.
7. PHRs permit easy exchange of information across healthcare systems.

FIGURE 16–1 • Attributes of an ideal personal health record

Markle's *Common Framework* offers valuable guidance for the development and deployment of patient-centered PHRs. The *Framework* identifies seven attributes of an ideal PHR. Shown in Figure 16–1, it includes key concepts such as security, privacy, transparency, and lifetime control of records.

While still at an early stage, the PHR enterprise races ahead, becoming more robust yet more complex. In 2006, there were over 80 PHR applications (Gearon et al. 2007). By 2008 over 200 were identified. While the full reach and impact of PHRs has yet to be understood, many stakeholders have adopted strong, positive beliefs about having patients connecting directly to their healthcare information using consumer-centered technology.

PHRs and Patient Engagement, Efficiency, and Quality

The drive for PHR development and use comes from inside and outside healthcare. While consumers increasingly demand relevant information to support their clinical decisions, healthcare payers and policy makers require that care become simultaneously less costly and achieve higher quality. The concept of patient access to information to improve healthcare quality is central to the Institute of Medicine's (IOM) landmark report, *Crossing the Quality Chasm: A New Health System for the 21st Century* (IOM 2001). In its "Ten Rules for Design" to improve care and quality, the IOM identified core principles that specifically engage patients in their own care, including:

1. Care is based on continuous healing relationships.
2. Care is customized according to patient needs and values.
3. The patient is the source of control.
4. Knowledge is shared, and information flows freely.
5. Transparency is necessary.

By harnessing technology to provide patients with personalized communication and services, fully functional PHRs help address each of these areas. As the number of people with chronic conditions such as diabetes, hypertension, and obesity increases, there will be a concomitant increase in patient and family need for help in managing these problems. Empowering patients is critical for chronic illness care. Consumer HIT tools can facilitate productive interactions between patients and their care teams, in keeping with recommendations to improve the overall quality of care delivered (Wagner, Austin, & Von Korff 1996). Giving patients and caregivers information through electronic tools will encourage self-care and enhance the patient experience.

Consumer demand for personal health information and PHRs appears to be growing. A national survey in 2010 showed that while PHR use remains low nationwide, use was twice as high as 2 years earlier. Importantly, among those who had used a PHR, 64% reported finding value in verifying that the information in their medical record was correct (California Foundation 2010). As demand increases for technology that is both convenient and meaningful, use will be stimulated further.

Interest in PHRs is not limited to consumers. At a time of rising health costs, PHRs are seen as a means to deliver care more efficiently and potentially to reduce utilization. In its report, *The Value of Personal Health Records*, the Center for Information Technology Leadership describes PHRs as potentially cost saving, with greater value accruing as rates of consumer use rise over time (Center for Information Technology Leadership 2008). Health insurance plans, that communicate frequently with their members for administrative and financial purposes, are eager to connect online with enrollees. Because of their extensive and detailed claims and diagnostic and utilization data, insurers can position themselves to create a "health-plan" PHR model. Employers are also interested in HIT solutions that improve population health and reduce employee health costs. Several large employers, for example, formed a consortium to develop a PHR system called *Dossia* (http://www.dossia.org).

It remains unclear who will most benefit from PHRs. Early experience suggests PHRs increase patient satisfaction (Ralston et al. 2007), reduce telephone calls and outpatient visits (Zhou, Garrido, Chin, Wiesenthal, & Liang 2007), and improve some health outcomes (Green et al. 2008; Ralston et al. 2009a). PHR use is consistent with health system shifts toward greater support of patient self-management of chronic conditions and moves away from episodic, in-person visits (Wagner et al. 1996; IOM 2001). Ultimately a leading motivation behind PHRs comes from consumers valuing improved access to their health information and 24-hour communication with their healthcare system.

In the remainder of this chapter we will examine the current and future landscape for PHRs. The Tethered, Nontethered, and Networked PHRs section describes broad categories of PHRs, and the Current PHR Use section provides information about PHR use. In the PHR Functions section you will read about common features of PHRs, such as medication lists, laboratory results, and secure messaging. In the Evidence of PHR Impact section, existing evidence about the value of PHRs in terms of satisfaction and health outcomes is presented. The PHRs and Transformation of Care section looks at how PHRs may play an important role in shifting traditional care delivery to a new model that includes engaged patients and family members to the forefront. Finally, in the Toward a Future of Networked Care section, we highlight some challenges from moving toward a networked model that includes PHRs, such as ensuring data security and bringing patient-entered data in the EHR.

TETHERED, NONTETHERED, AND NETWORKED PHRS

Precursors to Electronic PHRs

PHRs have existed before the invention of computers. Families keep paper files or a notebook listing medications, family health histories, and handwritten notes from doctor visits. A wall calendar can also provide some PHR functions, that is, reminding patients of upcoming appointments or medications to be taken or refilled. Individuals walk around with part of their health record, that is, memories of important health events. In many families keeping health information may be the responsibility of a single person. These systems can be woefully inadequate, however, when there are acute and complex chronic conditions in a single family, for example, ranging from appendicitis or breast cancer to depression and hypertension.

Early methods for PHRs between patients and providers included the use of paper booklets, and patients were expected to enter information such as diagnoses, hospitalizations, medications, provider information, and other medical history. One advantage of this type of record is that it allows aggregation of data from multiple sources. Major drawbacks of such records are that they require continual self-entry, are tedious to maintain, and have limited search capacity and challenges accessing data when traveling or in an emergency. Electronic PHRs have been developed to overcome many of these shortcomings.

Stand-Alone Versus Tethered PHRs

There have been several proposed PHR taxonomies (Tang, Ash, Bates, & Overhage 2006; Vincent et al. 2008). As definitions continue to evolve, a common distinction is whether the patient-accessible information is *tethered* to data in a specific health system's EHR or is *stand-alone*, that is, not tied to any particular healthcare system. Such descriptions can be problematic in the current dynamic environment of PHR development. Even some stand-alone applications are likely to become tethered to health data repositories and ultimately serve as patient portals that allow a consumer to pull his or her information from multiple sources.

Some fully stand-alone applications are available commercially through the Internet or other formats such as smart card, CD, or flash drive. These tools rely on an individual or caregiver to enter his or her own health information. Some allow information from a payer or provider to be uploaded or scanned into the system, but are not considered to be connected to electronic system holding that information. These systems usually allow users to add information so that the PHR can be customized to the individual. In the current health care environment standalone PHRs have the disadvantage of consumers having to self-enter, or at least to actively refresh, data to maintain a comprehensive and accurate record. Further, stand-alone PHRs such as those on thumb drive devices have been found to have significant security risks (Wright & Sittig 2007). As the market changes rapidly with vendors leaving or merging, it becomes problematic to offer stand-alone products.

In contrast, a *tethered* PHR is inextricably linked to a single entity or health system (Detmer, Bloomrosen, Raymond, & Tang 2008). In this common PHR model, an individual can view and access data stored by one institution or organization. This involves providing electronic access through a *patient portal,* ideally offering patients a longitudinal view of their record (Simons, Mandl, & Kohane 2005). Through a secure connection, select elements of the EHR can be accessed such as medication lists, test results, visit history, and after-visit summaries. Additional functionality may be provided with a tethered PHR, such as online medication refills or secure messaging with a provider or healthcare team. In essence, these tools are the patient-facing component of the EHR.

Examples of tethered PHRs include Kaiser's HealthConnect and the Veteran Health Administration's *My HealtheVet,* shown in Figure 16–2. Patients enrolled in Kaiser and authenticated with

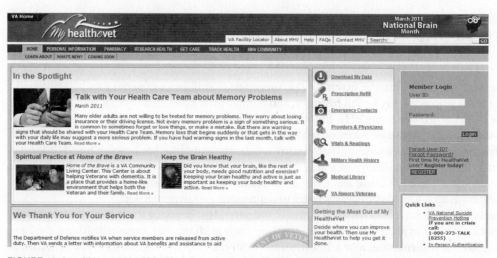

FIGURE 16–2 • Veterans health administration's *My HealtheVet* PHR

their PHR can find information related to their care such as medications, laboratory results, and summaries of clinic visits (Kahn, Aulakh, & Bosworth 2009; Pagliari, Detmer, & Singleton 2007). PHRs may also include asynchronous, secure communication between patients and clinicians. The degree to which online clinician-to-patient communication is reimbursed or integrated into the EHR varies, however. Other PHR tools may include health diaries and tracking logs for patients to self-enter measures such as blood pressure, physical activity, or weight.

Tethered tools offer considerable value for people who receive the bulk of their care from a single health system. Although PHRs vary, they have potential to engage patients in their health and improve self-management (Tang et al. 2009). From the standpoint of the health system, PHR services that are desirable, such as secure messaging, can attract and retain patients, as well as engage people to participate more in their own care. Many consumers, however, receive care from multiple healthcare systems. Tethered PHRs do not usually have mechanisms to export data out to other systems or to import data from elsewhere.

PHRs tethered to insurers and health plans, such as from Medicare (http://medicare.gov) or Aetna (http://www.aetnatools.com), offer consumers access to claims data generated from encounters, tests, and procedures. Some also provide options for tracking health, such as following blood pressure. Yet since these PHRs are not linked to a provider's EHR, this information does not flow back to clinicians (Grossman, Zayas-Cabán, & Kemper 2009). Insurers are adding features to these PHRs such as searching for a provider or a pharmacy, estimating costs for tests and medications, and connecting—through online chat—for assistance. Recently, a few have partnered with vendors to provide enrollees with 24/7 access to a physician. One example is Blue Cross and Blue Shield of Minnesota, collaborating with the company American Well, which provides telephone, online chat, or Web video visits with a physician for a fee. Summary notes from these encounters can be printed or e-mailed to a primary provider. These care services, while patient-centered and convenient, are not connected to EHRs or provider-based PHRs.

The untethered PHR is designed to accept and integrate information from many different sources, such as health systems, providers, insurers, and so on. It provides patients greater control over who has access to (e.g., family members, health providers from different health systems) and what kinds of information to put in them (e.g., ability to input nonprescription medications and alternative therapies). Examples of untethered PHRs are Microsoft's *HealthVault* and the now defunct *Google Health* (Figure 16–3). Proponents of untethered PHRs argue that they better meet patients' needs to access and control their health information (Mandl, Szolovits, & Kohane et al. 2001; Simons et al. 2005). Some health systems with tethered PHRs are making it possible for patients to export their personal health data into untethered PHRs. *Dossia*, created through a collaboration of Wal-Mart, Intel, Pitney Bowes, AT&T, and other large employers, is a PHR platform enabling employees and retirees to access health data consolidated from a variety of sources (e.g., health plans, pharmacies, and laboratories). *Dossia* also offers tools enabling individuals to self-enter information, as well as financial information about clinical services.

The Networked PHR

PHRs allow people to electronically view, collect, manage, or share their health information or process health-related transactions. As discussed earlier, a tethered PHR limited to a single provider presents barriers to a complete and accurate health record. A logical next stage of PHR development is to create PHRs that draw information from a network of data dispersed across multiple locations. Described as a networked PHR, the consumer can create a more comprehensive PHR. Markle Foundation has described the vision of a networked PHR.

Shown in a simplified schematic in Figure 16–4, consumers can access data residing in multiple locations, ranging from providers to health plans, to others such as health record banks or

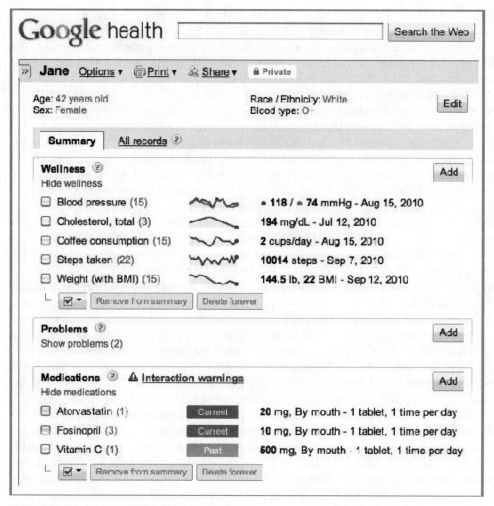

FIGURE 16–3 • Google health's PHR
Google Health. http://googleblog.blogspot.com/2010/09/google-health-update.html

laboratories. Connections occur through the use of *Consumer Access Services*. Such an entity would conduct authentication or identify proofing before allowing patient or proxy access to data from any source in the system. The entity may be separate from the PHR or may also provide a PHR or patient portal. In an ideal model, the consumer would be offered a "single sign on,", so that he or she would not be required to verify identify for each data source that was accessed.

Markle has articulated a set of core principles that serve as the foundation of networked consumer access to information (Table 16–1). While designed for networked PHRs, many of these principles apply equally well for PHRs in general. Principles focus on privacy and security, and an individual's control of his or her health information and how it is shared.

CURRENT PHR USE

The popularity of PHRs continues to expand. For over a decade, Web-based PHRs have been implemented by several large health systems. Kaiser Permanente, Group Health Cooperative, Palo Alto Medical Foundation, Geisinger Health System, and Beth Israel Deaconess Medical Center were early adopters of PHRs (Weingart, Rind, Tofias, & Sands 2006). A sizable number of patients served by those health systems currently use a tethered PHR on a regular basis. Over 3 million enrollees at Kaiser actively use HealthConnect (Kaiser Permanente HealthConnect

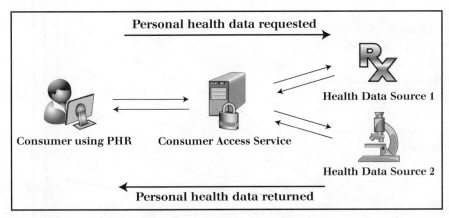

FIGURE 16–4 • Consumer networked to multiple data sources
Source: 2008 Markle Foundation. Connecting for Health Common Framework. Available at http://www.markle
.org/health/markle-common-framework

Electronic Health Record 2011). Among Group Health enrollees, the reach of *MyGroupHealth* nears 60% (Ralston, Coleman, Reid, Handley, & Larson 2010). Over 50% of patients cared for at Palo Alto Medical Foundation have registered for *My Health Online*. Figure 16–5 shows the steady growth over several years, in the percent of adult enrollees who registered to use Group Health's PHR.

TABLE 16–1	Connecting for Health Core Principles for Networked PHRs
1. Openness and transparency	Consumers should know what information has been collected about them, the purpose of its use, who can access and use it, and where it resides. They should also be informed about how they may obtain access to information collected about them and how they may control who has access to it.
2. Purpose specification	The purposes for which personal data are collected should be specified at the time of collection, and the subsequent use should be limited to those purposes, or others that are specified on each occasion of change of purpose.
3. Collection limitation and data minimization	Personal health information should only be collected for specified purposes and obtained by lawful and fair means. The collection and storage of personal health data should be limited to that information necessary to carry out the specified purpose. Where possible, consumers should have the knowledge of or provide consent for collection of their personal health information.
4. Use limitation	Personal data should not be disclosed, made available, or otherwise used for purposes other than those specified.
5. Individual participation and control	Consumers should be able to control access to their personal information. They should know who is storing what information on them, and how that information is being used. They should also be able to review the way their information is being used or stored.
6. Data quality and integrity	All personal data collected should be relevant to the purposes for which they are to be used and should be accurate, complete, and up-to-date.
7. Security safeguards and controls	Reasonable safeguards should protect personal data against such risks as loss or unauthorized access, use, destruction, modification, or disclosure.
8. Accountability and oversight	Entities in control of personal health information must be held accountable for implementing these principles.
9. Remedies	Remedies must exist to address security breaches or privacy violations.

Source: 2008 Markle Foundation. Connecting for Health. Available at http://www.markle.org/sites/default/files/Overview_
Consumers.pdf

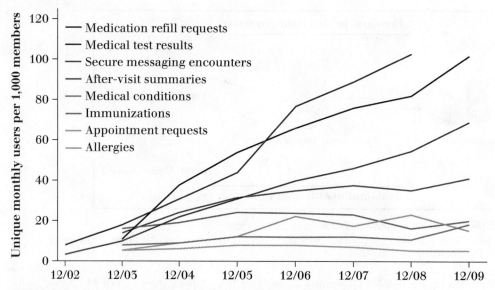

FIGURE 16–5 • Increase in *MyGroupHealth* enrollment since first offered

Source: Ralston, Coleman, Reid, Handley, & Larson (2010). Patient experience should be part of meaningful-use criteria. *Health Affairs 29,* 607–613.

Nationwide estimates of consumers using provider-delivered PHRs are reportedly 2.4 million (Halamka, Mandl, & Tang 2008). Perhaps the largest health system to deploy a PHR is the Veterans Health Administration (VA). In December 2010, over 1.2 million VA patients were registered for *My HealtheVet.* More than 18.5 million prescription refills have occurred online (http://www.myhealth.va.gov).

Among patient and enrollee populations who have registered for PHRs, the frequency of use is noteworthy. Among VA patients using *My HealtheVet,* approximately half report visiting the PHR Web site monthly and 30% say they visit weekly (Nazi 2010; Nazi & Woods 2008). Notably, over 30% of *My HealtheVet* patient users are over the age of 65. At Group Health, secure e-mail constitutes almost one-third of patient-provider contacts (Ralston, Coleman, Reid, Handley, & Larson 2010). Further, some studies have found that older users with chronic conditions have substantial use of PHRs and their functions. At Group Health, almost one-third of persons over age 65 with diabetes have used the PHR, most typically on a monthly basis (Weppner et al. 2010). Figure 16–6 shows PHR use among older patients having a diagnosis of diabetes.

PHR FUNCTIONS

Doctors and nurses are experts in clinical care; patients are experts in their daily experiences. Both need to share data from everyday life and can help bridge that gap.

Patricia Flatly Brennan, National Program Director, Project Health Design

In a relatively brief time span, PHRs have evolved from being a small window for patients to view parts of their EHR to being a suite of tools allowing patients to access and enter health information, and to communicate with providers and the health system. Here we describe five categories of PHR features: access to EHR-provided health information, secure messaging, self-entered data, proxy or delegation access, and administrative and financial data. Each of these categories, and salient features, is described next. These categories are also summarized in Table 16–3, which describes benefits, and potential concerns, of each feature.

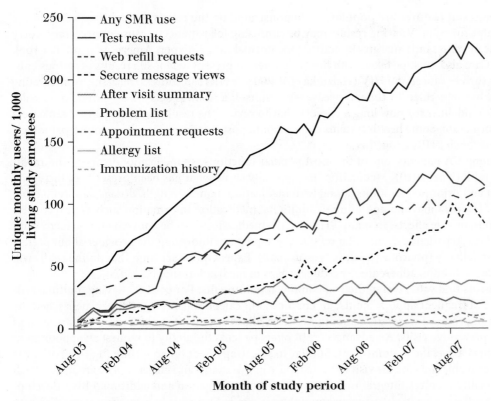

FIGURE 16–6 • Use of MyGroupHealth among patients aged 65 and older with diabetes
Source: Weppner (2010). *Diabetes Care 33*(11), 2314–2319.

EHR Personal Health Information

One of the simplest ways to offer a PHR has been to provide patients with access to elements of their medical record through a secure Web site. This shared medical record typically includes access to laboratory test results, a list of prescribed medications, and the ability to see future appointments.

Viewing laboratory and test results is the posting of test results for the patient to see. In the simplest form, the results appear much as the doctor sees them: the name of the test, the test value, and a normal range. More advanced PHRs link to information about each test: what the test is measuring, why the test is performed, the normal range of results, and what abnormal values may signify. Patients seem to like this feature, demonstrated by the fact that test views are the most common function used in PHRs. Table 16–2 shows a typical lab result posted on a PHR, providing the test name (abbreviated), the test value, the standard range, measurement units, and a column to indicate if the result is outside the normal range and may require follow-up (flag column).

Many patients may not know *TSH* is an abbreviation for thyroid-stimulating hormone. A PHR developed with a user-centered design would provide an information balloon, button, or hyperlink to more detailed information about the test, for example, stating the definition of TSH and the purpose of the test.

TABLE 16–2	Laboratory Test Result in a PHR			
Name	**Your Value**	**Standard Range**	**Units**	**Flag**
TSH	1.94	0.28–4.10	mIU/L	

Test result features are popular, as demonstrated by the relatively high frequency in the use of this function. Viewing results may be confusing for patients or cause unnecessary worry because of values only marginally outside the normal range (Pyper, Amery, Watson, & Crook 2004). Care also must be taken with how and when to present diagnostic results of serious conditions such as cancer and HIV (Halamka et al. 2008). PHRs can address this issue by integrating specific business rules for time to release test results. If a result is delayed for several days, rules become guidelines for how long a clinician has to review the results before a patient can access the information. Some health systems choose not to post certain results, for example, pathology, online through PHRs altogether.

Among VA patients, one of the most popular functions are medication list view and medication refill (Nazi 2010). Medication lists typically show what has been prescribed, including current and prior prescriptions, along with medication name, strength, dosage, and remaining refills. PHR data may include a link to additional medication information such as purpose, interactions, or side effects. In many PHRs, active medications can be conveniently refilled. With a few clicks, a patient can submit a refill request, possibly informing the provider about preference for delivery (pharmacy pick up versus mail). Expectations are high that online refills will enhance medication adherence, by reducing gaps in medication supply.

Patients find value seeing their upcoming appointments. For patients having multiple providers and frequent appointments, an appointment calendar can help manage their schedule. PHRs can provide information about past visits, allowing patients to keep track of care such as annual preventive visits. An advanced PHR offers patients the ability to request an appointment or confirm a specific appointment. Similar to selecting a seat on an airline flight, a patient is shown available slots for the visit (or care type, e.g., eye exam) and clicks on a desired time. Such functionality requires integration with a scheduling application and additional PHR development. An alternative to choosing an appointment is to use secure messaging to communicate an appointment request; the patient subsequently receives a reply.

It is believed that patients absorb only about half the information heard during a doctor visit (Ley, Bradshaw, Eaves, & Walker 1973). Reasons can include use of medical jargon, patient apprehension about asking questions, patient anxiety from health-related discussions, and too much information delivered. After-visit summaries are designed to improve information receptivity and include a narrative about the purpose of the visit and what was discussed. They may include vital signs, new and discontinued medications, preventive recommendations, advice made as a result of the visit, as well as laboratory, imaging, or other test orders. Visit summaries are not necessarily in electronic format; some provide them in paper form. The perceived value of after-visit summaries has steadily increased.

A step toward full transparency and open communication with patients is the concept of patient access to clinician visit notes. Some clinicians believe that progress notes are not meant to be read by patients, citing sensitive information and possible harm. Consumer health advocates argue that access to all notes is a right and a welcome and long-delayed action. Those supporting full transparency feel that patients and families will be better informed about clinician decision making and have an improved understanding of their clinical problems and treatment options (Burke et al. 2010). Importantly, the Health Insurance Portability and Accountability Act (HIPAA) of 2003 gives patients legal rights to copies of their medical record with a formal request. Few patients take advantage of these requests, as barriers are common such as lack of knowledge about release of information, hard-to-find medical records offices, printing charges, and delays; overall, this process can be onerous for patients (Fioriglio & Szolovits 2005). One project anticipated to make important strides in this area is the *Open Notes Project,* in which patients in three large health systems will be offered electronic access to complete notes through a PHR (Delbanco et al. 2010).

Tethered PHRs can play an important role in informing patients about needed or overdue preventive care and tests. Clinical reminders identified by an EHR can be transmitted to a patient

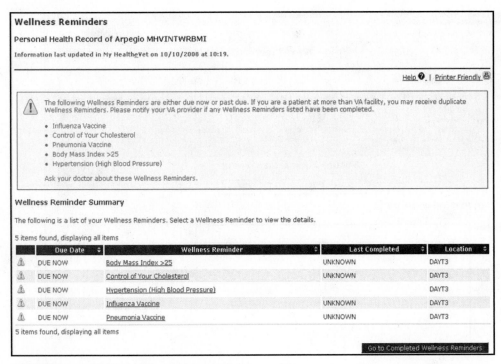

Wellness Reminders

Personal Health Record of Arpegio MHVINTWRBMI

Information last updated in My HealtheVet on 10/10/2008 at 10:19.

Help **?** | Printer Friendly 🖨

> ⚠ The following Wellness Reminders are either due now or past due. If you are a patient at more than VA facility, you may receive duplicate Wellness Reminders. Please notify your VA provider if any Wellness Reminders listed have been completed.
>
> - Influenza Vaccine
> - Control of Your Cholesterol
> - Pneumonia Vaccine
> - Body Mass Index >25
> - Hypertension (High Blood Pressure)
>
> Ask your doctor about these Wellness Reminders.

Wellness Reminder Summary

The following is a list of your Wellness Reminders. Select a Wellness Reminder to view the details.

5 items found, displaying all items

	Due Date ⬍	Wellness Reminder ⬍	Last Completed ⬍	Location ⬍
⚠	DUE NOW	Body Mass Index >25	UNKNOWN	DAYT3
⚠	DUE NOW	Control of Your Cholesterol	UNKNOWN	DAYT3
⚠	DUE NOW	Hypertension (High Blood Pressure)		DAYT3
⚠	DUE NOW	Influenza Vaccine	UNKNOWN	DAYT3
⚠	DUE NOW	Pneumonia Vaccine	UNKNOWN	DAYT3

5 items found, displaying all items

Go to Completed Wellness Reminders

FIGURE 16–7 • *My HealtheVet* wellness reminders

through a tethered PHR. Patient clinical reminders can prompt individuals to access specific care such as colon cancer screening, retinal exams, immunization, or attention to elevated blood pressure (Muller et al. 2009). Derived from reminders in the EHR, they can be triggered by patient sex, age, and data entered for the last encounter. Figure 16–7 displays a reminder sent to a patient using the VA's *My HealtheVet*. This patient is overdue for two vaccines and health screenings. If the patient clicks on the highlighted "Body Mass Index >25," another page will show more detail about the screening and why it is important and links to additional information.

Secure Messaging

PHR systems often include a function enabling patients to send secure, electronic messages to their health providers and care teams (see Figure 16–8). Secure e-mail differs from regular e-mail in that they have protections including encryption and authentication of users to prevent unauthorized parties from intercepting and viewing messages. Secure messaging is considered to be important for patient access, communication, and care coordination (Chen, Garrido, Chock, Okawa, & Liang 2009; Houston et al. 2004; Ralston et al. 2009b). The convenience and asynchronous nature of secure e-mail may lower barriers for patient use, so that they raise issues before they become acute.

Health systems may design secure messaging so that patient messages go first to a "triage team" prior to routing of messages to a provider or other clinician. Triage staff reviews the message, subsequently resolving the issue (e.g., changing an appointment) or have it assigned to the appropriate person. A clinical pharmacist may respond to a patient about a medication question, or a nurse may solicit additional information from a patient who has a nonurgent problem. Secure messaging communication between patients and health systems is part of the medical record. Depending upon the degree of integration of secure messaging with the EHR, messages may automatically be part of the EHR (Kaiser) and manually entered into the EHR depending upon message content (VA) or an information system entirely separate from the EHR.

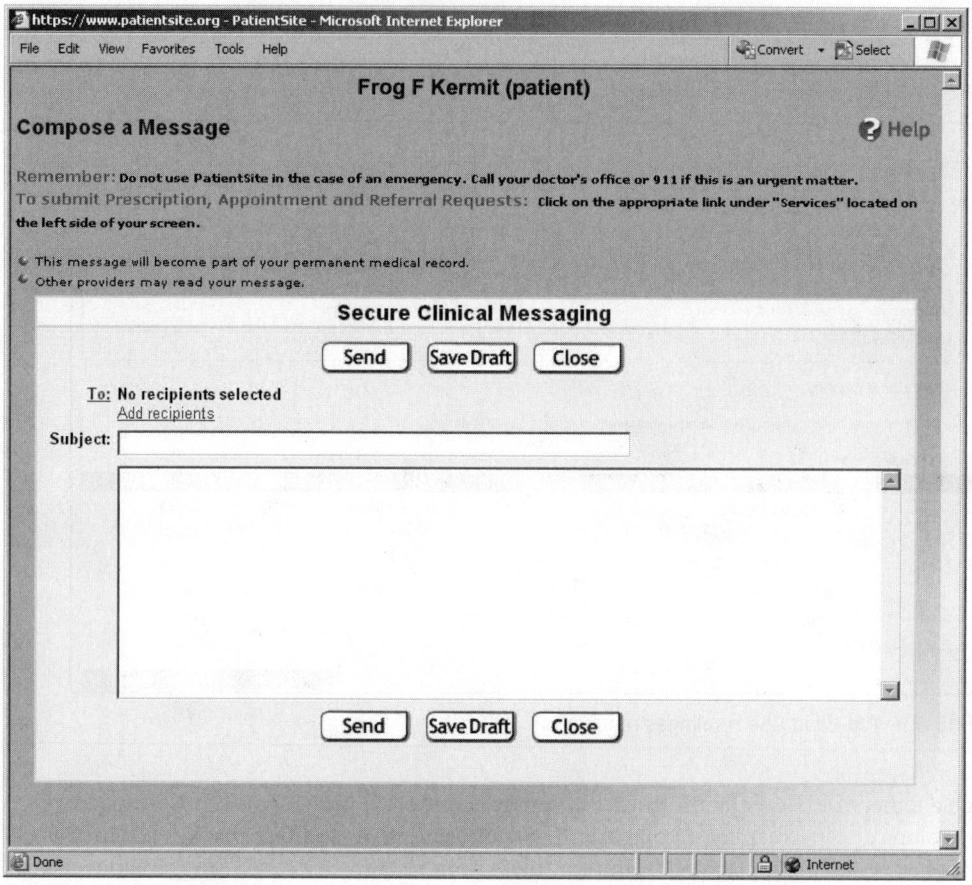

FIGURE 16–8 • PatientSite secure messaging, including language on appropriate use

Widespread adoption of secure messaging has been low but slowly increasing (Boukus, Grossman, & O'Malley 2010; Sciamanna, Rogers, Shenassa, & Houston 2007). Barriers are believed to be related to physicians' perceptions of difficulty delivering care online, beliefs that volume of messages will demand extra time, and fear of liability risk. Several large health systems have implemented secure messaging, and real-world observations have not borne such concerns (Byrne, Elliott, & Firek 2009; Sands & Halamka 2004). An unresolved issue related to secure messaging is financial reimbursement for clinician time spent responding to messages. Medicare and Medicaid do not currently reimburse for secure message consults in the same way they do for in-person and phone consultations (Halamka et al. 2008). As more providers and health systems adopt patient-centered medical home (PCMH) practice models, there will be greater need to seamlessly integrate virtual, secure patient communication into the structure and operations of care delivery (Zhou, Kanter, Wang, & Garrido 2010).

Patient-Entered Data

Some PHRs have the ability for a patient to enter information. As a complement to data in the EHR, patient-entered data can be of value to patients, caregivers, and providers. The patient can enter or modify this information, potentially providing a more comprehensive and accurate personal health information snapshot over time. Examples of self-entered information include prior medical history; major illnesses; health information on family members; as well as

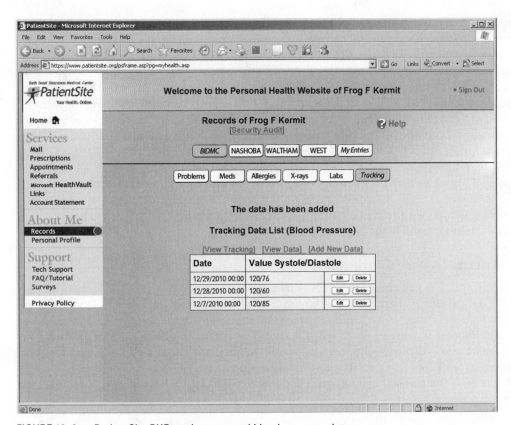

FIGURE 16–9 • PatientSite PHR: patient-entered blood pressure data

vitamins, supplements, or complementary and alternative medications, such as milk thistle or St. John's Wort. Patients are encouraged to track ongoing health and health-related behaviors through health logs or diaries. They typically include logs of food (types, amounts); exercise; as well as self-recorded health measurements such as weight, blood pressure, and blood sugar levels. Figure 16–9 shows *PatientSite* PHR screen allowing patients to enter self-recorded blood pressure values. These data can be graphed to show patients how measures change over time. Some systems encourage patients to complete a previsit questionnaire online. If a patient has a first appointment with a specialist, the patient may be asked to complete a questionnaire from the specialist prior to the visit.

There are several unanswered issues regarding patient-entered data, including what type of data patients should enter, as well as clinician responsibility to review and respond to the information. These issues are discussed further in the "Toward a Future of Networked Care" section.

Proxy Users (Delegation)

Many patients may have a family member or friend who serves as caregiver on their behalf. A PHR with an established process for proxy user, or delegation, allows the proxy person(s) to access many of the PHR features described earlier. A proxy can view information and use PHR functions such as secure messaging, refill medications, and obtain test results. Some systems enable a patient to adjust the level of access so that certain functions can be accessed and others are not available to the proxy (e.g., mental health information).

There are two situations for which PHR proxy function is well-suited. The first is where a patient requires assistance from others to manage health-related information and care. An elderly man, for example, may have physical limitations and is uncomfortable or unable (e.g., vision or manual dexterity) to use the PHR; his son can serve as his proxy, using the PHR for its convenience and information services. This proxy user can communicate to the patient's provider and gather information that will assist with care coordination. Second, a parent can obtain proxy PHR access on behalf of his or her child. Many systems offer parents proxy access until the child is 13 years of age. At 13, many states consider a child capable of making some of his or her own medical decisions, subject to a doctor's judgment. Conversations between the doctor and the teenager are considered confidential, even to the point of excluding the parent. This is especially evident with doctor visits and prescriptions relating to sensitive issues, such as sexual health or substance use ("*Teenagers' access to confidential reproductive health services*" 2005). For this reason, many PHR systems discontinue parent access when a child reaches age 13. Some systems, realizing that teenagers 13 or older may prefer to have parents as proxies, have allowed proxy access to continue. Software has been developed having administrative mechanisms ensuring that a teen voluntarily allows a parent to have proxy status, with blocks that can be put in place to keep selected health information confidential.

Administrative and Financial

Some PHRs provide patients access to financial, medical claims, and other health-related administrative information. Patients may have access to bills for recent services, including total charge, amount paid by insurer, co-pay, and remaining balance owed by the patient. If a PHR has data from a health plan or a managed care organization, the patient may be able to view details about coverage benefits such as visual, mental health, hospitalization, as well as coinsurance and premium information. Some PHRs may offer the feature to pay medical bills online.

Table 16–3 is a summary of various PHR functions, along with their associated expected value and possible concerns.

EVIDENCE OF PHR IMPACT

As PHRs have been deployed more widely, there is increasing research about their effectiveness, particularly related to the care of people with chronic disease. In general, PHR use is higher among insured patients and younger adults (Miller, Bandenbosch, Ivanov, & Black 2007); however, the proportion of older and publicly insured patients using PHRs are rising. We discuss available evidence on the acceptance of PHRs by patients and health providers, and the ability of PHRs to improve patient access and health outcomes.

Patient Satisfaction

An important benefit of PHRs would be to meet patients' needs. National surveys of Internet users indicate that most would like to interact remotely with their provider, by using secure messaging or scheduling appointments (California HealthCare Foundation 2010). An important consumer concern about PHRs relates to security and privacy (Markle Foundation Connecting for Health 2003). Yet, most people report that they would like access to their own health records and that the "benefits of electronic records outweigh the privacy risks" (Bright 2007).

When given access, patients appear to like PHRs. Group Health Cooperative found that over 90% of patients report satisfaction with *MyGroupHealth* (Ralston et al. 2007). Data suggest that high ratings are related to usability of the Web site as well as the services offered. Tethered PHRs offer a menu of transactions and services; frequently used features include viewing test results, medication refill requests, and secure messaging (Ralston, Coleman, Reid, Handley, & Larson 2010; Weppner et al. 2010; Zhou et al. 2007). In general secure messaging with healthcare teams receives high satisfaction ratings from patients, as does the ability to refill medications and view test results quickly (Ralston et al. 2007). Consumers report that the ability to communicate online with a provider is a factor that may affect their choice of provider and health system (Baldwin 2002). Timeliness

TABLE 16–3   PHR Functions, Potential Benefits, and Potential Concerns

PHR Component	Description	Potential Benefits (+) and Concerns (–)
EHR personal health information		
Laboratory and test results	Shows results of laboratory tests (e.g., blood sugar, urinalysis) or other tests (e.g., EKG, colonoscopy)	+ Reduces patient waiting time + Avoids letters and phone calls – May confuse and worry patients – Must ensure sensitive results (e.g., cancer or HIV diagnosis) are given in person or by telephone
Medication management (with refill requests)	List of currently prescribed medications (dose, instructions); often shows medications prescribed in the past	+ Allows patients to check and improve quality of medication list (medication reconciliation) + Encourages discussion with doctor to improve adherence + Patient can share medication information with other providers – May be incomplete or inaccurate if medications are from multiple prescribers
Appointment view (upcoming and history)	Time, date, and location of scheduled appointments, including tests and procedures	+ Keeps track of upcoming care + Reduces number of missed/cancelled appointments
Appointment request	Requests for appointments, which must be confirmed by the doctor's office. More advanced systems allow a patient to choose an appointment from those available	+ Greater patient control + Avoids tedious phone scheduling – May be challenging for the health system to offer open access – Appointment may not match the level or type of care needed
After-visit summary	A summary of what was discussed at a visit, including advice, vital signs, and prescriptions	+ Helps patient recall discussion during clinical encounter + Helps reinforce clinical advice + Information can be shared with caregivers
Clinician visit notes	The actual doctor write-up of the visit	+ Patients better understand clinician thinking and decision making + Patients better understand clinical issues and treatment options – Language may be confusing or misunderstood to patients – Clinicians may resist shared notes, citing patient harm and need to alter notes
Clinical reminders	Notice about recommended screening and preventive care (colon cancer screen, foot and eye exam, mammogram)	+ Increases patient adherence to preventive care
Secure messaging	Confidential and secure online communication between patients and their doctor or healthcare team	+ Convenient, 24/7 access + Avoids "telephone tag" + Can include in medical record – Fitting messages into workflow – Reimbursement lacking – Need patient education to prevent inappropriate use (urgent issues)
Self-entered data	May include family health history, diaries for diet and exercise, self-recorded vitals (e.g., blood pressure, blood sugar)	+ Important data complementary to EHR information + Helps patient see trends needing attention (rising blood pressure) – Patient may incorrectly assume provider is viewing the information – Unclear how to integrate with EHR
Proxy use (delegation)	Permits another person to have access to patient PHR	+ Allows sharing information and care with caregiver – Patient may inadvertently release information intended to be private
Administrative	Ability to view bills, co-pays, insurance benefits, etc.; May allow bill payment	+ Helps manage care and finances + Improves knowledge of benefits

of service is a likely factor affecting patient satisfaction. Surveys of patients using secure messaging found that levels of satisfaction decreased as response times increased from 1 to 3 business days (Liederman, Lee, Baquero, & Seites 2005).

Provider Satisfaction

Clinicians have voiced concerns about PHR functions that alter patient care or affect providers' daily work, such as secure messaging (Zhou et al. 2010). Some health professionals worry that patient-provider relationships may suffer if online communication replaces face-to-face encounters (Zickmund et al. 2008). After overcoming initial fears of using secure messaging, however, providers tend to be satisfied and report that the impact on their workload is minimal (Katz, Moyer, Cox, & Stern 2003; Kittler et al. 2004; Ralston et al. 2007; Tang et al. 2003). The asynchronous nature of secure messaging also allows nurses to batch and respond to messages easily, which has the potential to decrease interruptions and allow more time devoted to specific patients. Anecdotally, providers report that message volumes are less than expected, that they appreciate questions and information directly from patients, and that messaging can be more efficient than trying to reach patients by telephone. Ongoing provider concerns related to reimbursement, information security, and medical liability are expected to change as online communication becomes more prevalent.

Predictors of PHR Use

Early evidence suggested that PHR users have commonly been the "worried well," or relatively healthy, Internet-savvy patients (Weingart et al. 2006). In general, users of PHRs are more likely to be female, to be middle aged, have more healthcare needs, and have a provider who uses secure messaging; patients who live in low socioeconomic neighborhoods or have Medicaid insurance are less likely to use PHRs (Ralston et al. 2009b; Swartz, Cowan, & Batista 2004; Weppner et al. 2010). The use of the Internet continues to increase, particularly among older baby-boomers, aged 56 to 64 years of age, to 76% who were online in 2010 (Zickuhr 2010). There is likely to be increasing overlap between an individual's ability to use consumer technologies and the desire or need for health-related online services (Fox 2004). Recent studies show that users of PHRs are as likely or more likely to have more medical problems (Ralston et al. 2009b; Zhou et al. 2007). Among patients aged 65 and older and having a chronic illness such as diabetes, those who were sicker were more likely to use PHR services (Weppner et al. 2010). It is not clear how often caregivers (family and friends) use PHRs to help care for their family members or loved ones.

Several individual and environmental factors will play a role in PHR usage. Factors such as education, health literacy, race, income, and high-speed Internet access appear to impact PHR use (Roblin, Houston, Allison, Joski, & Becker 2009). For PHR usage to occur, a number of conditions need be met. Patients must be aware of the technology, be able to access, and further decide to "kick the tires" or try it for the first time. To gain a benefit from use, such steps cannot require a significant investment of time or money. Continuing use can follow if there is realized (or perceptions of) value (Rogers 2003). Different PHRs will have different challenges in access, ease of use, and value of services. For example, although a stand-alone PHR such as Google Health or Microsoft HealthVault is readily accessible, it may require additional input and work by the patient to collect sufficient information to make it useful. Conversely, tethered PHRs may provide important access to personal health information, but if there are cumbersome steps for patient identify-proofing, or ease of use is not high, patients may have little interest in their use.

Utilization and Efficiency

An important question is whether and how PHR use by patients will affect workflow and care delivery, such as outpatient visits and hospitalizations (utilization). This is of concern to busy health professionals, who are typically reimbursed based on the volume of encounters. This issue is also of interest to integrated health systems and insurance companies, who may need to develop and justify reimbursement for virtual communication and online visits. PHRs may help health systems achieve greater efficiency in delivering care. For example, managing chronic illness could be addressed by patients refilling medications, reviewing problem lists, and communication via secure messaging, possibly reducing visits or telephone calls.

Evidence on substitution of virtual care for face-to-face care focuses on secure messaging, with or without shared records. Early randomized, control trials of secure e-mail systems showed mixed results; some found no change in telephone calls, and others showed reduced outpatient visits (Bergmo, Kummervold, Gammon, & Dahl 2005; Katz et al. 2003). However, these were small studies using early electronic messaging systems largely independent of PHRs; therefore generalized observations cannot be made. Large observational studies (Kaiser, 2011) suggested that the use of secure messaging as part of a tethered PHR is associated with a 7% to 10% decrease in face-to-face office visits, as well as a 14% decrease in annual phone calls (Chen et al. 2009; Zhou et al. 2007). Another study of a tethered PHR indicated that the volume of messages per physician was approximately 20 per month for each 100 patients; this was offset by an equal reduction in the number of phone calls (Sands & Halamka 2004). Substituting care and communication using secure messaging is supported by patient surveys. At Group Health, when patients were asked what would occur if secure messaging were not available, almost two-thirds responded they would call their provider, and one quarter said they would schedule a visit. Only 7% believed they would not take action (*MyGroupHealth* Satisfaction Survey 2006, personal communication).

Quality of Care

While PHR features may lead to efficiency gains, an important impact would be improving the quality of care. The idea of sharing information to improve quality of care is not new. Years before the Internet, paper-based "shared medical records" were found to improve the quality of care for patients with chronic conditions (Greenfield, Kaplan, Ware, Martin, & Frank 1988). Studies have begun to shed light on how PHRs may facilitate better care and improve patient health. In one study, patients using a PHR had higher quality of care for diabetes, high cholesterol, and blood pressure than nonusers (Zhou et al. 2010). Another study demonstrated that a higher level of PHR use was associated with improved control of diabetes (Harris, Haneuse, Martin, & Ralston 2009). In this study, PHR users had higher rates of outpatient visits than nonusers. This finding conflicts with prior reports that PHR use, in particular secure messaging, improves care while reducing face-to-face visits. Two smaller trials studied the effect of PHRs and secure messaging on care for blood pressure and diabetes, demonstrating that patient users had better health outcomes than those randomized to usual care (Green et al. 2008; Ralston et al. 2009a). In both studies, clinical staff used secure messaging to actively engage patients.

Overall, research suggests that PHRs can improve care, particularly for those with chronic conditions. These improvements do not occur in isolation, and possibly reflect the integration of PHR functions into the daily work of nurses, providers, pharmacists, and other clinical staff. This assimilation is certain to accelerate in the coming years, with greater interest in use of patient-facing technologies and adoption of a PCMH model of care. "Medical Home" or PCMH is an enhanced model of primary care that puts the patients at the center of care by ensuring timely access, using technology to improve communication and information exchange, and using team-based care to coordinate care and effectively meet patients' needs (Berenson et al. 2008). Dissemination of medical home practices puts PHRs firmly in the center of quality, patient-centered care.

To ensure quality across the patient population, it will be critical to minimize disparities in PHR use and benefit. There is a concern that individuals with lower levels of education, literacy, or numeracy may have limited participation in PHRs, even among those having Internet access (Roblin et al. 2009).

Among those with chronic disease, disabilities may play a role in the capacity to use technology. Vigilant efforts are needed to mitigate this digital divide. First, development of PHRs and their functionality must attend to a user-centered design approach, ensuring testing and usability across a wide spectrum of education and health literacy levels. Second, interfaces can be created that improve usability, including variable font sizes, audio-assisted functions, and other techniques to enhance access. Last, extra effort must be made to promote PHRs for all potential users, with particular targeting for older individuals, those having lower levels of education, and rural residents.

PHRS AND TRANSFORMATION OF CARE

Healthcare has not kept pace with the digital revolution. Care delivery continues to be based on individual patients having face-to-face encounters with individual physicians or allied health professionals in a brick-and-mortar clinic space. Clinical workflows and payment models remain embedded in and dependent upon these in-person visits. Further, many health professionals continue to document by paper, and some are reluctant about using electronic records.

Yet it is a historic time, on the cusp of healthcare moving robustly into the digital age. How clinical information is collected, used, and exchanged is being transformed. Several factors are playing a role. In 2004, the U.S. government created the Office of the National Coordinator under Health and Human Services, setting a goal for most Americans to have EHRs by 2014 (Executive Order 13335, 2004). Surveys conducted by the National Center for Health Statistics showed that 48.3% of physicians now use full or partial EHR systems in their practice (Hsiao, Hing, Socey, & Cai 2010).

The American Recovery and Reinvestment Act (ARRA) of 2009 is stimulating adoption of EHR, offering incentives for Meaningful Use of electronic systems by eligible providers (Blumenthal 2009). In 2010, the Centers for Medicare & Medicaid Services (CMS) released the final rule on the definition of Meaningful Use. Referred to as *Stage 1* of the rule, CMS identifies three objectives for the first two years. While largely focusing on providers in this stage, 1 of 15 core objectives is "to provide patients with an electronic copy of their health information including diagnostic test results, problem list, medication lists and allergies."

The convergence of increasing EHR use and consumer demand for health information is poised to be a tipping point for integrating PHRs and patient portals into clinical care. The influence of **e-patients** and their impact on care delivery was heralded by Thomas Ferguson, MD, who since 1987 has focused on empowering consumers to use online resources and tools (Ferguson 1997, 1998). Ferguson, along with other pioneers including Gilles Frydman of *www.acor.org* (Association of Cancer Online Resources), studied and wrote about social networks to inform and support patients and achieve patient-clinician partnership toward better care (Ferguson 2000). An excerpt from the white paper, *e-Patients: How they can help us heal healthcare,* is shown in Box 16–1.

Services such as online medication refill, appointment scheduling, and secure e-mail will alter clinical workflows as they serve to enhance patient engagement. Such changes are part of a shift toward the delivery of care referred to as *participatory medicine*, or a "movement in which networked patients shift from being mere passengers to responsible drivers of their health, and in which providers encourage and value them as full partners" (Dyson 2009). As patients increasingly take advantage of virtual access to their personal health information, higher levels of patient engagement are certain to modify the patient-clinician relationship. PHRs offer significant promise to realize participatory care.

TOWARD A FUTURE OF NETWORKED CARE

The promise of eHealth and patient-facing HIT is to enhance the patient experience, improve health outcomes, and reduce healthcare costs. As healthcare journeys toward networked care, technology must meet the needs of patients and families. Consumer access to information will not replace the need for clinical experts in acute and ambulatory settings. HIT will supplement care provided by clinical teams and specialists, offering greater opportunities for patient self-care and "communities of care," such as condition-specific peer support and remote home monitoring.

What does a *future state* of patient-facing, networked personal health information systems look like? One way to envision this is to examine the types of services and information that

BOX 16–1   e-Patients: How They Can Help Us Heal Healthcare

Tom Ferguson and the e-patients Scholars Working Group. Whitepaper 2007.

"e-Patients are driving a healthcare revolution of major proportions."

"The old Industrial Age paradigm, in which health professionals were viewed as the exclusive source of medical knowledge and wisdom, is gradually giving way to the a new Information Age worldview in which patients, family caregivers and the systems and networks they create are increasingly seen as important healthcare resources."

"Something akin to a system upgrade in our thinking is needed—a new cultural operating system for healthcare in which e-patients can be recognized as a valuable new type of renewable resource, managing much of their own care, providing care for others, helping professionals improve the quality of their services, and participating in entirely new kinds of clinician-patient collaborations, patient-initiated research and self-managed care. Developing, refining and implementing this new open-source cultural operating system will be one of the principal challenges facing healthcare in the early decades of the 21st century. But difficult as this task may prove to be, it will pay remarkable dividends. For given the recognition and support they deserve, these new medical colleagues can help us find sustainable solutions to many of the seemingly intractable problems that now plague all modern healthcare systems."

http://e-patients.net/e-Patients_White_Paper.pdf

provide the greatest value for patients, families, and caregivers. Consumers, to get the best care and the best health, search for health information from health experts and from friends, families, and peers, or on their own. This has been the case long before the introduction of computers. With the advent of the Internet and "Health 2.0," patients, families, and caregivers can access expert information and the "community at large." Figure 16–10 shows a simple categorization of the types of functions to which a future consumer will be connected.

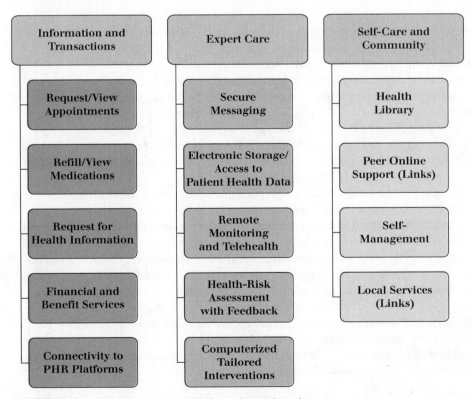

FIGURE 16–10 • Patient-facing health information and services

Source: Ahern, D. K., Woods, S. S., Lightowler, M. C., Finley, S., & Houston, T. K. (2011). Promise of and potential for patient-facing technologies to enable meaningful use. *American Journal of Preventive Medicine, 40* (Issue 5, Supplement 2), S162–S172.

In terms of health information services, people conduct transactions (such as request a refill) or obtain information—either from an expert or from the community. Other services can include peer-support, such as condition-specific social networking sites (PatientsLikeMe). Connecting patients to tailored, interactive Web-based interventions for chronic conditions brings opportunity to deliver evidence-based services shown to improve health (Jimison et al. 2008). An ideal PHR system would allow a user to readily connect to take advantage of all these functions and services. It is unlikely that a single PHR will provide all these services. Yet moving toward a "network of networks" will allow consumers and caregivers to avail themselves of valuable tools.

PHR Adoption

Evidence continues to mount that consumer HIT such as PHRs increases patient satisfaction and, in some instances, improves self-care and health outcomes (Halamka et al. 2008). Clinicians are likely to benefit from shared records by gaining knowledge about patients and enhancing therapeutic alliances. Implicit in these statements are several assumptions. First, patients and caregivers will proactively and purposefully seek PHRs to improve health. Second, they will have the capacity to use these tools and information as intended. Third, there will be usage of PHRs at a level sufficient to achieve real gains. Finally, clinicians and professionals will seamlessly integrate PHRs into their workflow, in a manner that does not impact quality or clinical performance. Therefore, successful adoption of PHRs and Meaningful Use can be realized only if certain barriers are mitigated or overcome. Specific potential barriers to PHR use are described here briefly, along with possible strategies that can improve patient adoption.

- *Access.* Ability to connect to the Internet is essential. Many rural communities remain "unwired." While this barrier goes beyond the scope of medical care, patients can be asked about access through friends, family members, work, and libraries. Some large health systems such as the VA provide computer access in libraries.
- *Awareness.* Patients and caregivers must know about PHR tools and understand their value. Promotion and marketing are important, including word of mouth, social networking, and clinician endorsement. Dedicated staff can help design promotional materials, demonstrating tools and disseminating through a variety of channels.
- *Usability.* How easy is the application to use? PHR systems that utilized, during their development, a user-centered design process, conducted usability testing, and were modified on user input can have greater ease of use and be more intuitive.
- *eHealth literacy.* Patients bring a wide variation in their capacity to use information technology. Those having lower levels of literacy and Internet abilities are likely to have greater challenges in using the PHR as intended. Ensuring a high level of usability, including easy navigation, simple functionality, and readability can enhance willingness and ability to use the PHR.
- *Meaningful Use.* PHR usage will be dependent upon users' perception of benefit. Patients must perceive that PHRs will be relevant to their health and beneficial to their lives. Incorporating features such as secure messaging, laboratory results, appointment, and medication requests will be most valuable to patient and caregivers.
- *Clinical integration.* Nurses, physicians, and other professionals providing care have an important role in the successful deployment and adoption of PHRs. As patients will continue to see health professionals as a source of expert information, encouraging and demonstrating use of these tools to patients and families will be important.

Emerging Issues

As use of HIT expands, a number of issues will likely play a role in PHR adoption and outcomes. A few are discussed briefly.

Change in Clinical Work Day-to-day clinical work will be modified by patient-facing functions that weave into the fabric of care delivery such as secure messaging and patient home monitoring. Some changes will create efficiencies, and some will not. Change is challenging in general, and some are certain to be welcomed more than others. Yet certain types of novel communication can potentially empower workers and improve job satisfaction. Secure messaging offers a new role and scope of practice for members of a healthcare team. Proactive use of messaging to patients can play an important role in care management, such as monitoring anticoagulation, heart failure, diabetes, and other chronic conditions. Nurse care managers and nurse specialists can use electronic tools to integrate patient self-monitoring into care in a wide variety of settings and specialties. Finding best practices and processes to deliver timely, personalized care will be an ongoing need for some time to come.

Patients—A Source of Data As PHRs and home monitoring functions expand, issues related to patients *as source of data and information* will emerge. While patient-centered care is the goal, concerns arise about (a) patients as accurate suppliers of data and (b) responsibility of data review. In-person encounters do not always lead to complete and accurate information in the record. Patients may hesitate to disclose information. Answers may reflect what patients feel clinicians care to know. As visits get shorter, discussions are limited. In addition, documentation may not incorporate all discussed in the visit. Evidence shows collecting data from patients electronically can be successful, sometimes more so than in-person. Compared to paper-based data collection, computerized data collection can be superior in quality and comprehensiveness (Lauteslager, Brouwe, Mohrs, Bindels, & Grundmeijer 2002; Lee & Kavanaugh 2007; VanDenKerKhof, Goldstein, Blaine, & Rimmer 2005; Waruru, Nduati, & Tylleskar 2005). Computerized screening can be particularly effective for sensitive issues such as substance use and sexual behaviors (Aiello et al. 2006; Turner et al. 1998). Therefore, patient data entry using PHRs could be valuable, particularly for those less likely to receive routine care—such as teenagers and young adults. A leader is Group Health, where members are asked to complete a health profile through *MyGroupHealth* PHR, and data is integrated into the EHR. Patients are given health summaries and reminders of recommended care, and healthcare teams can view this information in the electronic record, flagged as patient-entered data (Group Health Cooperative, personal communication).

Who is responsible for viewing and responding to the data? This is a second issue with patient-sourced data. One view is expressed by Paul Tang, who wrote (Tang et al. 2006):

> Although data provided by patients can inform providers' decision-making, not all patient-supplied data will do so, and the volume of "clinically irrelevant" information in patients' PHRs become overwhelming to review. While providers [use] the most recent blood glucose measurement in a diabetic's logbook, reviewing daily activities, detailed diet, exercise and sleep patterns and transient symptoms to find one crucial item of information becomes problematic.

Underlying this view are concerns about sufficient resources and liability. In effect, data should be collected only if there are adequate professional resources to review the information and explicit guidelines and policies for decision making related to clinically relevant data needing attention.

Clearly there is great opportunity to systematically integrate patient-entered information and self-monitoring data into clinical information systems. Biometric devices can automate data collection, providing valuable information on care management of chronic conditions. Using these tools can also enhance patient competency in self-care. Computerized screening is effective and can impact health promotion. The issue is not whether patients should submit information electronically. Key questions are *what* information will add value and improve patient outcomes and *how* health professionals can successfully integrate patient-sourced data into care delivery. The need for rigorous study will continue.

Consumer Protection of Privacy While the majority of adults in the United States would like access to their personal health information, there are public concerns about privacy of data and unauthorized disclosure (Markle Foundation 2006). These concerns may even have an effect on information patients share with clinicians (Bagchi, Moreno, & af Ursin 2007). The Privacy Rule of the HIPAA (U.S. Department of Health and Human Services n.d.) regulated the use and disclosure of personal health information held by "Covered Entities," including which are hospitals, health plans, and medical and other practices. A PHR that is tethered to an EHR or clinical information system and maintained by a health system or provider falls under HIPAA protections as a Covered Entity. A provider with a PHR from a commercial vendor, but maintaining the PHR for patients, has its content still considered protected health information.

These policies—and their limitations—become more critical in a vision of networked PHRs (Figure 16–4). HIPAA applies only to Covered Entities, and many PHRs and Consumer Access Services are not covered by the rule. If a provider contracts with a third party (e.g., Microsoft HealthVault or Google Health) to offer a PHR to patients, a Business Associate Agreement must be created that limits the third party's disclosure of health information. If an information breach occurs, the accountability may rest on the provider rather than on the vendor, depending upon "what the provider knew" prior to the breach. These policies and relationships are complicated and challenging to comprehend even among providers; understanding by consumers is certain to be even more difficult. At this point, details related to responsibility and liability continue to unfold.

Many state and regional Health Information Exchanges are using or planning to use a Consumer Access Service that is neither a Covered Entity nor a Business Associate of a Covered Entity. Personal health information can be exchanged if it comes from a provider, hospital, or laboratory (Covered Entity), in two ways. First, shown in Figure 16–11A, a consumer can authorize the information to be released (e.g., from a pharmacy) from a Covered Entity to the Consumer Access Service (noncovered). In Figure 16–11B, a consumer obtains a copy of health

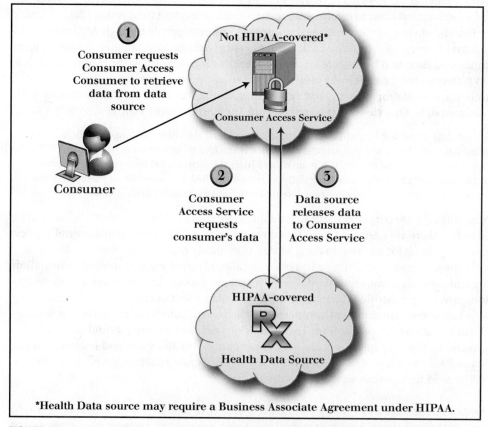

FIGURE 16–11A • Consumer authorizes data exchange from a covered to a noncovered entity

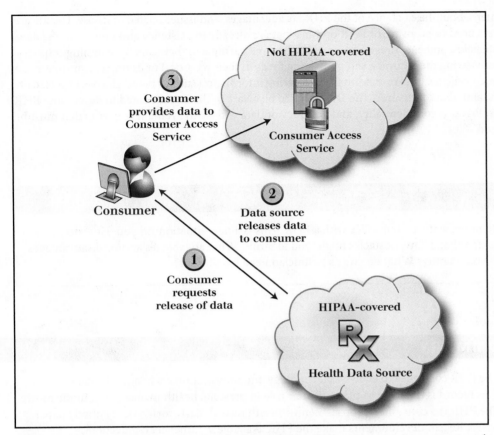

FIGURE 16–11B • Consumer requests data from a covered entity, provides copy to a non-covered entity

records directly from a Covered Entity, and then agrees to supply the data to the Consumer Access Service (noncovered). In both, the consumer plays a pivotal role in data exchange.

Consumers are increasingly positioned to benefit from the use of HIT. With healthcare's focus on delivering patient-centered, high-quality care that enhances the patient experience, PHRs play a critically important role. Access to health information including laboratory test results and after-visit summaries and online services such as appointment requests and medication refills are PHR functions that patient users frequently access. Secure messaging with healthcare team members offers a high level of patient access and care coordination in a personalized, timely manner. Health professionals' perception of online patient communication is generally positive; however, optimal integration into clinical workflow remains a challenge until virtual care is embraced as a mainstream model of care delivery. Younger consumers are more technology-savvy than ever, making online services increasingly relevant. Internet access is lower among older adults and those residing in rural areas; therefore ensuring PHR access and usage across patient populations remains important. PHRs will play a central role in networked health information and exchange. Policies related to protection of privacy continue to develop. A consumer-oriented approach is critical to ensure that people understand and accept both the opportunities as well as the risks.

FUTURE DIRECTIONS

The PHR will play an important role in helping to transform the healthcare delivery system as consumers make the shift to partners in care. The Informatics Nurse Specialist (INS) will facilitate the adoption and use of the PHR by educating other healthcare professionals and healthcare consumers about the existence of the PHR, its advantages, and issues related to its use. Healthcare providers need to be aware of PHR options that are already in existence and how to access data, populate fields, and encourage consumers to become partners in their care by assuming responsibility for viewing the accuracy and populating fields in their records. For example, consumers can manage chronic healthcare conditions by entering information such as blood glucose results, daily weights, and blood pressures. The INS needs to be aware of the issues related to developing PHR options. Privacy, confidentiality, and accuracy of data will always remain concerns that must be addressed.

CASE STUDY EXERCISE

A patient presents to your office with a PHR. This is a new situation for you. How do you access it? What, if any, obstacles might you identify? What advantages and/or disadvantages might you identify? What do you as a clinician need to consider?

SUMMARY

- The PHR continues to evolve as technology and information exchange advances.
- This record is expected to play a greater role in personal health management in the future.
- The PHR is a consumer-centric, lifetime health record. Early forms were entirely paper-based. Recent developments make the PHR available via Internet connections.
- Information in the PHR may be supplied from the individual, healthcare providers, pharmacies, third-party payers, therapists, laboratory tests, and radiology results, as well as other information deemed appropriate by the individual such as exercise routines and herbal supplements.
- The concept behind the PHR is that access and information are controlled by the consumer.
- Patients may use PHRs to better manage health conditions by entering their results for their own use as well as review by their providers.
- PHRs may also provide a means to verify and obtain authorization for treatment and to determine claim status.
- Portability, privacy, and accuracy of data populated by providers or payers constitute some of the big concerns related to PHR use.
- PHRs provide the potential to improve consumer health via the ability to generate reminders for appointments, blood tests, prescription refills, results, and wellness reminders.

REFERENCES

Ahern, D. K., Woods, S. S., Lightowler, M. C., Finley, S., & Houston, T. K. (2011). Promise of and potential for patient-facing technologies to enable meaningful use. *American Journal of Preventive Medicine, 40*, S162–S172.

Aiello, E. J., Taplin, S., Reid, R., Hobbs, M., Seger, D., Kamel, H., . . . Ballard-Barbash, R. (2006). In a randomized controlled trial, patients preferred electronic data collection of breast cancer risk factor information in a mammography setting. *Journal of Clinical Epidemiology, 59*, 77.

Bagchi, A., Moreno, L., & af Ursin, R. (2007, April). *Considerations in designing personal health records for underserved populations.* Mathematica Policy Research Issue Brief. Retrieved from http://www.mathematica-mpr.com/publications/pdfs/hlthcaredisparib1.pdf

Baldwin, F. D. (2002). The doctor is in. *Healthcare Informatics, 19*, 44–48.

Berenson, R. A., Hammons, T., Gans, D. N., Zuckerman, S., Merrell, K., Underwood, W. S., & Williams, A. F. (2008). A house is not a home: Keeping patients at the center of practice redesign. *Health Affairs (Millwood), 27*(5), 1219–1230.

Bergmo, T. S., Kummervold, P. E., Gammon, D., & Dahl, L. B. (2005). Electronic patient-provider communication: Will it offset office visits and telephone consultations in primary care? *International Journal of Medical Informatics, 74*(9), 705–710.

Blumenthal, D. (2009). Stimulating the adoption of health information technology. *New England Journal of Medicine, 360*(15), 1477–1479.

Boukus, E. R., Grossman, J. M., & O'Malley, A. S. (2010, October). *Physicians slow to e-mail routinely with patients. Center for Studying Health System Change* (Issue Brief No. 134). Retrieved from http://www.hschange.com/CONTENT/1156/#ib7

Bright, B. (2007, November 29). Benefits of EMRs seen as outweighing privacy risks. *Wall Street Journal Online.* Retrieved from http://www.medivoicerx.com/files/news/WSJ-Harris_Poll-eRx_11.29.07.pdf

Burke, R. P., Rossi, A. F., Wilner, B. R., Hannan, R. L., Zabinsky, J. A., & White, J. A. (2010). Transforming patient and family access to medical information: Utilisation patterns of a patient-accessible electronic health record. *Cardiology in the Young, 20*(5), 477–484.

Byrne, J. M., Elliott, S., & Firek, A. (2009). Initial experience with patient-clinician secure messaging at a VA medical center. *Journal of the American Medical Informatics Association, 16*(2), 267–270.

California HealthCare Foundation. (2010, April 13). *Consumers and health information technology: A national survey.* Retrieved from http://www.chcf.org/~/media/Files/PDF/C/PDF%20ConsumersHealthInfoTechnologyNationalSurvey.pdf

Center for Information Technology Leadership. (2008). *The value of personal health records, Healthcare Information and Management System Society.* Retrieved from http://tigerphr.pbworks.com/f/CITL_PHR_Report.pdf

Chen, C., Garrido, T., Chock, D., Okawa, G., & Liang, L. (2009). The Kaiser Permanente electronic health record: Transforming and streamlining modalities of care. *Health Affairs (Millwood), 28*(2), 323–333.

Connecting for Health Common Framework for Networked Personal Health Information. (2008). *Markle foundation.* Retrieved from http://www.markle.org/sites/default/files/Overview_Consumers.pdf

Delbanco, T., Walker, J., Darer, J. D., Elmore, J. G., Feldman, H. J., Leveille, S. G., . . . Weber, V. D. (2010). Open notes: Doctors and patients signing on. *Annals of Internal Medicine, 153*(2), 121–125.

Detmer, D., Bloomrosen, M., Raymond, B., & Tang, P. (2008). Integrated personal health records: Transformative tools for consumer-centric care. *BMC Medical Informatics Decision Making, 6*, 45.

Dyson, E. (2009). Why participatory medicine? *Journal of Participatory Medicine, 1*, e1. Retrieved from http://www.jopm.org/opinion/editorials/2009/10/21/why-participatory-medicine

Executive Order 13335. (2004, April 27). Incentives for the use of health information technology and establishing the position of the national health information technology coordinator. *Federal Register, 69*(84), 24059–24061. Retrieved from http://edocket.access.gpo.gov/2004/pdf/04-10024.pdf

Ferguson, T. (1997). Health online and the empowered medical consumer. *Joint Commission Journal Quality Improvement, 23*(5), 251–257.

Ferguson, T. (1998). Digital doctoring: Opportunities and challenges in electronic patient-physician communication. *Journal of the American Medical Association, 280*(15), 1361–1362.

Ferguson, T. (2000). Online patient-helpers and physicians working together: A new partnership for high quality health care. *British Medical Journal, 321*(7269), 1129–1132.

Fioriglio, G., & Szolovits, P. (2005). Copy fees and patients' rights to obtain a copy of their medical records: From law to reality. *American Medical Informatics Association Annual Symposium Proceedings, 251–255.*

Fox, S. (2004). *Older Americans and the Internet. Pew Internet & American life project.* Retrieved from http://www.pewinternet.org/Reports/2004/Older-Americans-and-the-Internet.aspx

Gearon, C., Barret, M., Brennan, P., Kibbe, D., Lansky, D., Nobel, J., & Sands, D. (2007, June). *Perspectives on the future of personal health records.* California Health Care Foundation. Retrieved from http://www.chcf.org/publications/2007/06/perspectives-on-the-future-of-personal-health-records

Green, B. B., Cook, A. J., Ralston, J. D., Fishman, P. A., Catz, S. L., & Carlson, J. (2008). Effectiveness of home blood pressure monitoring, web communication, and pharmacist care on hypertension control: A randomized controlled trial. *Journal of the American Medical Association, 299*(24), 2857–2867.

Greenfield, S., Kaplan, S. H., Ware, J. E., Martin, Y. E., & Frank, H. L. (1988). Patients' participation in medical care: Effects on blood sugar control and quality of life in diabetes. *Journal of General Internal Medicine, 3*(5), 448–457.

Grossman, J. M., Zayas-Cabán, T., & Kemper, N. (2009). Information gap: Can health insurer personal health records meet patients' and physicians' needs? *Health Affairs (Millwood), 28*(2), 377–389.

Halamka, J. D., Mandl, K. D., & Tang, P. C. (2008). Early experiences with personal health records. *Journal of the American Medical Informatics Association, 15*(1), 1–7.

Harris, L. T., Haneuse, S. J., Martin, D. P., & Ralston, J. D. (2009). Diabetes quality of care and outpatient utilization associated with electronic patient-provider messaging: A cross-sectional analysis. *Diabetes Care, 32*(7), 1182–1187.

Houston, T. K. (2004). Experiences of patients who were early adopters of electronic communication with their physician: Satisfaction, benefits, and concerns. *American Journal of Managed Care, 10*(9), 601–608.

Hsiao, C. J., Hing, E., Socey, T. C., & Cai, B. (2010, December). Electronic medical record/electronic health record systems of office-based physicians: United States, 2009 and preliminary 2010 state estimates. *National Center for Health Statistics Health e-stat.* Retrieved from http://www.cdc.gov/nchs/data/hestat/emr_ehr_09/emr_ehr_09.pdf

Institute of Medicine. (2001). *Crossing the quality chasm: A new health system for the 21st century.* Washington, DC: National Academies Press.

Jimison, H., Gorman, P., Woods, S., Nygren, P., Walker, M., Norris, S., & Hersh, W. (2008). *Barriers and drivers of health information technology use for the elderly, chronically ill, and underserved.* Rockville, MD: Agency for Healthcare Research and Quality, US DHHS. Contract No. 290-02-0024.

Jones, D. A., Shipman, J. P., Plaut, D. A., & Selden, C. R. (2010). Characteristics of personal health records: Findings of the medical library association/national library of medicine joint electronic personal health record task force. *Journal of the Medical Library Association, 98*(3), 243–249.

Kahn, J. S., Aulakh, V., & Bosworth, A. (2009). What it takes: Characteristics of the ideal personal health record. *Health Affairs (Millwood), 28*(2), 369–376.

Kaiser Permanente HealthConnect Electronic Health Record. (2011). *Kaiser Permanente news.* Retrieved from http://xnet.kp.org/newscenter/aboutkp/healthconnect/index.html

Katz, S. J., Moyer, C. A., Cox, D. T., & Stern, D. T. (2003). Effect of a triage-based E-mail system on clinic resource use and patient and physician satisfaction in primary care: A randomized controlled trial. *Journal of General Internal Medicine, 18*(9), 736–744.

Kittler, A. F., Carlson, G. L., Harris, C., Lippincott, M., Pizziferri, L., Volk, L. A., . . . Bates, D. W. (2004). Primary care physician attitudes towards using a secure web-based portal designed to facilitate electronic communication with patients. *Informatics in Primary Care, 12*(3), 129–138.

Lauteslager, M., Brouwe, H. J., Mohrs, J., Bindels, P. J. E., & Grundmeijer, H. G. L. M. (2002). The patient as a source to improve the medical record. *Family Practice, 19*, 167–171.

Lee, S. J., & Kavanaugh, L. (2007). Electronic and computer-generated patient questionnaires in standard care. *Best Practice & Research in Clinical Rheumatology, 21*, 637–647.

Ley, P., Bradshaw, P. W., Eaves, D., & Walker, C. M. (1973). A method for increasing patients' recall of information presented by doctors. *Psychological Medicine, 3*(2), 217–220.

Liederman, E. M., Lee, J. C., Baquero, V. H., & Seites, P. G. (2005). Patient-physician web messaging: The impact on message volume and satisfaction. *Journal of General Internal Medicine, 20*, 52–57.

Mandl, K. D., Szolovits, P., & Kohane, I. S. (2001). Public standards and patients' control: How to keep electronic medical records accessible but private. *British Medical Journal, 322*(7281), 283–287.

Markle Foundation. (2006). *Survey finds Americans want electronic personal health information to improve own health care.* Retrieved from http://www.markle.org/publications/1214-survey-finds-americans-want-electronic-personal-health-information-improve-own-hea

Markle Foundation Connecting for Health. (2003, July 1). *The Personal Health Working Group Final Report.* Retrieved from http://www.providersedge.com/ehdocs/ehr_articles/The_Personal_Health_Working_Group_Final_Report.pdf

Miller, H., Bandenbosch, B., Ivanov, D., & Black, P. (2007). Determinants of personal health record use. *Journal of Health Information Management, 21*, 44–48.

Muller, D., Logan, J., Dorr, D., & Mosen, D. (2009). The effectiveness of a secure email reminder system for colorectal cancer screening. *American Medical Informatics Association Annual Symposium Proceedings, 14*, 457–461.

Nazi, K. M. (2010). Veterans' voices: Use of the American customer satisfaction index (ACSI) survey to identify my HealtheVet personal health record users' characteristics, needs, and preferences. *Journal of the American Medical Informatics Association, 17*(2), 203–211.

Nazi, K. M., & Woods, S. S. (2008, November). My HealtheVet PHR: A description of users and patient portal use. *American Medical Informatics Association Annual Symposium Proceedings, 6*, 1182.

Pagliari, C., Detmer, D., & Singleton, P. (2007). Potential of electronic personal health records. *British Medical Journal, 335*(7615), 330–333.

Pyper, C., Amery, J., Watson, M., & Crook, C. (2004). Patients' experiences when accessing their on-line electronic patient records in primary care. *British Journal of General Practice, 54*(498), 38–43.

Ralston, J. D., Carrell, D., Reid, R., Anderson, M., Moran, M., & Hereford, J. (2007). Patient web services integrated with a shared medical record: Patient use and satisfaction. *Journal of the American Medical Informatics Association, 14*(6), 798–806.

Ralston, J. D., Coleman, K., Reid, R. J., Handley, M. R., & Larson, E. B. (2010). Patient experience should be part of meaningful-use criteria. *Health Affairs, 29*(4), 607–613.

Ralston, J. D., Hirsch, I. B., Hoath, J., Mullen, M., Cheadle, A., & Goldberg, H. I. (2009a). Web-based collaborative care for type 2 diabetes: A pilot randomized trial. *Diabetes Care, 32*(2), 234–239.

Ralston, J. D., Rutter, C. M., Carrell, D., Hecht, J., Rubanowice, D., & Simon, G. E. (2009b). Patient use of secure electronic messaging within a shared medical record: A cross-sectional study. *Journal of General Internal Medicine, 24*, 349–355.

Roblin, D. W., Houston, T. K., Allison, J. J., Joski, P. J., & Becker, E. R. (2009). Disparities in use of a personal health record in a managed care organization. *Journal of the American Medical Informatics Association, 16*(5), 683–689.

Rogers, E. M. (2003). *Diffusion of innovations* (5th ed., Vol. xxi, p. 551). New York: Free Press.

Sands, D. Z., & Halamka, J. D. (2004). PatientSite: Patient centered communication, services, and access to information. In R. Nelson & M. J. Ball (Eds.), *Consumer informatics: Applications and strategies in cyber health care.* New York: Springer.

Sciamanna, C. N., Rogers, M. L., Shenassa, E. D., & Houston, T. K. (2007). Patient access to U.S. physicians who conduct internet or e-mail consults. *Journal of General Internal Medicine, 22*(3), 378–381.

Simons, W. W., Mandl, K. D., & Kohane, I. S. (2005). Model formulation: The PING personally controlled electronic medical record system: Technical architecture. *Journal of the American Medical Informatics Association, 12*, 47–54.

Swartz, S. H., Cowan, T. M., & Batista, I. A. (2004). Using claims data to examine patients using practice-based internet communication: Is there a clinical digital divide? *Journal of Medical Internet Research, 6*(1), e1.

Tang, P. C., Ash, J. S., Bates, D. W., & Overhage, J. M. (2006). Personal health records: Definitions, benefits and strategies for overcoming barriers to adoption. *Journal of the American Medical Informatics Association, 13*, 121–126.

Tang, P. C., Black, W., Buchanan, J., Young, C. Y., Hooper, D., Lane, S. R., . . . Turnbull, J. R. (2003). PAMFOnline: Integrating EHealth with an electronic medical record system. *American Medical Informatics Association Annual Symposium Proceedings*, 644–648.

Tang, P. C., & Lee, T. H. (2009). Your doctor's office or the internet? Two paths to personal health records. *New England Journal of Medicine, 360*(13), 1276–1278.

Teenagers' access to confidential reproductive health services. (2005, November). *The Guttmacher Report on Public Policy* (Volume 8, Number 4). Retrieved from http://www.guttmacher.org/pubs/tgr/08/4/gr080406.html

Turner, C. F., Ku, L., Rogers, S. M., Lindberg, L. D., Pleck, J. L., & Sonenstein, F. L. (1998). Adolescent sexual behavior, drug use, and violence: Increased reporting with computer survey technology. *Science, 280,* 867–873.

U.S. Department of Health and Human Services (DHHS). (n.d.). *Health information privacy: The privacy rule.* Retrieved from http://www.hhs.gov/ocr/privacy/hipaa/administrative/privacyrule/index.html

VanDenKerKhof, E. G., Goldstein, D. H., Blaine, W. C., & Rimmer, M. J. (2005). A comparison of paper with electronic patient-completed questionnaires in a preoperative clinic. *Anesthesia & Analgesia, 101,* 1075–1080.

Vincent, A., Kaelber, D. C., Pan, E., Shah, S., Johnston, D., & Middleton, B. (2008). A patient-centric taxonomy for personal health records (PHRs). *American Medical Informatics Association Symposium Proceedings, 6,* 763–767. Retrieved from http://www.ncbi.nlm.nih.gov/pmc/articles/PMC2656090/?ool=pubmed

Wagner, E. H., Austin, B. T., & Von Korff, M. (1996). Organizing care for patients with chronic illness. *Milbank Quarterly, 74*(4), 511–544.

Waruru, A. K., Nduati, R., & Tylleskar, T. (2005). Audio computer-assisted self-interviewing may avert socially desirable responses about infant feeding in the context of HIV. *BMC Med Informatics Decision Making, 5,* 24.

Weingart, S. N., Rind, D., Tofias, Z., & Sands, D. Z. (2006). Who uses the patient internet portal? The PatientSite experience. *Journal of the American Medical Informatics Association, 13*(1), 91–95.

Weppner, W. G., Ralston, J. D., Koepsell, T. D., Grothaus, L. C., Reid, R. J., Jordan, L., & Larson, E. B. (2010). Use of a shared medical record with secure messaging by older patients with diabetes. *Diabetes Care, 33*(11), 2314–2319.

Who's online—Internet demographics, Pew Internet & American Life Project. (2010, May). Retrieved from http://pewinternet.org/Trend-Data/Whos-Online.aspx

Wright, A., & Sittig, D. F. (2007). Encryption characteristics of two USB-based personal health record devices. *Journal of the American Medical Informatics Association, 14*(4), 397–399.

Zhou, Y. Y., Garrido, T., Chin, H. L., Wiesenthal, A. M., & Liang, L. L. (2007). Patient access to an electronic health record with secure messaging: Impact on primary care utilization. *American Journal of Managed Care, 13*(7), 418–424.

Zhou, Y. Y., Kanter, M. H., Wang, J. J., & Garrido, T. (2010). Improved quality at Kaiser permanente through e-mail between physicians and patients. *Health Affairs (Millwood), 29*(7), 1370–1375.

Zickmund, S. L., Hess, R., Bryce, C. L., McTigue, K., Olshansky, E., Fitzgerald, K., & Fischer, G. S. (2008). Interest in the use of computerized patient portals: Role of the provider-patient relationship. *Journal of General Internal Medicine, 23*(Suppl. 1), 20–26.

Zickuhr, K. (2010, December 16). *Generations 2010. Pew Internet & American Life Project.* Retrieved from http://www.pewinternet.org/Reports/2010/Generations-2010.aspx

CHAPTER 17

Health Information Exchanges

After completing this chapter, you should be able to:

1. Define the concept of *health information exchanges*.

2. Discuss key factors in the infrastructure of an HIE.

3. Compare and contrast the different HIE models for their respective advantages and disadvantages.

4. Describe obstacles to HIE development and sustaining operation.

5. Describe the current status of the national health information network and HIEs in the United States.

6. Differentiate between clinical data networks and HIEs.

7. Describe the ways HIEs will impact healthcare delivery in the future.

A social networking society shares details to inform a select community interested in knowing the same information. Today, healthcare institutions and agencies strive to share more and more individual health information to make cost-effective and efficient decisions. The information can be stored within comprehensive, longitudinal electronic health records (EHRs). These repositories of health information hold allergy and medication profiles, problem lists, laboratory results, radiology images and interpretations, treatment plans for care, and much more. Repositories of information are extracted and held within centralized infrastructures for information exchange by state or regional organizations or within decentralized care delivery systems. The **health information exchange (HIE)** is defined as the electronic movement of health-related information among organizations according to nationally recognized standards (DHHS 2008, p. 6). The HIE is described as the process within a state health information organization or a regional health information organization (RHIO). The organization provides oversight to authorize the location of health information and the secure transfer and reuse of that health information electronically. The RHIO is defined as a health information organization that brings together healthcare stakeholders within a defined geographic area and governs HIE among them for the purpose of improving health and care in that community (DHHS 2008, p. 6). The HIE requires the exchange of health-related information according to nationally recognized standards to link into the **National Health Information Network (NHIN)**. The NHIN provides a standardized, secure, and confidential way to link information systems together for authorized users to share reliable health-related information (DHHS 2008, p. 27). In September 2010, the Office of the National Coordinator (2010) along with the Health Information Technology Standards Committee (HITSC 2010) proposed a standards and interoperability framework with principles and processes for the NHIN. The framework for the NHIN encompasses standards and practice and services development with functional requirements for technologies, laws, and policies for harmonization of core concepts and references. The activities include programs of tools and services to guide implementation that once completed will allow interoperable exchange of information (HIMSS 2009). The NHIN was first envisioned more than a decade ago.

A HIE infrastructure is a process for bidirectional sharing of patient health-related information among primary providers (nurse practitioners, physicians, and physician assistants), consulting specialists, hospitals, ambulatory centers, nursing homes, dentists, audiologists, optometrists, and occupational and school health professionals. Optimally each citizen contributes to the collection of health information. The EHR and personal health record (PHR) are tools that will provide background information on individual abilities and disabilities (e.g., vision, hearing, and mobility). The records will need to include common elements such as immunization status, allergies (foods, environment, and medications), values (preferences, and cultural and religious beliefs), social habits (alcohol or tobacco use), family history, advance directives, and insurance coverage or non-coverage that support decisions. The health record is not just for medical conditions or disease history but also for the patients' functional health patterns and health enhancement needs. A visit to the primary care or urgent care clinic allows providers to access information through a record locator application to obtain a patient's allergies or past history. This past health information once validated by a clinician helps ensure appropriate selection of interventions or medications for safe care.

KEY FACTORS

Health information exchanges can be useful for more than patient care and the uses are described at four levels (Proctor, Reid, Compton, Grossman, & Fanjiang 2005):

1. An individual level for care to enhance personal health outcomes
2. A professional level for clinical decision making to diagnose, plan interventions and surveillance, coordinate care, and evaluate patient outcomes

3. An agency/organization level for managing operations and fiscal resources and monitoring processes for quality and continuous improvement

4. A public health and national level for accreditation and regulatory bodies to evaluate population health and safety and recommend changes in policy

To accomplish exchanges for these four levels, an HIE infrastructure requires not only technology but an organizing structure for processes. The organizing structure establishes secure application and rules of operation, technical and content standardization for interoperable exchanges among entities, and outlines the use cases and workflow to obtain meaningful information use across the four levels. There are 11 key factors that are indispensable prerequisites to consider for the HIE organizing infrastructure (Iowa E-Health 2010).

First, data storage is necessary to enable the ability to aggregate data from disparate sources. Large health systems are often well positioned to store and share patient-protected information within secure structures with private access. This is not the case for many small clinics, community centers, schools, and occupational health staff for small businesses that need data storage to allow access to their health-related information for sharing when the agency closes on evenings and weekends. A central repository can temporarily hold information from small providers as it is collected for electronic medical or health record applications. This repository may also store data to serve as a core component for public health use of data registries for birth certificates, immunizations, work-related injuries, cancer, diabetes, trauma, or for monitoring communicable illnesses. The infrastructure for data storage may be consolidated with a centralized cooperative central data repository to push and pull data. The infrastructure may be decentralized or federated with access to information through multiple health systems. Finally, the HIE may be a hybrid infrastructure, which is a combination of the consolidated and federated models (CHPR 2009). A hybrid infrastructure model enables the access and exchange of data stored in existing provider networks and also through a central data repository maintained for smaller providers who would not be able to maintain 24/7 services for HIE access.

The second necessary factor for HIE process is a master person index (MPI). The MPI is a standard person identifier code to uniquely identify an individual and permit the correlation process to match the person's data from a variety of different sources of health providers (e.g., clinics, hospitals, pharmacies, nursing homes). Health systems often use enterprise-wide MPI applications and processes to maintain only one EHR for a person across many organizations within the system. When the MPI is not used or unknown for a patient, an algorithm of multiple identifiers (name, birth date, address, etc.) will need to be used to make a match with multiple external records. The risk in not matching records with a level of certainty can lead to either using information from another person's record or result in duplicate collection for the person when not found.

The third factor for the HIE process is a record locator service used to access and find health information that matches the identified individual. Some describe the record locator services as a map or pointer to search and locate the information. The record locator can point to specific types of information (e.g., laboratory results; medications from pharmacies; allergies, or continuity of care document [CCD] which is a summary of patient care).

The methods of authentication, the fourth factor, are necessary to identify who is allowed to access health information through the HIE record locator services. This individual will find important information for decision making about patient care and can download the information into the local record or simply document the original source of data used for local decisions. Valid users will include clinical professionals and public health professionals who use the healthcare data for patient and populations and information technology (IT) professionals who audit user access. Patients potentially can have access in the future.

Along with authentication, the fifth factor is to provide authorization for these users. This authorization process can occur through the healthcare organizations which already manage employment and professional appointments. The organizations are positioned to facilitate role-based security for a clinician user to gain access to the record locator service for HIE. This authorization process would include the steps to train individuals to locate and obtain correct patient-level information during their daily workflow of care or for public reporting.

The sixth HIE factor is the security policies and procedures necessary to ensure a person's privacy and confidentiality. The procedures clarify when information requests and reuse require patient consent. The operating rules include establishing data agreements among organizations to retrieve and reuse patient information previously collected and managed within other healthcare organizations. Additionally, each state or regional HIE establishes procedures to allow persons either to opt in (allow data to be shared) or to opt out (data are not to be shared) of health information from being exchanged. Current RHIOs and HIE organizations will vary in their procedures. The Health Information Security and Privacy Collaborative provides a framework, toolkit, templates for data agreements, patient consents, requests for opt-in and opt-out, public education materials, and interstate and intrastate policies and legislation. Entities will exchange information across HIEs via an NHIN that sustains a culture of respect for personal confidentiality and the integrity and accuracy of the information. For the NHIN, common security and privacy standards are critical for all. Regional and state organizations need to apply broad restrictions on access to specific health information to protect the confidentiality of patient information while permitting exchanges for both public safety and statistics. In the future, after the development of common request standards, a person may have the opportunity to specify limits to access specific health information (e.g., genetic code) or allow information to be shared (e.g., healthcare systems or clinical research). The Health Information Protection and Accountability Act (HIPAA) guidelines expand on meeting needs for exchange of protected health information for continuous care while requiring informed consent and tracking disclosure of other requests for information.

A seventh factor involves auditing and logging of HIE activities, both intentional and unintentional connections and disconnections to network services. These networking activities will allow improved configuration, generate alerts, and notify users during connection. The HIE organizations will monitor and report on activity and response levels to track thresholds for technical stability and for any security violation.

An eighth factor to exchange health information is the criteria-based standards for data transport, messaging, transfer of care, and other use cases to specify content formats and workflows for use of health information (HITSP 2010). A referral for consultation, discharge summary, and CCD are examples of using standardized formats for content exchange. The content needs will be developed from recognized taxonomies and classifications, and organized using approved information models which inform the user through uniform structures in health information technology (HIT) (Haley, Sensmeier, & Brokel 2009; HITSP 2010). The harmonization of concepts and data normalization are necessary to both achieve a level of interoperability and reuse of information for multiple uses. Certification Commission for Health Information Technology (2011) is another regulating body that certifies HIT using the American National Standards Institute HITSP standards and evolving HITSC standards. The technical standards for transport of health information to and from electronic destinations include industry-recognized transport types (e.g., Internet Protocol Version 6) and the recipient's technical capability (e.g., broadband access, electronic routing of files, fax, print mail to the patient's home or residence). The Federal Communications Commission (FCC) collaborates with the DHHS to ensure the connectivity bandwidth for download and upload speed requirements (upload greater than 200 kilobytes per second [bps] for broadband connections to support rural settings with HIT). A number of carriers are now offering download speeds of 1.5 Mbps and 3.0 Mbps and upload speeds as high as 768 kbps. Currently, the rural telemedicine program is funding the establishment of 16 additional broadband telehealth networks. For example, the Iowa Rural Health

Telecommunications Program for Iowa, Nebraska, and South Dakota supports the creation of a new statewide broadband network that will link approximately 100 healthcare facilities at speeds of 1 gigabyte per second (FCC 2010). HIT users must conform in order to exchange information within the statewide HIE. Requirements include data storage configurations and processes (e.g., edge servers, Web services), frequency for making data available through the HIE, and disaster recovery.

The standards and interoperability will need to support a range of HIE services for participating providers, consumers, payers, and personnel in public safety. The ninth factor for the HIE is the scope of services provided. The scope of services is determined by functionality to enable sets of standard types of data to be exchanged through the HIE. These data are exchanged through HIE using a push or pull function that may be triggered by user-initiated events. An example could include a request for a CCD being pulled in anticipation of receiving a patient in transfer from one facility to another. Examples for push functions are a push of final pathology results to update previously sent preliminary results, a push of new prescriptions or the changes in medications prescribed to a pharmacy, or a push to notify public health department about the occurrence of communicable illness. See Box 17–1 for examples of possible HIE services.

A tenth factor for participation in an HIE process is knowledge of the workflow among providers and other users for patient and public health outcomes. The Secretary of Health and Human Services approved and the Office of the National Coordinator (ONC) for Health Information Technology within the Department of Health and Human Services (DHHS) published multiple standard requirements. Publications include the Health Information Technology Standards Panel (HITSP 2007–2010) Use Case standards under the American National Standards Institute, which outline types of data necessary for HIE workflows. Tool kits are often used to promote adoption in clinical practices.

BOX 17–1   Types of HIE Services Provider Directory

- Provider to provider messaging
- E-prescribing
- Results delivery (e.g., laboratory or diagnostic study results)
- Discharge summary
- Continuity of care document (CCR/CCD summary)
- Radiology images
- Quality performance reporting for purchasers or payers
- Consultation/referral
- Personal health records
- Clinical documentation
- Alerts to providers
- Enrollment or eligibility checking
- Tracking immunizations status within registry
- Clinical decision support
- Disease or chronic care management
- Quality improvement reporting for clinicians
- Syndromic surveillance for communicable diseases

A final key factor for this discussion is the portal for access to enable authorized users a way to sign on to the HIE. Different portals may be necessary to support different types of information exchanges (or HIE services) required for continuous care delivery, public reporting, and quality monitoring. An example is a provider portal aligned with the EHR to query a patient and retrieve and download the CCD and laboratory results, or make a referral to a physician or nurse specialist or therapist with key data included. For a consumer and patient, the portal would allow going to a PHR to input self-monitored blood glucose levels, daily weight, responses to a previsit questionnaire, or log respiratory symptoms in the case of chronic diseases.

In summary, the constituents who set up regional or state health information exchange infrastructures need to engage consumers, providers, and public health professionals from the community to design processes (Adams 2009; Perez 2009). Consumer focus groups and healthcare professionals feedback sessions are important methods to dialog with providers and consumers to test ideas and develop procedures for the HIE and privacy protections. The providers will likely store data captured about the patient within a repository external to the active EHR. This storage (e.g., cache with edge server) will allow others to find and pull data from healthcare providers on an "as-needed" basis without disrupting the clinicians' workflow. Statewide tool kits and communication plans help guide entities and consumers on how to work together to standardize content, find it, and use it with the technology to exchange information. The implication is to educate the population in the state to allow information to be stored and shared, and thus accessible. However, before the HIE can accomplish these goals, the EMR and EHR adoption must first be broadly implemented.

DRIVING FORCES

The steps to information exchange began in 1965 when the Medicare and Medicaid programs required accurate and timely information for reimbursement procedures (Staggers, Thompson, & Snyder-Halpern 2001). In 2001 the National Committee on Vital and Health Statistics called for the creation of a national health information infrastructure (Overhage, Evans, & Marchibroda 2005). The Medicare Modernization Act of 2003 included provisions to support HIE related to e-prescribing. Later in the year, the Agency for Healthcare Research and Quality (AHRQ 2010) proposed opportunities to fund research on HIE in RHIO projects in Utah (Root 2008), Indiana (Overhage 2009), Tennessee (Frisse 2009), Massachusetts (Garber 2008), and New Mexico (Gunter 2008). In 2004, President G. W. Bush, with the DHHS, initiated federal HIT activities with an executive order to develop the ONC for HIT. The ONC would coordinate the work of multiple existing federal organizations and new private-public initiated panels (American Health Information Committee, Health Information Technology Standards Panel, Committee for Certification of Health Information Technology) to ensure that the developments for HIT were prioritized and coordinated to support interoperability necessary for information exchange. In 2005 and 2007, the ONC appealed for NHIN studies to exchange among nine HIEs (Kuperman, Blair, Franck, Devaraj, & Low 2010). In 2009 President Obama called for HIT to be operational nationwide by 2014 to improve healthcare quality and efficiency. The HITECH Act legislation, passed in 2009, has become the driving force for more state HIE programs initiating in the next 4 to 5 years. The July 2010 release of the final rule on Meaningful Use for achieving HIE includes clinical quality measures for hospitals and ambulatory settings (CMS 2010).

The impacts for HIE are to reduce duplication by sharing information often and at many different settings (clinics, pharmacies, ambulatory services, nursing homes, hospitals, schools, occupational health centers, public health centers). On average, persons have approximately 4 visits per year to clinics, emergency rooms, and hospital outpatient departments, and 60% of visits are to primary care clinicians (National Center for Health Statistics 2010). Those with chronic illnesses tend to access the delivery system more frequently than persons with diabetes, averaging 10–35 visits to primary care clinics per year. The costs of fragmentation in delivering healthcare have resulted in duplicated tests, quality gaps due to multiple records and discrepancies within these records, and increased costs to deliver. A person's complete longitudinal health record is important because a uniform holistic picture of his or her symptoms, conditions, and functional health patterns can impact his or her receipt of appropriate and timely care and treatment.

The HIE allows reuse of patient health information. The methods to transfer information across settings vary widely in format (e.g., letter, report, note) and method (e.g., e-mail, fax, portal to HIE record locator). When the information is not easily obtained, providers are forced to re-create the information or take action with incomplete information because the person or his or her caregiver does not remember. The primary goals of HIE facilitate access to and retrieval of clinical data to provide safe, timely, efficient, effective, equitable, and patient-centered care. The associated benefits of HIE are to save money, improve outcomes, and improve provider–patient relationships.

HEALTH INFORMATION EXCHANGE MODELS

The preparations for an HIE include organizing a governing body and establishing financial sustainability. There are several options for operational and business models that may be considered. The U.S. Internal Revenue Service Code Section 501 and its respective subsections stipulate criteria for organizations to qualify as tax-exempt. The subsections are the not-for-profit 501c(3) charitable organization, the 501c(4) social welfare organization, and the 501c(6) mutual benefit organization. There are also criteria for virtual business linked contractually but with no separate new entity form, quasi-governmental entity, state agency, partnership or limited liability corporation (LLC) pass-through entity, special joint powers authority, and cooperative (University of Massachusetts Medical School Center and for Health Policy and Research 2009). The tax-free status for a 501 organization applies to entities that reinvest in the development of services, but these models are not always sustainable due to the challenges of meeting evolving standards. Three of the conceptual public governance models are described as sustainable models (CHPR 2009) and the fourth model is considered as a possible new option.

- Government-led HIE with a direct government program that provides services for the HIE infrastructure, and oversight for the HIE has been used in states.
- Public utility HIE with government oversight where a public sector will serve an oversight role and regulate the private-provided services of the HIE.
- Private sector–led HIE with government collaboration where the government collaborates and advises as stakeholders in the private sector HIE services have been used.
- Public authority HIE with state government creating a public instrumentality of the state in the form of a nonprofit authority with comprehensive and extensive powers to operate the state HIE in a business-like manner.

This newer type of model is accountable to the people of the state through audits and legal oversight and financial disclosure. These models are the starting foundations for states or regions to provide oversight with or without a level of regulatory control by state governments to exert over the HIE infrastructure. The HIE has been local, community-wide, regional, statewide, and even a global enterprise such as the military operating sites (CHPR 2009). Integrated delivery networks (IDN) and health systems within multiple states are groups that predate the proposed models for HIE organizations. The IDNs with nursing homes, hospice, homecare, and clinics integrated with hospitals were able to exchange with standard content and identifiers adopted across settings. All IDNs experienced the challenges of adopting common information formats and learning new workflows for use cases. Current HIEs are becoming geographically defined and involve organizations that are led by multiple representatives from professional and healthcare entities to exchange information for the good of the individual and public services. Delaware had the first statewide-initiated HIE (Perez 2009), while many before were RHIOs.

The Department of Defense and the Veterans Administration healthcare settings exchange HIEs between them and collaborate with private healthcare organizations to achieve the same externally (AHRQ 2010). Other models are centered on the services with the PHR. Some PHRs are tethered to a hospital or physician office with Web-based portals to allow the patient or parent to document symptoms or status similar to a health record bank. The two parties upload and download information to help the patient continue care.

The challenge with HIE models is to sustain the process over time with funding. The University of Massachusetts Medical School Center and for Health Policy and Research (2009) suggests that governing bodies of any of these models should secure funding support from the public sector, nonprofits, and through grants. It also suggests three funding models for the HIEs to sustain services. A **Membership Fee Model** involves stakeholders paying to support shared services for all. The fees are tiered toward size or volume of activity or may be based on relative value to each type of participant. An HIE **Transaction Fee Model** involves the state-level HIE charging transaction fees for services or products on the basis of benefit to the participants. The fees could be for clinical result delivered, for covered life per month, for hour for technical assistance, or for monthly use of an HIE application. A **Program and Service Fee Model** involves charging stakeholders for participation in the HIE services or purchasing and implementing the HIE program. Several HIEs charge a fee to agencies that participate for information services that reduce administrative needs (de Brantes, Emery, Overhage, Glaser, & Marchibroda 2007). Physicians and nurse practitioners may not pay for access to patient information such as lab results, pathology reports, diagnostics reports, discharge summaries, consultation reports because the burden is generally on this group of professionals who collect patient data with little benefit back (Adams 2009; Perez 2009). However, this is not a universal practice with all HIE and professional providers may be charged a fee for transactions when using the HIE (NeHII 2009). When the data are used for group practice management, e-prescribing, EHR-lite, quality measures monitoring, biomedical devices, and pharmaceutical manufacturers, fees are considered for use. The secondary use of data for profit presents ethical concerns that consumers and participating providers will raise as HIPAA violations. The third-party payers have provided incentives for HIE participating providers by offering quicker reimbursements and payment for performance. Content management systems have outlined Meaningful Use incentives within the HITECH Act to encourage adoption and implementation of EHRs in small practices that lead to disincentives for nonuse of EHRs and HIE after 2014 (DHHS, ONCHIT 2009).

CURRENT STATUS

The community health information networks, which developed during the 1990s, have emerged into a few state HIEs as interoperable technology became available with a focus to improve healthcare safety and quality. The emerging state-initiated HIEs and regional HIEs are increasing rapidly and currently there are about 67 public entities and 161 private HIEs initiatives reported as operational in 2010 compared to 37 and 52 in 2009 (KLAS Research 2010). In 2009, all states were in the process of planning, developing, and implementing HIEs with the ONC-HIT (National Governors Association 2009) oversight to fund statewide plans in 2010–2014.

The success of HIEs will be determined by the level of responsiveness to what stakeholders need and want for improving patient-centered healthcare and population health. The HIE organization will evolve across time and seek stakeholder buy-in to be responsive to operations and technology issues. A quality HIE infrastructure is necessary to financially receive a return on investment (ROI) and achieve some savings in the healthcare industry. Financial sustainability is still uncertain, but ROI studies are under way and finding that not all stakeholders will likely see benefit from the services of an HIE (AHRQ 2010). Early ROI models suggest the federal and state governments may indeed benefit the most from HIE and NHIN exchanges by reducing duplicated tests and consultations and by reducing readmissions for the same medical condition, thus controlling the costs with Medicare and Medicaid reimbursements to providers (AHRQ 2010). With this expectation, the employers or purchasers of health insurance plans and the insurers themselves and even consumers should see declines in medical costs over time with the reductions in duplicated services. Hospitals can benefit as well with reduction of costs with fewer required test supplies and better coordination of patients who have shorter stays and prospective payment plans. Understanding this expected ROI forecast would mean that those collecting information electronically will see an increase in burden and costs associated with documenting aspects of care in standard formats, or they may see a decline in the use of necessary tests or decline in paperwork eventually when fully automated. In this picture benefits to individual physicians, nurses, and pharmacists are minimal because the burden to collect and validate more data to ensure safety and prevent errors increases.

OBSTACLES

Even successful HIEs have endured a variety of obstacles with policy, organizational structure, financial sustainability, legal procedures, technical designs and equipment, and operational processes (University of Massachusetts Medical School Center and for Health Policy and Research 2009). Preparing the workforce, motivating providers to adopt, implementing rules of operation, and planning communication to consumers and providers are necessary expenses. The obstacles to sustainability result from underestimating the size and scope of the project, identifying critical mass of data to exchange (e.g. standards for medication history, allergies, side effects, indications, weight/height), identifying critical mass of participants (e.g., pharmacies), the collaboration between common competitors in communities, the resistance to changes in workflow, and the numbers of unskilled workforce with HIT.

The challenge begins with identifying individuals for a governing board and an HIE workforce with the necessary health informatics knowledge and skills. The principal composition and structure for the governing body is an obstacle for HIEs because those who financially support the HIE effort may ask for greater representation in governance, while stakeholders who are intensely impacted by the technology and workflow exchange and not financially impacted are not available but need representation to evolve the services they use. The key is to ensure a composition of both. The governing board and leaders need to set strategy, secure funding, and exercise oversight of all operational work and use workgroups and subcommittees to see input from stakeholders. Stakeholder organizations should nominate their own representatives or pass the seat to other professional groups. The appointments are necessary on the basis of skills and competencies needed to carry out the work (Adams 2009; Perez 2009; University of Massachusetts Medical School Center and for Health Policy and Research 2009).

For the community of providers, the adoption of standardization in clinical data, new workflows, and new functions within the EHR/EMR technology is a time-intensive obstacle. The education and use of clinical terminologies, information models, evidence-based content, and redesigned workflows are requirements to accompany the technology to ensure the right clinical data is captured, stored, and retrievable for interpretation when needed. New skills are necessary to support these needs. In 2010, the ONCHIT proposed funding multiple grant opportunities to develop short-term informatics educational programs for six community college positions and six university-level positions. University positions included clinician/public health leader, health information management and exchange specialists, health information privacy and security specialists, research and development scientists, programmers and software engineers, and health IT subspecialists. The skills provided at the community college included developing trainers, technical/software support staff, implementation managers, implementation support specialists, clinician/practitioner consultants, and practice workflow and information management redesign specialists. The federal initiatives have funded nearly 70 regional extension centers across the country to support the adoption of EHRs and HIE.

NATIONAL HEALTH INFORMATION NETWORK AND STATE-LEVEL HIE

The NHIN is a structure that brings together the state-level HIE and regional HIOs when all stakeholders are using the evolving information exchange standards (DHHS 2008). In the early NHIN trial implementations to exchange information, each HIE participant had to represent data using content specifications to endorse both syntactic (structural) and semantic (meaningful) standards for interoperability (Kuperman et al. 2010). The state-level HIE programs have the responsibility to organize and facilitate the implementation of interoperability standards with stakeholders through statewide operational planning. The HIE initiatives are often started by research teams, advisory councils, and executive committees, which can serve as the steering committee to coordinate the communication, education, foundational planning, and adoption activities to initiate and sustain standards for a state-level HIE program. The key difference is a statewide network that ensures all stakeholders and communities are included rather than excluded and can legislate the standards to carry out functions through a single entity accountable to the citizens. The role of the state-level HIE program can adapt to the state's needs and priorities based on characteristics of providers from the evaluation of current HIT use. The agencies such as public health and Medicaid services within the state government are stakeholders and will be involved with HIE services. The success of the NHIN is dependent on the statewide HIEs.

Characteristics that greatly affect the statewide HIE initiative are stakeholders who drive the effort, the capabilities and availability of skilled human resources for the effort, the state HIE entity's ability to access sufficient financial resources, and the strength of leadership across the state; momentum could also determine the direction and role that the state-level HIE initiative assumes. The role may also change across time, and as circumstances dictate the skills and priorities must change. The overall role of the state-level HIE initiatives can be loosely grouped into three broad categories:

- *HIE enabler/readiness.* Focuses on coordinating and enabling ongoing regional HIE initiatives.
- *HIE outsourcing/technical partnership.* Focuses on the business and policy aspects of HIE, but outsources the technology implementation and services.
- *HIE operator.* Focuses on implementation and management of the technical and business operations of HIE (CHPR 2009).

FUTURE DIRECTIONS

Critical implications for the future of HIEs are the far-reaching adoption of interoperable standards at all levels (Halamka 2010). Dr. John Halamka, a physician, has led the federal HITSP standards panel with multiple technical committees' volunteer work to develop these interoperable standards. The Secretary of Health and Human Services has approved a number of interoperability standards. The standards are published for the Certification Commission for Healthcare Information Technology certification process and for state HIE programs. A process of adding recognized interoperability standards will be ongoing and state-HIEs will need tool kits for education and robust communication plans to guide implementation across a variety of healthcare entities. The published interoperability standards have been and will require more research in trial sites for the Nationwide Health Information Network (Kuperman et al. 2010).

CASE STUDY EXERCISE

Patient Emergency Room. A widowed 85-year-old male is transported to the emergency room for a fractured hip after found dazed and semi-oriented in his home by a visiting neighbor. The triage nurse receives the emergency medical service phone call that the patient is 20 minutes out. The nurse uses the patient's name to search within the HIE record locator service to access essential information. The nurse is able to find one unique patient based on the emergency medical service–reported patient name and address. After log in to the HIE, the emergency room nurse views information provided by from the patient's primary care physician and cardiologist, the patient's pharmacy, the public health registry, the laboratory results on last International Normalized Ratio INR, and chemistry and hematology results. An older hospital record is also found on this patient and this information is retrieved to help prepare for the patient. On the patient's arrival, the nurse and the emergency physician find the patient unable to state allergies and some of the medications, so they use the information from the HIE to verify past history. The nurse verifies with the patient the information and uses the provider data repository to contact the pharmacy on recent dosing protocols for the patient's anticoagulant. They are able to complete assessments and examine current status and route the patient to the radiology department for additional testing.

Describe the standard healthcare information the nurse will be able to find through the HIE. Describe the types of services the triage nurse and emergency physician could use after accessing the HIE.

Visit nursing.pearsonhighered.com for additional cases, information, and weblinks.

SUMMARY

- A health information exchange (HIE) infrastructure is a process for bidirectional sharing of patient health-related information among primary providers (nurse practitioners, physicians, and physician assistants), consulting specialists, hospitals, ambulatory centers, nursing homes, dentists, audiologists, optometrists, and occupational and school health professionals.
- Information will include common elements such as immunization status, allergies (foods, environment, and medications), values (preferences, cultural and religious beliefs), social habits (alcohol or tobacco use), family history, medication list, care plan, and insurance coverage or noncoverage that support decisions.
- HIE requires an organizing structure in addition to technology for exchange at individual, professional, organization, and public health and national levels.
- Key factors for consideration in creating the HIE infrastructure include data storage, a master person index (MPI) or code that can be used to uniquely identify an individual and his or her information from different sources, a record locator service used to access and find health information that matches the identified individual, authentication of allowed users, security policies and procedures to ensure privacy and confidentiality, audit trails of all activity, standards for transport and messaging, scope of services, knowledge of workflow, and portal for access.
- Regional or state HIE infrastructures need to be set up to engage consumers, providers, and public health professionals from the community to design processes.
- The impetus for HIE began with the inception of the Medicare and Medicaid programs.
- HIE has the potential to reduce duplication and provide reuse of patient health information.

- Preparations for an HIE include organizing a governing body and establishing financial sustainability.
- There are several models for HIE organization including not-for-profit, public utility, mutual benefit, for-profit, government-led initiatives, as well as permutations of these models.
- The public authority HIE is accountable to the people of the individual state through audits and legal oversight and financial disclosure.
- Integrated delivery networks (IDN) and health systems within multiple states predated the proposed models for HIE organizations.
- The Department of Defense and the Veterans Administration healthcare settings have HIE and are working to achieve HIEs with external enterprises.
- The challenge with HIE models is to be self-sustaining over time with funding. Many were started with public funds, some charge for access to patient information while others charge only for other services or generate revenue from the secondary use of data. Third-party incentives for HIE include quicker reimbursement payment for services.
- All states are in the process of planning, developing, and implementing HIEs with the ONC-HIT oversight.
- The success of HIEs will be determined by the level of responsiveness to what stakeholders need and want for improving patient-centered healthcare and population health.
- Even successful HIEs have endured a variety of obstacles with policy, organizational structure, financial sustainability, legal procedures, technical designs and equipment, and operational processes.
- The NHIN is a structure that brings together the state-level HIE and regional HIOs when all stakeholders are using the evolving information exchange standards.
- Characteristics that greatly affect the state-wide HIE initiative are stakeholders who drive the effort, the capabilities and availability of skilled human resources for the effort, ability to access sufficient financial resources, and the strength of leadership.

REFERENCES

Adams, L. (2009). *Rhode Island quality institute.* Retrieved from http://www.riqi.org/matriarch/ MultiPiecePage.asp_Q_PageID_E_61_A_PageName_E_BoardAdam

Agency for Healthcare Research and Quality (AHRQ). (2010). *National resource center for health IT.* Retrieved from http://healthit.ahrq.gov/portal/server.pt?open=512&objID=562&&PageI D=5531&mode=2&in_hi_userid=3882&cached=true

de Brantes, F., Emery, D. W., Overhage, J. M., Glaser, J., & Marchibroda, J. (2007). The potential of HIEs as infomediaries. *Journal of Healthcare Information Management, 21*(1), 69–75.

Center for Health Policy and Research (CHPR). (2009). *Public governance models for a sustainable health information exchange industry.* Report to the State Alliance for e-Health. University of Massachusetts Medical School in collaboration with the National Opinion Research Center (NORC) and the National Governors Association Center for Best Practices. Retrieved from http://0902ehealthhitreport.pdf, 1–65

Centers for Medicare & Medicaid Services (CMS). (2010). 42 CFR Parts 412, 413, 422 et al. Medicare and Medicaid Programs; Electronic Health Record Incentive Program; Final Rule. Retrieved from http://www.cms.gov/EHRIncentivePrograms/

Certification Commission for Health Information Technology. (2011). CCHIT Certified 2009 Health Information Exchange Certification. Retrieved from http://www.cchit.org/ node/2075

Federal Communications Commission. (2010, February 18). Rural telemedicine program funds 16 more broadband telehealth networks. *FCC News,* pp. 1–3. Retrieved from http://www.fcc.gov

Frisse, M. (2009). *Health information exchange links records for better health*. Retrieved from http://healthit.ahrq.gov/portal/

Garber, L. (2008). *Secure architecture for exchanging health information (SAFEHealth)* (UC1 HS 015220). Retrieved from http://healthit.ahrq.gov/portal/

Gunter, M. J. (2008). *New Mexico health information collaborative (NMHIC)* (UC1 HS 015447). Retrieved from http://healthit.ahrq.gov/portal/

Halamka, J. (2010). *The health care blog*. Retrieved from http://www.thehealthcareblog.com/the_health_care_blog/john-halamka/

Haley, E. C., Sensmeier, J., & Brokel, J. M. (2009). Nurses exchanging information: Understanding electronic health record standards and interoperability. *Urologic Nursing, 29*(5), 305–313.

Health Information Systems Society (HIMSS). (2009). *Definitions & acronyms*. Retrieved from http://www.himss.org/content/files/RHIO_Definitions_Acronyms.pdf

Health Information Technology Standards Panel. (2010). *Use cases and interoperability specifications*. Retrieved from http://www.hitsp.org/

HIT Standards Committee (HITSC). (2010). *Standards and interoperability framework: Principles and processes*. Retrieved from http://healthit.hhs.gov/

Iowa e-Health Executive Committee and Advisory Council. (2010). *Health information technology and exchange*. Iowa Department of Public Health. Retrieved from http://www.idph.state.ia.us/ehealth/default.asp

KLAS Research. (2010). *Total number of live HIEs exchanging data more than doubles in past year*. Retrieved from http://www.klasresearch.com/News/PressRoom/2011/HIE

Kuperman, G. J., Blair, J. S., Franck, R. A., Devaraj, S., & Low, A. F. H. (2010). Developing data content specifications for the nationwide health information network trial implementations. *Journal of the American Medical Informatics Association, 17*(1), 6–12. doi:10.1197/jamia.M3282

National Center for Health Statistics. (2010). *Health, United States, 2009: With special feature on medical technology*. Hyattsville, MD. 2010. Retrieved from http://www.cdc.gov/nchs/data/hus/hus09_InBrief.pdf

National Governors Association. (2009). *Preparing to implement HITECH: A state guide for electronic health information exchange* (pp. 1–31). Report from the State Alliance for E-Health. Retrieved from http://0908healthHITECH.pdf

Nebraska Health Information Initiative (NeHII). (2009). Retrieved from http://nehii.org/

Office of the National Coordinator. (2010). Retrieved from http://healthit.hhs.gov/blog/faca/indexphp/2010/12/10/onc-seeks-comment-on-standards-and-interoperability-framework-initiatives-by-december-23-2010/

Overhage, J. M., Evans, L., & Marchibroda, J. (2005). Communities' readiness for health information exchange: The national landscape in 2004. *Journal of the American Medical Informatics Association, 12*(2), 107–112. doi:10.1197/jamia.M1680

Overhage, M. (2009). *Nationwide Health Information Network (NHIN) Trial Implementations Indiana Health Information Exchange* (Contract No. HHSP23320074102EC). Retrieved from http://healthit.ahrq.gov/portal/

Perez, G. (2009). *Delaware health information network*. Retrieved from http://www.dhin.org/Home/tabid/36/Default.aspx

Proctor, P., Reid, W., Compton, D., Grossman, J. H., & Fanjiang, G. (Eds.). (2005). *Building a better delivery system: A new engineering/health care partnership* [for Committee on Engineering and the Health Care System, National Academy of Engineering, Institute of Medicine]. Washington, DC: National Academies Press.

Root, J. (2008). *Improving communications between health care providers via a statewide infrastructure: Utah Health Information Network (UHIN) Clinical State and Regional Demonstration Project* (Contract Number: 290-04-0002). Retrieved from http://healthit.ahrq.gov/portal/

Staggers, N., Thompson, C. B., & Snyder-Halpern, R. (2001). History and trends in clinical information systems in the United States. *Journal of Nursing Scholarship: An Official Publication of Sigma Theta Tau International Honor Society of Nursing/Sigma Theta Tau, 33*(1), 75–81.

University of Massachusetts Medical School Center and for Health Policy and Research. (2009). *Public governance models for a sustainable health information exchange industry.* Report to the State Alliance for e-Health. Retrieved from http://www.nascio.org/events/2009Midyear/documents/NASCIO-Himmelstein.pdf

U.S. Department of Health and Human Services (DHHS). (2008, April 28). *The national alliance for health information technology report to the office of the national coordinator for health information technology on defining key health information technology terms.* pp. 1–40.

U.S. Department of Health and Human Services (DHHS). (2009). HITECH and funding opportunities. Retrieved from http://healthit.hhs.gov/portal/server.pt/community/healthit_hhs_gov_hitech_and_funding_opportunities/1310

CHAPTER 18

Health Policy and Health Information Technology

After completing this chapter, you should be able to:

1. Comprehend factors that lead to the successful development, advancement, and deployment of policy.

2. Understand factors that led to the emergence of healthcare reform as a policy imperative.

3. Examine the potential benefits that health information technology can offer for healthcare reform.

4. Analyze the composition of health information technology policy advisory boards and discuss the potential ramifications of representation of special interest groups.

5. Examine the role of informatics groups, healthcare professionals, and informatics professionals in shaping local, state, national, and global policies for the integration of health information technology into healthcare delivery.

6. Consider future areas for health information technology policy development.

Health policy making is not an easy process. The availability of new treatments juxtaposed over established treatments leads to pressures to increase spending and adds to the complexity of care and ability of research to establish a base of evidence for safe, cost-effective treatment (Arrow et al. 2009). There are also multiple goals to address while considering the collective interests of all involved parties (Chernichovsky & Leibowitz 2010). Articulation of public interests is typically assigned to experts such as policy analysts, bureaucrats, and health professional groups. Realizing the benefits of medical breakthroughs and innovations requires the design of a better healthcare delivery system, however (Rouse & Cortese 2010).

Policy is developed through a multistage process that entails the following:

- Recognition of a problem or issue
- Agenda setting
- Policy formation
- Adoption
- Implementation
- Evaluation (WHO n.d.)

Each stage of the policy development process is important, but the initial recognition of the problem is critical as nurse leaders must be able to bring the problem to the notice of the organization or government in order to work toward action. Milstead (1999) likened the policy-making process to the nursing process in the following ways: Both are dynamic, and progression through either may not be linear or sequential. Good initial information is critical to the expeditious, correct identification of the issue so that it may be placed on the agenda for further discussion and decisive action. Public policy represents the collective wisdom of individuals, organizations, and various agencies that possess expertise or a special interest in the area. Policy moves from the sphere of private to public when the identified problem is felt to require government intervention. This move should not negate views from the private sector, however (Brailer 2009).

STATUS OF THE U.S. HEALTHCARE DELIVERY SYSTEM

While the U.S. healthcare delivery clearly does many things right, demonstrating world-renowned accomplishments, there are also a number of problems (Weil 2008). According to Knickman (2005) health policy may at times contribute to negative trends. Certain aspects of U.S. health policy have been blamed for creating or contributing to some of the health problems seen today (A recipe for disaster 2008; Berwick, Nolan, & Whittington 2008; Gruber 2009; Lefton 2008; Luft 2006). These include, but not limited to:

- Higher expenditures than those of other developed countries with outcomes that are no better, and in some cases worse
- A lack of clinical and administrative standardization
- Fragmented care
- Unequal access to care
- The creation of ill-health through the creation of large social and economic inequalities, promoting unhealthy eating and lifestyles
- Turning health problems into marketing opportunities
- Failure to curtail costs for services
- Less than optimal safety
- Poor evaluation of quality by patients
- Payment per services rather than maintaining wellness
- A lack of rewards for primary care
- An expensive collection of different providers and payers rather than a unified system
- The perception that technology is the driver of costs rather than a tool to better capture efficiencies

Skyrocketing costs are due in part to a reimbursement system built upon payment for services and disease management, rather than a more cost-effective, preventive approach (Novelli 2008). Clearly this is not a sustainable situation. While much may be learned from studying other health systems, the political and social culture, demographics, and government will ultimately shape the U.S. solution (Ginsburg, Doherty, Ralston, & Senkeeto 2008). Detmer (2009) talked about the need for public policy to support the infrastructure needed to foster value-driven healthcare. This includes the orchestration of harmony and balance across the knowledge, care and payment domains, and a greater dialog to develop policy supportive of health within society and within the healthcare delivery system.

HEALTHCARE REFORM

The need for healthcare reform has been obvious for some time but the implications of the broken U.S. healthcare delivery system were largely brought to the attention of the public via the classic Institute of Medicine (IOM) report *To Err Is Human: Building A Safer Health System* (1999). Since that time surveys have shown a growing demand on the part of the American people for a new direction and approach to healthcare with a more active role by the government to effect change (Gruber 2009; McInturff & Weigel 2008). Americans also want their doctors to be able to access all of their medical records in order to provide the best care possible (Goldstein & Blumenthal 2008). Experts observe that improving the U.S. healthcare system requires simultaneous efforts to improve the care experience, improve population health, and reduce per capita healthcare costs (Berwick et al. 2008). This calls for state and federal involvement with goal-setting based on best practices and redistribution of resources and an improved feedback to clinicians on the quality of care provided (Clancy, Anderson & White 2009; Weil 2008). According to Zaccai (2009) the goal should be to develop a system that provides for a better customer experience and improved health maintenance, bringing healthcare delivery system closer to the ideal, particularly when done in conjunction with science and technology. It was at this time that healthcare reform re-emerged as a policy imperative (Clancy et al. 2009; Crane & Raymond 2011). Health information technology (HIT) was seen as a tool to aid the reform process with recognition of its potential to improve the safety and efficiency of healthcare delivery, facilitate transparency, increase engagement, personalize healthcare, and facilitate the sharing of information needed to improve the quality of care as well as decrease costs and disparities (Goldstein & Blumenthal 2008). The technologies seen as having the greatest potential are electronic health records (EHRs), personal health records, and health information exchange (Clancy et al. 2009).

President George W. Bush initiated an important change in U.S. policy on HIT when he signed Executive Order 13335 in 2004, creating the position of National Health Information Technology Coordinator (Miller & West 2009). Bush also called for the development of an EHR for every American by 2014. In another executive order in 2006, Bush required providers of care to Medicare beneficiaries to make cost and quality data publicly available by January 2007, a move designed to increase transparency of information and HIT adoption.

President Obama supported the 2014 goal for the EHR by signing the American Recovery and Reinvestment Act (ARRA) and HITECH (Health Information Technology for Economic and Clinical Health) Act into law in 2009 (McDermott Will & Emery 2009; Walker 2010). HITECH provisions aligned with the goals of the Office of the National Coordinator and provided permanent designation to ONC as well as funds to develop a national HIT framework through HITECH. HITECH provided the Department of Health and Human Services with the authority to establish programs to improve healthcare quality, safety, and efficiency through the use of HIT that is inclusive of EHRs (ONC 2011a). Other provisions called for:

- An updated federal health IT strategic plan
- The integration and sharing of information across the healthcare delivery system—providers, third party payers, the government, and other appropriate parties
- Privacy and security provisions for electronic data exchange of personal health information

- Security measures for authentication and specified encryption technologies
- Strategies to enhance HIT use to improve quality of care, reduce errors, decrease health disparities, improve population health and resource utilization, and improve continuity of care.

NATIONAL HEALTH INFORMATION TECHNOLOGY POLICY

The United States has been slow to develop a national HIT policy, lagging behind many other nations, but policymakers are making important steps toward overcoming obstacles to HIT adoption (Goldstein & Blumenthal 2008). HHS secretary Mike Leavitt (Schaeffer 2008) noted that the introduction and use of HIT required leadership by the government to help organize efforts. Diamond and Shirky (2008) stated that one of the biggest obstacles to expanded HIT use was an overly narrow focus on ways to increase its adoption instead of an overall consideration of all of the related issues. HIT adoption must instead be guided through the development of policy. Policies provide purposeful plans of action to deal with issues in either the public or private sector (DePalma 2002). Policies help to provide the foundation for action and influence budget allocation and the quality of care provided. Policy is shaped using input from individuals, experts, organizations, and public values (Connecting for Health 2007). Public values guide the policies and technologies used to support quality reporting and other uses of health data. There are many organizations and foundations that follow healthcare policy formation and offer recommendations. eHealth Initiative (2011) is a group of more than 200 organizations representing all healthcare stakeholders and attempts to educate and help members navigate different healthcare issues, policies, and strategy. Box 18–1 provides a sample listing of some other groups that follow or attempt to shape healthcare policy. Policymakers require ample, quality data to develop solid policies. Even so policy requires periodic review to ensure that it is still appropriate. Ultimately widespread adoption of HIT requires economic incentives and policies that make quality improvement and cost reduction essential to providers in order to accomplish their financial and professional goals (Goldstein & Blumenthal 2008). Policy makers are expected to link investments in HIT infrastructure to the objectives of healthcare reform (Clancy et al. 2009).

STATUS

ARRA provided for the creation of an HIT Policy Committee under the auspices of the Federal Advisory Committee Act (FACA). The HIT Policy Committee is charged with making recommendations to the National Coordinator for Health IT on a policy framework for the development and adoption of a nationwide health information infrastructure, including standards for the exchange of patient medical information (ONC 2011b). The HIT Policy Committee subsequently formed several workgroups to enable it to meet its charge. The workgroups are comprised of stakeholder representatives and subject matter experts who make recommendation to the HIT Policy Committee on their respective areas of expertise. The HIT Policy Committee's workgroups include:

- Meaningful Use Certification/Adoption Information Exchange
- National Health Information Network (NHIN)
- Strategic Plan Privacy & Security Policy
- Enrollment
- Privacy & Security Tiger Team
- Governance
- Quality Measures
- The report of the President's Council of Advisors on Science and Technology (PCAST)

Some of the workgroups are further divided into teams. The Quality Measures Workgroup is divided into six teams, each focused on a different measure domain. The HIT Policy Committee is comprised of members chosen by the secretary of DHHS, as well as appointees of the majority

BOX 18–1 Sample Listing of Groups That Follow or Impact Healthcare Policy

Agency for Healthcare Research and Quality

Government agency whose research provides evidence-based information on healthcare outcomes, quality, cost, use, and access.

Alliance for Health Reform

Bipartisan, nonprofit that conducts health policy briefings on Capitol Hill for congressional staff and media. Publishes resource books on health policy topics, aids journalists to develop articles and broadcasts on health issues, and maintains a list of hundreds of healthcare experts.

American Federation of Labor and Congress of Industrial Organizations

Political voice for workers. Represents employees in policy reforms, including healthcare and employee benefits.

American Enterprise Institute for Public Health Research

Nonpartisan, nonprofit. Its research focuses on economics and trade; social welfare; government tax, spending, regulatory, and legal policies; U.S. politics; international affairs; and U.S. defense and foreign policies.

American Hospital Association

National organization representing hospitals, healthcare networks, patients and communities in national health policy development, legislative and regulatory debates, and judicial matters.

America's Health Insurance Plans

Trade association that conducts research and distributes information to the public on healthcare finance and delivery.

Bureau of Labor Statistics

U.S. Department of Labor agency that reports on a variety of issues, including data on national health expenditures.

Center for Studying Health System Change

Nonpartisan policy research organization that designs and conducts studies on the U.S. healthcare system to inform policymakers in government and private industry.

Center on Budget and Policy Priorities

Specializes in research and analysis oriented toward policy decisions that policymakers face at federal and state levels. Also examines data and research and produces analyses accessible to public officials, other nonprofit organizations, and the media.

Centers for Medicare & Medicaid Services

Administers several public health programs and produces quantitative information, inclusive of data on Medicare and Medicaid spending, enrollment, claims data, and estimates of future spending and program growth. Also prepares estimates and projections of national health expenditures.

Changes in Health Care Financing and Organization

Robert Wood Johnson Foundation program that provides public and private decision makers with information on healthcare policy, financing, and market developments.

Commonwealth Fund

Private foundation that supports independent research on health and social issues and provides grants to improve healthcare practice and policy. Committed to helping people become more informed about their healthcare, and improving care for vulnerable populations and the uninsured.

Congressional Budget Office

Provides Congress with nonpartisan research and analysis needed for economic and budget decisions.

(*continued*)

BOX 18–1 (*continued*)

Dartmouth Atlas of Health Care

Dartmouth Medical School online resource that provides information about the American healthcare system, inclusive of data on expenditures.

Employee Benefit Research Institute

Nonpartisan organization dedicated to data dissemination, policy research, and education on economic security and employee benefits.

Government Accountability Office

Audit, evaluation, and investigative arm of Congress.

Health Care Leadership Council

CEO-level task forces on healthcare quality and costs to discuss policy reform options and offer legislative and regulatory recommendations.

Henry J. Kaiser Family Foundation

Nonprofit, private operating foundation that focuses on major healthcare issues. Independent voice and source of facts and analysis for policymakers, media, healthcare professionals, and the public.

National Bureau of Economic Research

Private organization that researches issues related to economic policy, including health economics.

National Business Group on Health

Formerly the Washington Business Group on Health. Nonprofit that represents large employers on health policy, legislation, and regulations.

National Center of Policy Analysis

Nonprofit, public policy research organization that seeks to develop and promote private alternatives to government regulation and control.

National Coalition on Health Care

Nonprofit, nonpartisan, alliance working to improve America's healthcare, bringing together businesses, labor unions, consumer groups, religious groups, and primary care providers.

Office of Management and Budget

Executive branch agency that oversees the federal budget, prepares the president's annual budget proposal, and supervises its administration.

RAND Corporation

Conducts quantitative research on national issues such as health economics, disparities, aging, and mental health.

Robert Wood Johnson Foundation

Large philanthropy devoted to health and healthcare. Provides grants to assure access to quality affordable healthcare; to improve healthcare quality and support for the chronically ill, for healthy communities, and lifestyles; and to reduce harm caused by substance abuse.

Urban Institute Health Policy Center

Provides data analysis on major health policy topics, inclusive of insurance coverage, costs, health reform, Medicaid policy, welfare policy, and long-term care, aging and disabilities.

U.S. Chamber of Commerce

Represents businesses and business associations in national health policy reform issues and sponsors publications on issues that impact health benefits.

Source: Adapted from Keyser.edu.org. (n.d.). Key Organizations. Retrieved from http://www.kaiseredu.org/Issue-Modules/US-Health-Care-Costs/Key-Organizations.aspx

and minority leaders of the Senate and the speaker and minority leader of the House of Representatives, and appointees of the Acting Comptroller General of the United States.

The Health IT Standards Committee is another FAC charged with making recommendations to the National Coordinator for Health IT (ONC 2010). This committee focuses upon standards, implementation specifications, and certification criteria for the electronic exchange and use of health information. Initial work will examine the policies developed by the Health IT Policy Committee.

There have been other efforts that are critical to creating the national health information infrastructure (Clancy et al. 2009; Detmer 2009). These include, but are not limited to, the identification of the type of data most used in quality assessment, and the creation of unique clinician identifiers. ARRA and HITECH impose several requirements to both move HIT adoption forward and collect data to demonstrate the impact of HIT adoption.

Walker and Carayon (2009) called for the redesign of HIT to support improved, patient-centered care rather than the isolated tasks of specific healthcare professionals, noting that this approach has policy implications as HIT would mitigate the results of shortages of physicians. This would be achieved through the following:

- Requiring other healthcare providers and patients to learn new skills
- Increasing the numbers and use of clinical analysts, business-process managers
- Improved human factors design
- A shift to payment for improved patient well-being
- A shift from tasks to a patient-centered approach

The federal government is expected to save $34 billion in 10 years just through the requirement for healthcare providers to use HIT as a condition of participating in Medicare ("Health Care Reform and Health IT" 2009). More importantly, however, are the expected gains in the quality of care and improved population health. Common threads in both national and global HIT discussions include the need for strong workable policies, engagement of stakeholders, coordination of funding, the ongoing need to address standards and interoperability, and to learn from the experiences of others (Gerber 2009).

Education

Education goes hand-in-hand with policy. Health policy and health information technology policy requires informed policymakers, professionals, and an informed public. One of the many facets of the HITECH Act includes education components through the following initiatives (McDermott Will & Emery 2009):

- It required the DHHS to establish a research center, which will provide technical assistance and best practices to accelerate the adoption and best use of HIT in conjunction with regional extension centers (RECs). RECs will work with nonprofit organizations that apply for and receive financial assistance from DHHS to incorporate HIT and best practices.
- HHS awarded demonstration projects to integrate certified EHR technology into the clinical education of healthcare professionals and provide institutions of higher learning with informatics programs to ensure sufficient numbers of healthcare and IT professionals for the rapid and effective adoption and use of IT.
- The DHHS requirement of a designated person at each regional office to provide guidance and education on privacy and security requirements for privacy and security.
- The requirement for the Office of Civil Rights (OCR) to develop and maintain a national educational initiative to educate the public about the potential uses of their personal health information, the impact of the same, and individual rights related to PHI use.

Professionals According to the IOM's *Future of Nursing: Leading Change, Advancing Health* (2010a) report, one of the many competencies needed by nurses to delivery high-quality care is health policy. Healthcare professionals interested in health policy beyond the course content offered in formal nursing programs should explore educational opportunities offered through the IOM's Health Policy Educational Programs and Fellowships office. This office serves as the program office for the following programs (IOM 2010b, 2011a, 2011b):

- The Robert Wood Johnson Foundation's (RWJF's) Health Policy Fellows program
- The IOM/American Nurses Foundation (ANF)/American Academy of Nursing (AAN) Distinguished Nurse Scholar-in-Residence program
- The Norman F. Gant/ABOG Fellowship

The RWJF's Health Policy Fellows program provides an opportunity for midcareer health professionals to better understand the health policy process, contribute to the formulation of new policies and programs, and become leaders in academic health centers and in health policy. The Distinguished Nurse Scholar-in-Residence program seeks to help nurse leaders play a greater role in the development of national health policy. Participants are expected to produce a policy paper or work in an IOM study in their area of expertise. The Scholar-in-Residence program is supported by the AAN, the ANA, and the ANF. The Norman F. Gant/ABOG Fellowship is limited to obstetricians and gynecologists.

The Public At present there is a lack of public awareness of some major HIT issues such as medical identity theft. Policymakers need to educate the public about both the benefits and emerging risks associated with HIT (Rowe 2011).

The Role of Nursing

Nurses have a dual role in HIT policy. First and foremost, nurses always have a professional responsibility to act in the best interests of the public that they serve (Gorenberg, Alderman, & Cruise 1991). Nurses also need to understand the importance of the national HIT agenda and be prepared to influence the process to ensure the representation of nursing (Halley, Sensmeier, & Brokel 2009).

Nurses have long been underrepresented in the shaping of healthcare policy. Peters (2002) called for nurses to garner increased attention to the role of nursing in healthcare. Underrepresentation of nurses in policy-making decisions is felt to be a reason why there is a large-scale failure to understand the contributions that nursing makes to healthcare. Nurses need to become active in policy formation. They can do this by becoming involved and visible in the process (Kopanos 2008). State and national nursing organizations provide one means to do this through education and links to inform members of policy and legislation issues. The ANA (2011) maintains a Health Care Policy Web page that represents one example of this activity.

Wakefield (2002) noted that nurses are positioned to engage the public and policymakers to implement strategies to deal with costly healthcare challenges. The IOM's report *The Future of Nursing: Leading Change, Advancing Health* (2010a) was more explicit in its call for nurses to be full partners along with physicians and other healthcare professionals, in the redesign of U.S. healthcare, recognizing that this redesign requires better data collection and an improved information infrastructure. The report also called for effective workforce planning and policies for all U.S. nurses to exercise their power. Nurse must also work closely with government entities, businesses, healthcare organizations, professional associations, and the insurance industry to design a system that provides affordable, quality care with improved outcomes that is accessible to all.

Nursing leaders need to be involved at all levels of policy to facilitate the movement away from disease focus to wellness policies and procedures (Peters 2002). Nurse leaders must also be responsive to the big changes set into place with the passage of ARRA and Meaningful Use requirements (Walker 2010). According to the TIGER Initiative [n.d.] (*Revolutionary Leadership Driving Healthcare Innovation: The TIGER Leadership Development Collaborative Report*) transformation of the healthcare delivery system through the development of a national health

---

BOX 18–2   Activities That Nurse Executives Can Perform to Promote HIT Adoption and Use

- Develop ROI models for HIT related to patient safety imperatives
- Overcome financial and cultural barriers related to HIT
- Identify and acquire funding sources to support HIT projects
- Optimize interoperability by supporting an integrated HIT framework for all technology within the organization
- Support and provide leadership development on HIT-related topics
- Articulate the HIT vision and its alignment to the organization's objectives
- Support competency-based training of all nursing staff to use HIT effectively
- Incorporate HIT competencies into job descriptions and career ladders
- Improve patient safety through the use of decision-support tools at the point of care
- Use HIT as an *enabler* to develop a culture of safety and evidence-based practice
- Ensure visibility to measurable patient outcomes for all healthcare providers
- Contribute to research that substantiates the business case for nursing
- Insist on technological advances that *improve* nursing practice

Source: NURSING EXECUTIVE HIT-RELATED ACTIVITIES, p. 7
The TIGER Initiative. (n.d.). *Revolutionary leadership driving healthcare innovation: The TIGER leadership development collaborative team report.* Retrieved from http://www.thetigerinitiative.org/docs/TigerReport_RevolutionaryLeadership.pdf

---

information infrastructure requires that nurse leaders "understand, promote, own, and measure the success of health IT." This is best accomplished through:

- Education programs for nurse executives and faculty that stress the value of information technology and empower them to use HIT appropriately
- The expansion/integration of informatics competencies into nursing leadership development programs
- Sharing best practices using HIT effectively to improve the delivery of nursing care
- Alignment with the Magnet Recognition Program to demonstrate nursing excellence via technology to improve practice and delivery of safer, more effective care

Policy was one of the seven pillars identified in *The TIGER Summit Report Evidence and Informatics Transforming Nursing: 3-Year Action Steps Toward a 10-Year Vision* report (TIGER Initiative 2007). The *TIGER Leadership Development Collaborative Team* report (TIGER Initiative n.d.) noted that one of the top goals of the TIGER Initiative was to have more nurses play an active role in the development of a national healthcare information technology (NHIT) infrastructure and the development of leadership to drive, empower, and execute the transformation of healthcare. Box 18–2 lists activities that nurse executive can perform to promote HIT adoption and use.

ISSUES

There are numerous issues to consider in the development, implementation, and evaluation of HIT policy. One problem with the existing healthcare delivery system is the limited motivation to share information across institutions, particularly when there are concerns of competitive advantages (Diamond & Shirky 2008). Some experts also express concern that there is an overemphasis upon the adoption of standards when issues of privacy and trust must be addressed first. Privacy issues need to be addressed through a comprehensive approach that implements core privacy principles, adopts trusted design characteristics, and establishes mechanisms for oversight and accountability. This approach will require changes to existing legislation, new rules for entities outside the traditional health care sector, a more nuanced approach to the role of consent, and stronger enforcement mechanisms. Another area of concern is the potential dominance in the formulation and enactment of policies by stakeholders who have a vested interest in the process. Established constituencies, in particular, are resistant to change (Peters 2002).

Policymakers require good information to set policies. There is no perfect or complete knowledge, so waiting for that to develop can lead to disastrous delays, but one must also consider the possibility of bias (Jewell & Bero 2008; Knickman 2005).

There are even questions as to whether promoting the adoption of the EHR was the best U.S. approach at this time (Simborg 2008). EHRs have been promoted because of the assumption that they will promote quality, reduce costs, and result in more efficient care particularly with the use of decision support. Critics note that EHR systems actually slow physicians down and may increase opportunities for fraud.

FUTURE DIRECTIONS

Until recently most efforts to reform healthcare have been restricted to individual sites but changes in the capabilities of technology and policies make it possible to look at the entire system and effect changes (Berwick et al. 2008; Goldstein & Blumenthal 2008). More evidence of HIT efficiencies will help to advance the cause. Nurse leaders need to see nursing informatics and technology as essential to support everyday nursing functions (Walker 2010). This perception requires the development of core nursing informatics competencies for every nurse. Nursing leadership needs to become familiar with the TIGER Initiative and the long-range view afforded through HIT benefits to improve healthcare delivery, increase efficiencies, reduce costs, and provide personalized healthcare. Nurse leaders need to pave the way to enable necessary changes. Informatics nurses and informatics nurse specialists need to guide the process.

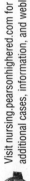

Visit nursing.pearsonhighered.com for additional cases, information, and weblinks.

CASE STUDY EXERCISE

You are asked to present a lecture on the importance of health policy in the adoption of HIT. What key points would you include? What would you say about the role of the nurse in the process?

SUMMARY

- Health policy is an important competency for all nurses at any point in time but particularly with the introduction of healthcare reform measures.
- Health information technology has been advanced as an integral part of healthcare reform.
- Nurses, particularly informatics nurses and informatics nurse specialists, have an obligation to represent nursing at the policy table and to educate the public on major HIT issues including benefits and risks.

REFERENCES

A recipe for disaster: Can US healthcare woes be turned around? (2008, October 18). *PharmacoEconomics & Outcomes News, 564,* 2.

American Nurses Association (ANA). (2011). *Health care policy.* Retrieved from http://www.nursingworld.org/MainMenuCategories/HealthcareandPolicyIssues.aspx

Arrow, K., Auerbach, A., Bertko, J., Brownlee, S., Casalino, L., Cooper, J., . . . Silber, B. (2009). Toward a 21st-century health care system: Recommendations for health care reform. *Annals of Internal Medicine, 150*(7), 493–495.

Berwick, D., Nolan, T., & Whittington, J. (2008). The triple aim: Care, health, and cost. *Health Affairs, 27*(3), 759–769. doi:10.1377/hlthaff.27.3.759

Brailer, D. J. (2009). Presidential leadership and health information technology. *Health Affairs, 28*(2), w392–w398. doi:10.1377/hlthaff.28.2.w392

Chernichovsky, D., & Leibowitz, A. (2010). Integrating public health and personal care in a reformed US health care system. *American Journal of Public Health, 100*(2), 205–211. doi:10.2105/AJPH.2008.156588

Clancy, C. M., Anderson, K. M., & White, P. J. (2009). Investing in health information infrastructure: Can it help achieve health reform? *Health Affairs, 28*(2), 478–482. doi:10.1377/hlthaff.28.2.478

Connecting for Health. (2007, July 30). *Connecting for health response. AHRQ request for information on national health data stewardship.* Retrieved from http://www.markle.org/sites/default/files/cfh_ahrq_aqa_rfi_073007.pdf

Crane, R. M., & Raymond, B. (2011). Roundtable on public policy affecting patient safety. *Journal of Patient Safety, 7*(1), 5–10.

DePalma, J. A. (2002). Proposing an evidence-based policy process. *Nursing Administration Quarterly, 26*(4), 55–61.

Detmer, D. E. (2009). Engineering information technology for actionable information and better health. *Information Knowledge Systems Management, 8,* 107–118. doi:10.3233/IKS-2009-0138 IOS Press

Diamond, C. C., & Shirky, C. (2008). Health information technology: A few years of magical thinking? *Health Affairs, 27*(5), w383–w390. (published online: 2008, August 19; doi:10.1377/hlthaff.27.5.w383)

eHealth Initiative. (2011). *About us.* Retrieved from http://www.ehealthinitiative.org/about-us.html

Gerber, T. (2009). Health information technology: Dispatches from the revolution. *Health Affairs, 28*(2), w390–w391. doi:10.1377/hlthaff.28.2.w390

Ginsburg, J. A., Doherty, R. B., Ralston, J. F., & Senkeeto, N. (2008). Achieving a high-performance health care system with universal access: What the United States can learn from other countries. *Annals of Internal Medicine, 148*(1), 55–75.

Goldstein, M. M., & Blumenthal, D. (2008, Winter). Building an information technology infrastructure. *Journal of Law, Medicine & Ethics, 36,* 709–715.

Gorenberg, B., Alderman, M., & Cruise, M. (1991). Social policy statements: Guidelines for decision making. *International Nursing Review, 38*(1), 11–13.

Gruber, D. (2009). Can consumers cure healthcare? *Studies in Health Technology and Informatics, 149,* 74–89.

Halley, E. C., Sensmeier, J., & Brokel, J. M. (2009). Nurses exchanging information: Understanding electronic health record standards and interoperability. *Urologic Nursing, 29*(5), 305–313.

Health care reform and health IT proposals remain top policy priority. (2009, March). *Magazine of Physical Therapy*, p. 12.

Institute of Medicine (IOM). (2010a). *The future of nursing: Leading change, advancing health.* Washington, DC: National Academies Press.

Institute of Medicine (IOM). (2010b, September 14). *Health policy educational programs and fellowships.* Retrieved from http://www.iom.edu/About-IOM/Leadership-Staff/Boards/Health-Policy-Educational-Programs-and-Fellowships.aspx

Institute of Medicine (IOM). (2011a). *IOM/ANF/AAN/ANA distinguished nurse scholar-in-residence.* Retrieved from http://iom.edu/Activities/Education/NurseScholar.aspx

Institute of Medicine (IOM). (2011b). *Robert Wood Johnson foundation health policy fellows.* Retrieved from http://iom.edu/Activities/Education/RWJFellows.aspx

Jewell, C. J., & Bero, L. A. (2008). "Developing good taste in evidence": Facilitators of and hindrances to evidence-informed health policymaking in state government. *Milbank Quarterly, 86*(2), 177–208. doi:10.1111/j.1468-0009.2008.00519.x

Knickman, J. R. (2005). Commentary on "when health policy is the problem." *Journal of Health Politics, Policy and Law, 30*(3), 367–373.

Kopanos, T. (2008, March). What is your power to influence healthcare policy? *Colorado Nurse,* p. 13.

Lefton, R. (2008). Healthcare reform. Reducing variation in healthcare delivery. *Healthcare Financial Management, 62*(7), 42–44.

Luft, H. S. (2006). What works and what doesn't work well in the US healthcare system. *Pharmaco Economics, 24,* 15–28.

McDermott Will & Emery. (2009, February 20). *Economic stimulus package: Policy implications of the financial incentives to promote health IT and new privacy and security protections.* Retrieved from http://www.mwe.com/info/news/wp0209e.pdf

McInturff, W., & Weigel, L. (2008). Déjà vu all over again: The similarities between political debates regarding health care in the early 1990s and today. *Health Affairs, 27*(3), 699–704.

Miller, E. A., & West, D. M. (2009). Where's the revolution? Digital technology and health care in the internet age. *Journal of Health Politics, Policy and Law, 34*(2), 261–284. doi:10.1215/03616878-2008-046

Milstead, J. A. (1999). Advanced practice nurses and public policy, naturally. In J. A. Milstead (Ed.), *Health policy & politics: A nurse's guide* (pp. 1–41). Gaithersburg, MD: Aspen Publishers.

Novelli, W. (2008). Transforming the healthcare system: A focus on prevention. *Healthcare Financial Management: Journal of the Healthcare Financial Management Association, 62*(4), 94–99.

Office of the National Coordinator for Health Information Technology (ONC). (2010, August 3). *Health IT standards committee (a Federal Advisory Committee).* Retrieved from http://healthit.hhs.gov/portal/server.pt/community/healthit_hhs_gov__health_it_standards_committee/1271

Office of the National Coordinator for Health Information Technology (ONC). (2011a, February 9). *Electronic health records and meaningful use.* Retrieved from http://healthit.hhs.gov/portal/server.pt?open=512&objID=2996&mode=2

Office of the National Coordinator for Health Information Technology (ONC). (2011b, November 22). Federal Advisory Committees (FACAs). Retrieved from http://healthit.hhs.gov/portal/server.pt/community/healthit_hhs_gov__federal_advisory_committees_%28facas%29/1149

Peters, R. M. (2002). Nurse administrators' role in health policy: Teaching the elephant to dance. *Nursing Administration Quarterly, 26*(4), 1–8.

Rouse, W., & Cortese, D. (2010). Engineering the system of healthcare delivery. Introduction. *Studies in Health Technology & Informatics, 153,* 3–14. doi:10.3233/978-1-60750-533-4-1

Rowe, J. (2011, April 28). *On HIT, public education is a policy issue.* HITECHWatch. Retrieved from http://hitechwatch.com/blog/hit-public-education-policy-issue

Schaeffer, L. D. (2008). Leading the way: A conversation with HHS Secretary Mike Leavitt. Interview by Leonard D. Schaeffer. *Health Affairs, 27,* w52–w59. doi:10.1377/hlthaff.27.1.w52

Simborg, D. W. (2008). Promoting electronic health record adoption. Is it the correct focus? *Journal of the American Medical Informatics Association, 15*(2), 127–129. doi:10.1198/jamia.M2573

TIGER Initiative. (2007). *The TIGER Summit Report evidence and informatics transforming nursing: 3-year action steps toward a 10-year vision report.* Retrieved from http://tigersummit.com/uploads/TIGERInitiative_Report2007_Color.pdf

TIGER Initiative (n.d.). *The TIGER leadership development collaborative team report.* Retrieved from http://www.tigersummit.com/uploads/TIGER_Leadership_Collaborative_Report.pdf

U.S. Department of Health and Human Services (DHHS). (2011a, March 25). *ONC seeks public comment on the federal health IT strategic plan: 2011–2015.* Retrieved from http://www.healthit.gov/buzz-blog/from-the-onc-desk/hit-strat-plan/

U.S. Department of Health and Human Services (DHHS). (2011b, April 29). Testimony Statement by David Blumenthal, National Coordinator, Office of the National Coordinator for Health IT (ONC) U.S. Department of Health and Human Services on Health IT adoption and the new challenges faced by Solo and Small Group Healthcare Practices before Committee on Small Business Subcommittee on Regulations and Healthcare United States House of Representatives. Retrieved from http://www.hhs.gov/asl/testify/2009/06/t20090624a.html

Wakefield, M. (2002). Health policy and politics. Turning up the volume to battle chronic disease. *Nursing Economics, 20*(5), 229–231.

Walker, J. M., & Carayon, P. (2009). From tasks to processes: The case for changing health information technology to improve health care. *Health Affairs, 28*(2), 467–477. doi:10.1377/hlthaff.28.2.467

Walker, P. H. (2010). The TIGER initiative: A call to accept and pass the Baton. *Nursing Economics, 28*(5), 352–355.

Weil, A. (2008). How far can states take health reform? *Health Affairs, 27*(3), 736–747.

World Health Organization (WHO). (n.d.). *Health service planning and policy-making: A toolkit for nurses and midwives. Module 4: Policy-development process.* Retrieved from http://www.wpro.who.int/NR/rdonlyres/1E08B706-D28E-4F42-BE5B-6D43E2ED4E9F/0/hsp_mod4.pdf

Zaccai, G. (2009). Designing the future of healthcare. *Studies in Health Technology and Informatics, 149,* 49.

CHAPTER 19

Legislation

After completing this chapter, you should be able to:

1. Review legislation impacting the protection of healthcare information.

2. Discuss legislative efforts to stimulate the adoption of healthcare information technology.

3. Relate issues arising from implementation of HITECH programs.

4. Analyze the impact of these laws on nursing informatics practitioners.

This chapter examines significant federal legislation affecting electronic healthcare information systems. These laws address many aspects of healthcare, including the dissemination of healthcare information, the protection of confidential personal health information, the adoption of electronic health records (EHRs) throughout the United States, the use of technical standards, and the legitimacy of electronic signatures. Some of these laws impact not only health and healthcare information but the structure of healthcare organizations as well.

LEGISLATION

The specific laws discussed in this chapter are **Electronic Signatures in Global and National Commerce Act (ESIGN) of 2000**, **Medicare Improvements for Patients and Providers Act (MIPPA) of 2008**, **Health Insurance Portability and Accountability Act (HIPAA) of 1996**, and **American Recovery and Reinvestment Act of 2009 (ARRA)**. First, key elements of each law are summarized. Then, the impact of each law on healthcare informatics and nursing informatics is discussed.

E-Sign

The Electronic Signatures in Global and National Commerce Act ("E-Sign or ESIGN") was signed into law by then-President Clinton on June 30, 2000. E-Sign gives electronic signatures the same legal status as hand-written signatures. From a legal perspective, this means that any contract signed electronically cannot be declared invalid on the basis of an electronic signature (Freeman 2004). Sausser (2002) noted the definition of electronic signature as "any electronic means to indicate consent to the content of a transaction (e.g., handwritten signatures that are recorded electronically or digital signatures) (p. 72). The main focus of this Act was the enhancement of e-commerce. The Act supports electronic records and electronic transactions but does not require them. Evans (2001) studied the impact of the Act and noted that it facilitates e-commerce and the use of electronic records and signatures, and enhances consumer confidence. The Act preserves the right to receive written information already established by state and federal law. ESIGN also discourages deception and fraud by those who might fail to provide consumers with information the law requires that consumers should receive.

A digital signature is a method of signing electronic documents that provides the recipient with verification of the sender's identity and the sender's authority. Additionally, a digital signature can determine that the content of the document has not been altered since it was signed. This capability prevents senders from repudiating the fact that they signed and sent the document.

MIPPA

The Medicare Improvements for Patients and Providers Act (MIPPA) of 2008 included a provision calling for financial incentives for e-prescribing. Positive financial incentives are provided for practitioners who use e-prescribing from 2009 through 2013. MIPPA requires the use of e-prescribing in 2011 and beyond through negative financial incentives—reducing Medicare payments to providers who do not e-prescribe. A 2% bonus was available in 2009 and 2010 for e-prescribing, and a 1% bonus was given in 2011 and will be given in 2012. The penalties for not e-prescribing will be –1% in 2012, –1.5% in 2013, and –2 percent in 2014 and beyond (American College of Cardiology 2008).

HIPAA

Individuals receiving healthcare and those delivering healthcare (e.g., nurses, physicians, therapists) have long held concerns over who gets access to recorded health and healthcare information. These concerns, however, may be alleviated by the use of EHRs. A Harris Poll of 2007 showed that 75% of the 2,153 U.S. adults surveyed believe better healthcare will result if healthcare professionals were able to share information more easily (Bright 2007). Over half (63%) agree sharing of healthcare records could decrease medical errors. Belief in reduced healthcare costs from such sharing was held by 55% of survey respondents. However, about 25% of adults were unsure whether EHRs can provide these benefits.

The Health Insurance Portability and Accountability Act (HIPAA) of 1996 created landmark legal protection for personal health information (PHI). PHI refers to individually identifiable health information such as demographic data; facts that relate to an individual's past, present, or future physical or mental health condition; provision of care; and payment for the provision of care that identifies the individual. Examples include name, address, birth date, Social Security number, allergies, claims data, lab results and other diagnostic history, prescription history, records about past visits to physicians, emergency rooms and other healthcare encounters, vaccination records, and prior in- and outpatient procedures.

Transactions are electronic exchanges involving the transfer of information between two parties for specific purposes (CMS n.d.[a]). When a healthcare provider sends a claim for payment of services, a transaction has taken place. HIPAA mandated the adoption of selected standard transactions for electronic data interchange (EDI) of healthcare data. These standard transactions are claims and encounter information, payment and remittance advice, claims status, eligibility, enrollment and disenrollment, referrals and authorizations, and premium payment. HIPAA also named specific code sets for use in all Medicare-related transactions. These standardized code sets are Healthcare Common Procedure Coding System for ancillary services/procedures, Current Procedural Codes, Version 4 for physicians procedures, Code on Dental Procedures and Nomenclature for dental terminology, International Classification of Diseases (ICD) for medical diagnosis and hospital inpatient procedures and National Drug Codes for drugs. The United States has been among the last of the industrialized nations to adopt ICD Version 10. Version10 provides additional codes that will facilitate the implementation of electronic health records by making more detail available in electronic transactions. The adoption of ICD-10 is required in 2013 (Monegain 2011).

ARRA

The American Recovery and Reinvestment Act of 2009 (ARRA) has specific provisions for information technology in general and health information technology (HIT) in particular. These provisions include funding for a Smart Grid Information Clearinghouse, the Small Business Administration, the Department of Education, the Veterans Administration, and other government agencies for improving information technology systems.

The stimulus legislation codifies the position of the Office of the National Coordinator for Health Information Technology (ONCHIT)—the position was created by HIPAA but was never funded. ARRA also provides $2 billion for ONCHIT discretionary spending and sets a goal that an EHR will be used for each person in the United States by 2014. Two federal advisory committees on HIT are established—on policy and standards. These committees work with the private sector and consumer groups on development of a nationwide health information network. Specific aspects design interoperable EHRs for seamless data exchange and methods for ensuring privacy and security of patient data.

Under HIPAA, every person has the right to examine and obtain a copy of protected information. Typically, requested copies have been in paper form. Under ARRA, every person now has the right to have an electronic copy of an EHR and to have a copy directly transmitted to any designated entity (Steinbrook 2009).

HITECH

Title XIII of ARRA is the Health Information Technology for Economic and Clinical Health Act (HITECH). The HITECH Act makes several significant changes to the current HIPAA Security and Privacy Rules and provides funds and incentives to increase the use of EHRs by physicians and hospitals that meet eligibility criteria (Tomes 2010).

EHR Incentives Beginning in 2011, Medicare and Medicaid will provide financial incentives from $40,000 to $65,000 per eligible physician and up to $11 million per hospital for Meaningful Use of HIT. These positive incentives will be paid over several years. Negative incentives will begin in 2015 for physicians and hospitals that do not use certified information technology meaningfully.

As noted earlier, the ONCHIT oversees information technology standards, implementation strategies, and impact assessment. The goals of the Office of National Coordinator are to achieve the use of an EHR for each person in the country by 2014 and to develop a nationwide HIT infrastructure in support of the first goal. A major role of the ONCHIT is certification of EHR products. To receive the positive incentives, physicians and hospitals must use EHRs certified by ONCHIT (Tomes 2010).

The HITECH Act also funds the establishment of 70 or more regional centers to help promote EHR adoption. These centers will offer technical assistance, guidance, and information on best practices.

The Centers for Medicare & Medicaid Services (CMS) published the final rule on the incentive program, including the objectives for Meaningful Use, in July of 2010. This rule can be found at http://edocket.access.gpo.gov/2010/pdf/2010-17207.pdf. Meaningful Use is a complex component of the EHR incentive program. Discussion of Meaningful Use is beyond the scope of this chapter. A summary of Meaningful Use requirements is provided next.

CMS explains that the Meaningful Use requirements include a core set of objectives and a menu set of objectives. These sets are specific to eligible professionals or eligible hospitals and critical access hospitals (CAHs). For eligible professionals, 20 of 25 Meaningful Use objectives must be met to quality for an incentive payment. Fifteen of these objectives are required core objectives. The rest (5) are chosen from 10 menu-set objectives. Eligible hospitals and CAHs must achieve 19 out of 24 Meaningful Use objectives, with 14 of these required and 5 selected from 10 menu set objectives (CMS n.d.[b]).

CMS has many pages of its Web site devoted to explaining the incentive program, Meaningful Use, and the certification process: http://www.cms.gov/EHRIncentivePrograms.

Privacy and Security Provisions There are significant areas of change in federal privacy and security provisions with major impacts for medical practices, hospitals, health plans, and their business associates. A brief summary of key aspects follows.

Healthcare entities, as well as their business associates, must notify individuals whose health information is breached within 60 days of that breach. The entity also needs to notify the DHHS and local news media if more than 500 individuals are affected by a breach of information security. If data are encrypted, notification of a breach is not required. However, an entity has to validate whether data encryption works and meets federal standards (Nelson 2010).

Patients can now restrict some disclosures of personal health information (PHI) in certain circumstances. These restrictions are limited in scope. If a medical practice uses EHRs, the practice has to respond to patient requests for an accounting of all PHI disclosures up to 3 years (Nelson 2010).

HITECH also increases penalties for violations of HIPAA and HITECH security rules. Healthcare entities face fines of up to $1.5 million for violating a single requirement multiple times in a calendar year.

Patient Protection and Affordable Care Act of 2010

The Patient Protection and Affordable Care Act (Affordable Care Act), signed into law in March 2010, brings major changes to the U.S. health system. It guarantees access to healthcare for all Americans, creates new incentives to change clinical practice to foster better coordination and quality of care, gives practitioners more information so they can improve their clinical practice, gives patients more information to help them become more value conscious, and changes the healthcare payment system to reward value.

One of the objectives of this act is to improve protection of healthcare-related information and create incentives to change clinical practice. To meet this objective, the Affordable Care Act encourages the establishment of patient-centered medical homes (PCMH) and accountable care organizations (ACO) that should allow healthcare practitioners to focus on coordinating care and preventing avoidable hospitalizations. The Act also expands access to data about practitioner, hospital, drug, and device quality and safety (Aaron 2010).

An ACO is a group of healthcare provider organizations that takes on the responsibility for the quality and cost of healthcare delivered to a specific population of Medicare enrollees. The entities in an ACO can be combinations of hospitals, primary care practitioners, and healthcare specialists.

The Affordable Care Act also creates the idea of the PCMH. Not a patient's actual home filled with medical equipment, a PCMH is a healthcare delivery practice that serves as a center or one-stop shop for information, primary care, and care coordination. Each PCMH has a defined group of patients. Each patient has a personal healthcare practitioner who leads a team. The team takes on the responsibility for all of a patient's healthcare needs, either directly or through coordinated referrals (Laine 2011).

IMPACT ON INFORMATICS

Running through most of the legislation just reviewed is an implicit assumption that functioning, effective, and ubiquitous EHRs, along with supporting information systems, will be present in all healthcare delivery settings. To meet the demands for PHI protection and compliance reporting, every healthcare practice and hospital will need these electronic systems.

A major problem is the absence of these perfect systems. There are few healthcare practices and acute care hospitals with nearly paperless systems. These are too few in number to meet government and public expectations. Thus, the entire healthcare delivery system is scrambling to acquire, install, and use EHRs and health information systems.

Even though most healthcare organizations have some capacity for implementing information technologies, most will have to expand their capabilities to support the transformation of clinical care. Infrastructure, including skilled personnel, will be needed to make effective use of increased data, redesign the delivery of patient care, and improve outcomes (patient, staff, and organizational) and the performance of both staff and organization (Arlotto 2010).

Bigalke (2009) reports on a recent survey in which 1.5% of the 3,000 hospitals responding claimed to have comprehensive EHRs in use. Until now, cost has been a major impediment to EHRs for hospitals and practices. The HITECH Act is expected to alleviate much of this impediment, setting off a buying spree among chief information officers.

With the numerous vendors offering information technology solutions, informaticists (medical, nursing, etc.) and information technology leaders should consider the following factors when making purchase decisions: ONCHIT certification, site visits, preparing clinical staff, decision-support tools, and value. As well, purchasing a comprehensive EHR system will not be enough. Unless that system also provides all the functionality of a healthcare information system, purchasers will need to add the ancillary and support systems that enable an EHR to obtain necessary data. Existing systems may need upgrading or complete replacement. Given the emphasis on comprehensive EHRs, the extent to which these purchases are covered by the incentives under HITECH is not immediately clear.

The availability of working technical standards is another challenge. While HIPAA and HITECH have designated some technical standards as mandatory, those standards are insufficient to enable collection, management, and exchange of the mandated data. Technical standards are needed to ensure that structured and codified terminologies, sufficiently comprehensive to capture all of healthcare, are widely available, that data can be securely and easily exchanged within and across organizations, and that a valid, safe, and reliable patient-centered community-care record can be created and maintained (Arlotto 2010).

The demand for well-prepared, clinically savvy informatics practitioners will increase. Nursing informatics, clinical informatics, and medical informatics are now essential elements of strategic planning for any healthcare organization (Arlotto 2010). Informaticists are needed to mine data, analyze data aggregates, help in care-process redesign—especially information workflows—and design functional and clinically valid decision support. This demand will increase the number of undergraduate and graduate programs in informatics as well as the enrollment in these programs.

FUTURE DIRECTIONS

Predicting the future is always risky. As of this writing, controversy still swirls around the ARRA, with proponents predicting success and detractors aiming for reduction, revision, or complete removal of the Act. Regardless of the ultimate outcome of these political activities, a spotlight has been focused on EHRs and HITs and the expected benefits to individuals and populations of large-scale adoption. It is unlikely that this emphasis will diminish significantly.

Healthcare organizations and the care-delivery processes will change. More patient data will be available, and will transform to support better decision making. Informatics practitioners face a future of wonderful opportunities.

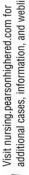

Visit nursing.pearsonhighered.com for additional cases, information, and weblinks.

CASE STUDY EXERCISE

You are teaching an undergraduate course titled Nursing Informatics. One class session is scheduled for a discussion on the protection of patient information stored in an electronic information system. How would you summarize the current status of legislative safeguards for this information in the United States? How would you help your students apply these concepts in their practice setting?

SUMMARY

- Legislation can and does shape the design and use of information systems.
- The Electronic Signatures in Global and National Commerce Act, also known as E-Sign, gives electronic signatures the same legal status as hand-written signatures.
- The Medicare Improvements for Patients and Providers Act (MIPPA) provides financial incentives for providers who use e-prescribing. The Health Insurance Portability and Accountability Act (HIPAA) provides legal protection for personal health information, set standards for electronic data interchange of claims data, and named specific code sets for use in all Medicare-related transactions.
- The American Recovery and Reinvestment Act of 2009 (ARRA) provided funds for the position of the Office of the National Coordinator for Health Information Technology (ONCHIT) and for the adoption of technology, and provides the right for every individual to receive an electronic copy of his or her EHR or to have a copy transmitted to any designated party.
- The Health Information Technology for Economic and Clinical Health Act (HITECH) strengthened HIPAA security and privacy protection and provides financial incentives for the user of EHRs.

- The Patient Protection and Affordable Care Act (Affordable Care Act) guarantees access to healthcare for all Americans and encourages the establishment of patient-centered medical homes and accountable care organizations to improve coordination of care.
- Informatics nurse specialists are key to ensuring the following:
  - successful acquisition and implementation of EHRs and health information systems' optimal use of aggregate data
  - re-design of resulting work processes

REFERENCES

Aaron, H. J. (2010, October 28). The midterm elections—High stakes for health policy. *New England Journal of Medicine*, 1685–1687. doi:10.1056/NEJMp1011213

American College of Cardiology. (2008). *The Medicare Improvements for Patients and Providers Act of 2008 (MIPPA). PL 110-275. ACC summary: Provisions impacting cardiovascular care.* Retrieved from http://stage.acc.org/advocacy/pdfs/ACC_Summary_MIPPA_07_08.pdf

Arlotto, P. (2010). 7 strategies for improving HITECH readiness. *Healthcare Financial Management, 64*(11), 90–96.

Bigalke, J. T. (2009, June). Filling the HIT gap by 2015. *Healthcare Financial Management,* 38–39.

Bright, B. (2007, November 29). Benefits of electronic health records seen as outweighing privacy risks. *Wall Street Journal.* Retrieved from http://online.wsj.com/article/SB119565244262500549.html

Centers for Medicare & Medicaid Services (CMS). (n.d. [a]). *Overview.* Retrieved from https://www.cms.gov/TransactionCodeSetsStands/

Centers for Medicare & Medicaid Services (CMS). (n.d. [b]). *Meaningful use.* Retrieved from https://www.cms.gov/EHRIncentivePrograms/30_Meaningful_Use.asp#BOOKMARK2

Evans, D. (2001). Electronic signatures in global and national commerce act. *The consumer consent provision in section 101(c)(1)(c)(ii).* Washington, DC: Federal Trade Commission. Retrieved from http://www.ftc.gov/os/2001/06/esign7.htm#ENDNOTES

Freeman, E. H. (2004). Digital signatures and electronic contracts. *Information Systems Security, 13*(2), 8–12. Retrieved from http://www.tandf.co.uk/journals/titles/1065898X.asp

Laine, C. (2011). Welcome to the patient-centered medical neighborhood. *Annals of Internal Medicine, 154*(1), 60. Retrieved from http://www.annals.org/

Monegain, B. (2011, November 3). Begin the ICD-10 climb now. *Healthcare IT News.* Retrieved from http://www.healthcareitnews.com/news/begin-icd-climb-now

Nelson, R. (2010, December). *Managing data security. AAOS now.* Retrieved from http://www.aaos.org/news/aaosnow/dec10/managing2.asp

Sausser, G. (2002). Digital perspectives. Use of electronic signatures: Past and present. *Healthcare Financial Management, 56*(6), 72–73.

Steinbrook, R. (2009). Health care and the American Recovery and Reinvestment Act. *New England Journal of Medicine, 360*(11), 1057–1060. Retrieved from http://www.nejm.org/

Tomes, J. (2010). Avoiding the trap in the HITECH act's incentive timeframe for implementing the EHR. *Journal of Health Care Finance, 37*(1), 91–100. Retrieved from http://www.aspenpublishers.com/product.asp?atalog_name=Aspen&product_id=SS10786767&cookie_test=1

CHAPTER 20

Regulatory and Reimbursement Issues

After completing this chapter, you should be able to:

1. Know which agencies govern the regulation of reimbursement for medical services at the federal, state, and local levels.

2. Demonstrate a basic understanding of Medicare Parts A, B, and C, and Medicaid.

3. Recognize the impact that Electronic Data Interchange (EDI) has had on the healthcare delivery system and the role that informatics nursing has played.

4. Discuss the ramifications of the Pay-for-Performance legislation, its pros and cons, and possible stumbling blocks.

5. Delineate potential problems and benefits involved in the transition to the ICD-10 and what will occur during the transition period.

6. Articulate a basic knowledge of billing codes and their effect upon reimbursement amounts, rejections, and appeals.

7. Appraise the impact that changes in Medicare physician payment in reimbursement and the expansion of the "do not pay" list will have on the healthcare delivery system.

8. Discuss the impact of the new regulatory and reimbursement laws passed in 2009–2010 on system use and design and when they will be integrated into the system.

9. Comprehend the financial incentives for implementing technology and the impact of the adoption of certified Electronic Health Records (EHR) systems on Medicare reimbursement procedures.

10. Explore the role of the informatics nurse in strengthening the Meaningful Use of EHR systems.

REGULATORY AGENCIES

Heath insurance regulation is visible at every government level. Each of the fifty states has the authority to regulate power not specifically deemed in the Constitution. Thus, the financial care of the poor and/or disabled citizens in each state is the responsibility of that state through Title XIX, or the Medicaid program of 1965. Regulation of insurance companies licensed to practice in that state and the monitoring of healthcare costs and reimbursements by those insurance companies also falls under Title XIX (Maurer & Smith 2005). Each state determines how it will fill this regulatory role mandated at the federal level.

Each state has a health agency, though the exact name may vary, which is the principal regulator of healthcare services for that state. That agency delegates the various health-related responsibilities to other agencies.

Since the ratification of the Title XVIII (Medicare) and Title XIX (Medicaid) Acts in 1965, the role of the federal government in regulating healthcare costs has continued to expand. The U.S. Department of Health and Human Services (USDHHS) is the umbrella under which all regulatory agencies eventually fall because the health and welfare of the citizens of the nation are ultimately deemed to be federal responsibility. That puts the U.S. government in a regulatory stance, delegating particulars to other agencies through organizations such as the Centers for Medicare & Medicaid Services (CMS) and the Health Care Finance Administration (HCFA).

Under the Health Maintenance Organization (HMO) Act (1973), and as a result of the McCarran-Ferguson Act (1945), regulation at the state level is reinforced but that does not preclude national involvement. Thus, the HCFA is responsible for overseeing any grievances involving Medicare recipients, but consumers who have complaints against Medicaid, HMOs, PPOs, POS, or other insurance plans must first seek assistance at the state levels (Free Advice n.d; Reutter 2005).

Most insurance companies' policies are found in the private sector and provided by agencies through employers or individuals. Premiums are paid by individuals or by employers on behalf of those individuals in order to fund the claims that are paid. State regulators then have the job of keeping tabs on the practices and policies of the insurance companies used by individuals and employers who reside in their state.

Workers' compensation is regulated by the states for injured workers who must receive medical care; however, Social Security Disability, which provides for healthcare for the permanently disabled, is governed by Medicare at the federal level. If a person is so severely injured on the job that she or he becomes permanently disabled, then he or she may well receive privately funded, state, and federal medical benefits.

Federal healthcare is provided for soldiers, veterans, and dependents under Tricare/Champus and the Veterans Health Administration. In different regions of the country, insurance companies bid to be Tricare/Champus providers.

The Federal Employees Health Benefits Program is a system of managed care benefits offered to civilian government workers and their dependents in the U.S. federal government. The government pays two-thirds of the cost of the insurance, and the employee pays the remaining one-third.

The Children's Health Insurance Program (CHIP) guarantees healthcare for every child that is a citizen regardless of income; however, it is administered by the states under their Medicaid programs. The federal government provides matching funds for the states to establish their own CHIP program to secure healthcare for children whose parents are in the gap between Medicaid and private insurance affordability and access. On February 4, 2009, President Barack Obama signed into law the Children's Health Reauthorization Act of 2009 (CHIPRA), thus expanding accessible healthcare to over 4 million previously uninsured children and pregnant women (Georgetown University 2009).

The Health Care and Education Reconciliation Act of 2010 (Pub.L.111-152, 124Stat.1029) amends the Patient Protection and Affordable Care Act (PPAC) signed into law on March 23,

2010 and further strengthens the federal grip on healthcare regulation in the United States. The Act is an effort to address the problems of the uninsured or underinsured in the United States. The PPAC authorized legislation to guarantee access to insurance for every citizen, with penalties for those who did not purchase coverage. Lower income families can receive up to 94% financial assistance in their premiums, while others can receive assistance based on a sliding scale. In addition, to help offset the influx of Medicaid policies expected under the PPAC, the federal government will pay all of the costs until 2016, then pay on a sliding scale as follows: 95% in 2017, 94% in 2018, 93% in 2019, and 90% thereafter. If states are already providing Medicaid benefits to children they will be provided more federal money through 2018 (Blankenship 2010).

Bridging the chasm between providing healthcare for all citizens and funding that effort leads to regulation. Taxes, together with funds from state and the federal governments, provide a finite number of dollars allocated for healthcare of citizens who qualify for federal and/or state assistance each fiscal year. This necessitates regulation of the costs of healthcare, although the PPAC Act has subsequently faced administrative, legislative, and legal challenges (Oberlander 2010).

Medicare and Medicaid

Medicare Medicare has several different parts, namely, A, B, C, and D. Medicare is age or disability based. Taxes taken out of the working population's paychecks help to fund this program. Medicare Part A *pays* for the facility-related expenses for inpatient, hospice, home health, or nursing home residency care. For the most part, individuals don't pay a premium for Medicare Part A coverage, but it does have an annual deductible that must be satisfied each year.

Medicare Part B is for medically necessary physician and outpatient expenses. This includes the fees for labs, x-rays, and so forth. It encompasses the cost of some supplies and DME (durable medical equipment) as well as some preventive measures such as pneumonia and flu shots. It also has an annual deductible and pays 80% of the allowed fee for any given service. Most people have supplemental policies or Medicaid, which pick up the remaining 20%.

Medicare Part C is called the *Advantage Plan.* An individual must be eligible for both Parts A and B to enroll. It combines the benefits of A and B as well as some additional benefits they exclude. A monthly premium is paid, similar to an employer-based or private insurance plan, as are co-payments.

Medicare Part D covers certain prescription drugs and medical supplies relating to the administration of those drugs.

While each state contracts with an insurance company to provide Medicare coverage, the reimbursement and fee schedules are regulated at the federal level. Services are reimbursed in accordance to the area of the country the provider practices and whether or not it is rural or urban. In order to further regulate and monitor costs, many Medicare programs are now HMOs.

Medicaid Medicaid eligibility is income based. Recipients must meet criteria based on their medical needs, income, and other resources, or lack thereof, to pay for those needs. Eligibility is regulated by each state based on criteria determined by each state. In some states, recipients pay co-payments on a sliding scale for some services.

Medicaid picks up the expenses approved, but not paid, by Medicare for Medicare beneficiaries who qualify. Therefore, Medicare deductibles, co-payments, and coinsurance costs may be covered by the state in which the elderly, indigent, or disabled person lives (CMS, Pub.11306, 2008).

State Health Departments

Healthcare within state-funded entities, such as schools, mental health facilities, and rehabilitation hospitals, falls under the jurisdiction of the state, not the federal government. There may be a myriad of agencies under the umbrellas of the state health department, including a regulatory commission in charge of overseeing the cost of healthcare premiums and reimbursements, insurance licensing, public health concerns and policies, and the enforcement of health laws.

The state health department oversees conditions in the marketplace and workforce as well, ensuring that companies follow OSHA (Occupational and Safety Health Administration) and CLIA (Clinical Laboratory Improvement Amendment) guidelines. Restaurants and other places where food is sold, cultivated, grown, and/or prepared are often under this department. Doctor's offices, labs, hospital and outpatient facilities, and long-term care centers and rehabilitation facilities are also under the regulatory realm of their state's health department.

Disease and contamination are two peas in a pod, so to speak, that must be regulated and also the cost for treating them. Again, the dividing lines between state and federal jurisdiction become blurred. Oftentimes, the federal government mandates regulation yet leaves the implementation of that regulation up to the individual states. Many states then pass the buck onto local and county levels. In the reimbursement world, the pecking order is usually private resources, local, then state or federal. In the regulatory realm, it is not so clear-cut.

The waters have been further muddied by the recent healthcare reform legislation. For example, in August 2010, $46 million in grants were offered to the states by the USDHHS to help them better regulate the escalating costs of health insurance premiums in preparation for transition to the federal health insurance law. In a recent article in the East Valley Tribune online, Fisher (2010) stated:

> But Arizona law sharply limits the ability of the state Department of Insurance to regulate what health insurers charge. And state lawmakers never gave the agency the power to help enforce the new federal healthcare law.
>
> Erin Klug, spokeswoman for the state insurance department, said her agency has absolutely no authority over what rates are charged by health maintenance organizations. And even with individual policies, state law requires only that companies pay out at least 50 to 60 cents in benefits for every dollar received in premiums, depending on the type of coverage. (p. 1)

For that reason, Arizona joined nearly two dozen other states in challenging the legality of the new healthcare reform legislation. In the meantime, Arizona lawmakers and the Arizona State Health Department have been working on a formula to determine the definition of "unreasonable insurance premium hikes" (Fisher 2010, p. 1).

This is just one example of the complicated inter-weaving of government regulatory agencies when it comes to healthcare issues. Healthcare in the United States also involves many entities that owned and operated in the private sector yet under the scrutiny of the states in which they are licensed to operate. Those state agencies, in turn, must follow federally mandated guidelines to the best of their ability without violating their state constitutions.

REIMBURSEMENT ISSUES

How healthcare professionals are reimbursed for their services in the care of the public is at the heart of any regulatory effort, and has been since the Carran-McFerguson Act of 1945. Ever since the Title XVIII and Title XIX Programs were launched in the mid 1960s, fair and reasonable charges and reimbursements have been an issue. At the center is the question of exactly what is the cost of healthcare. How do you put a price on the saving of a human life, or the taking of preventive measures to better ensure a quality of life? What should a physician be worth for 10 minutes of his or her time and expertise behind the closed doors of an examining room? What should he or she charge for supplies, the duties the staff performs, and so forth. Healthcare has overhead. How much profit is ethical?

The Balanced Budget Act of 1997 reduced the payment percentages Medicare would reimburse healthcare professionals. These were later revised in the Balanced Budget Reform Act of 1999 and the Budget Improvement and Protection Act of 2000. In an effort to regulate the skyrocketing costs of healthcare, the U.S. federal government, which funds the Medicare programs, continues to try and harness reimbursement issues (Doherty n.d).

Most insurance companies follow Medicare's lead in reimbursement percentage and regulation. Therefore, the way CMS interprets federal legislation affects all insured and to some extent noninsured citizens, not just Medicare beneficiaries.

Electronic Data Interchange

In this age of electronic information exchange, there are obvious challenges. How does one uphold the HIPAA (Health Insurance Portability and Accountability Act of 1996) while transmitting sensitive patient information over the fax, phone, or the World Wide Web? Confidentiality rules must be adhered to by all in the healthcare profession who have access to medical records.

The welfare of the person being treated depends on the accurate transference of information from one healthcare professional to another, and reimbursement is more and more dependent upon electronic data interchange. Great strides have been made in the technologies that allow medical necessity proofs to be piggy-backed with claims, avoiding delays in processing such claims.

The burden of medical necessity falls on the performer of the service. Failure to do so will lead to a denial for reimbursement. For example, in order to be reimbursed by Medicare Part A for the admission and per diem treatment on a SNF (Skilled Nursing Facility) unit, a patient must have first been hospitalized as an inpatient in a freestanding facility. All Part B and ancillary care are based on that criterion.

The Medicare, Medicaid, and State Children's Health Insurance Program (SCHIP) Balanced Budget Refinement Act of 1999 (BBRA) further clarified this burden of proof. For example, since 1998, the **Resource Utilization Group (RUG)** had been a patient classification of over 35 criteria that set the per diem reimbursement standards to care for a certain SNF qualifying diagnoses, including time and supplies needed (CMS 2006). Now, under The Patient Protection and Affordable Care Act (PPACA), enacted on March 23, 2010, in Section 10325 (Pub. L. 111-148), a self-implementing provision involving the SNF payment system is restructured (CMS Federal Register, 2010).

In order to regulate the conformity of electronic transmission of information, the CMS published a mandate that required all providers, insurers, and any middlemen involved in the healthcare industry to submit claims for reimbursement or for registering care, verifying eligibility, precertification of services, or any other client-related information, to adhere to a uniform format. This was to occur by October 2002 but Congress extended the date to October 2003. Though paper claims were exempt, this measure was intended to help phase out paper claims except under extensive appeal circumstances.

This action forced all providers to install EDI transmission programs in their billing and medical record systems by buying practice management systems or utilizing a clearinghouse that screened and then transmitted electronic claims and records to the various insurance companies.

Private sector insurance companies were forced in the 1990s to establish Common Procedural Terminology coding that was recognized by Medicare. Up until that time, Common Procedural Terminology and Healthcare Common Procedure Coding System (HCPCS) varied from company to company, especially with the use of modifiers. Claims were often denied due to incorrect coding, and those claims could not be properly processed through Medicare or Medicaid for reimbursement. The move to EDI further reinforced uniformity in coding.

In another effort to obtain uniformity, the HIPAA Administrative Simplification Provision directives declared all providers must have a National Provider Identifier (NPI) on each electronic or paper claim by May 2007. The referring physician's NPI must also be present on the CMS-1500 (HCFA) forms, which were revised to accommodate the digits. Billing software companies scrambled to update programs, as did insurance claims processing programs. This 10-digit NPI number is universal, replacing the need for provider ID numbers or Unique Physician Identification Numbers (UPINs) assigned by different insurance companies. Prior to this time, a healthcare provider could have up to 20 or more provider ID numbers, leading to confusion on secondary and tertiary claims (AASP 2006).

Each time legislation is passed a grace period is given to allow ample time for conversion. This does not mean transmissions go smoothly. This is why accurate and detailed record keeping of all EDI transmissions, whether they involve claims processing or not, is a must.

Confidentiality statements that meet HIPAA standards must be identifiable and clear on all facsimile transmissions. All phone calls, be they with insurance companies involving precertification and clarification of care, with patients' family members, or other third parties, must adhere to HIPAA and fall under EDI guidelines.

With the move toward more extensive monitoring of quality care and payment based on performance, Health Information Technology (HIT) is developing into a vast infrastructure of medical information exchange between hospitals, physicians, agencies, and Medicaid and CHIP programs on a nationwide basis. Such information distribution is vitally important because of each state's flexibility in the implementation of programs within Medicaid and CHIPS parameters. EDI will continue to play an important role in the uniform efforts to bring state programs within the guideline parameters mandated by federal legislation, from which reimbursements are determined.

Pay-for-Performance

What has been termed *ObamaCare* involves a system called **Pay-for-Performance** (P4P) otherwise known as Value-Based Purchasing (VBP). Accountable care organizations will be formed to police the quality of services healthcare professionals and facilities provide. This system rewards physicians and other healthcare professionals when patients receive good results from those services. At first, this seems logical. Consumers pay for performance when it comes to repairs and servicing of cars and electronics, for maid and janitorial services, for agents, entertainment, and so forth. If one does not care for the results, one either doesn't pay or ask for a refund.

However, humans are not products, so excellence in performance is, therefore, harder to judge. Success is not so easily measured tangible and universal means. Measuring the quality of performance of health-related services is similar to grading teacher and school performances in the educating of children. Through state-leveled testing of students, officials can see if a majority of students in a class mastered the level of education they were to achieve. Educators are then rated by their performance in helping those students achieve those goals. But the child's ability to learn, social factors that may affect his or her learning capability, and so forth, must also be taken into account.

In the same way, when measuring healthcare performances, several chronic diseases may influence an acute disease. How does one determine the result from any medically related care as good enough to be paid? CMS addressed this issue in an ePamphlet. In it, the CMS states the goals for VBP.

- Financial viability—where the financial viability of the traditional Medicare fee-for-service program is protected for beneficiaries and taxpayers.
- Payment incentives—where Medicare payments are linked to the value (quality and efficiency) of care provided.
- Joint accountability—where physicians and providers have joint clinical and financial accountability for healthcare in their communities.
- Effectiveness—where care is evidence-based and outcome-driven to better manage diseases and prevent complications from them.
- Ensuring access—where restructured Medicare fee-for-service payment system provides equal access to high quality, affordable care.
- Safety and transparency—where a value-based payment system gives beneficiaries information based on quality, cost, and safety of their healthcare.
- Smooth transitions—where payment of systems supports well-coordinated care across different providers and settings.
- Electronic health records—where value-driven healthcare supports the use of information technology to give providers the ability to deliver high quality, efficient, well-coordinated care. (CMS Goals For Value-Based Purchasing 2010, p. 4)

CMS changed roles "from a passive payer of services to a more active purchaser of high quality and affordable patient care" (Kuhn 2008, p. 1). Physicians will not be paid based on their volume of services but on the quality of those services. Per diems under Part A will be reevaluated for efficiency and performance. In fact, CMS has already begun the process of reporting data on the quality of hospitals, Home Health Agencies (HHAs), and physicians.

CMS admits that it will have to develop new strategies for physician self-referral rules. Payment will be based on broader bundles of service, not individual procedures. The patient's total care will be examined. The questions of how to fairly monitor clinical progress are vast. If a diabetic patient has cardio-pulmonary complications and goes into renal failure, how does one determine the efficiency and quality of each specialty's involvement in the care?

Patients will play a more active role in the determination of performance-based payment. But is this valid? Can an uneducated patient correctly judge his or her treatment as "good"? The Personal Health Record system will allow patients and their designated beneficiaries to have access to and input into their medical records repository. The ideal scenario is that patients will have a clearer understanding of their healthcare requirements and take a more active role in compliance. Transparency will equip the average patient to make more informed decisions. Also, their health information and medical history will be stored electronically and be more easily accessible in the future.

This is already being tried out in hospital settings throughout the country, where a patient voluntarily registers his or her medical history. But, who will monitor and collate the amount of information that is data entered? Will criteria be different for hospitals and doctor's offices? For primary care physicians versus specialists?

Hospital-Based Pay-per-Performance The Medicare Improvements for Patients and Providers Act provided for performance-based payments for End Stage Renal Disease facilities beginning in 2012. SNF, home health, and outpatient clinics will soon follow, as will physician offices.

In July 2003, CMS began the National Voluntary Hospital Reporting Initiative, also known as Hospital Quality Alliance Improving Care Through Information, in an effort to provide a viable means to measure and report on the quality of care in U.S. hospitals. One result of this has been a Web site tool called Hospital Compare (http://www.hospitalcompare.hhs.gov), which debuted April 1, 2005 (CMS Goals For Value-Based Purchasing 2010, p. 5).

For 4 years from 2006 to 2009, under a CMS program called Premier Hospital Quality Incentive Demonstration, which included over 250 hospital systems in 38 states across the nation, bonus incentives were given for the quality of patient services in five clinical areas—acute myocardial infarction (AMI), pneumonia, heart failure, Coronary artery bypass graft surgery (CABG), and hip/knee replacements. Each area received a composite quality score. In all areas, there was a measurable increase in quality of care over a 3-year period, according to CMS (2010b):

From 87.5 to 96.1 for AMI

From 84.8 to 97 for CABG

From 64.5 to 88.7 for heart failure

From 69.3 to 90.5 for pneumonia

From 84.6 to 96.9 for hip/knee replacement. (p. 8)

Physician-Based Pay-per-Performance CMS developed an effective and fair VBP for physicians. Under the Tax Relief and Health Care Act of 2006 (TRHCA-P.L. 109-432), a quality reporting system included a payment incentive to report accurate, quality-measured data for covered professional services. Reimbursements began in 2007. CMS dubbed this program Physician Quality Reporting Initiative (PQRI).

By 2008, there were 119 measures that the professional could choose to evaluate a patient's care; 117 were clinic and 2 were structural. Fifty-two more were added in 2009. requirements and measure specifications for each year are published in the Federal Register and may differ from the previous year (CMS 2011). Measure groups address care for osteoarthritis, rheumatoid arthritis, back pain, coronary artery bypass, CABG, chronic kidney disease, oncology, HIV/AIDS, and so forth.

CMS has also developed a Physician Group Practice (PGP) demonstration to determine the amount of monies saved in the Medicare program and, based on performance, the amount to share back to those physicians who complied. The bonuses are based on 32 quality measures, and the PGP is awarded up to 80% of what it saved Medicare in payments. The result so far, according to CMS (2010b) is as follows:

> All 10 of the participating physician groups achieved benchmark or target performance on at least 25 out of 27 quality markers for patients with diabetes, coronary artery disease, and congestive heart failure. (p. 13)

One example of the shift in emphasis to performance-based measuring is CMS's desire to become a more active partner with the states in the administration of the Medicaid and CHIP programs.

The CMS publication entitled *Medicaid and CHIP Quality Practices* (n.d.) stated:

> CMS defines quality as—The right care for every person every time. CMS is responsible for supporting State Medicaid and CHIP programs in their efforts to achieve safe, effective, efficient, patient-centered, timely and equitable care. CMS will partner with States to share best practices, provide technical assistance to improve performance measurement, evaluate current improvement efforts to inform future activities, collaborate with quality partners and coordinate Center activities to ensure efficiency of operations. . . .
>
> CMS recently developed a Medicaid/CHIP Quality Strategy. Key strategies include: (1) Evidenced-Based Care and Quality Measurement (2) Payment Aligned with Quality (3) Health Information Technology (4) Partnerships (5) Information Dissemination, Technical Assistance, and sharing of best practices. (p. 1)

It is evident that performance measurement will better ensure the success of this process for gleaning information on the quality of healthcare for Medicaid and CHIP eligible patients.

Transition to ICD-10

On October 1, 2013, the federal government will implement the mandatory transition to the *International Classification of Diseases, Tenth Revision* (ICD-10). The reasoning behind the move is to better manage the data that will be used in measuring the quality of healthcare in the United States through more precise and accurate diagnostic coding.

The ICD-10 will have more than 155,000 different code variations in comparison to the current ICD-9, which has 17,000 (ICD Common n.d.). Here is an example of the change courtesy of the AMA (2008), whose source is the CMS:

ICD-9 code was 599.7 Hematuria

ICD-10 code - Specify one of the following:

    R31.0 Gross hematuria

    R31.1 Benign essential microscopic hematuria

    R31.2 Other microscopic hematuria

    R31.9 Hematuria, unspecified

ICD-9 Code 896.2 Traumatic amputation of foot, complete or partial, bilateral

ICD-10 Code Specify one of the Following:

S98.011 Complete traumatic amputation of right foot at ankle level

S98.021 Partial traumatic amputation of right foot at ankle level

and one of the following

S98.012 Complete traumatic amputation of left foot at ankle level

S98.022 Partial traumatic amputation of left foot at ankle level

The ICD-9 is nearly 30 years old and has undergone numerous revisions, almost yearly. In August of 2008, USDHHS announced that the process of replacing the outdated coding. This was in an effort to keep up with electronic record keeping and monitoring, the measurement of quality care, and the new discoveries in medical disease and treatments. Along with the ICD-10 is the ICD-10-PCS for inpatient hospital procedural coding, which replaces Volumes 1 and 2 of the ICD-9 and Volume 3 for procedure codes (Evans 2008). The compliance deadline for adoption of ICD-10 is now set for October 1, 2013 (AMA 2011).

Will the transition be simple? Many physician organizations have emphatically stated they will not be ready.

> Before physicians, hospitals and others can use the new code sets, they must upgrade their electronic transaction systems to be compatible. (Trapp 2008, p. 1)

Although procedural codes (see Billing Codes and Reimbursement), which are used to define the service performed, will remain intact, electronic transmissions, such as verifying eligibility, requesting a remittance advice, or filing a claim, require diagnosis codes and thus will be affected by this ruling and also by an update in HIPAA standards for administrative electronic transmission, known as the 5010 revision, which was announced on January 16, 2009, by the USDHHS. The deadline for compliance with the new HIPAA standards is January 1, 2012 (AMA Physician Resources n.d.).

Currently, and since the year 2000, the 4010 version has been used. After January 1, 2012, any transmission using the 4010 will be rejected as not compliant with HIPAA standards. Thus, two new conversions must be implemented by physician offices—the 5010 and the ICD-10.

Private insurance companies will also have to upgrade their software to accommodate the new diagnostic codes on the electronic claims, as will clearinghouses that screen and file claims for many smaller physician practices. The cost of converting all these systems will be staggering. However, reimbursement rates are not increasing, and in fact, with new legislation to reduce the cost of healthcare, the transition may indeed leave many healthcare professionals in a bind. It is estimated that until proficiency in the new coding is achieved, physicians will see productivity losses anywhere from $50 million to $250 million nationwide. The workload in proper coding practices will increase 3–4% (Benson 2009).

Robert Tennant, senior policy adviser from the Medical Group Management Association, stated in an article to amednews.com, "CMS underestimates the proposed rules' impact, particularly on small physician practices" (Trapp 2008, p. 1).

However, both the American Hospital Association and the American Health Information Management Association are on public record that they support the transition. In a white paper by Wolters Kluwer, it is stated, "The ICD-10 mandate is driven by more than costs and benefits. Developed more than thirty years ago, the ICD-9 code set has simply outlived its usefulness" (Benson 2009).

It is clear that in the past 30 years there has been much change in the diagnosis and treatment of disease, and many were unknown when the ICD-9 first came out. Each year codes were revamped, added, subtracted, or deleted, causing confusion as well as misfiled and denied claims as insurance companies and medical billing programs scrambled to update. A new system seems warranted. However, will that all halt with the ICD-10? The prognosis is doubtful. Updates will continue as medical breakthroughs and diagnostic discoveries are found.

During the transition phase, IT companies, hospitals, and physicians will be in varying phases of conversion, necessitating a dual system of accepting either ICD-9 or ICD-10 by insurance companies for a period of time. Otherwise, too many claims will reject unnecessarily, putting further financial burden upon practitioners and other healthcare facilities.

There is one argument for the implementation of the ICD-10. In an ever-growing global society, medical care boundaries are blurring. Over 100 countries have already adopted the ICD-10 coding system (Benson 2009; WHO 2011). When U.S. healthcare providers come onboard no doubt the global consistency in diagnosing, exchange of treatment ideas, and communication of medical practices will improve. It will enhance and clarify technological advances in medicine as well as the transmission of electronic information through a common coding language. Language barriers may dissipate when everyone knows R31.0 is a gross hematuria.

The hope is the implementation of the ICD-10 will improve electronic procedure documentation and more accurate coding solutions as well as assure more uniformity and fairness in quality performance-based reimbursements and procedural precertifications.

Billing Codes and Reimbursement

Common Procedural Terminology-Healthcare Common Procedure Coding System Reimbursement is not just based on the diagnosis (ICD), but also on the corresponding treatment required to cure, alleviate, or monitor that ailment. Along with computerized claims processing came the development of coding for various forms of treatment. But each insurance company had a different code for an office visit, for a chest x-ray, and so forth. To elevate this problem, the **Common Procedural Terminology** codes were developed in 1966. These codes are the copyrighted property of the American Medical Association (AMA) and are monitored and updated by that organization in coordination with CMS. A Common Procedural Terminology Editorial Panel of 17 members meets quarterly to review the updates, deletions, and additions to the over 8,500 codes now in existence proposed by the Common Procedural Terminology Advisory Committee, which is made up of representatives from over 90 healthcare organizations and medical societies (marqpdx 2010).

Common Procedural Terminology codes also grouped into three categories. Category I is the most commonly referred to when someone speaks of Common Procedural Terminology codes. In that category are six subcategories:

1. Evaluation and management
2. Anesthesiology
3. Surgery
4. Radiology
5. Pathology and laboratory
6. Medicine

Category II Common Procedural Terminology codes, mainly used for measurement procedures, are four digits followed by the letter "F."

Category III codes are temporary codes under review. If they are not assimilated into the Category I codes within 5 years they are dropped. Most of these codes need supporting documentation to justify their billing and may not have set pricing.

Common Procedural Terminology codes were grouped into services by the first digit followed by four more digits that further described the procedure. For example, the number 9 is reserved for visits related to evaluation and management procedures.

Thus, the Common Procedural Terminology code 99211 is an office visit for less than 10 minutes and is often used when the patient only sees a nurse for an injection, blood pressure check, or some other simple procedure, which does not involve direct contact with the physician. Common Procedural Terminology codes 99212, 99213, and 99214 are all incremented as more one-on-one time between the patient and the medical professional is required. The diagnosis codes help justify the time spent with the physician.

Two-digit modifiers are also used to further distinguish services and procedures, such as repeated, same area but different procedure, left, right, assistant surgeon, etc. Each sub-category has appropriate modifiers. Incorrect use of codes and modifiers delays claim processing. Therefore, precise coding choice is paramount to timely reimbursement. The current revision is the 2005–2009 Common Procedural Terminology-4 codes.

Common Procedural Terminology codes were designed to universally assign a number to each conceivable task or service performed by a healthcare provider, be it medical, diagnostic, or surgical. Or so was the idea. However, it was not as complete as CMS wanted.

Thus, the development of the HCPCS came into play, which more thoroughly covered the Common Procedural Terminology-coded services and other services, such as DME, supplies, drugs, or ambulance services. HCPCS is in two levels. Level I is the same as the Common Procedural Terminology codes, whereas Level II is more extensively for supplies, equipment, and auxiliary services not normally passing through a physician's office (Torrey 2009).

Other Coding Systems

G-Codes As previously discussed under the P4P, measurement groups known as PQRIs are also coded. In 2006, the acting administrative head of CMS suggested the development of measurements for the quality of care physicians gave to their office patients. Physicians who complied with measurement reporting receive percentage initiative reimbursement. The outcome is a system called **G-codes**, which are a special set of nonpayable HCPCS codes. Also termed as **quality data codes** (QDC), the G-codes are used to supplement the claim data with supporting clinical data, so the quality of service can be measured. Each quality is assigned a corresponding G-code. The G-codes are submitted along with the Common Procedural Terminology/HCPCS codes. Physicians who voluntarily report three measures on at least 80% of their patients are paid a bonus of 1.5% of their allowable charges under the Medicare Fee Guidelines (Rogers 2007). The reporting period is January 1 through December 31 each year.

RUGs A per diem system of billing for skilled nursing facility (SNF unit) patients was developed in 1998 under a Prospective Payment System. Per diem payment was based on the patient's condition, which qualified them for SNF care, and classifications to qualify that care was divided into RUGs. This system was to help clarify that the level of care provided for each patient matched the per diem rate. There are upwards of 35 categories of RUGs. CMS (2007) states if the beneficiary met the level of care requirement, contractors shall also determine whether the furnished services and intensity of those services, as defined by the billed RUG group, were reasonable and necessary for the beneficiary's condition. To determine if the beneficiary was correctly assigned to a RUG group, contractors shall verify that the billed RUG group is supported by the associated provider documentation. (p. 1)

MSDRG When a patient enters the hospital, a PAO (present on admission) diagnosis is given and the patient is assigned to a **Medicare severity diagnosis related group (MS-DRG)**. There are 745 such classifications, and these determine the per diem rate as of May 2007 (Walters 2007).

In October 2008, Medicare determined it could not assign a higher MS-DRG upon inpatient discharge than was listed on the PAO, or admitting diagnosis ICDs. This means proper initial diagnosis is essential, as is well-organized and documented medical record tracking when complications arise while a patient is in-house. The proper reimbursement rate per diem of each inpatient person can have an enormous financial impact on a hospital system.

Changes in Reimbursement

With the move toward P4P in both hospital and outpatient settings, changes in the way healthcare professionals and facilities are reimbursed will be massive. Perhaps not since the initiation of the Title XVIII and Title XIX Acts has there been such rumblings as those produced over the past 5 or 6 years, especially with the 2010 passage of The Health Care and Education Reconciliation Act of 2010 and the PPACA under the Obama administration along with the decision to implement the ICD-10 by 2013.

Change is inevitable. The reimbursement process under CMS is in constant flux and always has been. Each attempt to improve the accuracy of reporting criteria for reimbursement is met with opposition, and revisions are made yearly to try and reconcile the opposing views.

Physician reimbursement has been based on service geographic area in which that service was performed. Cost of living expenses vary across the nation, from city to city and state to state. Physician Fee Schedules (PFS) were developed as part of the reimbursed profile.

The formula is complicated and is based on the 75% percentile of the prevailing charges of physicians of like specialty in any given area. Each year CMS updates and revises the PFS and adjusts for the medical inflation rate; however, due to the amount of data that must be accumulated to set the new rates, the PFS's are often years behind the cost of living indexes.

The calendar year 2011, PFS is available on the Federal Register as of June 25, 2010, and tries to reflect, according to CMS (2010a):

> Proposed annual updates to the relative weights of physician services and would implement key provisions in the Affordable Care Act of 2010 that expand preventive services for Medicare beneficiaries, improve payments for primary care services, and promote access to health care services in rural areas. (p. 1)

On June 25, 2010, the Preservation of Access to Care for Medicare Beneficiaries and Pension Relief Act was signed into law. Section 101 of Pub.L.111-191 of that Act provided for a 2.2 % update of the 2010 PFS, but only for dates of service June 1, 2010 through November 30, 2010 (CMS 2010a).

With such rapid changes in health legislation and healthcare reform, confusion in Medicare physician payment rules is obvious. According to an article in the *American Medical News*, the AMA and other influential physician organizations are supporting the proposal to review the key factors that determine how Medicare providers are reimbursed, known as the Medicare Economic Index (MEI). The AMA, along with the American College of Physicians and the Medical Group Management Association, wants to freeze all attempts of revisions to the MEI until a technical panel representing over 72 specialty societies and other healthcare professional organizations release their findings (Silva 2010).

The articles goes on to state that the AMA is putting pressure on CMS to improve the PQRI system in how it reports feedback to physicians and how it issues bonus payments to those physicians who meet the thresholds, as is required under the heath system reform law.

Silva, in the same article, quotes the AMA Executive Vice President and CEO Michael D. Maves, MD, MBA, as follows:

> To be effective, reports must be distributed at a point during the reporting period so as to allow physicians to assess their reporting performance status, and revise their reporting practices, if needed, to be a successful participant. (p. 1)

The AMA fears the MEI doesn't properly reflect the growing percentage of employment that is needed in physician office, especially in primary care. In 2002, the increase was 3.7%, whereas in 2009 it had grown to 18.4%.

Clearly, tighter and more frequent communication between federal levels and individual physicians will be necessary to facilitate fair reporting and reimbursement/performance bonus incentives under the new healthcare reform legislation. This may well mean physician office employment percentages will continue to climb, and AMA feels that should be reflected in the reimbursement factors.

Expansion of the Do Not Pay List In an effort to control the quality and cost of healthcare, Medicare developed a Do Not Pay list for preventable complications. Examples are poor control of blood sugar levels or the extra cost for treating blood clots after hip replacement surgery. Naturally, other insurance companies are following suit.

Under the Do Not Pay rules, if patients develop certain medical problems during their hospital stay, Medicare will not reimburse the hospital at the higher rate for the treatment of the complication. However, it will still pay for treatment related to the primary diagnosis and other complications not on the list. The physicians who provide that care are not under the rule.

Nevertheless, the AMA opposed this, stating there are better methods of control healthcare spending and reimbursement costs. Physicians fear the Do Not Pay expansion will have a reverse effect on the quality of care. Each patient's circumstances are unique and complications cannot always be prevented or explained (Medicare-Medicaid.com n.d.).

Patients may not receive proper treatment or services for fear that a complication could result and the finger of blame may be pointed. Medical care involves risks and the Do Not Pay does not effectively take into account certain patient risk factors that initial diagnostic tools do not uncover.

In 2008, the list expanded to 10 categories, which according to CMS would save over $21 million in Medicare costs per year (Trapp 2008). The goal, according to CMS officials quoted in the article, is not just an economic one but also a way to provide safer care for Medicare beneficiaries in hospital settings.

The 10 categories on the 2008 Do Not Pay list included:

1. Stage III, IV pressure ulcers
2. Fall or trauma resulting in serious injury
3. Vascular catheter-associated infection
4. Catheter-associated urinary tract infection
5. Foreign object retained after surgery
6. Certain surgical site infections
7. Air embolism
8. Blood incompatibility
9. Certain manifestations of poor blood sugar control
10. Certain deep vein thromboses or pulmonary embolisms.

In 2 years, that list grew substantially to 42 categories. Starting on October 1, 2010, Medicare's fiscal new year, CMS retired only one criterion and added these new measures:

- Heart failure 30-day risk standardized readmission measure
- Failure to rescue
- Surgery patients on a beta-blocker prior to arrival who received one during the perioperative period
- Death among surgical patients with treatable serious complications
- Adult collapsed lung
- Postoperative wound reopening
- Accidental puncture or laceration
- Abdominal aortic aneurysm mortality rate
- Hip fracture mortality rate
- Mortality for a composite of selected medical conditions
- Mortality for a composite of selected surgical procedures
- Complication and patient safety for a composite of selected indicators
- Participation in a systematic database for cardiac surgery.

IMPACT ON SYSTEM USE AND DESIGN

As discussed, the more federal and state-mandated healthcare cost reform legislation comes into play, the more burden of proof is placed on the healthcare community to justify their services and receive proper reimbursement for them. That means more man-hours in coding, medical records logging and storing, EDI, and the evaluation of systems and procedures. Extra man-hours cut into profit. In 6 short years, employment rose by almost 16% in physician offices alone to handle the load, as has been reported in a previous section. It is no wonder that many predict nursing informatics is on the rise more than hands-on care nursing.

Technological developments can be cost and time savers, but there is a learning curve involved, and with the rapid change in procedural methods, reimbursement criteria, and monitoring of care, nurses and other healthcare professionals are hard pressed to keep abreast of what is now law, what will be law, and what may be law.

Accountable care organizations are already being implemented. Soon, the bundling of services will be the norm rather than payment for individual procedures. The impact of these changes is already being felt. Even though much of the Health Insurance Reform Act, also known as the PPACA (Public Law 111-148), will not go into effect until 2014, the following is a list of points that were immediately put into effect when the final bill was signed in May, 2010 (Dymkova-Fuchs 2010):

- Young people can remain on parents' health insurance until age 26.
- There can be no discrimination against children with pre-existing conditions.
- No dropping people from coverage when they get sick.
- There will be no lifetime limits on coverage.
- New plans must offer free preventive care.
- There will be an expanded ability to appeal decisions made by the health plan. (p. 1)

The physician's office must adjust to these new rulings and put them into place in their office systems. Insurance companies must alter their criteria for claims eligibility.

Most of the rulings now in effect benefit citizens seeking medical care. This will translate into more people opting for care since their insurance company will potentially pay for it. It is safe to assume physicians will need to hire more staff, seek entrance into larger groups that can accommodate the increased access to care, and revise their office systems to facilitate the flow of patients.

Other, more subtle changes will have an impact on the physician's office as well as outpatient facilities, ancillary services, and hospitals. In order to become, or perhaps soon remain, a Medicare/Medicaid provider, a Medical Compliance Program must be in place.

According to the Fox Group's Web site (n.d., p. 1.) that includes:

- compliance with health and safety laws and regulations,
- compliance with environmental laws and regulations,
- compliance with human resources laws and regulations, and
- compliance with HIPAA laws and regulations.

Risk-based coding and medical documentation must be accurately implemented in order to be in compliance in these areas. Treatment criteria evaluation may need to be refocused, as will the procedural patterns within each office or facility. Further reliance on exact and detailed data entry, coding, and medical record input is evident, and the technology to sort and verify the new criteria must be mastered. The Fox Group Web site further states:

> Efficient and effective medical group operations have always been sought, but as reform measures bring about the above described scrutiny, be aware of how much more critical billing practices, personnel management, and general practice operations are going to be if you are to prosper in this new environment. (p. 1)

FINANCIAL INCENTIVES FOR IMPLEMENTING TECHNOLOGY

Adoption of Certified EHR Systems and Medicare Reimbursement

HHS adopted regulations regarding electronic health records (EHR) on August 1, 2006, which created two exceptions to the Stark Law. The overall purpose of the Stark Law was to prevent improper patient referrals by prohibiting physicians from referring patients receiving Medicare or Medicaid to facilities in which the physicians or their family members had financial interests whether that might be a salary or ownership (Hanson 2010; Paddock & Fornataro 2010; Stirewalt 2009). Hospitals and physicians can establish donation relationships in the interexchange of EHR technologies and not be in violation of the Stark Law. This was further solidified in April 2009.

The Office of the National Coordinator from Health Information Technology (ONC), a subsidiary of the USDHHS, released a temporary list of EHR products tested and certified by CMS as reliable and compatible with the Medicare system. According to Dr. David Blumenthal, ONC Director and Health IT National Coordinator, the final plan, which will certify which EHR products are to be in compliance with federal regulations, will be released in 2012 (Fernandez 2010).

This has all come about due to the passage of the American Recovery and Reinvestment Act (ARRA), otherwise referred to as the Economic Stimulus Bill, which allocated $19 billion to help healthcare professionals adopt EHRs guaranteed to be in compliance with HIPAA privacy of information laws. The funding especially targets healthcare in rural areas and for acute care facilities with at least 10% Medicaid volume.

The PPACA of March 2010 (PPACA) Section 1561 will, when fully activated by 2014 as discussed, extend affordable healthcare to an estimated 32 million more people. This will require more supplies, more staff, and more HIT coordination. An electronically transmitted system must be developed with "interoperable and secure standards and protocols that facilitate electronic enrollment of individuals in Federal and State health and human services programs" (ONC 2010a, p. 1).

HIT must include structured patient demographics as well as clinical information and interactive data retrieval for reporting to CMS, especially with the establishment of PQRI and Medicare pay incentives. The ONC has set up competitive grants for the states in the union who make loans for physicians to purchase the certified EHR systems.

This is all in an effort to improve the inter-transmitting of data electronically between the federal and state agencies and the healthcare professionals and facilities. With the implementation of the upcoming P4P legislation, EHR must be accurate and retrievable in a timely manner and accompany or piggy-back electronic claims for proper processing and reimbursement.

To date, a 20-member HIT Policy Committee has been established to pave the way for a national HIT system under the direction of the USDHHS (Kohn 2009).

In the above-referenced Section 1561 Recommendations, the ONC (2010a) under Recommendation 2.2, states:

> We recommend development of a Federal reference software model, implementing standards for obtaining verification of a consumer's initial eligibility, renewal and change in circumstances information from Federal agencies and States to ensure a consistent, cost-effective and streamlines approach across programs and State delivery systems. (p. 2)

The ONC (2010a) further suggests under Recommendation 3.2 of the same document that a system be developed that is collaborative in the exchange of pertinent information and that the federal government establish the necessary guidelines and rules to put the PPACA into practice for a seamless integration at all governmental levels of health and human services.

The Meaningful Use of EHR

In 2004, President George W. Bush, in his State of the Union address, spoke of the need to within 10 years establish an EHR for every American citizen in order to help avoid dangerous mistakes in medical records, as well as to reduce costs and improve healthcare. That is when the ONC was developed.

Funding through the USDHHS led to several organizations being established. In 2006, the Agency for Healthcare Research and Quality (AHRQ) launched a National Resource Center for Health Information Technology. The previous year, HHS established a HIT Standards Panel and the Certified Commission for HIT (a.k.a. CCHIT) for certifying EHR systems (Murphy 2010).

ARRA, which followed the PPACA, was signed in May 2010. Its adoption into law added even more reason for the establishment of a Meaningful Use for EHR.

The purpose is to establish an EHR system that will be patient-centered and abundant in up-to-date clinical and demographic information. Reimbursement incentives will be given, and have in fact already begun for hospitals and eligible providers that agree to take the necessary steps to become Meaningful Users of EHRs.

Another Congressional act in 2009, called the Health Information Technology for Economic and Clinical Health Act (HITECH) was passed in February 2009 as part of the Stimulus Bill. It authorized $147 billion to reform the healthcare industry (of which the aforementioned $19 million in grants to help set up EHRs was a portion). If hospitals and providers are not compliant with Meaningful Use EHRs by 2015, there will be monetary penalties. Those that do comply will be rewarded in higher Medicare and Medicaid reimbursements.

On July 13, 2010, the USDHSS released a final ruling after analyzing over 2,000 comments from hospitals and providers. It divided the criteria of Meaningful Uses into five initiatives:

1. To improve the quality, the safety, and efficient manner of record transmissions and sharing and thus reduce health disparities in medical records.
2. To engage patients and their families in their medial record maintenance and accuracy.
3. To improve care coordination between specialties, facilities, and ancillaries.
4. To improve the information of the population that seeks public health facilities and treatment.
5. To ensure privacy and security of electronically shared information in accordance to HIPAA standards. (Murphy 2010)

One of the Meaningful Uses of an effective EHR system is for hospitals and providers to report measurement results to CMS or the state agencies that show their compliance to the goals set out for 2011, 2013, and 2015 milestones under the ARRA and HITECH Acts. This is a massive undertaking and CMS is not expected to be fully ready to receive such data electronically until 2012. This doesn't relieve hospitals and providers from the responsibility to report, however through already established means.

Funding is available for the further development of informatics in nursing thanks to the ARRA. The National Institutes for Health has designated 200 grants of $1 million each to fund scientific and health research. The National Library of Medicine is offering applied informatics grants to organizations. The Strategic Health IT Advanced Research Program has allocated $60 million in funding to further the performance of HIT on a national level. Nineteen so-called Beacon Communities have been established through further funding to be the guinea pigs in the efforts to improve the measurability of healthcare quality, safety, and efficiency. Workforce education in EHRs is also being funded under the ARRA so more informatics training can be established in community colleges in all 50 states along with a universal HIT competency examination program (Murphy 2010).

In order to efficiently develop a nationalized EHR system, leading EHR vendors must work together instead of competitively to ensure compatibility in the transmission of each patient's demographical and clinical information. A network must be established between CMS and individual providers, and also between providers and facilities themselves. This will improve patient care because all involved in healthcare will have access to the pertinent information that is needed to treat a patient, especially when the patient is unable to speak for himself or herself due to language barriers, a medical condition, lack of knowledge, and so forth.

This will especially be true for the facilities and providers that treat patients who are in poverty-prone areas because they are the most reliant upon the Medicaid and Medicare programs. According to Dr. David Blumenthal of the ONC, in an article dated October 18, 2010, "racial and ethnic minorities remain disproportionately affected by chronic illness(es), a contributing factor to intolerably high mortality and morbidity rates" (ONC 2010b, p. 1). Thus, it is critical that a Meaningful Use of EHR be established in these regions specifically, and throughout the

United States generally, to enhance the improvement of patient care and give physicians the needed reimbursement incentives to care for them.

Achieving a nationalized EHR system also requires education of end users. Paper medical records are antiquated and will be more and more so in the upcoming years as the ARRA ramifications are seen. Providers will need immediate access to records in order to treat patients safely and effectively. This will take the guesswork out of diagnosing and medicating through the sharing of accurate, updated vital electronic information. Through Meaningful Use of EHR, patient care can be better coordinated between specialties, be it routine or emergency. More accurate treatment will be the result, which will not only lead to fewer errors, but will be cost saving and perhaps life saving (Murphy 2010).

Patients will be able to, if they opt to do so, view their medical records and take an active role in monitoring accuracies. That may help them take a more active role in their overall health. With permission, families can also become more active in the care of their loved ones (ONC 2010b).

Overall, the Meaningful Use of a nationally compatible EHR system will make our healthcare system more accurate, more accessible, and better able to effectively treat the American population.

FUTURE DIRECTIONS

Ever since the implementation of Titles XVIII (Medicare) and XIX (Medicaid) in 1965, the federal government has involved itself in healthcare for its citizens. That involvement has continued to grow, and has expanded with the passage of PPACA in 2010, which involves moving toward a national healthcare system.

P4P will require more closely recorded medical documentation and place even more reliability on accurate informatics nursing. EHRs and other HIT systems will become inner-coordinated between agencies, insurance companies, hospitals, care facilities, diagnostic centers, and physicians. The concern is that basing reimbursement and bonuses on P4P may lead healthcare providers to steer away from high-risk patients who need care for fear of not being compensated.

CMS pledged to continue to work with the AHRQ as well as the AMA and other organizations to develop standard evidence-based guidelines for Do Not Pay lists, P4P, and PQRI bonuses (Trapp 2008).

Private insurance companies and third parties will have to comply with these changes to stay in business. Their roles in the future of healthcare reform are nebulous and claims processing and timely reimbursement may suffer because of that fact.

According to some sources (Potetz 2008; Social Security 2011), Medicare will be insolvent in 2014 despite attempts to initiate budget cuts in reimbursement and establish cost reform. This is partially due to the influx of Baby-Boomers and a smaller base of employed persons paying taxes to support the program.

Zinger (2010) stated a bleak future:

> The medical industry will begin to reposition itself. Those providers that relied on MRI's, CT scanners, laboratories, pain centers, etc will begin to move/sell those assets to others as this will most likely be a key area of cost reduction in the future. Some providers will stop accepting Medicare patients due to the reimbursement rate. Some doctors will plan their retirement for 2015, but not to the high rate that many predict will leave. The medical colleges will see a large increase in applications for General Practitioners and there will be legislation to enable Licensed Practical Nurses to have a greater role in primary care due to the anticipated shortage in front line medical professionals. We will probably see one of the largest labor organizing movements in history as the unions target the health care workers. (p. 1)

No doubt, if history proves correct, there will be many bugs to iron out. However, due to the ARRA grants and incentives, the federal CMS system will survive. A metamorphic shift toward a national system of reporting and healthcare deliverance has already begun. The importance of accurate, detailed, and accessible medical record proof of service will be even more essential.

Physicians, hospitals, and other healthcare entities as well as regulatory agencies will depend more and more on HIT systems to work properly, timely, and efficiently.

As more patients flood the healthcare system mandated and monitored at the federal level, new challenges for nursing informatics will become evident, as will be its growing impact on healthcare regulation and reimbursement procedures.

Nursing Informatics' Vital Role

The more involved federal agencies become in healthcare, the more informatics will play a vital role, as will the nurses who utilize it as the liaison between physician and patient and physician and agency. EHRs and HITECH will soon become a part of the everyday medical care system of documentation, treatment, and practice decision making. Informatics nurses will play a key role in all aspects of regulatory and reimbursement issues (Murphy 2010).

The nurse who is HIT trained will be an asset to the medical community for the improvements in safety, privacy, and accuracy of patient information and care. It will fall on the shoulders of nursing staff to replace the burden of antiquated mounds of paperwork and files with a modern, electronic, patient-centered universal information system.

As Murphy (2010) states:

> Many nursing and heath care leaders agree that the future of nursing depends on a profession that will continue to innovate using HIT and informatics to play an instrumental role in patient safety, change management, and quality improvement, as evidenced by quality outcomes, enhanced workflow, and user acceptance. (p. 286)

As regulatory agencies become more involved in the monitoring and distribution of healthcare to U.S. citizens, nurses will no doubt be the guides to lead IT technicians, physicians, policy developers, researchers, and chief clinical information officers into the age of HITECH, evidenced and patient centered practices, and safer care. Nursing institutes across the country are developing career programs in informatics.

Since 1994, the American Nurses Association has recognized this HIT field as a specialty. Through recent regulatory legislation, the rest of the medical community as well as policy and lawmakers are seeing it as a necessity. Medical care reimbursements will be impossible without informatics. P4P is based on the accuracy of electronically transmitted information to government entities such as CMS. EHR systems will be even more so. And most of all so will the patients whom the medical professionals and facilities treat in the United Sates and around the world.

Visit nursing.pearsonhighered.com for additional cases, information, and weblinks.

CASE STUDY EXERCISE

You have been asked to work with your healthcare system's physician practices as they work to acquire and implement electronic records. How would you explain current incentives to adopt electronic record systems and the significance of selecting systems that meet CCHIT certification for reimbursement purposes.

SUMMARY

- Health insurance regulation and reimbursement impact all healthcare providers.
- The U.S. health insurance regulation and reimbursement system is quite complex and consists of a number of federal and state programs, federal programs that are administered at the state level, and the private insurance sector.

- Most insurance companies follow Medicare's lead in reimbursement percentage and regulation. Therefore, the way that CMS interprets federal legislation affects all insured and to some extent noninsured citizens, not just Medicare beneficiaries.
- Medicare Part A pays for the facility related expenses for inpatient, hospice, home health, or nursing home residency care.
- Medicare Part B is for medically necessary physician and outpatient expenses.
- Medicare Part C is available to persons eligible for Medicare Parts A and B providing the benefits offered by the first two as well as a few additional benefits for a monthly premium.
- Medicare Part D covers certain prescription drugs and medical supplies.
- The very complexity of healthcare regulation and reimbursement requires the use of information technology to ensure compliance and optimize reimbursement.
- The Health Insurance Portability and Accountability Act (HIPAA) of 1996 sought to reduce the complexity and attendant costs of the system by requiring electronic submission of reimbursement claims. Medical necessity proofs can be electronically piggy-backed with claims expediting processing and payment.
- HIPAA and a 2006 CMS mandate required all submission of claims for reimbursement or registering of care, the verifying of eligibility, the precertification of services, or any other client-related information to adhere to a uniform format forcing providers EDI transmission programs in their billing and medical record systems or to utilize a clearinghouse that would submit claims for them.
- Private insurance companies were forced in the 1990s to establish a Common Procedural Terminology coding that was recognized by Medicare.
- HIPAA required that all providers to have a NPI on each electronic or paper claim by May 2007 in order to receive reimbursement necessitating changes to electronic billing systems.
- Increased monitoring of quality care and payment based on performance require exchange of information between hospitals, physicians, agencies, Medicaid and CHIP programs, and private payers.
- Federal and state mandated healthcare cost reform legislation places a greater burden of proof on the healthcare community to justify their services and receive proper reimbursement resulting in additional time spent coding.
- Pay-for-Performance (P4P), also known as Value-Based Purchasing (VBP), will result in massive changes in the way healthcare professionals and facilities are reimbursed.
- Medicare's Do Not Pay list for preventable complications limits payments to facilities to the primary reason for admission, eliminating payment for care related to complications that occurred during the patient's stay.
- The transition to the International Classification of Diseases, Tenth Revision (ICD-10) slated for 2013 is designed to better manage data used to measure the quality of healthcare delivered in the United States but requires changes to information system software to accommodate the new format for ICD-10 code.
- Common Procedural Terminology codes assign a number for a task or service to submit claims for reimbursement of procedures. The HCPCS was developed to better meet CMS needs to describe additional services, equipment, and supplies.
- G-codes, also known as quality data codes (QDC), evolved as nonpayable system to supplement claim data with supporting clinical data to measure the quality of service delivered.
- Resource Utilization Groups (RUGs) represent a per diem system of billing for skilled nursing facility (SNF unit) patients.
- While healthcare reform is designed to improve the quality of care and decrease related costs, many of the attendant changes are labor intensive requiring additional use of technology and changes to current technology.

- Financial incentives have been created to encourage the adoption of EHR by providers to facilitate the collection of data required to measure patient outcomes.
- Informatics nurses have a vital role in the adoption and appropriate use of technology to collect data needed to measure the quality of care delivered and to ensure that maximum reimbursement for services can be obtained. This role includes the evaluation of software for purchase consideration as well as screen design that forces the collection of needed information.

REFERENCES

American Medical Association (AMA). (2011). ICD-10 code set to replace ICD-9. Retrieved from http://www.ama-assn.org/ama/pub/physician-resources/solutions-managing-your-practice/coding-billing-insurance/hipaahealth-insurance-portability-accountability-act/transaction-code-set-standards/icd10-code-set.page

AMA Physician Resources. (n.d.). *Version 5010 electronic administrative transactions. Solutions for managing your practice.* Retrieved from http://www.ama-assn.org/ama/pub/physician-resources/solutions-managing-your-practice/coding-billing-insurance/hipaahealth-insurance-portability-accountability-act/transaction-code-set-standards/version-5010-electronic.shtml

Association of American Physicians and Surgeons (AASP). (2006). *National provider identifier (NPI) frequently asked questions.* Retrieved from http://www.aapsonline.org/npifaq.php

Benson, S. (2009). *Easing the transit on to ICD-10; the role of automated procedure documentation and coding solutions* (Wolters Kluwer white paper). Retrieved from http://www.provationmedical.com/.../ProVation_RoleOfProcedure_WhitePaper_fFIN.pdf

Blankenship, J. (2010). *Getting your financial ducks in a row: Posts on retirement saving and advice on all things financial.* Health Care and Education Reconciliation Act of 2010. Blankenship Financial. Retrieved from http://financialducksinarow.com/legislation/health-care-and-education-reconciliation-act-of-2010/

CMS. (2006, January 1). Skilled nursing facility prospective payment system. *Payment system fact sheet series. Medicare Learning Network.* Retrieved from http://www.cms.gov/MLNProducts/downloads/snfprospaymtfctsht.pdf

CMS. (2007). *Medical review of skilled nursing facility prospective payment system (SNF PPS) bills 6.1* (Rev. 196, Issued: 03-30-07, Effective: 01-01-06, Implementation: 04-30-07). Retrieved from http://www.cms.gov/manuals/downloads/pim83c06.pdf

CMS. (2008, April). *CMS publication 11306.* Centers for Medicare and Medicaid Services Article. Retrieved from http://www.medicare.gov/publications/pubs/pdf/11306.pfd

CMS. (2009). *The 2009 physician quality reporting imitative.* Retrieved from http://www.cms.gov/MLNProducts/downloads/2009-PQRI-Booklet.pdf

CMS. (2010a). *Physician fee schedule formula.* Retrieved from https://www.cms.gov/PhysicianFeeSched/

CMS. (2010b, April 2). *Goals for value-based purchasing.* Retrieved from http://www.cms.org/QuailtyIniativesGenInfo/downloads/VBPRoadmap_OEA_1-16_508.pdf-2010-04-02

CMS. (2011, October 17). *Physician quality reporting system formerly known as the physician quality reporting initiative.* Retrieved from https://www.cms.gov/PQRS/

CMS. (n.d.). *Medicaid and CHIP quality practices: Overview.* Retrieved from http://www.cms.gov/MedicaidCHIPQualPrac/

CMS Federal Register. (2010, July 22). *Medicare program; prospective payment system and consolidated billing for skilled nursing facilities for FY 2011* (Volume 75, Number 140, Notices, pp. 42885–42942). Retrieved from the Federal Register Online via GPO Access: http://www.wais.access.gpo.govDOCID:fr22jy10-157

Doherty, M. S. (n.d.). *Colorado gerontological society and senior answers and services.* Retrieved from http://www.senioranswers.org/Pages/cgs.medbba.htm

Dymkova-Fuchs, G. (2010, October 7). Physicians already seeing impact of early healthcare reform: Are you prepared? *The Fox Group.* Retrieved from http://www.foxgrp.com/blog/physicians-already-seeing-early-impact-of-healthcare-reform-are-you-prepared/

Evans, B. (2008, August 18). *HHS announces timeline for transition to ICD-10-CM: Briefings on coding compliance systems.* Retrieved from http://www.healthleadersmedia.com/content/FIN-217198/HHS-announces-tieline-for-transition-to-ICD10CM.html

Fernandez, D. (2010, October 11). *ONC release certified EHR product list.* Retrieved from http://h184435wp.setupblog.com/2010/10/onc-releases-certified-ehr-product-list/

Fischer, H. (2010, August 16). *Despite health-care reform, AZ powerless to regulate premiums.* East Valley Tribune, Capital Media Services. Retrieved from http://www.eastvalleytribune.com/local/health/article_07b69b1e-a999-11df-8ca9-001cc4c03286.html

The Fox Group. (n.d.). *Compliance & HIPAA are now more important than ever.* Retrieved from http://www.foxgrp.com/services/compliance-hipaa/

Free Advice. (n.d.). Health insurance: Are there any government agencies that regulate how health insurance companies or plans operate? *Insurance Law, Health Insurance Regulation.* Retrieved from http://law.freeadvice.com/insurance_law/health_insurance-regulations.htm

Georgetown University. (2009). *The children's health insurance program reauthorization act of 2009: Overview and summary March 2009.* Retrieved from http://ccf.georgetown.edu/index/cms-filesystem-action?file=ccf%20publications/federal%20schip%20policy/chip%20summary%2003-09.pdf

Hanson Academic Medical Center. (2010, January 25). *The academic medical center exception to the Stark law: Compliance by teaching hospitals* (p. 376). Retrieved from http://www.law.ua.edu/lawreview/articles/Volume%2061/Issue%202/hanson.pdf

ICD Common. (n.d.). A primer on the ICD-10 transition. Retrieved from http://www.icd10prepared.com/ICDComon/basics/

Kohn, D. (2009). *Healthcare infonomics impact on ECM industry.* AIIM.org. Retrieved from http://www.aiim.org/healthcare/infonomics/impact-on-the-ecm-industry.aspx

Kuhn, H. (2008, May 8). *Testimony on medicare physician payments before small business committee U.S. House of Representatives.* Retrieved from http://www.hhs.gov/asl/testify/2008/05/t20080508a.html

marqpdx. (2010). *CPT codes getting billed.* Retrieved from http://www.webhealtharticles.com/web-health/cpt-codes-getting-billed/

Maurer, F. A., & Smith, C. M. (2005). Unit one: Role and context of community/public health nursing practice. In *Community/public health nursing practice: Health for families and populations* (3rd ed., p. 63). St. Louis, MO: Saunders Elsevier.

Medicare-Medicaid.com. (n.d). *Do not pay list expansion.* Retrieved from http://medicare-medicaid.com/medicare/medicare%e2%80%99s-do-nt-pay-list/

Murphy, J. (2010, July–August). The journey to meaningful use of electronic health records. *Nursing Economics, 28*(4), 283–286.

Oberlander, J. (2010). Beyond repeal—The future of health care reform. *New England Journal of Medicine,* 363(24), 2277-9. doi 10.1056/NEJMp1012779

ONC. (2010a). Patient protection and affordable care act section 1561 recommendations: Toward a more efficient, consumer-mediated and transparent health and human services enrollment process. *Office of National Coordinator for Health Information Technology—USDHHS* (p. 1). Retrieved from http://healthit.hhs.gov/pdf/electronic-eligibility/aca-1561-recommendations-final2.pdf

ONC. (2010b, October 18). *A letter to the vendor community: Health IT and disparities. A message from Dr. David Blumenthal, National Coordinator for Health Information Technology.* Retrieved from http://heathit.hss.gov/portal/server.pt/community/healthit_hhs_gov_home/1204

Paddock, M. W., & Fornataro, M. T. (2010). Health reform legislation promises significant limitations on new and continued physician ownership and investment in specialty and other hospitals. *ABA Health eSource, 6*(5). Retrieved from http://www.americanbar.org/newsletter/publications/aba_health_esource-home/Paddock.html

Potetz, L. (2008). *Financing Medicare: An issue brief.* Retrieved from http://www.kff.org/medicare/upload/7731.pdf

Reutter, M. (2005). State vs. federal rules at issue in regulation of HMOs. *News Bureau Illinois* (Blog. 12/1/05). Retrieved from http://news.illinois.edu/news/05/1201managedcare.html

Rogers, W. D. (2007). *CMS' medical officer explains PQRI.* Retrieved from http://www.medicarepatientmanagement.com/issues/02-03/mpmMJ07-PQRI_Rogers.pdf

Silva, C. (2010, September 6). *Doctor group seeks changes to 2011 Medicare fee rule* (AmedNews
.com). Retrieved from http://www.ama-asn.org/amednews/2010/09/06/gvsb0906.htm

Social Security and Medicare Boards of Trustees. (2011). A summary of the 2011 annual reports.
Retrieved from http://www.ssa.gov/oact/trsum/index.html

Stirewalt, K. (2009, December). *Changes to the Federal Stark Law that affect diagnostic imaging arrangements* (Minnesota Medicine). Retrieved from http://www.minnesotamedicine.com/PastIssues/
PastIssues2009/December2009/MedicineLawPolicyDec2009/tabid/3274/Default.aspx

Torrey, T. (2009, February). *What are HCPCS codes? Healthcare common procedure coding system–
billing codes: About.com patient empowerment.* Retrieved from http://patients.about.com/od/
costsconsumerism/a/hcpcscodes.htm

Trapp, D. (2008, August 25). *Final medicare no-pay rule targets 10 hospital-acquired conditions.*
Retrieved from http://www.ama-assn.org/amednews/2008/08/25/gvl10825.htm

Trapp, D. (2008, September 8). *CMS calls for transition to ICD-10 in 3 years.* Retrieved from
http://www.ama-asn.org/amednews/2008/09/08/gvsa0908htm

World Health Organization (WHO). (2011). International Classification of Diseases (ICD).
Retrieved from http://www.who.int/classifications/icd/en/

Zinger. (March 18, 2010). *The only score that matters is the final score: The future of health care,
implications of health care legislation, ObamaCare, Congress and Health Care, Election 2012,
President Obama.* Retrieved from http://blog.zingerking.com/2010/03/18/the-future-of-
health-care-implications-of-health-care-legislation-obamacare-congress-and-health-care-
election-2012-president-obama.aspx

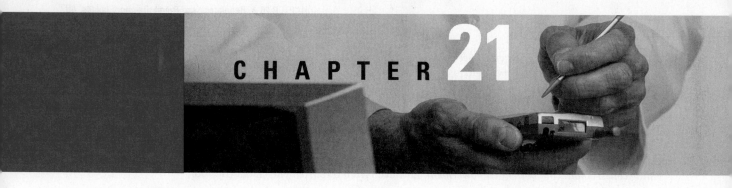

CHAPTER 21

Accreditation Issues for Information System Design and Use

After completing this chapter, you should be able to:

1. Review the accreditation process and major accrediting agencies in healthcare delivery.

2. Discuss the influence of major accrediting agencies on the design and use of healthcare information systems.

3. Examine ways in which information system support for Magnet Recognition resembles support for accreditation.

Healthcare institutions deal with an increasing number of accreditation issues daily. Some of the organizations that perform accreditation and establish standards for healthcare delivery in the United States are:

- The Joint Commission
- Commission for Accreditation of Rehabilitation Facilities (CARF)
- The National Committee for Quality Assurance (NCQA)
- Healthcare Facilities Accreditation Program (HFAP)
- Utilization Review Accreditation Commission (URAC)
- Accreditation Association for Ambulatory Healthcare (AAAHC)
- American Association for the Accreditation of Ambulatory Surgical Facilities (AAAASF)
- Accreditation Commission for Health Care (ACHC)
- Community Health Accreditation Program (CHAP)

Accreditation entails an extensive review process that monitors performance against predetermined standards. The accreditation process certifies to the public that the facilities involved meet nationally accepted standards through a recognized program. The amount of documentation required for compliance with these regulations and performance standards is voluminous. There is a growing recognition that information systems can and must be used to improve client safety and quality of care as well as enhance regulatory compliance through improved data capture and system prompts, thereby relieving demands on already overburdened healthcare providers. This capture should occur as a by-product of daily documentation activities.

ACCREDITATION

Accreditation determines whether providers receive funding. It also serves to enhance provider image, instills confidence in the quality of services rendered, and attracts qualified professionals. This process has direct implications for how documentation and information systems are structured. Several accrediting bodies exist. The Joint Commission and the Commission on Accreditation of Rehabilitation Facilities comprise two of the major accrediting bodies and will be addressed here in order to illustrate how information systems support the accreditation process. Box 21–1 lists some of the typical participants involved in the preparations for accreditation and for the accreditation process itself.

BOX 21–1 Typical Accreditation Participants

Administration

Nursing administration

Medical Records

Information systems and technology

Privacy and security officers

Compliance officers

Legal representation

Educators

Decision support staff

Quality assurance staff

Clinicians

Policy makers

Ancillary departments

The Joint Commission

The mission of the Joint Commission is "to continuously improve health care for the public, in collaboration with other stakeholders, by evaluating health care organizations and inspiring them to excel in providing safe and effective care of the highest quality and value" (The Joint Commission 2009, para. 1). The Joint Commission has focused on client safety and the safe administration of medications for several years. One example of this is the attempt to ensure consistent interpretation of medication dosages that fall within a range that is subject to nursing judgment (Manworren 2006). Once limited to acute care facilities, the Joint Commission standards now exist for ambulatory, long-term, home health, mental health, hospice care, managed care, health plans, and healthcare networks (healthfinder.gov 2010). The Joint Commission accreditation benefits providers by helping them to meet all, or portions of, state and/or federal licensure and certification requirements. Accreditation also expedites third-party payment and provides guidelines for the improvement of care, services, and programs. Other benefits include community confidence in the organization and improved staff recruitment and retention.

The Joint Commission standards and goals shape organization practice and documentation, thereby affecting information system documentation design (Ridge 2006). Each year specific target areas are selected, or refined, as safety goals. When accreditation standards change, documentation must reflect additional requirements. Hospital accreditation standards alone number more than 250, addressing everything from patient rights, patient education, and medication management and safety (Joint Commission 2011a). The Joint Commission introduced information management standards for healthcare organizations in 1994. Those standards addressed the following areas:

1. Measures to protect information confidentiality, security, and integrity, inclusive of:
   - Determination of user need for information and level of security;
   - Retrieval of information with ease in a timely fashion without compromising security or confidentiality;
   - Written and enforced policies restricting removal of client records for legal reasons;
   - Protection of records and information against loss, destruction, tampering, and/or unauthorized use.
2. Uniform definitions and methods for data capture as a means to facilitate data comparison within and among healthcare institutions
3. Education on the principles of information management and training for system use. This may include education about the transformation of data into information for subsequent use in decision support and statistical analysis.
4. Accurate, timely transmission of information as evidenced by the following characteristics:
   - 24-hour availability in a form that meets user needs
   - Minimal delay of order implementation
   - Quick turnaround of test results
   - Pharmacy system designed to minimize errors
   - Efficient communication system
5. Integration of clinical systems (i.e., pharmacy, nursing, laboratory, and radiology systems) and nonclinical systems for ready availability of information.
6. Client-specific data/information. The system collects, analyzes, transmits, and reports individual client-specific data and information related to client outcomes that can be used to facilitate care, provide a financial and legal record, aid research, and support decision making.
7. Aggregate data/information. The system generates reports that support operations and research and improve performance and care. For example, information may be provided by practitioner, client outcomes, diagnosis, or drug effectiveness.
8. Knowledge-based information. The system is capable of providing literature in print or electronic form.

9. Comparative data. The system can extract information useful to compare the institution against other agencies. Deviations from expected patterns, trends, length of stay, or numbers of procedures performed may be noted.

In 2006, the Joint Commission expanded information standards to include business continuity and disaster recovery planning, data and information retention, decision support, and specific documentation areas and formats. Information standards may be demonstrated through the presence of the following: planning documents, institutional and departmental policy and procedures, data element definitions and abbreviations, observations, continuing education outlines and records, interviews with administrators and staff, and meeting minutes. Subsequent updates to requirements may be found on the Joint Commission Web site. Some updates that directly or indirectly impact information systems include the following requirements:

- A reliable emergency electrical power source (Joint Commission 2011b)
- Availability of information when it is needed for care and services (Joint Commission 2011b)
- The ability to monitor social work services rendered in psychiatric units in accredited critical access hospitals (Joint Commission 2011b)
- The development of accountability measures to help hospitals to compare their performance against others and ultimately improve patient outcomes (Joint Commission Resources 2011a)
- The use of uniform data sets to standardize data collection throughout the healthcare delivery system (Joint Commission 2010)
- Medication reconciliation updates upon admission, changes (Joint Commission Resources 2011b)
- Automated identification technology in lieu of a second person for two-person verification for blood transfusions (Joint Commission 2010c).

A scoring system notes the degree to which each standard is met. Scoring criteria can be found in the Joint Commission's accreditation manual.

Commission on Accreditation of Rehabilitation Facilities

The Commission on Accreditation of Rehabilitation Facilities (CARF) is another healthcare accrediting body (CARF 2011a). In addition to its focus on the improvement of rehabilitative services to people with disabilities, CARF provides accreditation in the following health and human service areas:

- Aging services
- Behavioral health
- Opiod treatment programs
- Business and services management networks
- Child and youth services
- DMEPOS (durable medical equipment, prosthetics, orthotics, and supplies) (CARF 2011b)

CARF provides a template for operations as well as a tool for evaluation. CARF is a private, nonprofit organization that uses input from consumers, rehabilitation professionals, state and national organizations, and third-party payers to develop standards for accreditation. Although similar in purpose and structure to the Joint Commission, CARF places a greater emphasis on the following factors:

- Accessible services
- Comprehensiveness and continuity in individual treatment plan
- Input from consumers about CARF and its decision making

- Safety of persons with disabilities and their evacuation in the event of an emergency
- Post-discharge outcomes

CARF standards also shape institutional practices and documentation requirements. This may necessitate changes in automated documentation systems to comply with standards.

SPECIAL FACILITY/AGENCY ISSUES

Specialized facilities have unique needs with implications for automated documentation systems. In addition to accreditation requirements, state regulations, including mental health legislation, play an important role in dictating standards for information systems. No attempt is made here to address each type of facility, but pertinent considerations are noted.

Geriatric and Long-Term Facilities

Because of long stays and high client ratios for each nurse, documentation in nursing homes and long-term facilities must be concise, while addressing specific problems for this client population. Many institutions have developed their own forms to expedite this process and address required areas in accord with mandates for documentation. For example, monthly comprehensive summaries on each resident are required. Box 21–2 identifies areas that a monthly summary might include. Figure 21–1 displays a sample documentation screen from an automated summary. When long-term or skilled beds (beds occupied by clients who require specialized nursing care) are located within an institution with automated documentation,

---

BOX 21–2   Minimum Data Set for Nursing Home Resident Assessment and Care

- Identification and background information
- Cognitive patterns
- Communication/hearing
- Vision patterns
- Physical functioning and structural problems
- Continence in last 14 days
- Psychosocial well-being
- Mood and behavior patterns
- Activity pursuit patterns
- Disease diagnoses
- Health conditions
- Oral/nutritional status
- Oral/dental status
- Skin condition
- Medication use
- Special treatment and procedures
- Identification information
- Resident information
- Discharge information

Section B. Cognitive Patterns

1 Comatose
- ❏ Yes (skip to Section E)
- ❏ No

2 Memory
Short-term—recall after 5 minutes
- ❏ OK
- ❏ Problem

Long-term
- ❏ OK
- ❏ Problem

3 Memory/recall ability
- ❏ Current season
- ❏ Location of own room
- ❏ Staff names/faces
- ❏ That he/she is in a nursing home
- ❏ None of the above

4 Cognitive skills for daily decision making
- ❏ Independent
- ❏ Modified independence—some difficulty with new situations
- ❏ Moderately impaired—poor decisions, requires supervision
- ❏ Severely impaired—never makes decisions

5 Indicators of delirium/ disordered thinking
- ❏ Less alert, easily distracted
- ❏ Changing awareness of environment
- ❏ Episodes of incoherent speech
- ❏ Periods of motor restlessness or lethargy
- ❏ Cognitive ability varies over course of day
- ❏ None of the above

6 Change in cognitive status
- ❏ None
- ❏ Improved
- ❏ Deteriorated

FIGURE 21–1 • Sample screen shot from an automated summary for a nursing home resident

additional screens are needed to meet the special needs of this population. Automation can speed updates, provide prompts to ensure appropriate response, decrease entry errors on reimbursement codes, and generate automated plans of care. Screen design of documentation requires an increased emphasis on psychosocial functioning and several other areas. The requirements of the Joint Commission, Medicare, and Medicaid are driving forces in documentation design. Accurate completion of the minimum data set is necessary for compliance and reimbursement.

Psychiatric Facilities

Documentation must comply with Joint Commission requirements as well as state laws. Essential information for charting on the application of restraints, for example, includes date and time applied, reason for use, type of restraint applied, length of time the client remains in restraints, neurovascular status distal to the restraint, and frequency of assessments done on the client in restraints. Policy must be established that includes these areas and identifies a maximum length of time that a client may remain in restraints without a renewal order from a physician. This policy should be reflected in time limits on documentation screens. Seclusion policies should be basically the same. Figure 21–2 shows a suggested documentation screen for restraint use and seclusion.

Documentation of Restraint Application/Assessment

Time applied: __:__ (Maximum time policy identifies for removal automatically shown)
Time scheduled for release: __:__
Reasons for use: (indicate all that apply)
❑ Behavior harmful to self/to others
❑ Necessary to prevent injury
❑ Assaultive behavior
❑ Increased agitation
❑ Impulsive behavior
❑ Other (Specify): _____

Type of restraint applied:
❑ Soft wrist
❑ Waist
❑ Jacket posey
❑ Geriatric chair
❑ Locked leather wrist
✓ One
✓ Two
❑ Locked leather ankle
✓ One
✓ Two
Time restraints removed: __:__
Neurovascular status distal to restraints:
-Pulses: may select from predetermined responses or indicate "other" and describe
-Color: may select from predetermined responses or indicate "other" and describe
-Sensation: may select from predetermined responses or indicate "other" and describe
Frequency of nursing assessments: __:__

FIGURE 21–2 • Suggested screen design for restraint use in an automated documentation system

There also is a greater tendency for interdisciplinary documentation in psychiatric care, due to the need to provide adequate system and record access to many different personnel. Nursing staff, psychiatrists, psychologists, social workers, art therapists, music therapists, and play therapists require access to psychiatric client records regardless of the unit to which the client is admitted.

Assisted-Living Facilities

Both the Joint Commission and CARF provide accreditation for assisted-living facilities (ALFs). The scope of services provided by ALFs has increased according to what is allowed by state laws and community philosophies, blurring the distinction between ALFs and skilled care. As the number of persons residing in these facilities continues to increase, a commensurate number of new regulations and accreditation standards are expected.

Homecare Agencies

Homecare accreditation includes programs for home health, personal care and/or support, home medical equipment, hospice, and pharmacy activities. The Accreditation Commission for Health Care (ACHC) and the Joint Commission provide accreditation in this area. Given the wide variety of services that fall under the homecare umbrella—infusion services, skilled nursing, rehabilitation services—agencies juggle requirements from multiple entities. Incorporation of required data fields into information system design lessens the burden on agency staff while ensuring that appropriate data is collected to satisfy accreditation, reimbursement, and legal purposes.

QUALITY INITIATIVES

Hamm (2007), in a report prepared for Robert Wood Johnson Foundation, noted that it is the role of accrediting bodies to serve as change agents. That role has been demonstrated repeatedly over the years. A few examples will be noted here. The Joint Commission launched the ORYX initiative, a national program for the measurement of hospital quality, in 1998. Initially ORYX used nonstandardized data on performance measures (Chassin et al. 2010). By 2002, accredited facilities were required to collect and report data on performance for at least two of the following four core measure sets (acute myocardial infarction, heart failure, pneumonia, and pregnancy). Recently the Joint Commission announced a new approach to performance measurement in an endeavor to link quality performance with improved patient outcomes (Joint Commission Resources 2011a). The Joint Commission is also considering ways to integrate these into accreditation standards.

The Joint Commission was involved in a partnership with Centers for Medicare & Medicaid Services (CMS) on the Hospital Quality Initiative. This Medicare program initiated in 2001 measures how often clinical benchmarks are met and makes the information available via the Hospital Compare Web site (CMS 2008). CMS collaborated with the Hospital Quality Alliance (HQA) on hospital measurement and reporting. The Joint Commission was a HQA member.

The Joint Commission also plays an active role in quality initiatives through its Center for Transforming Healthcare (Joint Commission Center for Transforming Healthcare 2011). The Center provides links to current projects that include:

- Hand-off Communications, a project to improve the quality of hand-off reports on patients thereby decreasing medical errors and improving safety.
- Preventing Avoidable Heart Failure Hospitalizations
- Surgical Site Infections
- Wrong Site Surgery Project
- Hand Hygiene Project

The National Committee for Quality Assurance (NCQA) is a private, nonprofit organization dedicated to improving healthcare quality (NCQA 2011). NCQA accredits and certifies healthcare organizations and manages the evolution of the Health Plan Employer Data and Information Set, a set of standardized performance measures that health plans use to measure and report on their performance. NCQA introduced a Web-based Interactive Survey System that is expected to change the way in which healthcare organizations are reviewed, making the process faster and more efficient while providing organizations with more immediate feedback.

Magnet Recognition

The Magnet Recognition Program recognizes healthcare organizations that provide nursing excellence and provides a means for disseminating successful nursing practices and strategies (ANCC 2011). More specifically the program recognizes quality patient care, excellence in nursing, and innovations in nursing practice. While the pathway to Magnet Recognition is distinctly different from that of the accreditation process, both entail an extensive review process and both offer benefits to the institution, employees, and all those that the institution serves. Informatics and information systems support the process by providing aggregate data related to quality improvement. The Magnet Recognition Program uses the American Nurses Associations National Database of Nursing Quality Indicators (NDNQI). This database meets CMS reporting requirements for nursing sensitive care, and is the only database containing data collected at the nursing unit level (ANA 2011). Tangible benefits associated with Magnet Recognition include (Mueller 2002; Russell 2010; Steltzer 2002):

- Recognition of the worth of the nurse
- Recruitment and retention
- Increased public confidence in healthcare

- High quality physicians, specialists, and staff
- Positive collaborative relationships
- A positive environment
- Quality patient outcomes
- Improved communication among nurses, doctors, and administrators

The TIGER Initiative and Magnet Recognition Program have aligned their forces. Both organizations recognize the need for transformational leadership. The resulting document identified the force of magnitude, an illustration of how it is demonstrated within the organization, and corresponding TIGER efforts (TIGER Initiative 2008). The intent of the resulting model was to help transform organizations to meet the needs of the future.

FUTURE DIRECTIONS

Demands for quality will continue well into the future so that the accreditation process will continue to play an important role in the healthcare delivery system. The increased adoption of EHR technology secondary to Meaningful Use reimbursement will make it easier to provide data on patient outcomes. Informaticists will be needed to ensure that accreditation requirements are met through screen design and capture, guiding clinicians to complete all needed observations and measures. Hand-in-hand with the ongoing quest for quality, Magnet Recognition is another way to show that individual organizations are quality providers of care using NDNQI as a way to provide visibility for the work of nurses.

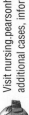

Visit nursing.pearsonhighered.com for additional cases, information, and weblinks.

CASE STUDY EXERCISE

You have been appointed to the Clinical Information Systems Committee, which is charged with looking at ways that automation can facilitate data collection for the next accreditation visit by the Joint Commission. List examples of how your community hospital demonstrates adherence to the Joint Commission information standards, and state your rationale for your decision that these examples display compliance.

SUMMARY

- Accreditation issues and quality initiatives place increased demands on healthcare providers to safeguard, track, provide, and manage information. Information systems can and must facilitate this process.
- Accreditation needs such as those imposed by the Joint Commission and CARF add to documentation requirements that must also address state and federal laws and reimbursement issues.
- Information systems and the design of automated documentation must incorporate standards for quality of care imposed by accrediting agencies.
- Automated documentation can facilitate the collection of data for accrediting bodies.
- Special care facilities documentation requirements may require additional screen design.
- The Magnet Recognition Program, while not an accrediting body, is very much like an accrediting body because it provides an assurance of quality and recognizes the essential role that information systems play in supporting that process.

REFERENCES

American Nurses Association, Inc. (2011). *The national database*. Retrieved from http://www.nursingworld.org/ndnqi2

American Nurses Credentialing Center (ANCC). (2011). *Program overview*. Retrieved from http://www.nursecredentialing.org/Magnet/ProgramOverview.aspx

CARF. (2011a). *About CARF*. Retrieved from http://www.carf.org/home

CARF. (2011b). *Who we are*. Retrieved from http://www.carf.org/About/WhoWeAre/

Centers for Medicare & Medicaid Services (CMS). (2008). *Hospital quality initiative overview*. Retrieved from https://www.cms.gov/HospitalQualityInits/Downloads/Hospitaloverview.pdf

Chassin, M. R., Loeb, J. M., Schmaltz, S. P., & Wachter, R. M. (2010). Accountability measures—Using measurement to promote quality improvement. *New England Journal of Medicine, 363*(7), 683–688.

Hamm, M. S. (2007). *Quality improvement initiatives in accreditation: Private sector examples and key lessons for public health. Prepared for the Robert Wood Johnson Foundation*. Retrieved from http://www.phaboard.org/wp-content/uploads/QIInitiativesinAccreditation.pdf

Healthfinder.gov. (2010). *The Joint Commission—JCAHO*. Retrieved from http://www.jointcommission.org/assets/1/18/Primary_Care_Home_Posting_Report_20110519.pdf

The Joint Commission. (2006). *Critical access hospital 2006 management of information*. Retrieved from http://www.jointcommission.org/NR/rdonlyres DD06404B-66AE-4C7F-9D67-6419734651D7/0/06_cah_im.pdf

The Joint Commission. (2009, August 15). *The Joint Commission mission statement*. Retrieved from http://www.jointcommission.org/the_joint_commission_mission_statement/

Joint Commission Center for Transforming Healthcare. (2011). Join the Partnership. Retrieved from http://www.centerfortransforminghealthcare.org/join_the_partnership.aspx

Joint Commission on Accreditation of Healthcare Organizations. (2010). *Joint Commission Perspectives, 30*(6), 13.

Joint Commission on Accreditation of Healthcare Organizations. (2010c). *Joint Commission Online*. Revised NPSG.01.03.01 EP. Retrieved from http://www.jointcommission.org/assets/1/18/jconline_Sept_22_10.pdf

Joint Commission on Accreditation of Healthcare Organizations. (2011a). *Joint Commission FAQ page*. Retrieved from http://www.jointcommission.org/about/JointCommissionFaqs.aspx?faq#293

Joint Commission on Accreditation of Healthcare Organizations. (2011b). *Joint Commission Perspectives, 31*(3), 3, 9–11.

Joint Commission Resources. (2011a). The Joint Commission sets the bar for performance measurement with accountability measures. *The Joint Commission Benchmark, 13*(5), 1–2. Retrieved from http://www.jcrinc.com

Joint Commission Resources. (2011b). Medication reconciliation: Complying with NPSG.03.06.01. *Joint Commission Perspectives on Patient Safety, 11*(3), 1–5.

Klein, S. R., & Keller, J. P. (2006). A new paradigm for medical technology procurement. *Journal of Healthcare Information Management, 20*(4), 14–16.

Manworren, R. (2006). A call to action to protect range orders. *American Journal of Nursing, 106*(7), 65–68.

Mueller, C. (2002). Demonstrating excellence, attaining magnet status. *Creative Nursing, 8*(2), 7.

National Committee for Quality Assurance (NCQA). (2011). *About NCQA*. Retrieved from http://www.ncqa.org/tabid/675/default.aspx

Ridge, R. A. (2006). Focusing on JCAHO national patient safety goals. *Nursing, 36*(11), 14–15.

Russell, J. (2010). Journey to Magnet: Cost vs. benefits. *Nursing Economics, 28*(5), 340–342.

Steltzer, T. M. (2002). The magnetic pull. *Nursing Management, 33*(1), 41.

TIGER Initiative. (2008). *Alignment of ANCC forces of magnitude and TIGER collaboratives*. Retrieved from http://www.thetigerinitiative.org/docs/AlignmentofANCCForcesofMagnitudeandTIGERCollaboratives.pdf

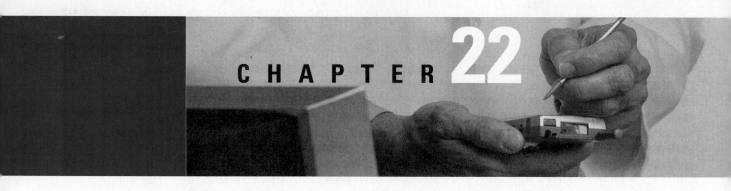

CHAPTER 22

Continuity Planning and Management (Disaster Recovery)

After completing this chapter, you should be able to:

1. Understand the continuity life cycle.
2. Provide the reasons why continuity planning is important.
3. Provide a rationale for developing a Business Continuity Plan (BCP).
4. Discuss the relationship between continuity planning and disaster recovery.
5. Outline the steps of the continuity planning process.
6. Review the advantages associated with continuity planning.
7. Identify events that can threaten business operation and information systems (IS).
8. Discuss how information obtained from a mock or an actual disaster can be used to improve response and revise continuity plans.
9. Discuss legal and accreditation requirements for continuity plans.

INTRODUCTION AND BACKGROUND

In the past, disaster recovery planning focused primarily on the recovery and restoration of data. However, as reliance on timely access to data has grown, so has the importance of continuity planning for all organizations that rely on continued operations for timely access to and the processing of information. This is especially true for healthcare provider organizations with respect to their information systems, networks, and freestanding personal computers (PCs). Lost or corrupted data have a negative impact on business processes, impede the delivery of timely and safe care, reduce productivity, and undermine public confidence in the organization. Lost or corrupted data are costly to re-create and threaten the survival of a business or healthcare delivery system in a highly competitive environment. An estimated 40% –90% of organizations suffering a significant system failure with data loss go out of business within 5 years (Kirschenbaum 2006; Lawton 2007). There is evidence that organizations do not invest enough time and resources into preparations for disruptive events based on disaster survival statistics. Fires permanently close another 44% of affected businesses (Naef 2003). In the 1993 World Trade Center bombing, 150 businesses out of 350 affected failed to survive the event. Conversely, the firms affected by the September 11 attacks with well-developed and tested business continuity plan (BCP) manuals were back in business within days (Stohr, Rohmeyer, & Shaikh 2004).

Since the primary focus of healthcare delivery is the care and well-being of the clients, it is essential to protect the technology and data that support client care. Information technology (IT) and its associated data must be viewed as a critical resource to support daily operations. Healthcare providers have an obligation to determine how a disaster may affect the delivery of services and identify strategies and related procedures to ensure the availability of information and the continuity of care on a 24-hours-a-day, 7-days-a-week basis. Disasters can be man-made or natural. Natural disasters include floods, hurricanes, tornadoes, earthquakes, volcanoes, wildfires, thunderstorms, and lightning strikes (Sandhu 2002). Man-made disasters can include terrorist attacks, bio-threats, acts of war, riots, explosions, train wrecks, chemical and toxic waste spills, mining accidents, and shipwrecks. Blackouts, brownouts, and pandemics are also disasters that can occur. The effect of any of the earlier mentioned disasters on a healthcare delivery system could potentially be disastrous. During Hurricane Katrina in New Orleans, patients were moved after the threat had occurred but a hospital should plan for moving patients before the event or be self-sustaining during and after such an event. The experience with Hurricanes Katrina and Rita demonstrated that critical emergency management capabilities must be increased from simply minimum disaster management levels. When a catastrophic disaster occurs, significantly more business continuity management (BCM) capabilities in relation to quantity and quality are needed. **Business continuity management (BCM)** is broadly defined as the process that seeks to ensure organizations are capable of withstanding any disruption to normal functioning (Elliott & Swartz 2002).

Medical facilities have become increasingly dependant on information technology services, which renders these facilities vulnerable to technology-related failure. Whenever a business is heavily dependent on information technology, all risks and threats need to be considered when preparing for recovery. If a disaster occurs and the organization cannot recover fast enough, the consequences can be devastating. Unfortunately, IT also has to consider disgruntled employees and social unrest; therefore, these must be added to the list of man-made disasters.

WHAT IS CONTINUITY PLANNING?

Continuity planning, usually called **business continuity planning (BCP)**, is the creation and validation of a practiced logistical plan for how an organization will recover and restore partially or completely interrupted critical functions within a predetermined time after a disaster or extended disruption. The logistical plan is called a **business continuity plan**. Continuity planning and **disaster recovery** are processes that help organizations prepare for disruptive events, whether the event is a hurricane or simply a power outage. Continuity planning is the process of ensuring the uninterrupted operation of critical services regardless of any event that may occur. This includes all critical applications, resident data, as well as Web, database, networks, and file servers utilized by an organization. A continuity plan is a critical aspect of an organization's risk management strategy and is instrumental to its survival should a disaster occur (Wainwright 2007). Tolerance for information technology downtime is rapidly declining, with a survey setting the figure at 5 hours or less (Lindeman 2007; Witty 2006).

Historically, BCP began as disaster recovery, but as dependence on automation has increased for nearly all daily operations it has created a need for more detailed planning to maintain daily operations under a wide array of potential disruptive events. Continuity planning is typically referred to as BCP or contingency planning. BCP now encompasses disaster recovery planning for IT and data as a component of the plan (Glenn 2006; G'Sell 2007; Wainwright 2007). Continuity planning and disaster recovery is the process by which an organization resumes business after a disruptive event. The event might be a disaster such as a huge earthquake or a terrorist attack or a smaller disruptive event like malfunctioning software caused by a computer virus.

Business continuity planning suggests a more comprehensive approach to making sure an organization can keep operating, not only after a natural calamity but also in the event of smaller disruptions, including the illness or departure of key staffers, supply chain problems, or other challenges that businesses are likely to face at some point in time. Disaster planning and recovery is primarily focused on the risks to IS and the data that they utilize. Information technology staff members are primarily responsible for this area of business continuity. Data recovery and protection are required for healthcare providers because rapid access to usable data is essential and can literally become a life and death situation. BCP has evolved into its own specialty, resulting in the formation of the Disaster Recovery Institute International and a certification process for its experts. The development of a continuity plan is the most difficult aspect of business continuity. The widening scope of continuity planning requires expertise from many different disciplines. Consultants may be hired to help develop a continuity plan, but its ultimate success requires the involvement of persons across the organization since they are in the best position to know its policies, standards, functions, data, clients, personnel, and operations (Glenn 2007). Developing continuity into the design of the organizational infrastructure helps prevent local events from disrupting the entire organization.

The BCP for IT needs to include servers, storage devices and media, networking equipment, connectivity links, vendors, suppliers, partners, and IT personnel, as well as air-conditioning and power supplies. The plan should ensure continued availability, reliability, and recoverability of all IT resources, including data as well as equipment, supplies, processes, personnel, and lines of communication. It should balance the costs of risk management with the opportunity cost of not taking action in preparing for disasters. The continuity plan should provide an enterprise-wide, risk-based approach, covering people, processes, technology, and the extended enterprise to ensure continued availability of operational support systems and minimize disruption risks. Disasters and system downtime can affect all aspects of a business, including facilities, workers, communications, clients, suppliers, partners, logistics, and data. Continuity of business is a back-up plan to ensure business as usual in the event of a natural or man-made disaster. Hospitals and other healthcare delivery organizations are businesses; the only difference is that the product is healthcare.

The processes and procedures a healthcare provider puts into place to avoid mission-critical business interruption or data loss during any type of disaster are essential to ensure that the right fail-over mechanisms are in place to continue operations. These fail-over systems are often in geographically dispersed locations, so that data access can continue uninterrupted if one location is disabled. Systems, data, and applications that can be impacted include electronic medical records, order entry, patient accounting, radiology/imaging services, reports, and distribution workflow. Other areas to be considered are emergency care, care management, patient monitoring, clinical profiles, lab dictaphones, physicians' portals, medical supplies, and a variety of other applications. Performance of IT is an area to be considered when establishing a continuity of business plan. Questions to be considered are:

- How will applications perform over a WAN or the Internet?
- What is the impact of distance on existing applications?
- How will the remote data center be managed?
- What are critical business continuity and disaster recovery applications?
- Should a separate business continuity and disaster recovery capability be devised for each application?
- If one application fails, how will it impact other applications?
- What are the points of failure?
- Will the plan scale to future requirements?
- What are the potential security threats created by the business continuity and disaster recovery plans that are in place?
- How can the integrity and privacy of the data be preserved?

A **disaster** is an event that disrupts or disables essential organizational functions and has the potential to disrupt and potentially destroy an organization by destroying financial, administrative, legal, contractual, personnel, inventory, and, in the case of healthcare organizations, clinical data needed for ongoing operations (Martin 2007). Disasters may strike without warning and require immediate action. For this reason, every organization needs to develop a plan that anticipates potential technology and data-related problems and provide implementation steps to avoid these problems by instituting policies and procedures to maintain the availability and security of client information under adverse or unexpected conditions. Continuity plans also address alternative means to support the retrieval and processing of information in the event that systems fail.

Disaster recovery plans enable the retrieval of critical business records from backup storage, restore lost data, and allow organizations to resume system operations. Unfortunately, in some cases, this process may take 48 hours or longer to complete. This time frame is unacceptable in today's information-driven and technology-dependent society. There is another difference between data and system restoration and business continuity (McCormick 2003; Price 2003): Restored data do not typically show the relationship between how and when information is created and used. One example may be seen in a physician's office when the daily backup does not occur, and the system loses pieces of information that are critical to a patient's treatment. Plans should ensure uninterrupted operation or expedite resumption of operation after a disaster while maintaining data access, integrity, and security. Business continuity plans must identify the scope and objectives, including multiple vendor platforms found in most organizations, and address the implications for other agencies when a system becomes inoperable (Price 2007). For example, if a healthcare IS is unavailable for a lengthy period of time, treatment of patients may be slowed and information will not be available to third-party payers and suppliers. A comprehensive plan consists of separate plans for each of the following areas:

- *The emergency plan.* This plan provides direction during and immediately after an incident. This may include a provision to switch to duplicate hardware and networks as a means to minimize disruption of services (Wainwright 2007).
- *The backup plan.* This plan outlines steps to ensure the availability of key employees, vital records, and alternative backup facilities for ongoing business and IS processing operations.
- *The recovery plan.* Restores full operational IS capabilities.
- *The test plan.* Uncovers and corrects defects in the plan before a real disaster occurs.
- *The maintenance plan.* This plan provides guidelines ensuring that the entire plan is kept up to date.

Consideration of each of these areas as separate plans may provide for better division of responsibility and increased awareness of significance for each area. An organization's security officer should have a key role in continuity and disaster planning, starting with a basic understanding of the plan development process to help direct the effort. Part of the security role is the protection of information. Data security is particularly important in order to comply with federal mandates and accreditation requirements.

STEPS IN THE BUSINESS CONTINUITY PLANNING PROCESS

Business Continuity Planning Life Cycle

Business continuity planning is not a one step or one time activity but is a set of successive stages that are repeated periodically and is best characterized as a life cycle as shown in Figure 22–1. A completed BCP life cycle results in a formal plan with a printed manual available for reference before, during, and after disruptions have occurred. The purpose of the documented plan and associated manual is to reduce adverse stakeholder impacts determined by both the scope of a disruption in terms of whom and what it affected and the duration of a disruption. A BCP

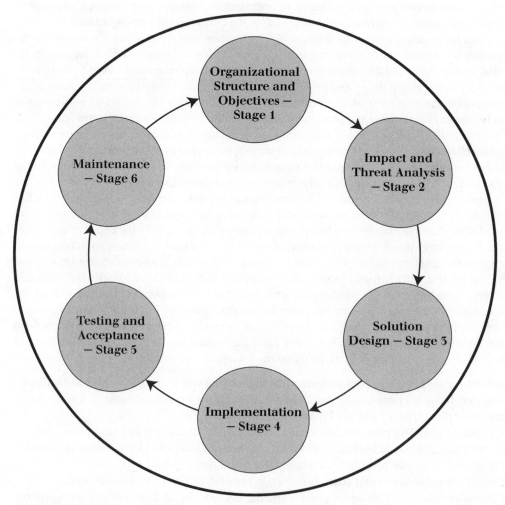

FIGURE 22–1 • BCP life cycle stages

manual for a small organization may simply be a printed manual stored safely away from the primary work location, containing the names, addresses, and phone numbers for crisis management staff, general staff members, clients, and vendors along with the location of the off-site data backup storage media, copies of insurance contracts, and other critical materials necessary for organizational survival. In its most sophisticated form, a BCP manual may outline a secondary work site, technical requirements and readiness, regulatory reporting requirements, work recovery measures, the means to reestablish physical records, the means to establish a new supply chain, or the means to establish new production centers. Organizations should make sure that their BCP manual is realistic and easy to use during a crisis. BCP should be considered as important as crisis management and disaster recovery planning and become a part of an organization's overall risk management strategy.

The stages in the life cycle of BCP are

- Organizational structure and objectives
- Analysis
- Solution design
- Implementation
- Testing and acceptance
- Maintenance

Organizational Structure and BCP Objective Stage

Create a BCP Workgroup

The business enterprise must create a business continuity workgroup within the organization, which can actively be involved in determining objectives, determining priorities, creating the BCP plan steps, documenting, implementing, testing, and maintaining the continuity plan. This group normally includes representatives from major business units, IT, functional experts in areas such as manufacturing, disaster planning experts, and often a legal representative. Their charter is to develop and document the specific risk areas the company faces, perform an impact and threat analysis, determine the mitigation responses to those risks, and develop testing and maintenance procedures. The activities for this stage include the following:

- *Secure top management support and commitment of resources.* This is critical because administrative support is essential to the development of a viable plan, which in turn can make the difference between an organization's demise and survival and provides a competitive advantage. Placing continuity planning within the business context of information technology makes the investment appear more palatable (G'Sell 2007). Administrators need to weigh actual costs against the potential cost and damage to the organization for failure to sustain operations.
- *Select the business continuity workgroup members.* Agency staff may develop a continuity plan, but consultant expertise on the team can develop a plan more quickly, objectively, and knowledgeably because no one individual can know everything needed to implement an effective plan for a large, complex system. For this reason, each section of the plan should be authored by the parties with the greatest expertise in the area. The chief information officer should play a role on the committee and in the development of the plan.
- *Perform a risk assessment.* During this phase, the business continuity workgroup identifies the following information:
  - Types and probabilities of various types of disasters; risks range from low to high (Croy 2007)
  - Potential impact of a particular disaster scenario
  - Estimated costs of lost/damaged information/records and lost time and customer confidence

- Costs to replace and restore records, equipment, and facilities, as well as to hire or replace staff, versus the costs to develop and maintain the disaster plan
- Risk of the worst-case scenario striking the organization
- *Set processing and operating priorities.* During this phase, the workgroup determines the equipment and telecommunication links and vital records needed to perform daily business functions and viable alternatives in the event that these are not available.
- *Collect data needed to support the plan.* This phase entails a determination of available resources. This includes external resources such as backup and duplication systems, recovery services, and internal resources. Internal assets include staff information; inventories of vital records, equipment, supplies, or forms; policies and procedures; contact lists for staff, vendors, and other service providers; a review of security systems; and an evaluation of facilities for potential problems.
- *Write the plan.* A common mistake is to assign the responsibility for writing the plan to an individual who already has a full workload or who lacks authority to confront managers about the criticality of information in their areas. If the task is tackled internally, it needs to be divided among persons with expertise in specific areas. A successful plan must be well organized, up to date, concise, and simple to follow. Software tools are available to aid the planning process; these include personal software or office productivity tools, enterprise software, and Web-based tools. Office productivity tools are readily available, but plans tend to get locked away on desktops with issues of version control and contact lists, and pager and telephone numbers that are not kept up to date. Enterprise software offers a proven track record but may be expensive, difficult to install and learn, and out-of-date in design. Web-based software is easy to use and provides version control and free access to extensive information and instant, interactive communication. It offers wide dissemination, the ability to incorporate questionnaires and surveys, automated contact management, and security.

The plan must catalog all strategies needed to sustain delivery of services and to test the plan. Well-documented systems and procedures are essential for the continuity of operations and disaster recovery. Although each organization and system is different, the plan should identify the following (Bermont 2007; Lindeman & Grogan 2007):

- Mission-critical systems are those in which failures directly affect the organization's revenue stream, have a safety and reliability impact, or could have significant legal impacts. Failure for a period of time would lead to nonrecoverable consequences, such as revenue loss or loss of life in the case of healthcare providers later.
- Mission-important systems are those that would require urgent repair to restore processes or operations. However, a short delay, such as hours, days, or weeks, depending on the system, would have recoverable consequences. The revenue stream or impact on patients would not be significantly impacted.
- Sustainable systems are those that will not impact the organization's operations if they fail for a period of time.

Each functional group or division within the organization will have its own set of priorities. For this reason, the final determination of criticality should be done at the top level of the organization so that there is a clear understanding of where resources and emphases should be placed. Priorities and associated recovery strategies are based on risk assessment.

BCP Planning Steps

The following steps should be taken by the BCP workgroup in creating an efficient and effective BCP that includes disaster recovery:

- Determine the objectives of the BCP—A statement of objectives including project details, on-site/off-site data, resources, and business type.

- Develop disaster recovery plan criteria—Documentation of the procedures for declaring an emergency, evacuation of site pertaining to the nature of disaster, active backup, notification of the related officials including team/staff as well as local, state, and federal disaster response officials, notification of procedures to be followed when a disaster occurs and alternate and location specifications. It is beneficial to be prepared in advance with impact scenarios and disaster recovery examples so that every individual in an organization is better educated on the basics. A workable BCP template or scenario plan should be available so that IT as well as other operational units in the organization can train employees with the procedures to be carried out in the event of a catastrophe.
- Define BCP workgroup roles and responsibilities—Documentation should include identification and contact details of key personnel in the disaster recovery team, their roles and responsibilities in the team.
- Develop a strategy for plan acceptance—No plan can be successful without the acceptance of the plan by all members of the organization. One way to ensure acceptance is to involve all members of the organization in the generation and approval of the plan. One of the most critical factors is to make sure all members of the organization understand their role when a failure or disaster occurs.
- Develop procedure to keep the plan and its associated manual current—A critical factor for a BCP is to make sure the manual for implementing the plan is complete and current.
- Document the procedures for each of the life cycle stages.

Analysis Stage The analysis stage in the development of a BCP plan is also referred to as a **Business impact analysis (BIA)** and consists of impact analysis, threat analysis, and impact scenarios, which results in the BCP plan requirements documentation. Analysis involves the examination of a business or problem situation and separating it into its components or elements in order to understand them and how they are related to the business situation. Measureable BIA areas in which hazards and threats reside include civil, economic, natural, and technical. The analysis of the business aspects of an organization is the process of determining the critical functions of the organization and the information vital to keeping these functions operational as well as the applications and databases, hardware, and communication facilities that use, house, or support this information (G'Sell 2007). This is critical in healthcare delivery because patient care requires timely access to accurate information. Interviews with employees in each area provide the data for the BIA.

Impact Analysis

An **impact analysis** results in the differentiation between critical (urgent) and noncritical (nonurgent) organization functions/activities. It will include at a minimum the following information:

- Description, purpose, and origin of the information
- Information flows
- Recipients, or users, of the information
- Requirements for timeliness
- Implications of information unavailability

The importance of information dictates the priority given to maintaining its continuity. A function may be considered critical if the impact of damage to a function is regarded as unacceptable to the organization. Perceptions of the acceptability of disruption may be modified by the cost of establishing and maintaining appropriate business or technical recovery solutions.

A function may also be considered critical if dictated by law. For each critical function, three values are then assigned:

- *Recovery point objective (RPO)*—The acceptable latency of data that will be recovered
- *Recovery time objective (RTO)*—The acceptable amount of time to restore the function
- *Recovery time actual (RTA)*—The actual amount of time to restore data and functionality based on testing

The Recovery Point Objective (RPO) must ensure that the Maximum Tolerable Data Loss for each activity is not exceeded. The RPO is the point in time to which you must recover data as defined by your organization. Typically, this is a determination of what an organization determines is an acceptable loss of data in a disaster situation. If the RPO of a company is 2 hours and the actual time it takes to get the data back into production is 5 hours, the RPO is still 2 hours and the process for restoration of the data must be modified so the data can be restored within 2 hours of a disaster. For example, if there is a complete backup of data at 9:00 AM and the system fails at 10:59 AM without a new backup, the loss of the data written between 9:00 AM and 10:59 AM will not be recovered from the backup. The data lost during this amount of time is considered acceptable because of the 2-hour RPO. This is the case even if it takes an additional 3 hours to get the site back into production. The system will be recovered from the 9:00 AM point in time. All data lost between 9:00 AM and 10:59 AM will have to be manually recovered through other means, which must be considered in the BCP. The RPO is usually measured in time such as seconds or dirty tracks, which are tracks that changed in the master copy but did not change in the backup image. Measuring the RPO for an entire data set that is stored as a database or file is more complex and requires using the lowest common denominator of all the physical elements protecting the logical data set. For example, calculating the RPO for an Oracle or SQL Server database that resides on 10 storage volumes requires understanding which storage volume(s) contain the database, requesting the RPO information for each of those volumes, and using the highest number for calculating the RPO. Additional complexity arises when not all physical volumes were backed up at the exact same time.

The Recovery Time Objective (RTO) must ensure that the Maximum Tolerable Period of Disruption for each activity is not exceeded. This includes the time for trying to fix the problem without a recovery, the recovery itself, testing, and communicating with users. The decision time for a user's representative is not included. The business continuity timeline usually runs parallel with an incident management timeline and may start at the same or different points in time. In accepted BCP methodology the RTO is established during the BIA by the owner of a process (usually in conjunction with the business continuity planners). The RTOs are then presented to senior management for acceptance. The RTO is documented as part of the business process in the BCP and not as part of the resources required to support the business process. The RTO and the results of the BIA in its entirety provide the basis for identifying and analyzing viable strategies for inclusion in the BCP. Viable strategy options would include any which would enable resumption of a business process in a time frame at or near the RTO. This would include alternate or manual workaround procedures and would not necessarily require computer systems to meet the RTOs. Once the RTO has been established, it is conveyed to the technology support team for infrastructure design and implementation that reflects the recovery time frame that is required by the business.

The RTA is established during an exercise, actual event, or predetermined based on the recovery methodology the technology support team develops. This is the time frame the technology support group takes to actually deliver the recovered infrastructure for the business. The business continuity workgroup then records the length of time that was taken to recover the function and its data. The business continuity workgroup coordinates the testing of that infrastructure with the business line that established the RTO and the IT staff. If testing is successful, then the initial RTA is valid. If the functional recovery testing by the business line and IT staff is not successful due to infrastructure recovery issues, then the recovery issues are turned over to the IT staff for further analysis of the recovery methodology and a new test is performed. If the business line verifies the recovered function as successful, then the business continuity workgroup reconciles the difference between the RTO and the RTA. Any gap is noted as a follow-up item and tracked accordingly through resolution.

After determining the RPO, RTO, and RTA, the impact analysis must determine the recovery requirements for each identified critical function. Recovery requirements consist of the following information:

- The business requirements for recovery of the critical function, and/or
- The technical requirements for recovery of the critical function

If the organization has an asset management program it can be used for quick identification of available and re-allocateable resources. The business requirements for recovery of a critical function include the following elements:

- The numbers and types of desks, PCs, telephones, functional-related equipment such as beds, medical supplies, medical equipment, and whether they are dedicated or shared; that are required outside of the primary business location at the secondary disaster recovery location
- The individuals involved in the recovery effort along with their contact information and technical details
- Business partners and vendor contact information and technical details
- The applications and application data required from the secondary location to support each critical business function
- The manual workaround solutions for each critical function
- The maximum outage time allowed for each application
- The peripheral equipment requirements such as printers, copier, fax machine, calculators, paper, pens, and so forth.

Some business environments that include production, distribution, warehousing, and so forth will need to cover these elements, but are likely to have additional issues to manage following a disruptive event. The technical requirements for a critical function include things such as:

- Names and location (primary and secondary) of application programs used for the function
- Names and location (primary and secondary) of files and databases used for the function
- Names, services, products, and contact information of vendors, suppliers, or partners who are involved with the function
- Equipment vendor, model, and types utilized for the function
- Communications equipment and networks used by this function
- IT personnel responsible for maintenance and enhancements for this function

Risk assessment is an important part of the impact analysis stage. The BCP workgroup needs to identify the following information:

- Types and probabilities of various types of disasters; risks range from low to high (Croy 2007)
- Potential impact of a particular disaster scenario
- Estimated costs of lost/damaged information/records and lost time and customer goodwill
- Costs to replace and restore records, equipment, and facilities, as well as to hire or replace staff, versus the costs to develop and maintain the disaster plan
- Risk of the worst-case scenario striking the organization

Threat Analysis

After identifying the critical functions and defining the business and technical recovery requirements for the functions, it is necessary to document the potential threats to help in developing the details of the specific disaster's unique recovery steps. This stage identifies threats and risks and includes a workflow analysis to determine interdependencies. Some common threats and the nature of damage they may cause include the following:

- Disease—reduces key personnel availability
- Earthquake—structural, utility, media, and equipment damage
- Fire—structural, utility, media, and equipment damage
- Flood—structural, utility, media, and equipment damage
- Cyber attack—data, application, and operating system damage
  - White hat—breaks security for nonmalicious reasons
  - Gray hat—has ambiguous ethics and/or borderline legality
  - Black hat—uses technology for vandalism, credit card fraud, identity theft, piracy, or other types of illegal activities
  - Script kiddie—breaks into computer systems by using pre-packaged automated tools written by others, usually with little understanding
- Sabotage—obstruction, disruption, and/or destruction of buildings, data, equipment, media, or availability of personnel
- Hurricane—structural, utility, media, and equipment damage plus availability of key personnel
- Utility outage—equipment, media, data, and application failure
- Electrical—blackout or brownout
- Telecommunications—wire line or wireless
- Terrorism—structural, utility, media, and equipment damage
- Equipment failure—application, media, and data damage
- Operating system failure—application, media, and data damage
- Application system failure—data, media, and operational failure
- Social upheaval—union strike, social protests, and so forth reduce the availability of personnel and supplies

All the threats listed above share a common impact: the potential of damage to organizational infrastructure—except for disease and social upheaval. The impact of diseases and social upheaval can be regarded as purely human and may be alleviated with technical and business solutions. However, if the humans behind these recovery plans are also affected by the disease or social upheaval, then the recovery process can fail. During the 2002–2003 SARS outbreak, some organizations grouped staff into separate teams, and rotated the teams between the primary and secondary work sites, with a rotation frequency equal to the incubation period of the disease. The organizations also banned face-to-face contact between opposing team members during business and nonbusiness hours. With such a split, organizations increased their resiliency against the threat of government-ordered quarantine measures if one person in a team contracted or was exposed to the disease. Damage from flooding also has a unique characteristic. If an office environment is flooded with nonsalinated and contamination-free water (e.g., in the event of a pipe burst), equipment can be thoroughly dried and may still be functional. Social upheavals usually deny access to a facility thereby eliminating access by key personnel and supplies needed for daily operations. The best defense against cyber attacks is prevention by using anti-virus and malware software but hackers sometimes slip through the anti-virus and malware database updates thereby requiring a plan to deal with such situations.

Impact Scenarios

After defining potential threats and their impact, documenting impact scenarios that form the basis of the business recovery plan is required. Defining the impact scenarios for the most serious disasters or disruptions is preferred over defining scenarios for smaller-scale problems since nearly all smaller-scale problems are part of larger disasters. A typical impact scenario such as "building loss" will encompass all critical business functions, and the worst possible outcome from any potential threat. A BCP may also document additional impact scenarios if an organization has more than one building. Other more specific impact scenarios such as the temporary or permanent loss of a specific floor in a building should also be documented. Organizations frequently underestimate the space necessary to make a move from one venue to another; therefore, it is important that organizations consider space requirements during the planning process so they do not have a problem when making the move. Table 22–1 lists threats to normal IS operation.

Some examples of scenarios based on an impact analysis that are reasonable to construct are discussed here.

TABLE 22–1 Threats to Normal System Operation	
Threat	**Examples**
Accidents	Brown-outs and power outages/grid failures
	File corruption
	Transportation accidents
	Chemical contamination
	Toxic fumes
Natural disasters	Avalanche
	Floods
	Earthquakes
	Tsunamis
	Hurricanes
	Tornadoes
	Blizzards
	Pandemics
Internal disasters	Hardware or software errors
	Water line breaks
	Construction accidents
	Fire
	Sabotage
	Theft
	Ex-employee violence
Malicious or violent acts	Hackers
	Bombs
	Terrorism and bioterrorism
	Electromagnetic pulse
	Civil unrest
	Armed conflict

- *Disease.* Design a plan that groups the staff into separate teams, and rotate the teams between the primary and secondary work sites, with a rotation frequency equal to the incubation period of the disease. Ban face-to-face contact between opposing team members during business and nonbusiness hours. This will increase an organization's resiliency against the threat of government-ordered quarantine measures if one person in a team contracted or was exposed to a disease.

- *Natural or environmental disaster.* Damage from earthquakes, hurricanes, flooding, lightening strikes, and fires can result in a wide array of damage to structures, equipment, media, utilities, and human life. Implementation plans need to be in place for each of these contingencies. Damage from flooding has a unique characteristic. If an office environment is flooded with nonsalinated and contamination-free water, equipment can be thoroughly dried and may still be functional. Environmental disasters may be natural or man-made. Plans must anticipate the predictable and the unpredictable, inclusive of climate, location, building features, internal hazards such as fire, water or smoke damage, and utility service. Many hospitals and providers lack the infrastructure to accommodate and support IS. Often, key clinical services, computers, and data are housed in areas threatened by floods, potential plumbing leaks, or exposure to dangerous materials, such as oxygen, anesthetic agents, or other hazardous chemicals. Both the security of the IS power supply and the availability of backup power to sustain uninterrupted computer operation, ventilation, and cooling of the data center must be considered. Excessive heat can shut computers down and cause processing errors (Barry 2007). Power capabilities must be kept up to date as data center consumption has increased (Johnston 2006; Komoski 2007; Rizzo 2006). Enough fuel should be on hand to power generators for at least 1 week. Hospital utility lines may be at risk because of their location, particularly if construction is under way and if power or telephone lines have not been marked and protected from inadvertent damage.

- *Power and telecommunication outages.* These are very common types of disruptions because of weather, vehicle collisions, construction damage to lines, or maintenance mistakes. These outages can last from minutes to days and the implementation plan must account for a range of time periods. Backup electrical and battery generators are required for long-term electrical power outages, but most computers and power strips can tolerate short-term power outages without damage to equipment or data.

- *Fire.* Man-made fires can be caused by everything from electrical short circuits to inadequate disposal of smoking materials. The implementation plan should require smoke detectors throughout a building along with fire extinguishers. All personnel should be taught how to use a fire extinguisher.

- *Flood.* Flooding may occur because of severe weather, broken pipes, or failure of flood control structures. The simplest preventative measure for flood protection from weather or flood control structural damage is to never locate information technology centers on a first floor or basement. Locating equipment on a platform inside computer rooms is a sensible preventative measure against broken water pipes. Also equipment rooms should have a drain into the building sewer system.

- *Cyber attacks.* The use of anti-virus software, firewalls, periodic password changes, encryption, and other preventive measures such as intrusion detection and monitoring must be in place to prevent cyber attacks.

- *Sabotage.* Protection from external physical attacks by nonemployees can be prevented by using video cameras with monitoring, windowless equipment rooms or window protection covers, and so forth. Protection from internal physical attacks by employees can be avoided by using keypad access devices to rooms or bio-sensory devices such as retinal scans or fingerprints.

- *Equipment failure.* The simplest protection against equipment failure is periodic maintenance and duplicate equipment. This is necessary for servers, switches, routers, and disk storage units.

- *Software failure (operating system or application).* Rigorous testing and running parallel versions of software are the best approaches for avoiding software-related problems.
- *Workforce disruption and bioterrorism.* In the event of a major disaster—such as the terrorist attacks of September 11, Hurricane Katrina, a pandemic, or bioterrorism—there will be problems securing and maintaining sufficient resources to carry out critical operations. An unanticipated problem after Katrina was the loss of qualified healthcare professionals and knowledgeable IT staff, who chose not to return or were unable to return post disaster (Martin 2007; Picking up the pieces 2006). A shortage of workers can also result from direct casualties, morbidity, problems getting to work sites, travel restrictions, fear, and family obligations (Epstein & Nilakantan 2007; Zirkel 2007).
- *Pandemic.* A pandemic is the emergence of a new communicable disease, such as bird flu, that infects humans, creates serious illness and death, and spreads into a global outbreak (Chandler, Wallace, & Coombs 2006). In the event of a pandemic, managers must assume that at least 40% of their workers will be unavailable for a period of between 6 and 8 weeks (Meyers 2006). Good planning and frequent communication take on even more importance under these circumstances to safeguard the safety of human resources and retain a sense of community. Consideration must also be given to the family and loved ones of the workforce. The implications of this type of situation call for major changes in the way that key applications are supported and the ability to run services remotely (Glenn 2007). In planning for pandemics, managers must devise strategies that address the need for providing employees with laptops with extra batteries, connectivity from home, and some form of wireless communication. Planning for pandemics is a relatively new event in continuity planning. On a related note, a recent Health Information Management Systems Society (2007) poll of chief information officers rated external threats such as bioterrorism low (3.1%) on their list of IT priorities. The U.S. Centers for Disease Control and Prevention has several emergency plans posted on its Web page for an array of disasters. The Agency for Healthcare Research and Quality of the Department of Health and Human Services posted a sample disaster recovery plan on its Web site to help organizations plan for pandemics and other health emergencies (*www.ahrq.gov/research/health/happk.htm*).
- *Human error.* Human error is the largest factor contributing to data loss, followed by mechanical failure. Both account for 75% of all data loss (Margeson 2003; Sussman 2002). Examples of human error include accidental file deletion, failure to follow proper backup procedures, unintended overwriting of files, the introduction of viruses or vandalism, theft, and loading flawed programs. Flawed programs are more commonly referred to as programs having bugs. This comes from the programmer jargon of debugging a software application as it is written to ensure that it works as designed. Commercial software that is distributed without being tested adequately first may include bugs. Bermont (2007) noted that several studies cite human error as the primary cause of problems in the data center, an area routinely responsible for the completion of file backups and for the support of hardware that runs major enterprise-wide applications. Training, fully tested documented procedures, and comprehensive maintenance records are suggested strategies to protect against human error in the data center. Nurses in the clinical area should be certain to save their documentation after entry because data may not be saved to the permanent record otherwise. Nurses and other healthcare professionals in clinical settings should also avoid downloading software from the Internet to hospital computers because this may have unintended consequences, such as poor computer performance and interference with institutional software.
- *Sabotage, cybercrime, and terrorism.* Both current and former employees pose the greatest risk to IS in terms of their capabilities to change data and damage systems because of their special knowledge and access. For this reason, random, unannounced background investigations of employees with access to sensitive and critical IS organizational information should be

considered as a means to avert sabotage, inadvertent disclosure of PHI, and wrongful system use, such as identity theft and credit card fraud (Marcella 2004). In the clinical area, personnel who note suspicious behaviors, such as changes in computer performance, deviant co-worker online behavior, and increased spam or e-mail traffic, should alert the information service department. On a national and international level, it is essential to consider the impact of terrorism and bioterrorism on the delivery of care and the potential effects on all services, not just information services. Threats that once seemed remote are now considered high risk. These include explosions, radiation, biological warfare, and electromagnetic pulses, which can kill and damage unshielded electronic devices (Maggio & Coleman 2007). Events associated with September 11 demonstrated what happens when infrastructure is destroyed, leaving organizations without power, communication, and water thereby and the workforce devastated (Ballman 2006). Since the September 11 attacks, efforts to improve responses to emergencies include the adoption of the Incident Command System (ICS) by the Department of Homeland Security. The ICS provides a unified approach for multiple agencies to use when responding to a disaster with the goal of improving communication and coordination of people and other resources. It has since been adopted by the healthcare industry as well and is mandated by the Joint Commission (Koch & Marks 2006). Another outcome of September 11 is the emergence of building vulnerability criteria (Kemp 2007). These criteria include visibility, criticality, significance of the site outside of its immediate location, public accessibility, presence of possible hazards, height of the edifice, type of construction, total capacity, and potential for collateral casualties. While many of these areas have no obvious connection to health information technology, there are questions as to whether IS and support personnel could sustain operations in the face of an attack.

- *System or equipment failure.* System or equipment failure may occur in the absence of any of the preceding environmental disasters. System failure may result from the failure of a component part or parts. Central processing unit (CPU) crashes, cabling and software problems, and even loose plugs may cause difficulties. When feasible, additional hardware such as hubs, patch cables, extra printers, PCs, and servers and trained support staff should be available to troubleshoot system problems, avert downtime, and initiate recovery. Redundancy in system design raises the initial system cost but increases IS reliability. A well-executed physical system prevents many problems or makes them easier to discover. A review of the facility, system, policies and procedures, and disaster plan conducted quarterly can identify vulnerable areas.

Solution Design Stage The goal of the solution design stage is to identify the most cost effective disaster recovery solution that meets two basic requirements based on the results of the impact and threat analysis stages. For information system applications recovery, solution design will include:

- The minimum set of applications and application data requirements
- The time frame in which the minimum applications and application data must be available

Disaster recovery plans may also be required outside the IS application domain such as preserving hard copy information, loss of skilled staff management personnel, or the restoration of embedded technology used in many machines. This BCP stage overlaps with disaster recovery planning methodology. The solution phase for a disaster should specify:

- The crisis management command structure
- The location of a secondary work site (where necessary)
- Data replication methodology and telecommunication architecture between primary and secondary work sites
- The applications and software required at the secondary work site

- Physical data requirements at the secondary work site
- Minimum application and application data requirements
- Time frame for availability after a failure or disaster
- Crisis management command structure
- Location(s) of secondary work site(s)
- Application, database, utility, and system software required at secondary work site(s)
- Physical requirements of the workspace at the secondary work sites
- General policy and procedures, hardware and software, troubleshooting, backup, training, testing, and overall costs must be weighed in determining solutions to potential threats. Interviews with department heads will help identify the most appropriate strategies to be used to maintain or recover business functionality and the steps necessary for restoration.
- Data and entity relationship flowcharts help to ensure that all critical processes are documented.

Each organization must determine its criteria for business recovery time frames based on its own perspective (Croy 2007). Typically the faster that an entire organization, division, or department needs to recover, the more the recovery will cost (Lawrence 2007). Even after information critical to system users has been identified, it is important to realize that critical information is more than the information required for direct client care. Individual areas within an organization have vendor contracts, personnel files, financial or claim documents, e-mails, permits, building blueprints, regulatory compliance documentation, equipment manuals, and reporting data in a variety of formats and locations. Approximately 60% of an organization's valuable information is not protected because it resides in PCs, laptop computers, and personal digital assistants (PDAs); on remote sites that are not backed up regularly; or only in paper format (Moore 2006). Much of this information would be difficult or time consuming to replace.

Implementation Stage The implementation stage is the execution of the design processes, procedures, and policies defined in the solution design stage. Individual component testing must take place during the implementation of the solution but implementation component testing does not take the place of organizational level testing. During the implementation stage, the outputs from previous stages are reviewed so that recovery plans can be developed that contain all the details an organization needs to survive a disaster and restore normal services. This stage also defines the actions necessary to prevent, detect, and mitigate the effects of potential disasters. One of the activities conducted in this stage is developing implementation plans, including the emergency response plan, the damage assessment plan, and the salvage plan.

Implementing standby arrangements includes defining, creating, and signing any contracts with standby providers and secondary backup locations. This includes contracts with external suppliers that support the IT organization in its delivery of services. This contract could be a support or maintenance agreement, and it should be capable of supporting targets agreed to in service level agreements (SLAs). Once completed, these contracts should be listed in the configuration management database and linked to the recovery plan and the associated SLAs. Necessary equipment and associated supplies also need to be purchased as part of the implementation stage. Implementation also involves developing procedures that detail what each member of the business continuity workgroup and the disaster recovery team must do if the plan is invoked. An example may be documenting the exact steps for immediately transferring operations to the backup site when a disaster occurs. The implementation stage also includes undertaking initial tests of the proposed solutions. Undertaking initial tests typically involves performing some initial testing of procedures before they are finalized. Final testing occurs in the formal testing stage.

By performing each of these activities, organizations can be sure that they have successfully completed the solution design stage of the business continuity life cycle. After implementation has been completed, the process needs to be formally tested and maintained as part of normal operating procedures.

As part of the implementation stage a complete inventory of information must be taken and recorded. This inventory should specify:

- Volume and description of information
- Format; for example, whether information is maintained on paper, CDs, DVDs, tapes, or removable drives
- When the information was created, its use, and how it relates to other records
- When the information is transferred to storage or destroyed
- Equipment used to store critical information
- Consequences for the loss of this information

An inventory of all information bearing records or documents should be created for each identifiable record in each department or function. Figure 22–2 provides an example of the type of information to be recorded for information bearing records or documents.

Test and Acceptance Stage The purpose of the test is to achieve organizational acceptance that the business continuity solution satisfies the organization's recovery requirements. The BCP may fail to meet expectations due to insufficient or inaccurate recovery requirements, solution design flaws, or solution implementation errors. Testing may include:

- Crisis command team call-out testing
- Technical switch from the primary work sites to the secondary work locations
- Technical switch test from secondary locations to the primary work sites
- Testing applications with backup data
- Testing business processes to ensure that all required functionality works correctly

Testing includes consideration of the reliability, adequacy, compatibility, and appropriateness of backup systems, facilities, and procedures. The BCP plan itself should be evaluated periodically and when major changes occur in system processes. Training of workgroup team members should occur at this time. An actual test of the BCP should be done in sections after peak business hours and evaluated for effectiveness. Strategies and methods must then be determined to test and evaluate the plan periodically to determine if it is workable, documentation is appropriate, and staff are trained. Testing twice a year, with a 6-month period in between, is recommended (Sheth & McHugh 2007). Offsite service providers and vendors should be included in tests. Actual disaster or outage situations provide an excellent test opportunity (Kirchner & Ziegenfuss 2003). Problems identified in the initial testing phase must be resolved during the maintenance stage and retested.

Maintenance Stage Maintenance of a BCP involves three periodic activities. The first activity is the confirmation and verification of information in the plan and the BCP manual and distribution to all staff for awareness and specific training for individuals whose roles are identified as critical in the response and recovery effort. The second activity is the testing and verification of technical solutions established for recovery operations. The third activity is the testing and verification of the documented organization's recovery procedures. A biannual or annual maintenance cycle is typical. All organizations and their operating environment change over time and as a result a continuity plan and its manual must change to stay relevant to the organization and its environment. This includes ensuring that data completeness and accuracy are verified and conducting a contacts call test to evaluate the notification plan's efficiency as well as the accuracy of the contact data. Some types of changes that should be identified and updated in the plan and associated manual include:

- Staffing changes
- Staffing personal

Make one copy of this page for each record listed. When parentheses appear, select one response from within them.

Record name:
Scheduled and Unscheduled Meds Due lists/Parenteral Therapy lists

Purpose of record:
Used to administer medications to patients

Who is responsible for this record:
HIS*-generated document based on MD orders

Media (paper, fiche, mainframe, etc.):
HIS paper document

Where is the record stored:
HIS system, on nursing units for 24 hours

Volume/frequency of change:
Many times/day

Retention requirement:
24 Hours

Originating office:
Nursing units

Location of any copies:
Nursing units/outdated copies

The record is: (irreplaceable, unique/difficult to replace/not hard to replace)

The record is: (essential for business/not essential but important/not important)

How would you obtain this record if your copy were destroyed?
If HIS system available, reprint; if not, go through each patient's chart

How would you re-create the information on this record?
Through patient's chart and current hard copy of Patient Care Plans

How long after a disaster could you work without this record?
Few hours—would use documents available

How is this record protected from destruction? (not protected, sprinklered office area, fireproof cabinet, duplicates kept in other locations, sprinklered warehouse, mainframe computer files, easily re-created, etc.)
HIS backups—paper documents not protected

Duplication and off-site storage is: (already being done/should be done/is not necessary)
Already being done—HIS

Are you prepared to supply input data, or work in progress, to allow the rerun of your critical applications from the last off-site backup?

Who is in charge of removing/restoring this record if it is damaged? What provisions have been made to restore/remove damaged records? What is the relocation destination? Who will transport damaged records and what is this person's 24-hour telephone number and security clearance?

* HIS, hospital or healthcare information service.

FIGURE 22–2 • Example of a physical vital records inventory sheet

- Changes to important clients and their contact details
- Changes to important vendors/suppliers and their contact details
- Departmental changes like new, closed, or fundamentally changed departments
- Changes in company investment portfolio and mission statement
- Changes in upstream/downstream supplier routes

During the maintenance stage, all technical solutions must be tested and verified. As a part of ongoing maintenance, any specialized technical deployments must be checked for functionality. These checks may include:

- Virus definition distribution
- Application security and service patch distribution
- Hardware operability check
- Application operability check
- Data verification

As organizations and their environment change over time, work processes change as well and the previously documented organizational recovery procedures may no longer be suitable. Verification of work processes against the BCP manual includes the following questions:

- Are all work processes for critical functions documented?
- Have the systems used in the execution of critical functions changed?
- Are the documented work checklists meaningful and accurate for staff?
- Do the documented work process recovery tasks and supporting disaster recovery infrastructure allow staff to recover within the predetermined recovery time objective?

There is a direct relationship between the test, maintenance, and impact stages. When developing a BCP plan and associated manual, there may be recovery infrastructure problems found during the testing phase, which may need to be reintroduced to the analysis phase. Box 22–1 lists areas that should be reviewed periodically, as part of maintenance, to avert system disasters.

BOX 22–1   Suggested Areas for Review to Avert System Disasters

- Organizational continuity plan
- Documentation
- Vital records
- Vendor service and maintenance agreements
- Vendor continuity plans
- Backup procedures
- Recovery procedures
- Network access controls
- Physical security
- Archived data
- Backup equipment
- Backup facility
- Network diversity
- Communications links
- Spare parts inventory
- Backup services
- LAN configurations
- Off-site storage
- Personnel availability
- Operations personnel
- Technical personnel
- Antivirus updates

Content of the Continuity Plan Manual

The continuity plan documentation must be explicit because staff changes occur and details get lost. Information cannot be confusing or lack detail in order to avoid problems when a disaster occurs. For example, instructions should provide details on responsibilities and where staff will report in an emergency (Lindeman & Grogan 2007). Key information, such as persons responsible for implementing the plan and their roles, must be kept up to date. Consideration must also be given to whether human resources are intact. Documentation should include goals for the implementation of suggested and/or required changes. Box 22–2 lists items that should be included in the continuity plan manual.

BOX 22–2   Suggested Content for the Continuity Plan Manual

- Planning process description
- Purpose of the plan
- General system policies and procedures, including who can declare a disaster, the mechanism for calling a disaster, and the distribution and maintenance of the plan
- The mechanism for calling a disaster, and the distribution and maintenance of the plan
- Persons for emergency notification (this may include a traditional calling tree/call schedule with telephone, cell phone, and pager numbers or utilize software specific for this purpose) and the length of time required for each identified person to arrive, whether the person is an employee, or any other individual key to the recovery process
- Responsibilities for each administrator and key employee
- Floor plans for water, gas, and oxygen lines and exits
- Cable, electrical, and telecommunication diagrams
- System configurations inclusive of server configurations and port connections
- Schematics for backup systems and schedules
- Software specific for this purpose
- System configurations inclusive of server configurations and port connections
- Schematics for backup systems and schedules
- Outline of what users should do in the event of a disaster, including their responsibilities with manual systems and restoration efforts
- Identification of people who will arrive, whether the person is an employee, or any emergency personnel
- Identification of individuals key to the recovery process
- Projected timeline for system restoration
- Troubleshooting and problem resolution
- Data backup, security, and restoration procedures
- Insurance documents
- Repair procedures
- List of basic resources required to perform services, including equipment and software vendors and restoration and storage services
- Vital record inventory that includes, but is not limited to, vendor/service provider and warranty information
- Provisions for nonclinical vital record access, backup, and, if needed, appropriate restoration techniques for each type of storage medium used
- Vendor service agreements along with identification numbers
- Mechanism to store and retrieve passwords and software from a protected site
- Locations of all operations
- Auditing procedures
- Evacuation plan

ADVANTAGES OF CONTINUITY PLANNING

It is not always possible to avoid a disaster or to provide 100% protection against every threat, but a satisfactory plan can anticipate problems and minimize losses incurred by damage (Pelant 2003). A good plan is clear and concise and should at a minimum provide the following (Miano 2003; Midgley 2002):

- Identifies strategies for correction of vulnerabilities within the organization
- Provides a reasonable amount of protection against interruption in services, downtime, and data loss
- Ensures continuity of the client record and delivery of care
- Expedites reporting of diagnostic tests
- Captures charges and supports billing and processing of reimbursement claims in a timely fashion
- Ensures open communication with employees and ensures customers of availability of services or interim arrangements
- Provides a mechanism to capture information needed for regulatory and accrediting bodies
- Helps to ensure compliance with HIPAA legislation and requirements of the Joint Commission
- Establishes backup and restoration procedures for systems, databases, and important files
- Allows time for restoration of equipment, the facility, and services

Basically, an effective disaster plan saves patients from unnecessary delays in treatment and avoids redundant procedures. It also saves money upfront and over time by limiting loss of data, equipment, and services. Any organization that requires a high level of information integrity and availability cannot afford to be without a continuity plan that provides for disaster recovery. A good plan can make the difference between an organization's survival and demise. Data has shown that the likelihood of bankruptcy increases with each increment of time that data are unavailable to an organization during a disaster.

DISASTERS VERSUS SYSTEM FAILURE

Hazards come from a variety of sources, including environmental disasters, human error, sabotage and acts of terrorism and bioterrorism, high-tech crime, operating system or application software bugs, viruses, overtaxed infrastructure, power fluctuations and outages, and equipment failure (Midgley 2002; Wiles 2004).

A thorough appraisal by information services personnel can minimize the risk of damage from various hazard situations. The impact scenarios provide a means to understand the impact of a disaster versus a system failure. A review of the impact scenarios should be performed and the scenarios updated because not only does the organization change but so does the technology and the environment in which it operates. An IS failure is something IT staff members typically have measures in place to correct, with, for example, redundant equipment and data backups, but a disaster affects an entire organization, all its systems, equipment, processes, personnel, clients, partners, and information in all media and formats.

CONTINUITY AND RECOVERY OPTIONS

The 24/7 operations of healthcare providers make continuity of services essential. Although continuity planning must encompass all aspects of daily operations, the focus on information should guide the selection of computer services, hardware and software for day-to-day operations, backup, and recovery. Problems are magnified by the fact that an estimated 60% of critical business data resides at remote sites away from IT staff with backups and testing of backups frequently hampered by limited and busy staff, slow WAN connections, and constantly increasing data storage requirements (Moore 2006).

Hardware redundancy is the first line of defense in providing continuous system operations because this allows operations to continue even when individual components fail. This redundancy may be accomplished via redundant processors and disk arrays in one location or at two separate locations of the same organization or another facility. An increasing number of organizations now split their IT infrastructure between two locations for added protection. A second data processing site requires sufficient space for equipment and staff, especially if it may double as a backup data center.

Functional requirements include mainframe and/or server capacity, printers, storage devices, network and communication equipment and services, sufficient cabling, power, an uninterrupted power source, air conditioning and space for a help desk, and an operations center and test room. Online replication of data is an integral part of business continuity, providing data availability, averting disaster, and reducing costs and recovery time. Redundant network storage provides multiple data paths, preventing damage and loss. Advances in technology in recent years help organizations to be better prepared in the event of a major disaster. These include improvements in data replication hardware, servers, and other equipment that require less electricity and better battery backup systems for small businesses. Improved software and equipment options for emergency notification make it easier and quicker to contact key administrators, employees, vendors, and suppliers (Ballman 2006; Veldboom 2007). Automated emergency notification applications expedite the traditional calling tree to contact personnel within a span of minutes, using methods that range from interactive voice response phone calls to e-mail, freeing personnel for other tasks in the process. Managed hosting services with Internet access also provide an option for a secondary site for backup and recovery.

A managed hosting site eliminates the need to purchase server and networking equipment, disk and tape storage hardware and media, telecommunications lines; perform backups; rent space; and purchase anti-virus and firewall software and is available wherever there is an Internet connection using Remote Desktop software or Virtual Private Network software. The latest versions of most Database Management Systems, such as SQL Server or Oracle, provide for database replication across a network as well as incremental and full backup capabilities. Using replication across a network, a secondary site database can be kept current with the production database in the organization's main site because each transaction that takes place for the production database also occurs at the replicated database site. The connection between the primary site and the replication site can be either leased lines or the Internet. Redundancy of communication capabilities is important for replication.

Backup and Storage

Data availability, recovery time, disaster avoidance, retention requirements, and costs determine the best backup and storage options for a given organization (Lindeman 2007). Continuous delivery of services is the goal, but solutions to achieve zero downtime are expensive and not always possible. For these reasons, organizations must determine data storage requirements and acceptable recovery time on a system-by-system basis. These decisions help to determine media choices for storage. Media choices include magnetic tape, hard disk, optical disc (CD and DVD), solid state storage (flash memory, thumb drives) as well as RBSs. CDs, DVDs, and solid state storage devices are convenient for backing up stand-alone PCs.

Common anti-disaster protection methods include the following: automated backups, off-site media storage, data mirroring, server replication, remote data replication, a virtual tape library that emulates multiple tape drives (by backing up data to disks with later conversion to physical tapes for off-site vaulting), and snapshots of data at prescribed intervals (Lindeman 2007). Virtual disaster recovery pools IT resources, masking boundaries between hardware to increase capacity. Data mirroring is the creation of a duplicate online copy. This technique eliminates wait time but may also replicate corrupted data.

Best practices for long-term data retention include the selection of standardized file formats, good management of **metadata**, the selection of media intended for long-term storage and proper housing, and regular inspection and maintenance of stored media. Metadata is a set of data that provides information about how, when, and by whom data are collected, formatted, and stored (Morgenthal & Walmsley 2000). File metadata describes each file's permissions, owner, group, ACLs, size, and so forth. System metadata is configuration information and each operating system has a different way of storing such information. Metadata is essential to the creation and use of data repositories.

Backup allows restoration of data if, or when, they are lost. Losses may occur with disk or CPU crashes, file deletion, and file corruption due to power or application problems, or overwritten files. Fast data recovery minimizes the worst consequences of downtime, including a tarnished image and financial losses. Networked storage area networks and electronic vaulting provides the type of protection needed to ensure business continuity.

Server replication is recommended for the most widely used applications because it ensures continuity by providing a reliable secondary infrastructure. Electronic vaulting sends backups over telecommunication links to secure storage facilities. This approach eliminates labor costs and the need to physically transport tapes. It also improves data integrity and shortens recovery efforts. Electronic vaulting may be provided by commercial enterprises that provide backup services for customers. Customers receive backup software at their site and at a central, remote file server. The customer connects to the remote server to back up data. Each customer has a separate account, and file access is limited to authorized persons.

Remote backup service (RBS) staff protects both data and data integrity. Data retrieval, when needed, is limited only by the speed of the communication link. RBSs also provide reports to show which files have been backed up. Tape and other older media do not support fast data recovery efforts. Recovery may require 12 to 48 hours depending on recovery location and the number of critical systems that must be rebuilt before applications and data can be loaded (Lindeman 2007).

Backups may fail because of faulty software, bad network connections, worn tapes, or poor storage conditions. For this reason, backup should be verified and periodically tested. Advancements in technology and changes in the costs of backup options and storage media provide more options to maintain business continuity and backup and storage. Newer tape drives have well-developed error correction, eliminating the need to verify backup copies but not the need to test stored media.

Storage conditions must be climate controlled and free from electromagnetic interference to avoid degradation of media. Agencies may opt to outsource storage to cold sites. A cold site is a commercial service that provides storage for backup materials or the capacity to handle the disaster-stricken facility's computer equipment (Wold & Vick 2003). Often, backup materials are found on a combination of different media. Materials are shipped from the institution to the cold site, where backups from multiple organizations are kept in protected vaults under controlled conditions. Organizational personnel are responsible for backup, dating, and labeling materials for storage. Cold sites should be located in areas free from floods and tornadoes and at least 5 miles away from the agency to avoid disaster conditions. Commercial cold sites provide environmental controls and possibly communication links and uninterrupted power sources. They are relatively inexpensive but cannot be tested as a backup facility unless equipment is shipped there and communication links are installed. There are commercial firms that offer managed hosted site as a backup, which provide the servers(s), storage facilities, backup facilities, and communication links at reasonable costs.

A traditional backup process writes data to a storage medium for transfer to another site for storage and, if needed, system restoration. While magnetic tape is still used, higher-capacity forms of media and faster processes are preferred, although tape may be used in combination with other media (Taylor 2007). The newer solid-state Blu-ray discs provide significant increases in the capacity of a single optical disc up to 50 GB for a dual layered disc. Tape dumps for off-site storage start off with a gap between creation and pickup/delivery time. Data may be lost in this gap and recovery from tapes can be unreliable and time consuming. Increasingly, critical data are stored on disk for quick restoration. For these reasons, backup reporting and analysis software is an emerging field of data protection management (McDonald 2007). Storage media differ but should permit permanent or semi-permanent record keeping. Magnetic tape is still used as a relatively inexpensive storage medium. Optical disks are another storage option with a longer shelf life but a higher cost. Electronic transfer over high-speed telephone lines to another site is a faster, more reliable means of backup that eliminates transportation concerns. When electronic transmission is not an option, a second set of backup media should be made and transported separately to ensure against accidental loss or destruction. Archived data must be inspected regularly to ensure that they can be processed and that the medium has not deteriorated or become outdated in light of current backup systems. The criteria for good backup system include the following four points:

- Backups must contain the requested data;
- Backups must complete within the prescribed time frame;
- Backups must occur as scheduled—full backup on some days and incremental on others; and
- Backups must be set to expire at the correct time.

Personal and Notebook Computers Although the primary focus of an IS continuity/disaster recovery plan is on the major systems in an organization, large amounts of information that is important for daily operations are also found on PCs, notebook computers, and PDAs. This is particularly true as mobile workers and telecommuters, who increasingly comprise a greater percentage of the workforce (McKilroy 2003). Mobile workers spend at least 50% of their time at a location outside of the main organization's site, using notebooks or PDAs. Homecare personnel exemplify one such group of mobile workers. Other healthcare professionals telecommute using the Internet and remote connections to access and transmit information. Telecommuters face IS threats that do not affect internal employees, such as firewall maintenance and denial of service attacks, and lost productivity when network connections are not available. For these reasons, IS disaster plans need to include notebook computers, PDAs, mobile devices, and remote users. Routine maintenance prevents many problems faced by mobile users. Box 22–3 lists maintenance tasks recommended for PC/notebook computers.

Organizations should not assume that users know how to perform the above tasks or that they will perform them regularly. Instruction and assistance should be provided for PC/notebook users. For example, computer support personnel should perform periodic backups using standardized backup procedures and media.

Manual Versus Automated Alternatives

The decision to use manual alternatives when a system has failed or is otherwise unavailable has implications for the delivery of care, the cost of care provided, record management, and employee system training. A backup alternative is a different means to accomplish a common task than what is ordinarily used. An example of a manual backup alternative is the completion of paper requests for laboratory tests that are then delivered to the laboratory, instead of selecting ordered tests from menus on computer screens. Implementation of a backup alternative may delay delivery of services for several reasons. First, personnel are less familiar with the alternative procedure and will take longer to accomplish their work thereby delaying results reporting and processing requests for services. Second, manual forms may no longer exist or may not be current in terms of displaying the newest available tests or test names. Third, because automation eliminated personnel who supported the manual process, there may be few people available who know the manual alternative.

> **BOX 22–3   Recommended PC/Notebook Maintenance**
>
> - Keep original software handy in the event that it must be reinstalled.
> - Establish a secure place for backup media away from the PC, preferably in a fire-proof safe or file cabinet. Backup media stored under poor conditions or kept in the same area as the PC are vulnerable to the same threats. Another backup option is online backup. This may be accomplished through the information services department or a vendor.
> - Do an incremental backup daily, a full backup weekly, and a full system backup monthly and back up/store files on network drives whenever possible. This is particularly important for remote sites not covered by IS staff.
> - Test backup media to ensure that they are good. Establish a policy for routine replacement of backup media.
> - Periodically delete files from the hard drive that are no longer needed.
> - Defragment all hard drives monthly.
> - Maintain air flow around the PC/notebook to allow cooling.
> - Keep storage media away from magnetic fields, including electronic devices.
> - Periodically clean PCs/notebooks.
> - Run virus protection software regularly and obtain updated versions as available.

Automated backup alternatives may also be available. For example, staff may be able to access information through a different screen than the one they generally use. Despite these potential problems, implementation of backup alternatives permits ongoing delivery of care, even if it is somewhat slower. Calculation of backup costs goes beyond initial setup costs and ongoing expenditures. Recovery costs can be high for several reasons:

- The personnel cost for hiring and training staff to use backup alternatives; additional costs for dual entry of data;
- Costs for cleanup, repair, or replacement of computer equipment; and
- Payment for backup computing or recovery services.

Another cost is the impact on the quality of services rendered during the time a system is not available. The expense for manual versus automated alternatives varies according to the length of time that the system is unavailable, the type of backup alternatives employed, and the resources required. Because implementing a backup alternative is costly, administrators must decide if the anticipated time a system is not available merits initiating the alternative. Extremely short periods of system unavailability are usually not worth the additional time and trouble. Costs for a manual alternative include additional labor for IS and other personnel, increased potential for error, and space requirements. Data entry into the system following a manual backup requires additional personnel and a place for them to work. For example, laboratory tests that were requested but not completed before the system became unavailable must again be requested by nursing manually. During the time a system is down, laboratory staff must try to match manual requisitions against those that were entered but not processed before the system failed. When the system is restored (goes live), laboratory tests that were ordered and completed during the time the system was down, along with test results, must be entered so that the client record is not fragmented.

Staff Training

The successful implementation of a manual alternative plan hinges on the cooperation and support of everyone in the organization. One way to ensure this success is through training. Detailed instructions on every aspect of the system, the plan, and the implementation of manual alternatives should be incorporated into initial computer training. However, this approach requires a longer

BOX 22–4   Ways to Ensure Business Continuity and Successful Recovery

- Display continuity plans in conspicuous places, and post revised versions as soon as they are available.
- List key contact people responsible for implementing continuity and recovery plans.
- Review staff responsibilities periodically.
- Provide clear step-by-step reference aids for staff to guide them through continuity and recovery options including manual alternatives.
- Emphasize the importance of disaster preparedness by incorporating mock disaster situations into training.
- Review the continuity and recovery plans at least twice each year.
- Schedule at least two mock disasters per year—one of which is community wide.
- Test backups periodically.
- Label backup materials and include explicit directions with them.
- Provide up-to-date hot and cold site information to persons responsible for recovery.
- Test the emergency notification periodically. This may include a calling tree, but more likely it will rely upon special software that provides almost instant, simultaneous notification of all key persons.
- Emphasize the need for emergency care arrangements for dependents and pets to personnel involved in disaster and recovery plan implementation.

training period and refresher training periodically. Recall of manual procedures is often poor when long periods elapse between instruction and execution. A more effective strategy entails posting plans in conspicuous places, yearly review of continuity plans, mock disasters, and the provision of step-by-step reference guides to help staff implement manual alternatives. Other measures to increase disaster awareness and ensure successful recovery efforts are listed in Box 22–4.

When it is not possible to maintain IS continuity, recovery is the next option. Recovery is not a simple undertaking and requires detailed and tested procedures. Few organizations have actually reconstructed IS from their backups, and few IT staff are equipped to deal with data recovery (Margeson 2003). The recovery process requires a safe place for employees to meet/work and a means for them to get there during times of travel restrictions (Lindeman 2007). Even when it would appear that equipment and storage media are damaged, assumptions should not be made that data are permanently lost, nor should persons unacquainted with salvage recovery techniques attempt to restore equipment or storage media (Olson 2002). For these reasons, it is best to call in recovery specialists when significant data loss has occurred. Successful recovery requires stabilization of the affected system and good problem-solving skills, staff preparedness, and good backups. Recovery is complicated when backups are not verified, delaying the detection of problems until restoration is attempted. Also, large organizations typically have data stored in many locations, on many different devices, on many different media, and in several different formats.

Most organizations use a combination of backup formats and software programs. Restoration of system operation may result from one of several approaches. First, materials stored at a cold site can be shipped back to the organization and reloaded onto the system. Second, information may be restored from RBSs or electronic vaulting. A third option is the use of hot sites such as a commercial managed hosted site. Commercial hot sites are fully equipped with uninterrupted power supplies, computers, telecommunication capabilities, security, and environmental equipment. Hot sites may accept transmission of backup copies of computer data, allowing restoration of operations using backup media. This is accomplished at another location served by a different power grid and central telephone office to avoid the effects of the disaster that affected the healthcare enterprise. The organization may develop its own hot site or outsource for services. When possible, hot sites should be close enough for practical employee travel, with sufficient space, power, cabling, parking, and satellite dish accommodations to support IS function. Hot sites are expensive and it may be difficult to get employees to the hot site location (Martin 2007).

A dedicated hot site usually sits idle when not needed but is available in the event of an emergency and is compatible with agency systems for ease of system restoration and updates. The creation of redundant computer capabilities and the acquisition of a dedicated hot site are costly. At one time, it was common to share the center with other healthcare alliance partners. A tenant would have to agree to relinquish the site in the event of a disaster. Sharing a site presumes that it is unlikely that two or more partners at separate locations would have a disaster at the same time. Shared arrangements are no longer practical because most systems now have extensive online processing. Hot sites may not be adequate to process critical applications or be able to provide for special equipment needs such as unique laser printers and forms handling equipment.

Mobile hot sites are also available. Another option is the creation of a backup facility onsite in another building owned by the organization. This option reduces real estate costs but still requires system redundancy. Internal hot sites can continue to provide processing for critical business functions, although typically this occurs at a reduced level of service. When not in use as a hot site, it can be used for other processing activities thereby eliminating certain types of fees. Commercial hot site services or managed hosting services charge monthly reservation fees in addition to restoration charges but are less costly than establishing an independent site. When using a commercial hot site there is a risk of being bumped by another client who requires services at the same time, particularly during a regional disaster when several organizations are affected by the same event (Martin 2007). This cannot occur when using a managed hosting service since an organization can have a server that is not shared with anyone else. Commercial vendors should be able to offer the assurance of a proven track record for mainframe recovery. Unfortunately, the uniqueness of most client–server environments made commercial recovery services unprofitable and unavailable until recently, forcing institutions to develop their own internal recovery options. Although clinical staff have no involvement in the establishment of hot and cold sites, it may have relevance for them in terms of possible delays in information access.

Vendor Equipment

Vendors may offer processing capability through their equipment either at their location or at the location of the disaster. This solution may work for a select few applications but does not address the needs of an entire organization. There are also issues related to costs, software versions and customizations, availability, and testing. Sending equipment from other locations can take days before the equipment arrives, the software is loaded, and the data are recovered from backup media. This option can be problematic in a regional disaster in which several organizations need the same type of services at the same time (Martin 2007). An alternative to system restoration is distributed processing. Distributed processing uses a group of independent processors that contain the same information, but these may be at different sites. In the event that one processor is knocked out, information is not lost because remaining processors can continue IS operation with little or no interruption. Distributed processing is more expensive upfront but eliminates the time a system is not available. Rapid replacement of equipment is yet another recovery strategy, but it is not always feasible because it is costly to maintain extra hardware.

Salvaging Damaged Equipment and Records

Once alternative arrangements have been made to maintain business options, restoration of the equipment and required data records becomes the focus. Few IS personnel possess the skills necessary to salvage damaged records and equipment, but internal personnel should know how to act quickly and effectively to limit damage and to obtain outside help. Quick action and a

> **BOX 22–5 General Salvage Rules**
>
> - Stabilize the site.
> - Pump any standing water out of the facility.
> - Decrease the temperature to minimize mold and mildew growth and damage.
> - Vent the area.
> - Do not restore power to wet equipment.
> - Open cabinet doors, remove side panels and covers, and pull out chassis to permit water to exit equipment.
> - Absorb excess water in equipment with cotton, using care not to damage pins and cables.
> - Call in professional decontamination specialists when hazardous chemicals or wastes are present.
> - Initiate salvage options within 48 hours.

basic knowledge of recovery techniques can expedite the return to full operation and minimize loss of equipment, records, as well as costs. Whether the information center was without climate control or was physically damaged by an event that exposed it to heat, humidity, and/or smoke damage, there are guidelines to follow to salvage materials. Some of these guidelines are provided in Box 22–5.

The first rule is to stabilize the site. In most scenarios, internal staff does not participate in the actual recovery process. Many processes require the use of hazardous and dangerous chemicals or knowledge of detailed salvage methods. Disaster recovery experts can best ensure data recovery from damaged media, particularly from magnetic media. Fires, heat, and floods leave residues that damage electronic equipment and storage media. Additional damage may occur when media are improperly stored and handled after the disaster and with the passage of time. Degradation of media also impedes recovery efforts. Data integrity is compromised when storage media are damaged. Recovery specialists must verify data on a bit-by-bit basis and reconstruct files before data can be recorded onto new media. It is important to have written agreements with restoration companies in times of widespread disasters, such as earthquakes or floods, when many organizations will be seeking help at the same time. Box 22–6 provides some recovery suggestions for both paper-based records and magnetic media.

Recovery Costs

The cost for recovery is frequently overlooked in developing the continuity/disaster recovery plan. Recovery costs should be determined as part of the continuity plan because unanticipated expenses during recovery are never well received and it can be an extremely expensive process, involving the following cost factors:

- Lost consumer confidence
- Financial loss
- Temporary computer services, including space rental, equipment, furniture, extra telephone lines, and temporary personnel
- Shipping and installation costs
- Post-disaster replacement of equipment, repairs, and costs associated with bringing the building up to new codes
- Recovery and possible decontamination
- Overtime hours for staff during the disaster for the implementation of manual alternatives, and after the disaster for entering data into the system that was generated during system downtime
- Reconstruction of lost data

BOX 22–6   Recommended Storage Media Recovery Techniques

General efforts recovery methods for paper-based materials:

- Have record salvage professionals on retainer. Initiate recovery within 48 hours of the disaster for best results.

- Consult recovery specialists before attempting any record salvage!

- Separate coated papers such as ECG tracing and ultrasound records to prevent them from permanently fusing together.

- Remove noncoated documents from file cabinets or shelves in blocks—do not pull each page apart, as this increases mold growth.

- Store paper documents in a diesel-powered freezer trailer until proper drying arrangements can be finalized.

- Remove excess mud and dirt before freezing documents.

- Pack wet files or books in a box with a plastic trash liner and allow room for circulation of air.

- Place files with open edges facing up and books with spines down.

- Label all boxes precisely and create a master inventory.

- Freeze-dry priority documents and sterilize and use fungicide as needed.

General magnetic media recovery techniques:

- Freeze-dry tape cartridges, then use recovery software to recover and copy information to new tape cartridges.

- Dry reel-to-reel tapes on a tape-cleaning machine, using warm air to evaporate moisture. Use recovery software to recover and copy information to new storage media.

Insurance coverage is recommended as a means to help pay for information system disasters. It is imperative that a complete inventory with photographs, replacement values for equipment, and all other documentation be finalized prior to submitting a claim (Baldwin 2007). Table 22–2 lists types of available coverage.

TABLE 22–2   Types of Insurance Coverage

Coverage	Purpose
Business interruption	Provides replacement of lost profits as a result of a covered loss. Must be certain that insurance covers the same period as the event.
Extra expense	Provides financial recovery for out-of-the-ordinary expenses such as a temporary office or center of operations, and additional costs for rent, staff, and rental of equipment and furniture while regular facilities cannot be used.
Code compliance	Often overlooked. Insurance will normally reimburse only for expenses associated with repair or replacement of a damaged building, but not additional costs associated with building code changes implemented since the building was built. This coverage provides for those additional costs.
Electronic data processing	Replaces damaged or lost equipment and media from a covered incident such as storm damage not covered in normal property insurance. May also include coverage for business interruption and extra expenses.

Source: Adapted from Cox, L. P. (1996). Disaster recovery: How do you pay for it? *Disaster Recovery Journal, 9* (2), 19–20; Baldwin, W. (2007). After a disaster strikes. *Disaster Recovery Journal, 20* (1). Retrieved from http://www.drj.com/articlees/winter07/2001–10.pdf.

One person should be designated to interact with the insurance company and a mechanism should be identified for how disaster-related costs will be documented. Insurance will normally reimburse only for expenses associated with repair or replacement of a damaged building, but not additional costs associated with building code changes implemented since the building was built. This coverage provides for those additional costs.

PLANNING PITFALLS

Continuity plans are subject to the following pitfalls:

- *Insufficient IT budgets.* Few IT budgets have sufficient funding for business continuity efforts. Continuity plan budgets need to be spread across the organization.
- *Lack of access to the plan.* If the plan is available online, measures must be taken to ensure that the computers that house the plan are accessible. All employees responsible for implementing any part of the plan should have a copy at home, at work, and in their briefcase. These copies may be on paper, PDAs, and/or notebooks. CD-ROM, DVD, or thumb drives may also be an acceptable distribution method. Everyone should be aware of their roles and responsibilities (Stephens 2003).
- *Failure to include all information and devices in the plan.* Businesses evolve and institute new processes. Many plans lag behind the technology that is being used. An increasing amount of important information is found on laptops, desktop PCs, PDAs, and even in paper format. Many plans fail to consider the importance of e-mail, enterprise resource planning systems, and Web-based transactions to daily operations. Many healthcare providers also have separate databases for various populations. Information services may not be aware of these separate databases until problems arise. There are also applications supported by application service providers. One such example might include a renal database for dialysis patients. Continuity plans must consider how services will be provided in the event that the vendor's database is unavailable due to failure on the vendor's end or because of an inability to access the database due to inoperable Internet or telephone connections (Bannan 2002). Another example might be the failure to consider the multivendor environment seen in most healthcare systems today. Data are frequently housed on several computers.
- *Failure to plan for regional disasters.* The 2005 Gartner survey (Witty 2006) showed that the majority of organizations planned for a single facility outage rather than a regional disaster. Subsequent events surrounding September 11 and Hurricane Katrina demonstrate the inadequacy of plans that focus on a single facility (Ballman 2006).
- *Failure to incorporate data growth into the plan.* Unprecedented data growth is a threat to recovery plans. Organizations need to focus on critical data to ensure business continuity and reduce recovery time. This can be done by separating inactive from active data as a means to keep operating databases at a manageable size and improve application availability (Lee 2003).
- *Failure to update the plan.* The continuity plan is a dynamic document that is subject to change as operations and personnel change and determinations are made that some portions of the plan do not work well. The BCP workgroup should control the change process and should print review and revision dates on each page. A change manual can be used to note changes, including the date and reason for each change. While not specific to the healthcare industry, a 2005 survey by AT&T found that one in four companies that had a continuity plan had not updated it in the past 12 months (Ballman 2006).
- *Failure to test the plan.* A significant percentage of organizations that have continuity and disaster recovery plans have never tested them, do not know if they have been tested, or have not tested them within the past year (Ballman 2006).
- *Failure to consider the human component* (Kirschenbaum 2006; Mitchell 2007; Zirkel 2007). Preservation of human life is the top priority in any disaster, followed by preservation of critical business functions. In any disaster, the loss of personnel is a distinct possibility. In times of disaster, the organization should be prepared to assist employees and their families, including

communication links to check on employees and provide such amenities as transportation to work and possibly temporary housing. Restoration of peace of mind for employees and families is just as important as recovering data from a computer system and maintaining business continuity. This includes reestablishing user confidence once normal operations are restored and addressing the emotional impact that the disaster has had on employees.

USING POST-DISASTER FEEDBACK TO IMPROVE PLANNING

Post-disaster feedback is invaluable in revising disaster plans for future use and should be an integral part of continuity planning (Price 2007). Personnel input after mock disasters or prolonged downtime should be used to identify what worked and what did not. Systems, technology, society, and organizations change over time. Plans that looked adequate before a disaster may not prove adequate after a disaster has occurred. Recovery expenses usually exceed anticipated costs, leading to a change in recovery strategies for future use. Figure 22–3 shows a checklist that can be used to evaluate the success of a business continuity disaster and recovery plan.

Checklist Item	Yes	No
Are backup(s) available? tested?	❏	❏
Are disaster/recovery plan copies available/accessible?	❏	❏
Are duplicate processors or storage options in place?	❏	❏
Are hot-site contract copies available/accessible?	❏	❏
Do key personnel have emergency care arrangements for dependents? pets?	❏	❏
Is home-site staffing coverage adequate?	❏	❏
Are the hot-site locations and access procedures known?	❏	❏
Are the cold-site storage sites and procedures for retrieval of backups known/arranged?	❏	❏
Is travel to the cold and hot sites feasible?	❏	❏
Has authorization for recovery-related expenses been confirmed?	❏	❏
Are contracts with record salvage services in place?	❏	❏
Is shipping information accurate for backup tapes from cold to hot sites and back again?	❏	❏
Is documentation accurate for tape restoration available with starting and ending tape numbers?	❏	❏
Are backup media labeled accurately?	❏	❏
Have network/communications persons been sent to the hot site?	❏	❏
Do restoration procedures agree with current software?	❏	❏
Have previous arrangements been made to have persons stay after hours at the remote site?	❏	❏
Are communications links for backup confirmed, appropriate, and available?	❏	❏
Are phone numbers available for all vendors and services?	❏	❏
Are stored supplies intact/usable?	❏	❏
Is a timeline for anticipated restoration of operations identified and appropriate?	❏	❏
Are packing materials and labels available to ship media from cold to hot sites and back again?	❏	❏
Is an extra container for reports among supplies?	❏	❏
Are human needs for food and rest adequately included in the plan?	❏	❏

FIGURE 22–3 • Checklist for successful implementation of an IS disaster and recovery plan

Another option for the development, revision, and management of continuity plans for organizations with limited resources is the use of a managed hosting service provider (Midgley 2002). Managed hosting service providers offer continuous data backup, safeguarding against data loss while allowing for immediate recovery and restoration of services in the event of a disaster. Organizations using managed hosting service providers retain control of data processing operations while the managed hosting service provides the resources. Customers can manage their data processing through a personalized Web management interface that allows them to initiate recovery from any location. Challenges for the future include:

- Finding ways to protect the growing amount of information, no matter where it is stored or used; and
- Finding ways to make sure people can stay connected to their data, no matter what the disruption.

Without addressing and linking these two elements, a plan may fall far short of its goals.

LEGAL AND ACCREDITATION REQUIREMENTS

A 2005 Gartner survey on business continuity and disaster recovery that spanned various types of industries including healthcare found that an increasing number of regulatory bodies require a documented methodology for conducting business continuity and disaster recovery activities (Witty 2006). The HIPAA security rule requires continuity planning and disaster recovery processes (Averell 2003; Bogen 2002; Miller & Lehman 2002; Zawada 2003). All healthcare organizations must have a data backup plan, a recovery plan, an emergency mode of operation plan, and testing and evaluation procedures. Although HIPAA does not specify the exact processes or procedures for compliance, it does demand safeguards for the security of protected healthcare information while operating in both normal and emergency modes. These safeguards encompass the creation, access, storage, and destruction of manual records. The final continuity planning component of the HIPAA regulations required compliance by April 2006. The Federal Information Privacy and Security Act of 2002 established a minimum standard of performance for the protection of information and information systems managed by federal agencies, their contractors, and other agencies acting on their behalf, and required the institution of continuity plans for information systems supporting the operations of the agency (Collmann 2007). Other federal legislation also exists that requires current access to information for organizations (Lindeman 2007). The Pandemic and All-Hazards Preparedness Act (PAHPA) was enacted in 2006 at the end of the 109th Congressional session (Goedert 2007). The purpose of this law was to improve the nation's public health and medical preparedness and response capabilities for emergencies, whether deliberate, accidental, or natural. This law authorized development of a national, near-real-time information network to coordinate federal and state response to public health emergencies within 2 years of enactment. The Secretary of Health and Human Services was charged with leading the federal response to these types of emergencies, usurping the role previously accorded to the Department of Homeland Security. Similar legislation focused upon hospital readiness to deal with disasters.

The Joint Commission set disaster preparedness standards as a requirement for hospital accreditation more than 30 years ago (Cutlip 2002). Until 2000, standards focused on disasters and accidents such as power plant failures and chemical spills. In 2001, the Joint Commission introduced new emergency management standards for hospitals, long-term care facilities, and behavioral health and ambulatory care that focus on the concept of community involvement in the management process. These guidelines address information security, disaster preparedness, and recovery planning. The Joint Commission has since added bioterrorism to the list of events that organizations must consider in their plans (McGowan 2002).

The Joint Commission suggests that organizations conduct at least two emergency drills per year with one community-wide drill. Accreditation standards mandate that healthcare organizations have an emergency plan that identifies potential hazards, their impact on services, and measures to handle and recover from emergencies. Accredited organizations must demonstrate a command structure, emergency preparedness training for staff, and a mechanism to enact an emergency plan, and they must identify their role in community-wide emergencies. The 2008 emergency management standards for hospitals, critical access hospitals, and long-term care facilities call for planning and testing plans during conditions when the local community cannot support the healthcare organization. It is no longer sufficient to plan for a single, simple event (The Joint Commission 2007).

Together, the Joint Commission and HIPAA require that healthcare providers perform a BIA and crisis management analysis; conduct employee training; implement ongoing continuity plan reviews; plan for information technology disasters and recovery; and audit their continuity plan processes (Zawada 2003). Several other accrediting bodies require disaster plans, though their focus is personnel safety rather than information safety. There are other groups that demonstrate varying levels of interest in BCM; these include the Food and Drug Administration, the Federal Emergency Management Agency (FEMA), the National Institute of Standards and Technology, the Disaster Recovery Institute International, the Bioterrorism Task Force of the Association for Professionals in Infection Control and Epidemiology, and the Bioterrorism Working Group of the Centers for Disease Control and Prevention. Recommendations from these other groups provide voluntary guidelines for better BCM that help continuity planners to achieve HIPAA and compliance with the Joint Commission.

There has been a move toward voluntary compliance with the Sarbanes-Oxley Act by not-for-profit healthcare organizations in recent years (Giniat & Saporito 2007; Greene 2005; Peregrine & Schwartz 2002). The Sarbanes-Oxley Act of 2002 was enacted by the federal government as a means to legislate corporate accountability and responsibility. While it applied only to publicly traded corporations, Sarbanes-Oxley impacts the healthcare industry by increasing the demand for fiscal responsibility, accountability, and accurate financial reporting and disclosure. Voluntary compliance with Sarbanes-Oxley is widely seen as a part of enterprise risk management and an opportunity to demonstrate good governance to the community. It requires the creation of audit functions and the presence of an expert in accounting on a corporate audit committee. Auditors must clearly see that a plan exists to protect and recover financial data. Voluntary compliance with Sarbanes-Oxley helps not-for-profit entities justify their not-for-profit status and maintain their reputation in the community. Compliance with Sarbanes-Oxley requires continuity of records.

FUTURE DIRECTIONS

Continuity planning in healthcare organizations will continue to receive greater attention for a variety of reasons as listed below:

- Consumers have come to expect a level of service that requires immediate access to data.
- Wait time decreases satisfaction and can diminish quality of care.
- Healthcare organizations are catching up with other industries in understanding the business case for continuity of operations.
- Compliance will become a larger issue, particularly as more legislation and regulatory bodies require the presence of a workable continuity plan.
- More professional organizations are now focused upon various aspects of continuity planning and response to disasters.
- The creation of a national network that will allow improved monitoring of the population's health for suspicious symptoms or early onset of epidemics will make it more imperative to maintain all links in the process.
- As the national monitoring of disease outbreak and bioterrorism activities improves, healthcare organizations can stockpile supplies, bring in additional staff, delay vacations, make bed space available, and put into place plans for remote and backup options to ensure continuity of overall operations (Goedert 2007).

Visit nursing.pearsonhighered.com for additional cases, information, and weblinks.

It is only a matter of time before another disaster occurs. The preparation provided by an effective business and continuity plan can minimize loss of life and data and can support ongoing operations. Healthcare organizations must be able to effectively deal with crises. The availability of disaster preparedness programs at schools of higher education such as those at Penn State University and the University of North Carolina along with certification programs by private and public organizations such as the Association of Public Treasures of the United States and Canada indicate the growing importance as well as the rigors of disaster preparedness and recovery and business continuity.

CASE STUDY EXERCISE

As the clinical representative for your unit on the Disaster Planning Committee, you are charged with identifying all forms in your area that require completion of a physical vital records inventory sheet. What forms would you list and why?

SUMMARY

- Business continuity planning is the process of ensuring the continuation of critical business services regardless of any event that may occur. It includes IT disaster planning. Continuity planning consists of several steps that are best defined as life cycle stages.
- The first stage of the life cycle requires that the organization develop a business Continuity workgroup, select members for the workgroup; define roles and responsibilities, develop a disaster recovery infrastructure, and develop priorities and a plan of action.
- The second stage of the life cycle is to gather data by conducting a BIA and a determination of vital organization functions and information. The BIA should be done as soon as possible. This stage determines the probabilities of all types of disasters, their impact on critical functions, and factors necessary for restoration of services. This second stage in continuity planning process is the development of the plan itself.
- The third stage of the continuity plan is to develop solutions based on the requirements developed in stage two. This includes procedures, processes, and policies that will minimize risks and be cost effective.
- The fourth stage in continuity planning is the implementation of the solutions and strategies identified in stages two and three to maintain business continuity, deliver patient services, and restore lost or damaged data. This includes policies and procedures and contracts with vendors and various service providers.
- The fifth stage of continuity planning is testing and evaluation of the plan and its policies, procedures, and processes.
- The sixth stage of the continuity life cycle is maintenance, which requires three periodic activities; namely:

  1. Confirmation and verification of information in the plan and the BCP manual and distributing it to all staff for awareness, and specific training for individuals whose roles are identified as critical in the response and recovery effort.
  2. Testing and verification of technical solutions established for recovery operations.
  3. Testing and verification of the documented organization's recovery procedures. A biannual or annual maintenance cycle is typical.

- Disasters that threaten IS operation may be natural or man-made. Continuity plans help to ensure uninterrupted operation or speedy resumption of services when a catastrophic event occurs. The identification of information vital to daily operation is best determined through interviewing system users. The purpose, flow, recipients, need for timeliness, and implications of information unavailability must be considered in this process. Not all information used in daily operations is automated. A vital records inventory should be conducted to identify additional information that requires protection.

- Documentation is essential to the development and successful implementation of a disaster plan. Plans must be detailed, current, and readily available to be useful.
- Careful attention to backup and storage helps ensure that information may be retrieved, or restored, later. Backup may be handled internally or outsourced. Commercial backup services provide transport or electronic transmission of backup media and special storage conditions until materials are needed.
- Manual alternatives to IS ensure ongoing delivery of services, although it is at a slower rate. Staff must receive instruction and support as they resort to manual methods.
- Restoration of information services post-disaster is not simple because backup media may be faulty and some information kept on other media is lost forever. System restoration may reload backup media stored at cold sites or resort to RBS or hot sites. Distributed processing and rapid replacement of equipment are other alternatives. Restoration is costly because it generally requires outside professional services, additional equipment, and extra hours from support staff. Expenses may be partially recouped through insurance coverage. Salvage of damaged records is an important aspect of recovery that is best handled by experts.
- System restarts require planning to avoid system overload as users try to catch up on work. Administrators must consider what functions should be restored first and how to integrate backup paper records with automated records. Post-disaster feedback is a major factor for the design and implementation of a better plan for future use.
- Continuity planning also needs to consider legal and regulatory requirements.

REFERENCES

Averell, H. (2003, June 1). Disaster recovery, HIPAA style. *ADVANCE for Health Information Executives*. Retrieved from http://www.advanceforhie.com/

Baldwin, W. (2007). After a disaster strikes. *Disaster Recovery Journal, 20*(1). Retrieved from http://www.drj.com/articlees/winter07/2001-10.pdf

Ballman, J. (2006). September 11—5 years later. *Disaster Recovery Journal, 19*(4). Retrieved from http://www.drj.com/articles/fall06/1904-01p.html

Bannan, K. J. (2002, January 29). Building your safety net—Every company needs a disaster recovery plan, but e-businesses have some special needs to guarantee they're running around-the-clock. *PC Magazine, 21*(1), 2.

Barry, S. (2007). Heat—The death knell for hard drives. *Disaster Recovery Journal, 20*(2). Retrieved from http://www.drj.com/articles/spr07/2002-11.pdf

Bermont, T. (2007). Ensuring your data center is in compliance. *Disaster Recovery Journal, 20*(2). Retrieved from http://www.drj.com/articles/spr07/2002-05.pdf

Bogen, J. (2002). Implications of HIPAA on business continuity and disaster recovery practices in healthcare organizations. *Healthcare Review, 15*(5), 14.

Chandler, R. C., Wallace, J. D., & Coombs, W. T. (2006). Current state of pandemic disaster preparedness. *Disaster Recovery Journal, 19*(4). Retrieved from http://www.drj.com/articles/fall06-1904-10.html

Collmann, J. (2007, January). The Federal Information Security Management Act of 2002 title III—Information security, electronic government act, public law (PL). pp. 107–347. *Health Information Management and Systems Society (HIMSS)*. Retrieved from http://www.himss.org/content/files/CPRIToolkit/version6/v6%20pdf/D68_FISMA.pdf

Croy, M. (2007). Enterprise, know thyself! *Disaster Recovery Journal, 20*(2). Retrieved from http://www.drj.com//articles/spr07/2002-02.pdf

Cutlip, K. (2002). Strengthening the system: Joint commission standards and building on what we know. *Hospital Topics, 80*(1), 24.

Elliott, D., & Swartz, E. (2002). *Business continuity management*. New York: Routledge/Taylor & Francis.

Epstein, K., & Nilakantan, C. (2007). Double jeopardy in a "slow" disaster. *Disaster Recovery Journal, 20*(2). Retrieved from http://www.drj.com/articles/spr07/2002-07.pdf

Giniat, E., & Saporito, J. (2007, August). Sarbanes-Oxley impetus for enterprise risk management. *Healthcare Financial Management, 61*(8), 64–70.

Glenn, J. (2006). Business continuity vs. protecting data. *Disaster Recovery Journal, 19*(4). Retrieved from http://www.drj.com/articles/fall06/1904-04p.html

Glenn, J. (2007). Planning for the pandemic. *Disaster Recovery Journal, 20*(3). Retrieved from http://www.drj.com/articles/sum07/2003-09.pdf

Goedert, J. (2007, February). The biosurveillance evolution. *Health Data Management.* Retrieved from http://www.healthdatamanagement.com/issues/20070201/14633-1.html

Greene, J. (2005). Looking harder: Not-for-profit hospitals use Sarbanes-Oxley to strengthen their boards' financial accountability. *Hospitals and Health Networks, 79*(6), 52–54, 56, 58.

G'Sell, D. M. (2007). From the beginning. *Disaster Recovery Journal, 20*(3). Retrieved from http://www.drj.com/articles/sum07/2003-04.pdf

Health Information Management Systems Society. (2007). *HIMSS leadership survey, CIO Results Questionnaire Index.* Retrieved from http://www.himss.org/2007Survey/DOCS/2007Healthcare_CIO_questionnaire_index.pdf

Johnston, E. (2006). Business owners are reminded of the perils of power loss. *Disaster Recovery Journal, 19*(4). Retrieved from http://www.drj.com/articles/fall06/1904-06p.html

Joint Commission. (2007, May). *Joint commission online.* Retrieved from http://www.jointcommission.org/Library/jconline/jo_05_07.htm

Kemp, R. L. (2007). Assessing the vulnerability of buildings. *Disaster Recovery Journal, 20*(2). Retrieved from http://www.drj.com/articles/spr07/2002-11.pdf

Kirchner, T. A., & Ziegenfuss, D. E. (2003). Audit's role in the business continuity process. *Disaster Recovery Journal, 16*(2). Retrieved from http://www.drj.com/articles/spr03/1602-11.html

Kirschenbaum, A. (2006). The missing link in business continuity. *Disaster Recovery Journal, 19*(4). Retrieved from http://www.drj.com/articles/fall06/1904-09p.html

Koch, R., & Marks, C. (2006). Prepare for the next wave of BC planning. *Disaster Recovery Journal, 19*(4). Retrieved from http://www.drj.com/articles/fall06/1904-12.html

Komoski, E. (2007). Is power your weakest link in data center flexibility? *Disaster Recovery Journal, 20*(3). Retrieved from http://www.drj.com/articles/sum07/2003-13.pdf

Lawrence, D. (2007). Hurricanes, floods and fires. *Healthcare Informatics, 24*(8), 37–39.

Lawton, S. (2007). When protecting an SMB image is everything. *Disaster Recovery Journal, 20*(3). Retrieved from http://www.drj.com/articles/sum07/2003-17.pdf

Lee, J. (2003). Effective strategy for meeting disaster recovery SLAs for mission-critical applications. *Disaster Recovery Journal, 16*(2). Retrieved from http://www.drj.com/articles/spr03/1602-15p.html

Lindeman, J. (2007). The next level of disaster recovery. *Disaster Recovery Journal, 20*(3). Retrieved from http://www.drj.com/articles/sum07/2003-01.pdf

Lindeman, J., & Grogan, J. (2007). Beyond disaster recovery. *Healthcare Informatics, 24*(8), 72, 74.

Maggio, E. J., & Coleman, K. G. (2007). A new face for an old threat. *Disaster Recovery Journal, 20*(3). Retrieved from http://www.drj.com/articles/sum07/2003-05.pdf

Marcella, A. J. (2004). CYBERcrime: Is your company a potential target? Are you prepared? *Disaster Recovery Journal, 17*(1). Retrieved from http://www.drj.com/articles/win04/1701-04p.html

Margeson, B. (2003). The human side of data loss. *Disaster Recovery Journal, 16*(2). Retrieved from http://www.drj.com/articles/spr03/1602-08p.html

Martin, Z. (2007). Disaster recovery. *Health Data Management, 15*(1), 30–32, 34, 36, 38, 40.

McCormick, J. (2003). Picking up the pieces: To prepare for a disaster, whether natural or man-made, you will need both backup and recovery applications—And a plan. *Government Computer News, 22*(5), 42.

McDonald, J. (2007). Successful backups are not enough for disaster preparedness. *Disaster Recovery Journal, 20*(3). Retrieved from http://www.drj.com/articles/sum07/2003-06.pdf

McGowan, B. (2002). The board's role related to disaster preparedness. *Healthcare Review, 15*(2), 15.

McKilroy, A. A. (2003). Connecting the islands: Disaster recovery planning for teleworking environments. *Disaster Recovery Journal, 16*(1). Retrieved from http://www.drj.com/articles/win03/1601-07p.html

Meyers, J. (2006). Preparing for the worst. *Healthcare Informatics, 23*(7), 44–45.

Miano, B. (2003, Fall). Key considerations for proactive planning. *Disaster Recovery Journal, 16*(4). Retrieved from http://www.drj.com/articles/fall03/1604-04p.html

Midgley, C. (2002). Protecting your data, protecting your business. *Disaster Recovery Journal, 15*(3). Retrieved from http://www.drj.com/articles/sum02/1503-09p.html

Miller, V., & Lehman, K. (2002). Assessment of HIPAA security requirements on disaster recovery planning. *Disaster Recovery Journal, 15*(1), 62–64.

Mitchell, V. J. H. (2007). Take your own pulse first. *Disaster Recovery Journal, 20*(3). Retrieved from http://www.drj.com/articles/sum07/2003-07.pdf

Moore, R. (2006). Living on the edge: Remote site back up. *Disaster Recovery Journal, 19*(4). Retrieved from http://www.drj.com/articles/fall06/1904-15p.html

Morgenthal, J. P., & Walmsley, P. (2000, February). Mining for metadata. *Software Magazine.* Retrieved from http://www.findarticles.com/cf_0/m0SMG/1_20/61298805/print.jhtml

Naef, W. (2003, October). Business continuity planning—A safety net for business. *Infocon Magazine* (Issue one). Retrieved from http://www.iwar.org.uk/infocon/business-continuity-planning.htm

Olson, G. (2002). Recovering data in a snap. *Disaster Recovery Journal, 15*(4). Retrieved from http://www.drj.com/articles/fall02/1504-12p.html

Pelant, B. F. (2003). Business impact analysis. *Disaster Recovery Journal, 16*(1). Retrieved from http://www.drj.com/articles/win03/1601-03p.html

Peregrine, M. W., & Schwartz, J. R. (2002, December). What CFOs should know—and do—about corporate responsibility. *Healthcare Financial Management, 56*(12), 59–63.

Peterka, A. (2007). Influenza pandemic presents unique challenges. *Disaster Recovery Journal, 20*(3). Retrieved from http://www.drj.com/articles/sum07/2003-08.pdf

Picking up the pieces. (2006). *American Journal of Nursing, 106*(9), 102.

Price, E. S. (2003, Summer). Application-aware solutions: The building blocks of business continuity. *Disaster Recovery Journal, 16*(3). Retrieved from http://www.drj.com/articles/sum03/1603-20p.html

Price, J. O., Jr. (2007). Planning to exercise or planning to recover. *Disaster Recovery Journal, 20*(3). Retrieved from http://www.drj.com/articles/sum07/2003-11.pdf

Rizzo, S. (2006). Aligning operational resilience to business requirements. *Disaster Recovery Journal, 19*(4). Retrieved from http://www.drj.com/articles/fall06/1904-08p.html

Sandhu, R. J. (2002). *Disaster recovery planning.* Cincinnati, OH: Premier Press.

Sheth, S., & McHugh, J. (2007). CIOs! How good is your disaster recovery plan? *Disaster Recovery Journal, 20*(2). Retrieved from http://www.drj.com/articles/spr07/2002-08.pdf

Stephens, D. O. (2003, January–February). Protecting records in the face of chaos, calamity, and cataclysm: Even organizations that do not think they are prime targets for terrorists do not have the luxury of considering themselves exempt from disaster planning. *Information Management Journal, 37*(1), 33.

Stohr, E., Rohmeyer, P., & Shaikh, M. (2004, August 16). *Business continuity in the pharmaceutical industry.* Report submitted to the AT&T Foundation. Retrieved from http://howe.stevens.edu/fileadmin/Files/research/ReportAllSep1004_v3.pdf

Sussman, S. (2002). Securing windows workstations in real time. *Disaster Recovery Journal, 15*(4). Retrieved from http://www.drj.com/articles/fall02/1504-15p.html

Taylor, C. (2007). Is tape dead? *Disaster Recovery Journal, 20*(3). Retrieved from http://www.drj.com/articles/sum07/2003-14.pdf

Veldboom, K. (2007). Emergency notification in a time of crisis. *Disaster Recovery Journal, 20*(2). Retrieved from http://www.drj.com/articles/spr07/2002-09.pdf

Wainwright, V. L. (2007). Business continuity by design. *Health Management Technology, 28*(3), 20–21.

Wiles, J. (2004). *Auditing your disaster recovery plan: A closer look at high tech crime. Will this be your most likely disaster in the 21st century?* Retrieved from http://www.disaster-resource.com/cgi-bin/article_search.cgi?id='93'

Witty, R. J. (2006). 2005 BCM/DR survey results from Gartner, DRJ. *Disaster Recovery Journal, 19*(4). Retrieved from http://www.drj.com/articles/fall06/1904-03p.html

Wold, G. H., & Vick, T. L. (2003). Comparing & selecting recovery strategies. *Disaster Recovery Journal, 16*(2). Retrieved from http://www.drj.com/articles/spr03/1602-05p.html

Zawada, B. J. (2003). Regulatory pressure on technology for business continuity. *Risk Management, 50*(7), 20.

Zirkel, S. (2007). Ensuring workforce continuity during a pandemic. *Disaster Recovery Journal, 20*(3). Retrieved from http://www.drj.com/articles/sum07/2003-10.pdf

CHAPTER 23

Integrating Technology, Informatics, and the Internet Into Nursing Education

After completing this chapter, you will be able to:

1. List ways computer technology may be used to support and enhance nursing education in clinical and academic settings.

2. Identify career opportunities for nurse informaticans in education.

3. Define virtual learning environments, distance learning, and e-learning.

4. List advantages and disadvantages of Virtual Learning Environments (VLE).

5. List advantages and disadvantages of Web-based instruction.

6. Compare and contrast e-learning with other educational strategies.

7. Provide examples of how computer technology supports education in formal nursing programs and continuing education.

8. Compare and contrast Web 2.0 applications; describe their use in nursing education and professional collaborations.

9. Explain mobile learning technologies applicable to nursing education.

INTRODUCTION

Technology provides educational opportunities for nurses at the point of care as well as in the academic setting. In the academic setting, course or learning management systems (C/LMS) not only replace traditional classroom instruction in distance learning opportunities, they supplement both classroom and clinical education by providing online resources. Videos on how to perform a physical assessment are easily posted for students on a C/LMS "classroom" site and can be viewed 24/7. Approximately a decade ago, Bradley (2003) noted that educational applications of computer technology were revolutionizing nursing education in all settings due to their capability to:

- enhance presentation of course content;
- ease barriers associated with updating and customizing in-service training for diverse groups of nurses and ease challenges related to acquiring current and reliable information;
- erase geographic boundaries;
- make learning opportunities available anytime anywhere;
- tailor instruction to individual learning needs;
- improve learning outcomes and provide a safe learning environment;
- satisfy regulatory and accreditation requirements;
- ease disruption caused by changes in personnel;
- provide a cost-effective alternative.

Needs assessment, well-developed learning objectives, good planning and design, and wise use and evaluation by educators and administrators are still required to realize the potential benefits identified above. Technology is increasingly prevalent in today's mobile society and dynamic workplaces and can readily be integrated into the education process if there is a match with the objectives of the learning module or curriculum. Proper use of technology can facilitate the learning process. Educators must become adept in the evaluation and use of technology that they plan to use.

INSTRUCTIONAL APPLICATIONS OF COMPUTER TECHNOLOGY

Technology-Based Strategies to Support Education in Clinical Setting

Computer technology is being used to support nursing practice. Educational applications are being deployed for hospital in-service presentations, conferences, and skills-development workshops. There are limitless online opportunities to obtain continuing education units (CEUs). While mandatory nursing education requirements vary from state to state (Nurse.com 2010), obtaining CEUs and record keeping can be simplified using computer technology.

Hospital Information Systems

Information management systems are used by hospital nurses to organize patient information data, monitor laboratory and imaging test reports, and for clinical decision support, computerized order entry, and medication administration (Lapinsky, Holt, Hallett, Abdolell, & Adhikari 2008). Information management systems are used to track budgets and supplies and enhance compliance with standards for quality improvement, regulatory requirements, and best practice recommendations. Nurse managers use data from electronic health records and patient census records to efficiently organize patient care and monitor patient safety. Significant time and cost savings have been attributed to the deployment of information management systems (Gugerty et al. 2007). Nursing leaders must receive proper education in using these resources to extract data and maximize use of the available technology.

Nurses at the point of care are among the primary stakeholders using these systems and should be engaged early in development to provide input into design. One role of the nurse educator is to ensure this happens, and that nurses participating in architecture and design are knowledgeable about the potential of computer information systems. Nursing education regarding information management systems needs to incorporate content regarding data protection, data security, and patient confidentiality with both initial implementation and on-going educational updates.

Academic Applications Connectivity with real hospital information systems (HIS) is an important use of computers in nursing education in the academic clinical setting. According to Hansen (in Hebda & Czar 2009), who has published widely on informatics applications in nursing, the incorporation of hospital and nursing information systems into nursing school curricula promotes professional socialization, helps students see the effects of their decision-making, and decreases orientation time for new graduates. Computer-generated care plans, or maps, enable nursing students to devote time for analysis of data that was once spent writing care plans. Information system use during clinical experiences ensures that graduates have exposure to a variety of applications in healthcare settings.

By using the software that they will encounter at the workplace, the student acquires marketable job skills. Students may receive live training sessions in system use by faculty or by hospital-based trainers. Alternatively, students may use computer-based training. Training may occur at the university, college, or healthcare facility enabling students to retrieve information for use in preparing for assignments. Security and privacy issues would need to be addressed to prevent changes in information to actual client records.

Health information systems connectivity provided at schools of nursing requires negotiation with the vendor for permission. Alliances between vendors and schools of nursing have resulted in the creation of a training hospital with fictitious patients to not only expose students to how information systems work but also make simulations more realistic.

Other concerns from the perspective of the clinical agency include increased demands upon the information system and confidentiality of client information under HIPAA regulations (Price n.d.). Access to HIS as a learning tool in schools of nursing offers the many benefits listed here (Doorley, Renner, & Corron 1994; Hebda & Czar 2009; Kennedy 2003; Poirrier, Wills, Broussard, & Payne 1996):

- Time to analyze clinical information, especially adequate time to compose care plans or review critical pathways
- Enables review of plans of care with faculty or hospital nursing staff prior to entry into the system
- Increases knowledge and proficiency when students enter the actual clinical setting
- Enables greater familiarity with students' assigned clients
- Poses fewer interruptions for staff from students requesting information
- Opportunity to retrieve diagnostic results, vital signs, admission assessment data, and nursing documentation for review in real time

In summary, incorporation of hospital and nursing information systems at schools of nursing facilitate role transition from student to graduate nurse, makes graduates more attractive to prospective employers, and may enable hospitals to better utilize orientation time for graduates with prior HIS training.

Competency-Based Training

Competency-based training is becoming increasingly important in the clinical setting. Healthcare organizations need to demonstrate that staff can perform skills safely. Computer-based competency training and testing have the potential to free instructor time, streamline instruction and testing, and eliminate costs associated with employee travel.

In a well-constructed, systematic review to identify whether working registered nurses (RNs) in the United States had sufficient informatics knowledge and computer competencies, Hart (2008) concluded that the evidence demonstrated that the need still exists for job-specific nursing competency development. Three areas of competencies were identified, which included nursing science, computer science, and information science. While the focus was on working RNs and bringing this population up to a competent level for evidence-based practice and overall informatics skills, the implications for nursing educators was evident.

In subsequent research on graduate baccalaureate nurses, Fetter (2009) found students reported more confidence in word processing skills and system operations skills than in care documentation and informatics knowledge. While newer graduates may not need as much emphasis in competency-based training as nurses in the current workforce for keyboarding and basic computer competency, they still require intensive nursing informatics education to keep pace. A good example of use of computer-assisted instructional technology to develop competency is provided by Telles Filho and Cassiani (2008), who described the development of a computer module to teach and learn about medication administration.

Computer-assisted instruction that is designed to enhance competency can be offered as anywhere, anytime learning. It is as appropriate for the current nursing workforce and will no doubt become increasingly useful for a new generation of nursing graduates who are citizens of the twenty-first century. The International Society for Technology in Education (http://www.iste.org) identifies the following competencies for students in an "ever-increasing" technological world (NETS for students 2007):

- Creative thinking and knowledge construction
- Communication and collaboration
- Application of digital tools
- Gather, evaluate, and use information
- Conduct research
- Understand legal and ethical behavior as it relates to technology and good "digital citizenship"

Simulation

Simulation technology is being incorporated across the curriculum in nursing education and in hospitals. Simulation technology enables users to learn and then demonstrate skills. There is a rich history of the use of simulation in nursing education for task training. The Chase Hospital Doll, first manufactured in 1911, is an example of low-tech simulation (Rogers 2007). By the 1960s, life-size mannequins had developed and progressed from "Mrs. Chase" to Resusci Anne, a simulator created by Laerdal to teach resuscitation skills. Laerdal also created Sim-Man, a portable and advanced patient simulator, for team training (http://www.laerdal.com). Sim-Man has been employed in both nursing clinical and academic sites internationally. Educational innovations using more sophisticated technology are seen with hi-fidelity simulators. These simulators are realistic, precise representations (Tuoriniemi & Schott-Baer 2008). These simulators are designed to:

- standardize student learning opportunities;
- develop collaboration, communication, and co-operation;
- provide a safe learning environment;
- augment clinical scenarios and faculty resources;
- present unusual or high-risk clinical situations;
- validate mastery of skills.

Patient physiologic responses can be re-created by the hi-fidelity simulator in the nursing skills lab to reinforce lecture and help develop clinical judgment. Strengths and weaknesses of simulation use were identified by Lasater (2007). These ranged from ethical considerations to the importance of crafting well-defined scenarios, and providing comprehensive de-briefing. Simulation technology is being used beyond the skills lab. For example, multimodal simulation is being used to enhance skills in mental health nursing (Edward, Hercelinskyj, Warelow, & Munro 2007). Another creative application of simulation is a simulated home visit described by Yeager and Gotwals (2009) in a community health-nursing course.

An international example of hi-fidelity simulation and case-based learning lab in nursing comes from the University of Tasmania School of Nursing and Midwifery (2007). Different scenarios can be tested without negative consequences. Research indicates highly positive effects of simulation on skill and knowledge acquisition (Ravert 2002, 2008; Rhodes & Curran 2005; Schlairet & Pollock 2010).

Simulation labs are popular in all disciplines of healthcare education. It has been demonstrated to be useful in promoting interdisciplinary learning. Florida International University's simulation lab is utilized across all departments of the school of nursing and health sciences, including the schools of nursing, physical therapy, occupational therapy, communication sciences and disorders, athletic training, health sciences, and health information management (Sudasassi 2010). Despite the increased investment in and use of simulation labs, caution must be exercised so that they do not totally replace clinical education (Hansen 2009).

INTEGRATION OF TECHNOLOGY THROUGHOUT THE EDUCATIONAL EXPERIENCE

Didactic Tools

In nursing education a variety of resources integrate technology into the curriculum. Didactic tools are available and delivered via the C/LMS and include Web resources (Weblinks, Weblogs, wikis, etc.). Learning materials may be prepared by either university professors or other experts in the educational area. Resources may also be developed from a traditional school context (articles, case studies, presentations). Participant-created materials (PowerPoints, videos, e-mails, social networking, blogs) are additional resources which can be accessed and even digitally archived.

Using Computer Technology to Support Education in the Academic Setting: Course/Learning Management Systems

Universities, colleges, and other educational institutions are accelerating their utilization of a variety of C/LMS. Products include open-source materials, commercial products, community source products, and specific locally developed product models. Examples of C/LMS systems include Stellar, an MIT developed product; Sakai, a subscription-based community source; Segue, an open-source system; and Blackboard, a commercial product (Massachusetts Institute of Technology 2006).

The platform for an online learning environment is defined in a Massachusetts Institute of Technology (MIT) Peer Comparison as being a platform "enabling the management, delivery and tracking of online and blended learning" (Massachusetts Institute of Technology 2006, p. 3).

Effective integration of C/LMS can be for legal, organizational, and administrative purposes such as posting a course syllabus, organizing course registration lists, mailing lists, maintaining grade books, or posting grades. Meaningful instructional use of C/LMS includes distributing course content, readings, and learning modules, providing a discussion forum, and providing a location for synchronous learning events including Webinars, surveys, and chat room spaces.

Clinical Tools

Technology is being integrated into clinical nursing education. Clinical and administrative systems are in use by nurses at the point of care in acute care settings, ambulatory, academic, and community-based settings. Birz (2009) reported that the majority of all clinical information system users of electronic documentation, Electronic Health records (EHRs), and picture archiving and communication systems are nurses. This technology is integral to patient care activities, and is taught to nursing students and seasoned nurses alike as described earlier.

Korte, Bopp, Kendall, Carlson, Saxton, Bopp, and Smith (2006) reported on an award-winning clinical performance assessment tool developed by faculty at Monroe Community College in Rochester, NY. By using a series of Excel spreadsheets, faculty were able to make use of a scoring rubric that allowed for standardized comments regarding clinical outcomes, and provided a space for personalized comments.

A notable innovation gaining considerable interest is the use of technology for clinical nursing education offered via online course offerings. These Web modules provide practicing nurses a convenient way to obtain CEUs. For example, the U.S. Department of Health and Human Services Centers for Disease Control and Prevention (CDC) (2011) education and training resource page for immunization lists courses, descriptions, and format for educational materials, some of which may be completed for CEU credit. Neonatal nurses can take advantage of free educational and informational resources offered by NIC University, a Web-based, multi-disciplinary education center (http://www.nicuniversity.org/lectures.asp). Many other CEU offerings may be found by visiting organizational Web sites or through Web searchers.

INSTRUCTIONAL SUPPORT APPLICATIONS

Multimedia

Education has always employed multimedia strategies, whether that included chalkboard diagrams, overhead transparencies, slide presentations, video, or skill demonstrations. The advent of computer-based instruction, interactive video disks, compact discs (CDs), digital video discs (DVDs), and streaming video have enriched educational media, and nursing education has benefited from these changes (Batscha 2002; Billings 1995; Calderone 1994; Gleydura, Michelman, & Wilson 1995; Simpson 2002; Smith-Stoner & Willer 2003; Sternberger & Meyer 2001). Formerly associated with "entertainment," virtual reality is emerging as a new educational strategy that will be discussed later in this text.

The term *multimedia* today refers to presentations that combine at least two of the following: text, voice or sound, images, and video, or hardware and software. Different technological strategies are used to deliver a message. NASA has a site devoted to multimedia presentations, many with interactive features (NASA 2010). The *New York Times*, leading provider of "information," also maintains a multimedia site (*New York Times* n.d.) that is updated frequently.

Regardless of the "media" used to deliver educational content, specific learning objectives need to be in place to guide both the content and selection of media. Interactive multimedia may be an excellent approach for nurses required to learn and communicate complex issues to clients; however, it is the responsibility of the twenty-first century teacher to become competent in both the use of and selection of the media that will serve best. Hansen (2009) noted that research on learning retention can be facilitated with an approach that incorporates seeing, hearing, doing, interactivity, and repetition, citing studies by Mayer (2001); Barrett, Lacey, Sekara, Linden, and Gracely (2004). Multimedia has been found to be at least as effective as traditional instruction. It has the additional advantage of providing greater satisfaction and added value as an adjunct to a more traditional learning strategy and an additional learning resource (Maag 2004; Palmer & Devitt 2007). Group-paced instruction with multimedia has the potential to decrease costs ordinarily incurred with both individual instruction and traditional classroom teaching.

Quality multimedia potentially reduces labor costs and participant time if self-paced. Recorded classes can be shown multiple times, without the actual educator being present. Additionally when groups work together, comfort with computers is increased and learning enhanced, however, both the environment and the content must be conducive to group use (Hansen 2009). Hansen also suggested that multimedia and use of technology has the potential to improve overall instructional effectiveness and foster productivity through user satisfaction and enjoyment. Cuellar (2002) and Ross and Tuovinen (2001) advised that nurse educators need to select and use multimedia well and creatively to realize its benefits. Multimedia can be incorporated into formative and summative evaluation as well (Hansen 2007b; Rossignol & Scollin 2001).

Hansen (2009) noted the value of changing technology that can now tailor multimedia presentations via the use of compact discs, digital video discs, and video clips on the Web (Calderone 1994; Gleydura et al. 1995; Goodman & Blake 1996; Smith-Stoner & Willer 2003). The tools to produce streaming video are increasingly available. Streaming video can be uploaded to Web pages or Course Management Systems. Streaming video may also be reproduced and distributed on CDs. Video is converted to a digital format for use on the Web or CD. DVD drives are standard equipment on PCs that support CDs as well as DVDs. Multimedia enhances VLE by using the interactivity, information management, and decision-making capabilities of computers (Billings 1995; Cambre & Castner 1993; Goodman & Blake 1996). Skiba (2007a) reported that students entering higher education are "digital natives" as opposed to their older colleagues who are "digital immigrants" (Prensky 2001; 2004). Digital natives are characterized by their understanding of multimedia and sophisticated skill with computer technologies. They prefer multimedia and the "multi-tasking" it requires and are quite comfortable using technology. In light of the needs and preferences of this twenty-first century student, engaging these students and new employees requires the nurse educator to begin exploring the use of strategies like YouTube and Second Life. YouTube "is a place for people to engage in new ways with video by sharing, commenting on, and viewing videos" (Web 2.0 Innovations 2008). Second Life will be discussed later in this section.

Authoring tools are software applications that enable those with little or no programming expertise to create instructional programs. For an example, see the Alice Web site (http://www .alice.org/). These tools require time for mastery: From 50 to 200 hours may be needed to prepare 1 hour of instruction. Hansen (2009) noted that authoring tools can enable program design to match learning objectives and foster higher cognitive development. Educators can exercise creativity in the design of multimedia. Older technology, like slide presentation software, for example, can be used to house streaming video presentations or narrate audio (Batscha 2002; Smith-Stoner & Willer 2003). Faculty comfortable with the various forms of multimedia are better prepared to integrate these strategies into their instruction. Figure 23–1 depicts an online tutorial on arterial blood gases, developed by a faculty member.

Video Teleconferencing   A videoconference, also known as a video teleconference, is "a set of interactive telecommunication technologies that allow two or more locations to interact via two-way video and audio transmissions simultaneously" (http://en.wikipedia .org/wiki/Videoconference). Another, more descriptive term for videoconference is visual collaboration. This technology was first deployed commercially by AT&T during the early 1970s. Videoconferencing uses both audio and video to bring people at different sites together for a meeting. This can be as simple as a conversation between two people at different sites as in a chat room, or it may involve many sites, which is the more traditional application of videoconferencing. Besides the audio and visual transmission of meeting activities, videoconferencing can be used to share documents, computer-displayed information, and whiteboards. Wolfe (2007) found that communication and informal interaction dynamics found in broadband videoconferencing supported knowledge creation and transfer.

The Centers for Disease Control and Prevention (CDC) training site (n.d.) defines a videoconference as "a meeting, instructional session, or conversation between people at different

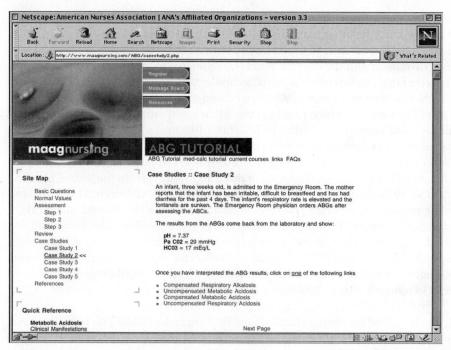

FIGURE 23–1 • An example online educational offering (Reproduced by permission of the author Dr. Margaret Maag)

locations relying on video technology as the primary communication link. Communication is two-way audio with either one-way or two-way video." The term *videoconference* is sometimes used to refer to conferences via compressed video, conferences via land lines, and broadcasts via satellite. To avoid confusion, using the term or phrase that uniquely describes the communication technology is recommended. In simple teleconferencing, learners at one site view and interact with an instructor and other learners at separate locations. Participants can be at multiple sites; hence, resources are pooled to establish collaborative programs. Resources are maximized through shared classes, instructors, and instructional materials.

Hansen (2009) advised that since video teleconferencing is now possible from desktop computers graduate and doctoral students, as well as staff nurses, can make use of this technology to bring educational opportunities to any number of areas. Content may be clinically oriented or focus on nursing informatics. On a larger, more polished scale video teleconferencing requires start-up funds and an investment in equipment, transmission media, and adaptation in communication methods, particularly when used in conjunction with traditional on-site classes. Classes, assignments, and feedback may be offered entirely online, "anytime, anywhere," extending the reach of educational programs and continuing education courses, accommodating students who would otherwise be unable to attend programs because of distance, family obligations, or work commitments. Drawbacks associated with video teleconferencing include sacrificing eye contact; appearance self-consciousness arises as well. Advanced technology is capable of addressing the problem of eye contact as clearer pictures and more real presentation enable more authentic interaction. Feelings of self-consciousness before a video camera will begin to subside as people become more adapt with the technology.

Free to the public is Skype, a peer-to-peer Internet telephony network that enables the callers to see one another as they speak. This computer-based technology requires a microphone and video camera, which are becoming standard on newer computers. Its popularity is rising around the globe. According to Wikipedia (2011a) there were 663 million users as of September 2011. The program offers instant messaging, file transfer, short messaging, video phone, as well as video teleconferencing. Nurse educators may benefit from using Skype as an educational and collaborative tool.

Educators may wish to consider guidelines before embarking on videoconferencing. Broadband is requisite as well as equipment that is easy-to-use with cross-platform capability. Videos produced for educational purposes may need editing for unique situations. Some may prefer still photos as the video portion of the production. Hansen (2009) advised that participants should be made aware of any other information technology (IT) or software that is needed during the videoconferencing or presentation.

Clickers

Classroom response systems (CRS) are increasingly being deployed to facilitate learning via the use of handheld transmitters. This hardware and software makes use of a "clicker" that beams information showing the response to specific, real-time questions projected overhead to a group of students to a receiver on the instructor's computer which transforms the data into a chart detailing the responses. Some CRS work via other mobile devices such as student cell phones, PDAs, or laptops (Turning Technologies 2010). Poll Everywhere is an example of an alternative audience polling site which offers free services for responses of 30 people or fewer per poll (http://www.polleverywhere.com). Classroom polling typically might consist of a brief two-to-three-question quiz on the homework at the beginning of a class session. The polling closes shortly after class begins. The quiz session has the twofold benefit of encouraging students to arrive on time and prepare for the lecture.

Clicker technology has long been used in the entertainment industry to ascertain audience responses. Bruff (2011) points out many useful applications of clicker technology in the classroom:

- Quiz delivery: Questions to ascertain recall of facts or conceptual understanding
- Questions which relate to knowledge application and critical thinking
- Gauge learner confidence level and metacognition
- Data collection for classroom experiments
- Multiple choice questions
- Classroom tasks such as taking attendance and homework collection
- Formative and summative assessment tasks
- Discussion promotion

As with any technology teachers should be prepared for obstacles relating to CRS use. Common challenges include technical difficulties, learning curves, adaptation of established lesson plans to include multiple choice answers/discussions, and the logistics associated with change. Well-designed content delivery, combined with carefully constructed questions, is key to proper clicker use.

Virtual Reality and Second Life Virtual reality is a form of multimedia that fully envelops learners in an environment. It has been used with medical students and surgeons to develop skills in a variety of areas including procedures such as the insertion of urinary catheters and surgical procedures (Ford 2010; Go Virtual Medical 2007; St. Jude 2011). Virtual reality applications are finding their way into nursing education. As an example Schmidt and Stewart (2010) report its incorporation into their baccalaureate-level community health courses. Use of this technology is now being explored within nursing education (Billings & Kowalski 2009a; Kilmon, Brown, Ghosh, & Mikitiuk 2010). Virtual reality offers the next best option to performing the skill on a real person but without risk to the learner or the patient. Doherty, Hansen, McCann, Oosthuizen, Hardy, Greig, Pasley, and Windsor (2007) reported at an EdMedia conference on an in-progress research to determine if a carefully engineered integrated simulator and an iPod video for male and female urinary catheter insertion would increase student confidence levels and enhance skill acquisition and retention.

Interactive technological tools that facilitate different forms of online communication, learning, and collaboration among educators, students, and colleagues are contained in a media known as Web 2.0 technologies which are discussed in chapters 4 and 5. Second Health: The Future of Healthcare Communication (n.d) reported on an online interactive learning tool that employed virtual reality. This three-dimensional virtual world of Second Life is an exciting online tool that allows healthcare students and professionals to interact with other visitors in a virtual hospital and help shape future healthcare.

Second Life is an innovative, Internet-based strategy that has been implemented into an accelerated online nursing program (Schmidt & Stewart 2010). It has demonstrated usefulness in engaging students in active learning and provides an opportunity to use simulation in a safe environment (Skiba 2007b). With Second Life, experiential learning is enhanced, allowing students to practice skills, try new ideas, and learn from mistakes. Anywhere, anytime education is enabled by Second Life, as students and educators work together from anywhere, facilitating a global network in the virtual classroom environment. This is but one example of how Second Life is being integrated into healthcare education. Beard, Wilson, Morra, and Keelan (2009) surveyed health-related activities on Second Life. Great examples of the use of Second Life in education can be found on the Internet. Some of these examples may be found via a simple search on YouTube for "Second Life nursing education."

EDUCATIONAL OPPORTUNITIES IN NURSING INFORMATICS

Opportunities for technology use in nursing education range from hospital in-service presentations, to conferences and workshops, to individual noncredit classes. College courses integrate technology at every level of nursing education from associate degree programs through advanced degrees. Educators must become adept in the evaluation and use of technology that they plan to use. There are a growing number of programs that prepare advanced practice nurses at the graduate level with degrees in informatics.

Basic Competencies

Nursing curriculum reform has placed an emphasis on computer proficiency along with patient care technology knowledge (Forbes & Hickey 2009). Technology-driven information management, communication tools, clinical equipment knowledge, and information literacy have been recognized by the Quality and Safety Education for Nurses Project (2010). Basic competencies for nurses incorporate attitudes, knowledge, and skills (Ainsley & Brown 2009) that include:

- habit of lifetime learning of information and technology;
- word processing skills, spreadsheet application;
- capability to use electronic documentation;
- ability to retrieve electronic data, including bibliographic information;
- capacity to protect patient privacy and confidentiality when using EHRs;
- aptitude to interpret and respond to technical equipment used at the point of care;
- data mining skills;
- ability to evaluate Internet resources and critically appraise Web sites.

Career Opportunities

Becoming a specialist in nursing informatics has two avenues. Increasingly, masters level nursing informatics programs are being developed. Working in the field of informatics in a clinical agency can also qualify an RN for status as a nurse informatician. The American Nurses Credentialing Center offers certification in nursing informatics (http://www.nursecredentialing.org/NurseSpecialties/Informatics.aspx).

The Healthcare Information and Management Systems Society (HIMSS) (2011) reported that the 2011 average salary of an informatics nurse was $98,702, with higher salaries for individuals holding certification in nursing informatics ($119,644). As EHR adaptation is accelerated by hospitals, clinics, and private practices, the demand for nurses with IT skills grows. Opportunities exist in a wide-range of workplaces from large hospitals and clinics, to vendors and systems development. Informatics nurses also find employment opportunities as consultants because of relevant work experiences. Relevant work experiences and competencies often include:

- Collaboration and communication skills
- Organizational and interpersonal skills
- Ability to review, critique, and evaluate evidence available through clinical practice guidelines and research
- Capacity to synthesize evidence as the basis for best practice
- Aptitude for translating clinical practice recommendations into algorithms
- Proficiency to disseminate research findings
- Clinical experience in the venue of current project need (e.g., for acute care phenomena, experience in a medical-surgical, or critical care area working with adult patients in an acute care hospital is required)
- Experience within a fully digital EMR system
- Strong nursing leadership and management skills
- Ability to articulate the vision for clinical workflow through technology that benefits patient care

VIRTUAL LEARNING ENVIRONMENTS, DISTANCE LEARNING, AND E-LEARNING

Evolution of the Concept of Virtual Learning Environments

A virtual learning environment exists whenever a learner and a teacher do not meet face to face, but rather communicate "at a distance" to enable learning. A good example of a popular virtual learning environment that is growing in acceptance for academics is the "wiki." Wikipedia (http://en.wikipedia.org/wiki/History_of_virtual_learning_environments) provides an extensive listing of events that led to the development of the phenomenon of virtual learning environments and has verifiable and credible references. Virtual learning environments began with "distance learning."

Distance Education

The term *distance education* dates back to 1892 (http://www.uwex.edu/ics/design/disedu2.htm). In the guise of correspondence courses, distance education preceded the virtual learning environment. Print media, both inexpensive and low tech, was the distance learning medium of choice prior to the development of the World Wide Web (WWW). Television took its place in 1953, when the University of Houston offered the first televised college credit classes via the first public television station in the United States. (http://www.houstonpbs.org/site/PageServer?pagename=abt_history). This mechanism of delivering education at a distance set the precedent for what has become known today as the virtual learning environment. While distance education encompasses more than computer-generated courses, it is discussed here in the context of its connection to technology.

Distance education in this context is the use of audio, video, computer, television, teleconferencing, or the WWW to connect educator and students who are located at a minimum of two different locations. Increasingly, the learners are spread out throughout different geographic locations, and, in some cases, in different time zones. Course or learning management systems compose a large portion of the distance learning movement.

Print media was less likely to engage a learner than are newer strategies that employ the use of the Internet, such as hyperlinks, interactive software, and online discussions. Both the Internet and the C/LMS, such as Blackboard and Lotus, have replaced the old paper-pencil correspondence school formats and TV for providing instructional material in distance education programs. Distance education broadens opportunities, eliminates long commutes and conventional "9 to 5" time frames. Many institutions of higher learning see this as a recruitment and retention strategy for nursing and other healthcare workers. It can provide access to experts and cut costs by paying faculty to teach at one site rather than multiple sites, or even from their homes. Killam and Carter (2010) discussed distance education as a means to support student clinical placement in rural settings with the end result of potentially increasing recruitment to these classically underserved areas. Mancuso (2009) noted that distance education is an important strategy to prepare future nurse educators and the nursing shortage.

Videoconferencing, as described earlier, plays a major role in distance learning and creating the virtual learning environment. Audio conferences may take place over the telephone or via Skype, which is a computer-mediated service that provides voice as well as video feed over the Internet as described earlier in this chapter. Video and teleconferencing have been popular in recent years and improved Internet capabilities, telephone use, and teleconferencing have eliminated the barriers faced by nurses in remote locations who wish to further their education via formal study or through continuing education programs, or who require additional job training (Corwin 2000; Kozlowski 2002; Southernwood 2008).

Synchronicity influences instructional design, delivery, and interaction. Distance education may occur in real, or synchronous, time or via a delay. In real time, all parties participate in the activity at the same time; this may include a classroom session or chat. With the delayed, or asynchronous, approach, the learner reviews material at a convenient time, which is generally not at the same time as other participants. This is particularly useful in nursing education, where shift work is common. Prior to the development of television, asynchronous strategies were the only possibility for distance learning. Today, asynchronous learning can be enhanced with the incorporation of ongoing electronic discussion to aid the clarification of ideas, promote retention, and aid critical thinking (Cartwright 2000; Harden 2003; Plack, Dunfee, Rindflesch, & Driscoll 2008).

Since the beginning of the twenty-first century, institutions of higher learning have increasingly offered some form of distance education as a means to improve student access, meet student demands, extend geographic boundaries, remain viable, and keep students on the cutting edge of technology (Bentley, Cook, Davis, Murphy, & Berding 2003; Charp 2003; Cuellar 2002). Careful consideration must be given to the marketplace, course objectives, choice of software platform, staff training, design of active learning, quality, technical and administrative issues, finances, and the fit with the overall institution (Hansen 2009). Distance education has rapidly become an acceptable mode of both nursing and medical education. Hansen (2009) documented the surveys by the American Association of Colleges of Nursing that demonstrated some involvement in distance or online education (Faison 2003; Sapnas et al. 2002). In a statement endorsed by the American Association of Colleges of Nursing Board of Directors and the Association of American Medical Colleges Council of Deans Advisory Board, a "Vision for Continuing Education and Lifelong Learning" was identified (see the report *Lifelong Learning in Medicine and Nursing* of the American Association of Medical Colleges and the American association of Colleges of Nursing 2010). The panel defined lifelong learning by identifying key competencies, one of which is "familiarity with informatics and literature search and retrieval strategies" (p. 6). The Institute for Higher Education Policy prepared a report sponsored by the National Education Association and Blackboard Inc. that identified 24 benchmarks deemed essential to ensure excellence in Internet-based distance education (IHEP 2000). These benchmarks included:

- Institutional support
- Guidelines for course development, review, and evaluation

- Teaching/learning guidelines for faculty-student interaction, feedback, and instruction on methods of effective research and evaluation of resources
- Course structure guidelines inclusive of student orientation, supplemental materials, and expectations
- Structured student support measures
- Extensive faculty support structures and guidelines
- Evaluation and assessment strategies inclusive of faculty development programs to promote new skills and teaching methods suitable for distance education

The growth of distance education programs also has implications for specialized nursing-related library services. Academic libraries must demonstrate the ability to provide equivalent resources and services electronically or through some other means to both on-campus and distance learners to meet customer demand and accreditation requirements. Some institutions have distance education librarians who work closely with faculty teaching distance education courses to meet student needs. This may be done through digitizing reserve materials and placing them on electronic reserves accessible only to students enrolled in the course. Restricted access, along with a prominent display of copyright notices on all readings, help to ensure compliance with copyright and fair use laws.

Distance education requires additional course preparation and organization by faculty and a concerted effort on the part of students to remain active participants. Learners in educational programs offered at a distance must assume responsibility for their learning needs. Box 23–1 lists key points for distance education students. Faculty must acquire new skills and teaching methods for distance education (Fetter 2009; Geibert 2000; Im & Lee 2003; Kozlowski 2002, 2004; McKenna & Samarawickrema 2003; Southernwood 2008). Today, online learning has virtually replaced the older methods of distance learning that were dependent on mail and telephone communication.

Another difference with distance education is that Internet-savvy students request automatic "push technology" instead of "pull technology." This entails a change in how course materials are provided. Traditionally faculty expect students to obtain data from the course management system via downloads "pulling" the information. Students now request that educators set up tools that will automatically disseminate (or "push") the information out to them. An example of this "push" technology is iTunes University. Podcasting lectures have become a mainstay over the past few years (Kaplan-Leiserson 2005; Lane 2006; Maag 2006; Malan 2007; Murray & Maag

---

BOX 23–1   Key Points for Students Involved in Distance Learning

- Reception sites may be in students' homes, workplaces, or recreational areas.
- Increases educational opportunities by eliminating long commutes.
- Class rosters with phone numbers and addresses may be distributed to all class members (pending individual approval) as a means to encourage interaction among students.
- Faculty may hold office hours online and provide feedback by telephone, electronic posting, instant messaging, e-mail, and Skype as well as during class time.
- Students may remain online after class to ask questions.
- The sponsoring agency notifies students of information pertaining to hardware and software requirements, reception sites, parking, and technical support.
- Additional effort is required from both students and faculty to maintain interactive aspects of the education process.
- Some modifications may be required in the use of audiovisual aids. Additional attention must be given to how well audiovisual aids transmit and whether they are visible to persons at other sites.
- Successful offerings are the result of a team effort that involves instructional designers, graphic artists, faculty training, and technical support.

2006). Distance education is integral to and has given rise to a growing phenomenon, the virtual "classroom" available in a "virtual learning environment."

Definitions of Virtual Learning Environments

There are many definitions of "virtual learning environment" (VLE) in the literature. The differences reflect emphasis that goes beyond semantics. The term is composed of three concepts—virtual, learning, and environment. A VLE can be viewed as the underlying concept for instruction delivered outside the boundaries of the traditional classroom in which instructor and instructed do not meet face to face. It is the virtual, or nonphysical, nature of the environment that sets the tone and direction for learning. The term *virtual*, defined as "being something in effect even if not in reality; or hypothetical" (Encarta World English Dictionary 2009), has come in our culture to be associated with "generated by a computer." This gives the sense that the learning is not real or authentic. This is not the case. The learning is real; it is the environment that is virtual. It has been suggested that "a virtual environment for learning" may be a more precise phase as this removes ambiguities. Educational applications of computers adapt well to a diversity of settings and learners. The flexibility of educational applications of computer technology makes them suitable for use in formal healthcare education programs, in workplace settings for in-service and competency testing, as well as for continuing professional education.

The definition of a VLE is by no means homogeneous. Wikipedia (2007) defines VLE as a system that uses the Internet to assist the educator in developing, managing, and administering educational materials for students and notes that the term is often used interchangeably with Course Management System (CMS), Managed Learning Environment, and Learning Management Systems (LMS). These programs facilitate electronic learning (e-learning) in an academic setting, providing for the tracking of students' progress in a course. They are generally run on the organization's servers. Examples of this definition of VLEs are Moodle Learning Management System, CyberExtension Virtual Managed Learning, Blackboard, and WebCt and CLOSE.

The *Handbook for Economics Lecturers*, a source from the UK, provides this definition of a VLE: "A package to help lecturers create a course website with a minimum of technical skill, including tools for discussion and document sharing" that reflects the emphasis on an academic setting.

What is it?.com (http://whatis.techtarget.com), a site that defines itself as "the leading IT encyclopedia and learning center," defines the virtual learning environment as "a set of teaching and learning tools designed to enhance a student's learning experience by including computers and the Internet in the learning process," extending the exclusive use of VLE beyond academia.

And finally, this definition was derived from Pimentel's (1999, p. 75) early work in the evolution of virtual learning environments, an environment "that allows learners to perceive the environment, assess situations and performance, perform actions and proceed through experiences and lessons that will allow them to perform better with more experience on repetition on the same task in similar circumstances."

Although originally designed to promote individualized learning, VLE applications can enhance group learning as well (Calderone 1994; Maag 2006). Studies have been conducted comparing the efficacy of virtual environments for learning and traditional classroom instruction. While additional research is called for, virtual environments prove to be at least as effective as traditional instruction (Shih-Wei & Liu 2005; Swan 2003). Virtual learning environments can serve to introduce technology into the curriculum, and this has become our current educational reality. A virtual classroom can also supplement traditional classroom instruction known as "blended learning."

Virtual learning environments have been purported to offer the following advantages (Hansen 2009, p. 394):

- *Improved reading habits.* Learners can proceed at a pace conducive to comprehension.
- *Convenience, learning offered at any site that has computer access.* Programs available for single users on freestanding PCs or via network connections.

- *Reduced learning time.* Learners can proceed at their own pace; they can skim through familiar content and focus on weak areas.
- *Increased retention.* Related to the active nature of the media that facilitates learner participation.
- *Twenty-four-hour access.* "Anywhere anytime access."
- *Consistent instruction in a safe environment.* Allows learners to practice new skills without fear of harm to themselves or others.
- *Flexibility of faculty schedules.* Makes it easier to teach around clinical instruction.

Three major variables influence the effectiveness of virtual learning environments: quality of the software, the environment of computer use, and characteristics of the learner. The following elements can lead to negative attitudes toward this process for delivering educational material:

- *Poor instructional design.* Many virtual applications do nothing more than automate page turning.
- *Lack of feedback.* This can be frustrating to learners.
- *Lack of control.* Control encompasses the ability to advance, repeat, or review portions of the program, or to quit at any point.
- *Lack of intellectual stimulation.* Programs that fail to maintain interest may cause learners to feel that they wasted their time.

Drug calculation programs are a common application used in a virtual environment in nursing schools. These programs are popular because drug calculation is a basic skill needed by all nurses, and, as such, drug calculation programs fit well into the curriculum, while programs on other content areas may not match curriculum objectives. An example of such an interactive program that assists students and nurses with drug dosages was the "Med-Calc Tutorial" (Hansen 2007a). Telles Filho and Cassiani (2008) also developed and tested a computer-assisted instruction module in drug administration that demonstrated positive outcomes.

Collaborative Instruction

Nurse educators have identified many challenges that prevent more widespread adaptation of e-learning. A collaborative approach has been advocated as a facilitating factor for transforming nursing and healthcare education (Kiteley & Ormrod 2009). E-learning development that remains sustainable, responsive, and multidisciplinary can only be achieved by adapting a team line of attack to the problem of ever changing technology, the unique aspects of online learning, and the qualities of a virtual learning community. Collaboration is not just limited to faculty, library, and technical support staff (Schutt & Hightower 2009). In virtual classrooms, nursing students collaborate to improve learning and learning outcomes.

Web 2.0 Applications in Professional Healthcare Education

The term *Web 2.0* has yet to be defined; however, it has been described as consisting of a set of "core characteristics" including user-centered design, crowd-sourcing, Web as platform, collaboration, power decentralization, dynamic content, SaaS (Software as a Service), and rich user experience (Sharma 2008). No formal updates to the WWW technical specifications have occurred. The term merely denotes the evolution in WWW use and versatility, which according to WWW inventor, Tim Berners-Lee, is precisely what he intended in the first place.

The term *Web 2.0* was first used in an article by Darcy DiNucci (1999), information architect since 1994. She described the Web we know now as "only an embryo of the Web to come" identifying "the first glimmerings of Web 2.0" in that year. "The Web will be understood as a transport mechanism, the ether through which interactivity happens" (DiNucci 1999). According to O'Reilly (2005), the concept Web 2.0 grew with a conference brainstorming in which O'Reilly and Web pioneer Dale Dougherty participated. They concluded that the WWW was "more important than ever, with exciting new applications and sites popping up with surprising regularity," designating this burgeoning change as "Web 2.0" (O'Reilly 2005). The term has since grown in popularity. Examples of what are considered Web 2.0 technology include Web-based communities, hosted services, Web applications, social-networking sites, video-sharing sites, wikis, blogs, mashups, and folksonomies sites, that allow users to interact with other users or to completely change content (Al-Khalifa & Davis 2006; Kaminski 2009; Wikipedia 2011b). These technologies may be used equally well in formal educational programs or informal learning opportunities.

Boulos (2007) wrote that Web 2.0 is now considered the read-write-listen Web. It offers venues for users to comment, annotate, create, mix, and share content related to health education. This presentation is a wonderful example of Web 2.0 technology and provides a comprehensive explanation of the Web 2.0 applications.

Applications for Professional Continuing Education

Hansen (2009) noted that interactive technological tools are becoming popular in healthcare education and clinical practice. Applications that facilitate online communication, learning, and collaboration among educators, students, and colleagues across international borders include blogs, podcasts, Webinars, and wikis. These are all considered part of Web 2.0 applications.

The term *mobile learning* or *m-learning* denotes the use of mobile technologies, such as the mobile phone, the PDA, and the iPod. The most well-known and popular, the PDA. There is grant funding available for healthcare educators who wish to pursue this area of educational research (Cell Phone 2007).

Wikis A wiki is a Web site that allows anyone to contribute and edit content. Perhaps the best-known wiki, Wikipedia (2010), defines a **wiki** as "a Web site that allows the easy creation and editing of any number of interlinked Web pages via a Web browser using a simplified markup language." In nursing education, wikis offer many possibilities as a tool to disseminate information, foster collaboration, share resources, and assist research teams (Kardong-Edgren et al. 2009).

Batista, McGrath, and Maude (2010) discuss the application of wikis and offer examples and suggestions about how this technology can benefit mental health nursing practices. Similarly, Billings and Kowalski (2009b) described how wikis can be used across a wider spectrum of healthcare settings to facilitate teaching and learning. The use of technology such as wikis may soon be part of every nurse's lifelong learning and clinical practice. Cobus (2009) advocates the use of wikis but cautions that health professionals must assume responsibility to critically appraise Web content that has not undergone rigorous peer review.

Podcasts Hansen (2009, p. 409) postulated that "educating the Net Generation requires educators to know and understand their audience prior to developing learning objectives and the delivery of educational materials." This is as true of brick and mortar teaching as it is with e-learning; hence, applications such as the use of podcasting and iPods to deliver educational material is quite applicable to the twenty-first century educator.

Podcasting has been described as "a portmanteau of 'broadcasting'" (Hansen 2009, p. 408). The iPod (Apple Computer's MP3 player) is an example of an Internet-based technology that allows for an audio event, a conversation, a lecture, a presentation, a speech, a group-learning occurrence, a video, or a song to be distributed via Really Simple Syndication (RSS). A desktop computer or an MP3 player offers venues for listening to podcasts, and software packages (iPod Touch 3.1 2010) enable educators to create enhanced podcasts. "As more cities around the globe become wireless" (Hansen 2009, p. 408), "learners will be able to access podcasts with great ease in a car, train, bus, or subway."

A new wave of learning and flexibility is available to learners and students through podcasting and iPods; hence they need not be anchored to desktops in computer labs. The ability to create interactive material is an important step toward mobile learning. Mobile technology is finding a place in the education for healthcare students (see Box 23–2). Students attending Harvard University stated a lecture podcast was used for review rather than as an alternative to attendance according to Malan (2007). In addition, 71% of the students in the study were more inclined to listen to or watch lectures on their desktop computers versus 19% of the participants relying on audio-only or 10% on video iPods. The use of podcasting and MP3 technology in nursing education is providing portability for listening to lectures (Maag 2006). Podcasts to reach to the public at large can be created using the step-wise instruction on how to create a podcast by Maag (2006). Australian educators and researchers, Palmer and Devitt (2007) demonstrated how case studies and anatomical images may be viewed via an iPod. The results of a student survey conducted after students viewed the interactive case indicated a favorable shift in student attitudes with the percentage of those who felt podcasting was useful to learning increasing from 9% to 41%. They concluded, however, that there was no evidence at this point to suggest greater effectiveness of learning in this way, identifying this as a fertile area for future research.

Walls, Kucsera, Walker, Acee, McVaugh, and Robinson (2010), for example, found that students may not be as ready or eager to use podcasting for repetitive or supplemental educational purpose.

Many universities subscribe to iTunes University (Apple 2011) making it easier for educators to make their lectures, presentations, and students' work available on the Internet. iTunes U uses the power of the iTunes store to distribute information. The technical components and interactions of podcasting are presented in Carnegie Mellon's teaching with technology white paper (2007).

Webinars Webinars and Webcasts are two related applications that are proving useful for professional education. Webinars are generally intended for a specific audience and number of people. A Webcast, on the other hand, is visible to everyone who chooses to watch it. Webinars are frequently used in business settings (Cruz n.d.).

Webinar is a contraction of the term *Web-based seminar*, forming a neologism that describes a specific type of Web conference. There are Web conferencing technologies on the market that incorporate the use of VoIP audio technology, to allow for a completely Web-based communication; however, some still reply on the telephone for two-way communication.

Like a physical conference room–based seminar, Webinars enable participants to view a presentation and to interact. The presentation, however, is delivered through a Web browser, while the audio may come through the telephone. The transmission of the audio and visual media file is scheduled at a particular time and is live. At a later date, it can be viewed over the Internet as well; however, Webinars are generally interactive, in contrast to Webcasts, in which data transmission is one way with no interaction between the presenter and the audience. Webinars may be used to conduct live meetings, training, or presentations via the Internet (Wikipedia 2011c). Usually a live presentation, it happens in real time as users participate through chats. Participants are able to ask the instructor questions and get answers in real time. Some Webinars have the capacity to conduct polls and ask questions. Participants often receive course materials by e-mail prior to the seminar. These types of online courses are very popular for continuing education offerings and have a large nursing market. One example is Pearls Nursing Review (http://www.pearlsreview.com/nurses.aspx), which offers a full line of certification review Webinars. The impact is greater than simply reading material on the Web. Webinars offer convenience and are very cost-effective, avoiding travel time.

A Webcast is a media file over the Internet using streaming media technology that may be distributed either live or on demand (Wikipedia n.d.). Webcasting is another way of saying broadcasting over the WWW by use of a webcam. The term *Webcasting* usually refers to noninteractive linear streams or events. Information is spread over the Internet using push technology (Wikipedia 2011d). This process broadcasts sound and/or video online and can deliver live or prerecorded information. The largest "Webcasters" include existing radio and TV stations, who "simulcast" their output. Internet broadcasting has also been described as the process of capturing, encoding, hosting, and delivering multimedia events such as training, infomercials, and concerts.

Virtual Meeting Spaces Virtual meetings are made possible by Web conferencing applications. Webinars and Web conferencing are sometimes used interchangeably; however, the latter describes conducting live meetings or trainings via the Internet. This would prove important for educators who must collaborate on educational initiatives. The availability of collaborative Web browsing and file transfer applications as well as application sharing make this an ideal tool for nursing educator's tool kit.

There are Web conferencing technologies on the market that have incorporated the use of Voice Over Internet Protocol (VoIP) audio technology, to allow for a completely Web-based communication; however, some depend on the telephone for two-way communication. Web conferencing offers advantages over traditional room-based videoconferencing. Web conferencing first appeared in the late 1990s with products such as PlaceWare, Microsoft's NetMeeting, and IBM's Sametime. In a Web conference, each participant can sit at his or her own computer. There is no travel time to the conference site. Participants are connected via the Internet, either through downloaded software or a Web-based application. The download application generally enables virtual meetings at one site. The application must be loaded on the computers of each attendee. Web-based applications enable attendees to access the meeting through an e-mail "meeting invitation" and can connect attendees at distant sites who click on the link provided in the invitation. Examples of virtual meeting software in use today include: IBM Lotuslive Engage and Adobe Acrobat ConnectPro. Web-based commercial virtual meeting products include: Fuze, Webex, and GoToMeeting.

BOX 23–2   Mobile Applications for Healthcare Education

Any discussion of today's mobile technology should begin with a bit of history, just to allow for an often much-needed dose of perspective ("much needed" in the sense that technology changes so fast, it's often hard to understand—even see—those changes occurring).

With this idea of perspective in mind, the first machine to come with the designation of mobile computer is usually identified as the Osborne I released in 1981. Weighing in at nearly 26 pounds, the Osborne I came "fully equipped" with a 5" CRT screen, a 300 baud modem, and a dual-floppy disk drive capable of storing 102K bytes of information. And it came with all these features for the bargain-basement price of $1795.00.

To put the Osborne into even more specific relief, consider its functionality (which was quite good for its day) compared to what is common in our modern devices: For example, the 300 baud modem in the Osborne I could transmit 600 bits of information a second; the high-speed Internet connection you have in your home might transmit at 32,000,000 bits of information per second. The Osborne floppy drive could store a total of 102K bytes of data as compared to a 5 gigabyte (GB) thumb drive you probably have on your keychain, the thumb drive has a storage capacity of 10,000,000,000 bytes. And you probably bought that thumb drive at your local Wal-Mart or Target for less than $20.00.

Yet perhaps what's even more impressive than rate of change in the speed and storage capabilities of technology is the size of the technology itself. In today's world, regardless of your discipline, a mobile device is often an absolutely essential business tool. But even the term "mobile technology" can mean different things. Table 23–1 looks across six mobile technology platforms, comparing/contrasting their various features.

Of the devices listed in this table, the smart phone and tablet are probably of most interest to nursing professionals in the clinical setting. The tablet—and especially the iPad—has certainly gained an enormous amount of attention since its (iPad) launch in the spring of 2010. As of this writing, millions of iPads have been sold in less than a year of availability, with the expected release of the "iPad 2" in late spring/early summer 2011 to undoubtedly increase these numbers. Features/functionality of the iPad 2 are still undetermined, but it is wildly believed the device will include both a front and rear-facing camera, and possibility some type of expansion slot (SD card, USB).

Questions to Think About when Choosing a Mobile Device

There are several questions you should keep in mind when choosing (or helping your department/organization to choose) a mobile device:

1. *Is pervasive access an absolute requirement?* As noted in Table 23–1, some devices offer pervasive access while others offer the possibility of such access (e.g., an iPad equipped with both WiFi and 3G capability, thus allowing it to connect to a service provider network, such as AT&T or Verizon). It's important to note that pervasive access, even with the most robust device and the best data service plan, can remain a relative term, as you have probably experienced physical locations that, for a number of reasons, have limited wireless network connectivity and/or none at all. There are often support options for improving access in such locations—for example, placing additional wireless hubs to strengthen signals. However, the possibility for "dead spots" to occur is an important consideration.

2. *Does the size of the mobile device make a difference?* At first glance, this may seem like an obvious question, but in practice the answer becomes more difficult. In a recent workshop with nursing professionals, it was noted by several attendees that while they were impressed with the functionality of the iPad, the fact it would not comfortably (if at all) fit into a lab coat made it an impractical device in a clinical setting. Also, the type of content you want to display on the device can be greatly impacted by its size. For example, if you wanted to show a patient video vignettes highlighting steps of a procedure, having a device with a larger screen (e.g., iPad) would be preferable to that of a smartphone.

3. *Do I need to use the device as a presentation tool?* More than likely, you will be in a situation at some point where you need to present information in a group setting and will want to use your device as the presentation tool. However, not every device connects, for example, to a digital

BOX 23–2   *(continued)*

projector in the same fashion, if at all: An iPad, for example, utilizes a proprietary Apple cable to connect to a digital projector, and not every iPad application (at least at the time of this writing) is written to provide support for video output.

4. *Is the application I need available on the device I want?* There are tens of thousands of applications (apps) available for the iPhone and iPad on the Apple "App Store," with a growing number of apps available for other smartphone devices. That said, your device can quickly prove worthless (or at the very least, far less functional) if the app you really need is not available for your device platform. Also, keep in mind that while some apps may appear to run across multiple devices, they may do so with limited functionality on one device compared to another. For example, the iPad does not support the popular "Flash" video/multimedia component used in thousands of Web sites.

5. *Beyond the size of the device, what other physical specifications of the device should I be concerned with?* While the difference between 2 pounds and 1 pound might not seem significant, carry the two devices around for an entire day and then see if you can find a (big) difference—more than likely, you will. In addition to weight, the heat a device outputs can be an issue. As devices get smaller and smaller, and their processing power continues to increase, heat is generated, and that heat has to go somewhere. Better designs allow for the heat to dissipate around/out of the device in an otherwise unnoticeable fashion; however, small laptops can get very hot very fast, some to the point of being uncomfortable even when placed on top of covered skin. Ultimately, there may not be anything you can do around this heat issue, but you might include it as part of your device evaluation, especially laptops and netbooks.

6. *How many devices do I want to carry?* This is another question that might seem strange when you first consider it, but—depending on the answer to any one of the questions mentioned earlier—you may find yourself in a situation where you need to carry more than one mobile device. For example, you might love the functionality of the iPad, and even though you have a model with 3G (i.e., access to a nationwide network) capability, the size of the device makes it impractical to utilize it as a phone; therefore, you also need to carry a smart phone. While it's unlikely you would need to carry more than two or three devices, the possibility of facing this situation is certainly not unheard of.

TABLE 23–1   Comparison of Mobile Technology Devices and Platforms

Device Type	Example	Typical Weight	Advantages	Disadvantages
Laptop	Dell Latitude E4200	1.5–10 lbs[1]	"Fully functional" (i.e., is a true desktop replacement), some models can be very lightweight	Weight (compared to other mobile devices), cost, not always capable of pervasive connectivity (i.e., constant Web access)
Netbook	Dell Mini	1.5–2.0 lbs	Lightweight, possibility for full functionality (with docking station/peripherals), possible pervasive connectivity	Form factor (especially small keyboard), not always capable of pervasive connectivity, price (relative to full-featured laptop)
PDA[2]	HP iPAQ	100–500 grams	Form factor, possible pervasive connectivity	Price (relative to other mobile devices, in context of functionality, outdated technology)
Smart phone	RIM Blackberry	100–300 grams	Pervasive connectivity, form factor, unique functionality (e.g., apps)	Pricing/confusing options and restrictions, interoperability, limited functionality (depending on use)
eText Reader	Amazon Kindle	8–10 ounces	Weight, unique functionality, pervasive connectivity	Limited ability to mark-up text, limited presentation ability, the "pagination problem"[3]
Tablet	Apple iPad[4]	1.5 lbs	Unique interface, enhanced functionality, possible pervasive connectivity	Limited interoperability, "unique interface," price (relative to other mobile devices)

[1] Laptop weight will vary significantly, depending on screen size, battery, inclusion of internal drive bays (e.g., CD-DVD), and other factors.
[2] At this point, a PDA could be considered a deprecated device at least compared to other mobile devices.
[3] As print texts are converted to eText format, page numbers between the two versions don't always match up, therefore making it potentially difficult to cross-reference specific pages.
[4] At the time of this writing, the Apple iPad remains the dominant (in terms of sales) tablet device, but offerings from Motorola, HP, Dell, Blackberry, and Samsung will soon challenge the iPad's dominant market position.

(continued)

BOX 23–2 *(continued)*

7. *What is the type and volume of data I'm expected to enter on a regular basis, and how does the device support said input?* More than likely, you would not want to type a dissertation on your iPad (unless you had the available external keyboard, but even then it would be a challenge). Or, if you were required to enter extensive numerical data, then the small keys of a Blackberry might be inconvenient. Given that some type of data entry is part of your profession, it's imperative that you take some time and "play around" with the input features of the various mobile devices. For example, the iPad's on-screen keyboard takes some getting used to, but is actually quite functional; however, in order to access different characters/numbers, you have to shift screens, type that symbol, and then shift back to the main keyboard. You should also consider devices that support other types of data input (e.g., voice input) and the apps available for each device that support said input. Many apps are customized as to make the entry of process-specific data easier, as the screen layout and common options are presented in a direct, easy-to-read/access format. Again, this will vary from device to device and from app to app.

8. *Can I live without the device?* That might sound like an ominous question, but more and more of our lives are integrated with our mobile devices, so you should be prepared with a "Mobile Plan B" should your device be lost, stolen, or broken. Keep in mind, too, that not all major wireless service carriers will replace/repair all devices under all conditions. For example, water damage—even if accidental—is not usually covered under your service carrier's basic warranty plan, so you would need to have purchased additional warranty coverage at the time of purchase of the original device in order for it to be replaced (and even then, usually with some deductible).

Locating Mobile Apps

Apps are available across a variety of platforms and devices. If you type in the search term "Nurse" on the Apple App Store, you'll see that (as of this writing), there are 54 apps written specifically for the iPad, and over 330 for the iPhone (note that most iPhone apps will run on the iPad, but the screen display will be smaller given it was designed for the smaller iPhone display). Not every one of these apps has to do with nursing care (e.g., the iPhone app, "The Nurse with the Red Clown Nose" is a storybook app), but the majority of the apps are focused on specific aspects of nursing care, including some apps focusing on a specific specialty. For example:

- **Pocket Lab Values:** A perfect app for nurses, med students, and other medical professionals, this app provides answers to common lab values, along with corresponding support information.

- **eFilm:** Use your iPad to view radiographic images, as well as download for sharing/offline viewing.

- **Clinical Orthopedic Exam:** This app includes over 250 different patient maneuvers, along with a step-by-step exam procedure guide.

- **Mediquations Medical Calculator:** This app, designed for nurses, includes over 200 formulas and scoring tools, along with an easy-to-use interface. Designed by a four-year medical student.

Note that these and many, many other nursing-related apps are also available at the Blackberry "App World" and for other devices/platforms.

Mobile Devices and eTextbooks

Electronic textbooks (or eTexts) continue to be a developing arena for content producers, instructors, and students. There is obvious functionality in having all your material available on a single, often very lightweight device; moreover, with device battery life continuing to improve (e.g., it is uncommon to get ten full hours of activity on an iPad, from a single charge), the utility of being able to study your materials whenever and wherever you want is a real advantage. Also, as the cost of printed textbooks continues to rise, the potential cost savings is significant.

Despite these advantages, there are several outstanding issues and questions that still remain around the broad adoption of eTexts:

- **The "pagination problem":** As mentioned in Table 23–1 the "pagination problem" continues to plague the eText arena, especially if, for example, only part of a class is utilizing an eText, while the other half is using a traditional printed textbook. When printed texts are converted to electronic format, the page numbers between the electronic and printed version don't always match, which can result in confusion/difficulty in trying to locate specific material.

- **Ability to electronically annotate:** Scribbling notes in the margins is a time-tested method of study, and there's no real reason why this can't carry over to the electronic format. And, with electronic notations, there's often the ability (depending on the app/software being utilized) to search across/organize those annotations in a variety of ways. Still, typing those comments—especially on a mobile device—can be tedious, depending on the device's input method, and traditional highlighting/underlining of text can also prove less intuitive. It should be noted, however, that this "disadvantage" is probably more of user preference than a limitation of the eText, as some users will find these features compelling and beneficial.

- **Licensing of content:** While traditional textbook publishing can often present maddeningly complex licensing rules, the move to eTexts does not necessarily eliminate those concerns; in fact, in some cases (e.g., supplementary handouts), it can be just as if not more difficult, especially if the content is to be made available across multiple device platforms.

BOX 23–2 (*continued*)

- **Integration with learning management systems (LMS):** The use of some type of LMS (BlackBoard, Desire2Learn, open-source solutions like Sakai, etc.) are pervasive across higher ed landscape. As these systems continue to offer more interoperability with third-party tools (e.g., ability to publish content directly from an LMS to iTunes U), having eText information accessible/interoperable with an institution's LMS will be a growing requirement for large-scale adoption.

- **Access on a mobile device remains, at the moment, somewhat limited:** The majority of vendors have made eText material accessible on a computer with a Web browser. While access on the types of mobile devices listed in this supplement is forthcoming, the interoperability of said content across multiple device platforms could continue to present a problem in the short term.

- **Ability to access eText information both on/offline:** Depending on the type of device being utilized to access eText information, as well as the location of the user (i.e., connected to a network via WiFi or national service carrier), having the ability to access text information both on and offline is essential.

Supporting Your Mobile Device

There are a large number of challenges to the IT professional in supporting the mobile environment. However, nearly all of these challenges also directly impact the actual user of the mobile device, and you should be prepared to accept some responsibility for the "care and up-keep" of your own device:

- **Acceptable use:** This can vary tremendously depending on when/where the device is utilized, but clear policies must be set forth on the type of content that can be accessed (personal versus company data), especially if that content is in some way sensitive in nature.

- **Data back-up/recovery:** Far too often, the user of any device (be it mobile or otherwise) falls under the dangerous assumption that their sensitive/critical information is being backed-up by someone else, usually their IT staff. While this is often the case, at least in terms of data that is stored/access from a central server, data that is stored locally on the device itself is usually not automatically backed-up, therefore putting the user at extreme risk for catastrophic data loss.

- **Virus/malware protection:** As with data back-up/recovery, devices used on a company network will usually be configured with some type of virus/malware protection. Still, it is the user's responsibility to understand common "tricks" utilized by malicious software (e.g., spam messages with inviting subject lines, asking the user to visit a specific Web site or to open an infected attachment) and to guard against them.

- **Secure access:** The level of security will vary depending on the sensitivity of information being accessed. However, physical security of a device is also critical, that is, if it contained sensitive information stored locally on the device itself, and in turn the device is stolen. Clearly, HIPAA regulations will govern sensitive information access, and may be more difficult to enforce given the ability to access such sensitive information from a variety of locations.

- **Support (hardware/software)—when and how that support is provided:** More and more IT support organizations are required to provide 24/7/365 support to their users. While this type of ubiquitous support may be available, it should remain the user's responsibility to under-stand basic functionality of his/her device and to recognize (to some degree) a problem may be occurring, so that it can be addressed in the timeliest manner possible.

FUTURE DIRECTIONS

It is critical that nurse educators identify skill sets that the next generation of nurses will need in order to prepare them for the ever-changing dynamics of modern healthcare. Emerging tech-nologies have implications for clinical competence, healthcare costs, and continuing education. Consumer demands and government initiatives further drive the market. Hospital information systems, multimedia, and course management systems are all part of the now. Decision support systems, monitoring devices, robots doing surgery, and virtual reality are all indicators of a future world. The future is now; nurse educators need to prepare themselves so they can prepare others.

Visit nursing.pearsonhighered.com for additional cases, information, and weblinks.

CASE STUDY EXERCISE

Locate and evaluate at least one online continuing education offering.

SUMMARY

- Computer technology can help revolutionize education in formal healthcare programs, continuing education, and consumer education. It also provides informal opportunities for networking among professionals via e-mail and social networking systems, such as wikis, blogs, and podcasts.
- Successful use of computers for education requires careful planning, specific learning objectives, orientation to the technology, convenient access, opportunities to question what is not understood, instructional design, and sound evaluation of learning outcomes.
- Formal nursing education is a logical place to introduce or expand basic informatics skills.
- Educational applications of technology should be subject to the same review criteria applied to other instructional materials before their adoption and following student use.
- Connectivity to HIS from schools of nursing allows students more opportunity to analyze client information before scheduled clinical experiences and facilitates professional socialization.
- Virtual learning environments are examples of the use of a computer to teach a subject other than computing. A VLE offers the following advantages: convenience, decreased learning time, and increased retention.
- Teleconferencing is the use of computers, audio and video equipment, and high-grade dedicated telephone lines, cable, or satellite connections to provide interactive communication between two or more persons at two or more sites. It may occur via desktop computers or via larger systems with multiple persons participating at one time.
- Distance education is the use of print, audio, video, computer, or teleconference capability to connect faculty and students located at a minimum of two different sites. Distance education may take place in real time or on a delayed basis. It expands educational opportunities without the need for a long commute.
- Web-based instruction uses the attributes and resources of the Internet to deliver and support education. It may be used as a stand-alone course or to supplement traditional classes.
- E-learning uses electronic media to present instruction. It is often suggested for corporate training because it is considered to be efficient. It allows users to skip material that they already know.
- Multimedia refers to the ability to deliver presentations that combine text, voice or sound, images, and video. Multimedia presentations tend to improve learning by actively engaging the senses.
- Technology expands educational opportunities via its 24/7 availability from any device with Internet capability.
- Simulation use is growing both as a means to develop skills and demonstrate competencies.
- Integration of technology tools may be done within course/learning management systems as well as within traditional face-to-face classroom settings.
- Videoconferencing and various Web 2.0 technologies foster student engagement and presence.
- Virtual reality applications are growing as a means to foster skill development in a safe setting and replicate hard-to-guarantee experiences.
- Distance education and virtual learning requires additional skills sets for faculty.

REFERENCES

Ainsley, B., & Brown, A. (2009). The impact of informatics on nursing education: A review of the literature. *Journal of Continuing Education in Nursing, 40*(5). doi: 10.9999/00220124-20090422-02. Retrieved from http://www.acteonline.org/uploadedFiles/About_CTE/files/The Impact of Informatics on Nursing Education.pdf

Al-Khalifa, H. S., & Davis, H. C. (2006). Folksonomies versus automatic keyword extraction: An empirical study. *Iadis International Journal on Computer Science and Information Systems, 1*(2), 132–143.

American Association of Medical Colleges and the American Association of Colleges of Nursing. (2010). Lifelong learning in medicine and nursing—Final conference report. Retrieved from http://www.aacn.nche.edu/Education/pdf/MacyReport.pdf

Apple Inc. (2011). *iTunes U.* Retrieved from http://www.apple.com/support/itunes_u/

Barrett, M. J., Lacey, C. S., Sekara, A. E., Linden, E. A., & Gracely, E. J. (2004). Mastering cardiac murmurs. *Chest, 126,* 470–475.

Bastida, R., McGrath, I., & Maude, P. (2010). Wiki use in mental health practice: Recognizing potential use of collaborative technology. *International Journal of Mental Health Nursing, 19*(2), 142.

Batscha, C. (2002). The pharmacology game. *CIN Plus, 5*(3), 1, 3–6.

Beard, L., Wilson, K., Morra, D., & Keelan, J. (2009). A survey of health-related activities on second life. *Journal of Medical Internet Research, 11*(2). Retrieved from http://www.jmir.org/2009/2/e17/

Bentley, G. W., Cook, P. P., Davis, K., Murphy, M. J., & Berding, C. B. (2003). RN to BSN program: Transition from traditional to online delivery. *Nurse Educator, 28*(3), 121–126.

Billings, D. M. (1994). Effects of BSN student preferences for studying alone or in groups on performance and attitude when using interactive videodisc instruction. *Journal of Nursing Education, 33*(7), 322–324.

Billings, D. M. (1995). Preparing nursing faculty for information age teaching and learning. *Computers in Nursing, 13*(6), 264, 268–270.

Billings, D. M., & Kowalski, K. (2009a). Teaching and learning in virtual worlds. *Journal of Continuing Education in Nursing, 40*(11), 489–490. doi:10.3928/00220124-20091023-04

Billings, D. M., & Kowalski, K. (2009b). Wikis and blogs: Consider the possibilities for continuing education. *Journal of Continuing Education in Nursing, 40*(12), 534–535.

Birz, S. (2009). Report outlines trends in technologies used by nurses. *Nurse Zone.* Retrieved from http://www.nursezone.com/printArticle.aspx?articleID=32220

Boulos, M. N. K. (2007). *e-Health and web 2.0: Looking to the future with sociable technologies and social software.* Retrieved from http://www.slideshare.net/sl.medic/ehealth-and-web-20the-3d-web-looking-to-the-futurewith-sociable-technologies-and-social-software-121698

Bradley, C. (2003). Technology as a catalyst to transforming nursing care. *Nursing Outlook, 51*(3), S14–S15.

Bruff, D. (2011). Classroom response systems ("clickers"). *Vanderbilt Center for Teaching.* Retrieved from http://www.vanderbilt.edu/cft/resources/teaching_resources/technology/crs.htm

Calderone, A. B. (1994). Computer-assisted instruction: Learning, attitude, and modes of instruction. *Computers in Nursing, 12*(3), 164–170.

Cambre, M., & Castner, L. J. (March 1993). The status of interactive video in nursing education environments. Presented at FITNE: Get in Touch with Multimedia, Atlanta, GA.

Carnegie, M. (2007). *Podcasting: A teaching with technology white paper.* Retrieved from http://www.cmu.edu/teaching/technology/research/index.html#podcasting

Cartwright, J. (2000). Lessons learned: Using asynchronous computer-mediated conferencing to facilitate group discussion. *Journal of Nursing Education, 39*(2), 87–90.

Cell phone as a platform for healthcare request for proposals 2007. (2007). *Microsoft research.* Retrieved from http://research.microsoft.com/ur/us/fundingopps/RFPs/CellPhoneAsPlatformForHealthcare_RFP.aspx

Charp, S. (2003). Technology for all students. *Technological Horizons in Education Journal, 30*(9), 8.

Chou, S. -W., & Liu, C. -H. (2005). *Learning effectiveness in web-based technology-mediated virtual learning environment, HICSS* (Vol. 1, p. 3a). Proceedings of the 38th Annual Hawaii International Conference on System Sciences (HICSS'05)—Track 1. Retrieved from http://doi.ieeecomputersociety.org/10.1109/HICSS.2005.385

Cobus, L. (2009). Using blogs and wikis in a graduate public health course. *Medical References Services Quarterly, 28*(1), 22–32.

Corner, S. K. (n.d.). Podcasting: Why should I bother? Power point presentation in nursing program at Governors State University circa 2008. Retrieved from http://www.govst.edu/uploadedFiles/eLearning/Events_News/Comer_Podcasting.pdf

Corwin, E. J. (2000). Distance education: An ongoing initiative to reach rural family nurse practitioner students. *Nurse Educator, 25*(3), 114–115.

Cuellar, N. (2002). Tips to increase success for teaching online: Communication! *Computers, Informatics, Nursing Plus, 5*(1), 1, 3–6.

Di Cruz, T. (n.d.). *Webinars vs. webcasts.* Retrieved from http://ezinearticles.com/?Webinars -Vs-Webcasts&id=2301921

DiNucci, D. (1999). Fragmented future. *Print, 53*(4), 32. Retrieved from http://www.cdinucci.com/ Darcy2/articles/articlesindex.html

Doorley, J. E., Renner, A. L., & Corron, J. (1994). Creating care plans via modems: Using a hospital information system in nursing education. *Computers in Nursing, 12*(3), 160–163.

Edward, K., Hercelinskyj, J., Warelow, P., & Munro, I. (2007). Simulation to practice: Developing nursing skills in mental health: An Australian perspective. *International Electronic Journal of Health Education, 10.* Retrieved from http://74.125.155.132/scholar?q=cache:I-hybZvgPOEJ: scholar.google.com/+hi+fidelity+simulation+in+nursing+education+psychiatric+nursing+&amp ;hl=en&as_sdt=8000000000

Encarta World English Dictionary. (2009). *Virtual.* Retrieved from http://encarta.msn.com/encnet/ features/dictionary/DictionaryResults.aspx?lextype=3&search=virtual

Faison, K. A. (2003). Professionalization in a distance learning setting. *The ABNF Journal: Official Journal of the Association of Black Nursing Faculty in Higher Education, 14*(4), 83–85.

Fetter, M. S. (2009). Curriculum strategies to improve baccalaureate nursing information technology outcomes. *Journal of Nursing Education, 48*(2), 78–85.

Forbes, M. O., & Hickey, M. T. (2009). Curriculum reform in baccalaureate nursing education: Review of the literature. *International Journal of Nursing Education Scholarship, 6(1),* Article 27. doi: 10.2202/1548-923X.1797. Retrieved from http://www.bepress.com/ijnes/vol6/iss1/art27

Ford, O. (2010). Researchers developing new virtual surgeon training tool. *Medical Device Daily, 14*(140), 1–8.

Geibert, R. C. (2000). Integrating web-based instruction into a graduate nursing program taught via videoconferencing: Challenges and solutions. *Computers in Nursing, 18*(1), 26–34.

Gleydura, A. J., Michelman, J. E., & Wilson, C. N. (1995). Multimedia training in nursing education. *Computers in Nursing, 13*(4), 169–175.

Goodman, J., & Blake, J. (1996). Multimedia courseware: Transforming the classroom. *Computers in Nursing, 14*(5), 287–296.

Go Virtual Medical Ltd. (2007). Welcome to Go Virtual Medical.com. Retrieved from http:// www.govirtualmedical.com/

Gugerty, B., Maranda, M. J., Beachley, M., Navarro, V. B., Newbold, S., Hawk, W., … Wilhelm, D. (2007). *Challenges and opportunities in documentation of the nursing care of patients.* Documentation Work Group, Maryland Nursing Workforce Commission, Baltimore. Retrieved from http:// www.mbon.org/commission2/documenation_challenges.pdf

Hansen, M. (2007a). *Med-calc tutorial.* Retrieved from http://www.m2hnursing.com/

Hansen, M. (2007b). *ECG activity.* Retrieved from http://www.m2hnursing.com/flash/ecg_activity.html

Hansen, M. (2009). Using the computer to support health care and patient education. In T. L. Hebda & P. Czar (Eds.), *Handbook of informatics for nurses & healthcare professionals* (4th ed.). Upper Saddle River, NJ: Pearson Hall.

Hansen, M., Doherty, I., McCann, L., Oosthuizen, G., Hardy, K., Greig, S., … Windsor, J. (2007). *Medical interns' clinical skills acquisition and self-confidence levels: Enhanced via iPods?* Paper submitted for EdMedia 2008 Conference, Vienna, Austria.

Harden, J. K. (2003). Faculty and student experiences with web-based discussion groups in a large lecture setting. *Nurse Educator, 28*(1), 26–30.

Hart, M. D. (2008). Informatics competency and development within the US nursing population workforce: A systematic literature review. *Computers, Informatics, Nursing, 26*(6), 320–329.

Healthcare Information and Management Systems Society (HIMSS). (2011). *2011 nursing informatics workforce survey.* Retrieved from http://www.himss.org/content/files/2011HIMSSNursing InformaticsWorkforceSurvey.pdf

Hebda, T., & Czar, P. (2009). *Handbook of informatics for nurses & healthcare professionals* (4th ed.). Upper Saddle River, NJ: Prentice-Hall, Inc.

Kaminiski, J. (2009, Summer). Folksonomies boost web 2.0 functionality. *Online Journal of Nursing Informatics, 13*(2), p. 1. Retrieved from http://ojni.org/13_2/june.pdf

Kennedy, R. (2003). The nursing shortage and the role of technology. *Nursing Outlook, 51*(3), S33–S34.

Im, Y., & Lee, O. (2003). Pedagogical implications of online discussion for preservice teacher training. *Journal of Research on Technology in Education, 36*(2), 155.

International Society for Technology in Education (ISTE). (1997–2010). Retrieved from http://www.iste.org/

iPod touch. (2010). *iPod touch 3.1 software update.* Retrieved from http://www.apple.com/ipodtouch/software-update.html

Kaminski, J. (2009). Folksonomies boost web 2.0 functionality. *Online Journal of Nursing Informatics, 13*(2), 1.

Kaplan-Leiserson, E. (2005). Trend: Podcasting in academic and corporate learning. *Learning Circuits.* Retrieved from http://www.learningcircuits.org/

Kardong-Edgren, S. E., Oermann, M. H., Ha, Y., Tennant, M. N., Snelson, C., Hallmark, E., … Hurd, D. (2009). Using a wiki in nursing education and research. *International Journal of Nursing Education Scholarship, 6*(1), 848–923. Retrieved from http://www.bepress.com/ijnes/vol6/iss1/art6/

Killam, L., & Carter, L. (2010). Challenges to the student nurse on clinical placement in the rural setting: A review of the literature. *Rural & Remote Health, 10*(3), 1–14.

Kilmon, C. A., Brown, L., Ghosh, S., & Mikitiuk, A. (2010). Immersive virtual reality simulations in nursing education. *Nursing Education Perspectives, 31*(5), 314–317.

Kiteley, R. J., & Ormrod, G. (2009). Towards a team-based, collaborative approach to embedding e-learning within undergraduate nursing programmes. *Nurse Education Today, 29*(6), 623–629.

Korte, P., Bopp, A., Kendall, M., Carlson, S., Saxton, R., Bopp, A., & Smith, C. (2006). Technology in nursing education: Clinical evaluation, assessment, and resources at the point of care. *Nursing Education Perspectives.* Retrieved from http://findarticles.com/p/articles/mi_hb3317/is_2_27/ai_n29262109/

Kozlowski, D. (2002). Using online learning in a traditional face-to-face environment. *Computers in Nursing, 20*(1), 23–30.

Kozlowski, D. (2004). Factors for consideration in the development and implementation of an online RN-BSN course: Faculty and student perceptions. *Computers, Informatics, Nursing, 22*(1), 34–43.

Lane, C. (2006). *Podcasting at the UW: An evaluation of current use.* Retrieved from catalyst.washington.edu/research_development/papers/2006/podcasting_report.pdf

Lapinsky, S. E., Holt, D., Hallett, D., Abdolell, M., & Adhikari, N. K. (2008). Survey of information technology in intensive care units in Ontario, Canada. *BMC Medical Informatics and Decision Making, 8*(5). doi:10.1186/1472-6947-8-5

Lasater, K. (2007). High-fidelity simulation and the development of clinical judgment: Students' experiences. *Journal of Nursing Education, 46*(6). Retrieved from http://131.193.130.213/media//Lasater_JNE2007.pdf

Maag, M. (2004). The effectiveness of an interactive multimedial learning tool on nursing students' math knowledge and self-efficacy. *Computers, Informatics, Nursing, 22*(1), 26–33.

Maag, M. (2006). Podcasting and MP3 players: Emerging education technologies. *Computers, Informatics, Nursing, 24*(1), 9–13.

Malan, D. J. (2007). Podcasting computer science E-1. *SIGCSE'07,* 389–393.

Mancuso, J. (2009). Perceptions of distance education among nursing faculty members in North America. *Nursing & Health Sciences, 11*(2), 194–205. doi:10.1111/j.1442-2018.2009.00456.x

Massachusetts Institute of Technology. (2006). *Peer comparison of course/learning management systems, course materials life cycle, and related costs.* Retrieved from http://web.mit.edu/emcc/www/MIT-WCET-C-LMS-Final-Report-07-19-06.pdf

Mayer, R. E. (2001). *Multimedia learning.* New York: Cambridge University Press.

McKenna, L. G., & Samarawickrema, R. G. (2003). Crossing cultural boundaries: Flexible approaches and nurse education. *Computers, Informatics, Nursing, 21*(5), 259–264.

Murray, P. J., & Maag, M. (2006). Towards health informatics 2.0: Blogs, podcasts and web 2.0 applications in nursing and health informatics education and professional collaboration. A discussion paper.

NASA multimedia page. (2010, March 4). Retrieved from http://www.nasa.gov/multimedia/index.html

NETS for students. (2007). *From the international national society website.* Retrieved from http://www.iste
.org/content/navigationmenu/NETS/forstudents/2007standards/nets_ for_students_2007.htm

New York Times. (n.d.). Retrieved from http://www.nytimes.com/pages/multimedia/

NIC University Website. (2010). http://www.nicuniversity.org/lectures.asp

Nurse.com. (2010). *Nursing continuing education requirements by state.* Retrieved from http://
ce.nurse.com/RStateReqmnt.aspx

O'Reilly, T. (2005). *Design patterns and business models for the next generation of software retrieved from
the internet.* Retrieved from http://oreilly.com/web2/archive/what-is-web-20.html

Palmer, E. J., & Devitt, P. G. (2007). A method of creating interactive content for the iPod, and its
potential use as a learning tool: Technical advances. *BMC Medical Education, 7*(32). Retrieved from
http://www.ncbi.nlm.nih.gov/pmc/articles/PMC2174451/

Pimentel, J. R. (1999). Design of net-learning systems based on experiential learning. *Journal of Asynchronous Learning Networks, 3*(2), 64–90. Retrieved from http://www.aln.org/publications/jaln/v3n2/
v3n2_pimentel.asp

Plack, M. M., Dunfee, H., Rindflesch, A., & Driscoll, M. (2008). Virtual action learning sets: A model for
facilitating reflection in the clinical setting. *Journal of Physical Therapy Education, 22*(3), 33–42.

Poirrier, G. P., Wills, E. M., Broussard, P. C., & Payne, R. L. (1996). Nursing information systems: Applications in nursing curricula. *Nurse Educator, 21*(1), 18–22.

Poll Everywhere. (2010). *Live audience polling.* Retrieved from http://www.polleverywhere.com/

Prensky, M. (2001, October). Digital natives, digital immigrants. *On the horizon* (Vol. 9, No. 5), MCB
University Press.

Prensky, M. (2004). *The emerging online life of the digital native: What they do differently because of technology, and how they do it.* Retrieved from http://www.marcprensky.com/writing/default.asp

Price, J. (n.d.). *Implementing an EHR in your curriculum.* Retrieved from www.laerdaltraining.com/
sun/2011/local/.../ppt/ehr_curriculum.ppt

Quality and Safety Education for Nurses Project. (2010). *Quality/safety competencies.* Robert Woods
Johnson Foundation. Retrieved from http://www.qsen.org/definition.php?id=6

Ravert, P. (2002). An integrative review of computer-based simulation in the education process.
Computers, Informatics, Nursing, 20(5), 203–208.

Ravert, P. (2008). Patient simulator sessions and critical thinking. *Journal of Nursing Education, 47*(12),
557–562.

Rhodes, M., & Curran, C. (2005). Use of the human patient simulator to teach clinical judgment skills in a
baccalaureate nursing program. *Computers, Informatics, Nursing, 23*(5), 256–262.

Rogers, D. (2007). High-fidelity patient simulation: A descriptive white paper report. *Healthcare
Simulation Strategies.* Retrieved from http://sim-strategies.com/downloads/
Simulation%20White%20 Paper2.pdf

Ross, G. D., & Tuovinen, J. E. (2001). Deep versus surface learning with multimedia in nursing education.
Computers in Nursing, 19(5), 213–223.

Rossignol, M., & Scollin, P. (2001). Piloting use of computerized practice tests. *Computers in Nursing,
19*(5), 206–212.

Sapnas, K. G., Walsh, S. M., Vilberg, W., Livingstone, P., Asher, M. E., Dlugasch., & Villanueva, N. E. (2002).
Using web technology in graduate and undergraduate nursing education. *Computers, Informatics,
Nursing Plus, 5*(2), 1, 33–37.

Schlairet, M. C., & Pollock, J. W. (2010). Equivalence testing of traditional and simulated clinical experiences:
Undergraduate nursing students' knowledge acquisition. *Journal of Nursing Education, 49*(1), 43–47.

Schmidt, B., & Stewart, S. (2010). Implementing the virtual world of second life into community nursing
theory and clinical courses. *Nurse Educator, 35*(2), 74–78.

Schutt, M. A., & Hightower, B. (2009). Enhancing RN-to-BSN students' information literacy skills
through the use of instructional technology. *Journal of Nursing Education, 48*(5), 248.

Second Health: The Future of Healthcare Communication. (n.d.). Retrieved from http://secondhealth
.wordpress.com/clinical-scenarios/

Sharma, P. (2008). *Core characteristics of web 2.0 services.* Retrieved from http://www.techpluto.com/
web-20-services/

Shih-Wei, C., & Chien-Hung, L. (2005). *Learning effectiveness in web-based technology-mediated virtual
learning environment, HICSS* (Vol. 1, p. 3a). Proceedings of the 38th Annual Hawaii International

Conference on System Sciences (HICSS'05)—Track 1. http://doi.ieeecomputersociety
.org/10.1109/HICSS.2005.385.

Simpson, R. L. (2002). Virtual reality revolution: Technology changes nursing education. *Nursing Management, 33*(9), 14–15.

Skiba, D. J. (2007a). Nursing education 2.0: YouTube. *Nursing Education Perspectives, 28*(2), 100–102.

Skiba, D. J. (2007b). Nursing education 2.0: Second life. *Nursing Education Perspectives, 28*(3), 156–157.

Smith-Stoner, M., & Willer, A. (2003). Video streaming in nursing education. *Nurse Educator, 28*(2), 66–70.

Southernwood, J. (2008). Distance learning: The future of continuing professional development. *Community Practitioner, 81*(10), 21–23.

St. Jude Medical opens tech center for physicians in Beijing. (2011). *Medical Device Daily, 15*(56), 1–8.

Sternberger, C., & Meyer, L. (2001). Hypermedia-assisted instruction: Authoring with learning guidelines. *Computers in Nursing, 19*(2), 69–74.

Sudasassi, M. (2010, February 1). College of nursing and health sciences to dedicate new $34 million building Feb. 4. *Florida University News.* Retrieved from http://news.fiu.edu/2010/02/college-of-nursing-and-health-sciences-to-dedicate-new-34-million-building-feb-4/

Swan, K. (2003). Learning effectiveness: What the research tells us. In J. Bourne & J. C. Moore (Eds.), *Elements of quality online education, practice and direction* (pp. 13–45). Needham, MA: Sloan Center for Online Education.

Telles Filho, P. C., & Cassiani, S. H. (2008). Creation and evaluation cycle of a distance module for nursing undergraduates, named "medication administration." *Latin American Journal of Nursing, 16*(1), 78–85.

Tuoriniemi, P., & Schott-Baer, D. (2008). Implementing a high-fidelity simulation program in a community college setting. *Nursing Education Perspectives, 29*(2), 105–109.

Turning Technologies. (2010). *Response technology for mobile devices, laptops, and desktops.* Retrieved from http://www.turningtechnologies.com/

University of Tasmania School of Nursing and Midwifery. (2007). Retrieved from http://www.m2hnursing.com/

U.S. Department of Health and Human Services Centers for Disease Control and Prevention (CDC). (2011). *Education & training: Immunization courses: Broadcasts, webcasts, and self study.* Retrieved from http://www.cdc.gov/vaccines/ed/courses.htm

U.S. Department of Health and Human Services Centers for Disease Control and Prevention (CDC). (n.d.). *Public health training network glossary of selected distance learning terms and phrases.* Retrieved from http://www2.cdc.gov/phtn/lingo.asp

Walls, S. M., Kucsera, J. V., Walker, J. D., Acee, T. W., McVaugh, N. K., & Robinson, D. H. (2010). Podcasting in education: Are students as ready and eager as we think they are? *Computers & Education, 54*, 371–378. doi:10.1016/j.compedu.2009.08.018

Web 2.0 innovations. (2008). *2008's most popular web 2.0 sites ranking has been released.* Retrieved from http://web2innovations.com/

Wolfe, M. (2007). Broadband videoconferencing as knowledge management tool. *Journal of Knowledge Management, 11*(2), 118–138.

Wikipedia (2007). Virtual learning environment. Retrieved September 17, 2007, from http://en.wikipedia.org/wiki/Virtual_learning_environment/en.wiktionary.org/wiki/Special:Search?search=push+technology+&go=Go

Wikipedia. (2010, April 16). *Wiki.* Retrieved from http://en.wikipedia.org/wiki/Wiki

Wikipedia. (2011a, December 4). *Skype.* Retrieved from http://en.wikipedia.org/wiki/Skype

Wikipedia. (2011b, June 3). *Web 2.0.* Retrieved from http://en.wikipedia.org/wiki/Web_2.0

Wikipedia. (2011c, December 1). *Web conferencing.* Retrieved from http://en.wikipedia.org/wiki/Web_conferencing_

Wikipedia. (2011d, November 23). *Push technology.* Retrieved from http://en.wikipedia.org/wiki/Push_technology

Yeager, S. T., & Gotwals, B. (2009). Incorporating high-fidelity simulation technology into community health nursing education. *Clinical Simulation in Nursing.* doi:10.1016/j.ecns.2009.07.004

CHAPTER 24

Consumer Education and Informatics

After completing this chapter, you should be able to:

1. Appreciate the role that online health information seeking plays in health management for consumers.

2. Acknowledge consumer health informatics as a subspecialty of medical informatics.

3. Recognize driving factors behind the development of consumer health informatics.

4. Compare and contrast ways that consumer health informatics is changing the way that health advice and care is sought and delivered.

5. Demonstrate familiarity with issues associated with consumer health informatics that have the potential to negatively impact access to care or the ability to self manage care.

6. Distinguish key features as well as relative advantages and disadvantages between various consumer health informatics applications.

7. Examine the role that the informaticist plays in the design, adoption and use of consumer health informatics applications.

Imagine that you get a call from your Aunt Mary asking you to help her decide about whether to keep taking her blood pressure medicine. Your aunt receives daily e-mails from a women's health Web site and recently has read that the medication that her doctor recommended for her can cause "a foggy brain." She "googled" "high blood pressure remedies" and found that garlic pills are recommended as a natural alternative to prescription medication. Your aunt has tried to reach her physician, but can't get a visit appointment for another 4 weeks.

If this scenario seems far-fetched, guess again. In 2007, a survey by the Center for Studying Health System Change noted that approximately 56% of all American adults, approximately 122 million people, reported seeking online information about a personal health concern during the previous 12 months, up significantly from 38% (about 72 million people) in 2001 (Tu & Cohen 2008). This explosion of online healthcare information seeking has been propelled by the general public's adoption of Internet technologies. The 2007 Pew Internet and American Life Report found that 74% of American adults (ages 18 and older) use the Internet, 60% of American adults use broadband connections at home, and 55% of American adults connect to the Internet wirelessly, either through a connection via their laptops or through their handheld device like a smart phone.

Your Aunt Mary is one of a growing number of **e-patients** or individuals who assume access to healthcare information 24/7 and expect to be a partner in healthcare decision making. It is clear that healthcare delivery is changing to include an increased emphasis on this partnership through consumer healthcare services that link information technologies, business structures, strategies, processes, and people. A new field termed *consumer health informatics (CHI)* has emerged as "a subspecialty of medical informatics which studies from a patient/consumer perspective the use of electronic information and communication to improve medical outcomes and the healthcare decision-making process" (American Medical Informatics Association, Consumer Health Informatics Working Group 2009). This chapter describes the evolution of CHI and further discusses existing and emerging applications, associated issues, and the evolving role of the healthcare professional in a consumer-driven and technology-centric healthcare delivery system.

EVOLUTION

Gunther Eysenbach (2000), a pioneer in **consumer health informatics (CHI)**, described a paradigm change in healthcare delivery from clinical medicine in the Industrial Age to public health in the Information Age. Fueled in part by the consumerism-movement in the 1970s, the proliferation of self-help programs of the 1980s, the growing use of the Internet in the 1990s (McDaniel, 2006), and the recent emergence of evidence-based medicine (Eysenbach, 2000), there has been a shift in healthcare decision-making practices from clinicians to patients (consumers). This movement to consumer-driven healthcare decision making has resulted in a greater need for consumer-centric healthcare information.

As a result, consumers are increasingly using information technology tools that facilitate interactive and personalized communication with their healthcare practitioners. Technology tools have the capability to assist in the creation of consumer-centric healthcare information that can be specifically customized or tailored for each individual patient. Eakin, Brady, and Lusk (2001) described the factors that contribute to a truly tailored message:

- Data are collected from individual consumers regarding their healthcare characteristics and behaviors and health profile is created.
- Healthcare information containing evidence-based practices must be available in an electronically retrievable format.
- A set of decision-making rules created from the information collected from the consumer is used to craft tailored messages to fit the consumer's specific needs.
- A process is established for easily sending the message (practitioner) and receiving the message (consumer) in a way that is clear to each individual.

TABLE 24–1   Messaging Types, Definitions, and Examples

Messaging Type	Definition	Example
Standard	Describes the usual care an individual might receive	You'll likely have your blood pressure taken as part of a routine doctor's appointment.
General	Expresses health behavior that is considered to fit everyone	Ask your doctor for a blood pressure reading at least every two years starting at age 20.
Targeted	Includes information that is directed to a specific subset of the general population	The doctor will likely recommend more frequent readings if you've already been diagnosed with high blood pressure, pre-hypertension, or other risk factors for cardiovascular disease.
Personalized	Contains general care for a specific condition	If you have kidney disease that can cause a sudden rise in blood pressure, also known as secondary hypertension, you may need your blood pressure checked more frequently. Ask your doctor how often you should have your blood pressure.
Tailored	Consists of information that has been specifically adapted to an individual based on their healthcare behaviors and unique characteristics	You have been taking corticosteroid medications to treat your arthritis, your cortisol levels are high, you are complaining of being excessively fatigued, and you are experiencing an increase in your blood pressure from your normal of 116/80 to 150/110. These symptoms are consistent with the symptoms that may indicate Cushing's syndrome; see your doctor for an evaluation.

Reprinted from Schlachta-Fairchild, L., and Elfrink, V. (2004). Models of Health Care and the Consumer Perspective of Telehealth in the Information Age. In *Consumer Informatics: Applications and Strategies in Cyber Health Care*. R. Nelson & M. J. Ball (Eds.) (95–105). New York: Springer, by permission of Springer.

To better understand the power of this made-to-order approach to healthcare decision making, examples of messaging types are provided in Table 24–1 (Schlachta-Fairchild & Elfrink 2004). The examples are adapted from the Mayo Clinic consumer health Web site for high blood pressure (Mayo Clinic Staff 2011).

As consumer health has evolved, the personal health information needs of the consumer have also expanded. Ferguson (2002) outlined 10 levels in which online healthcare consumers or e-patients access and use health-related information.

Level 1. Search for health information: Consumers engage in "search and rescue" missions related to their newly diagnosed diseases and disorders. They prepare for doctors' appointments by searching for information on the drugs and other treatments. These activities are not limited to themselves but are also geared toward helping others. According to the Pew Internet and American Life Survey, more e-patients search for medical information for friends and family members (81%) than for themselves.

Level 2. Exchange e-mail with family members and friends: Consumers use e-mail to communicate with loved ones, about their healthcare issues, and to further seek feedback, advice, and support. In a true network, loved ones respond with care and concern and may further recommend specific alternative healthcare resources.

Level 3. Seek guidance from online patient-helpers: When confronting a new healthcare issue or condition, consumers may seek out and communicate online with another patient who has experienced the same condition. Sometimes referred to as patient-helpers, these folks can offer support and point a newly diagnosed patient to the best online information.

Level 4. Participate in online support groups: Many healthcare consumers participate in online support. There are Web sites devoted to a single medical condition (e.g., HIV or diabetes) that allow individuals to share stories and ask questions through communications on Web site forums or electronic mailing lists.

Level 5. Join with other online consumers to research their shared concerns: Some consumer support groups organize themselves into online work groups and examine the healthcare literature, while other groups carry this mission further and actually conduct informal or more formal research studies.

Level 6. Use online medical guidance systems: Online healthcare consumers can access Web sites where they can enter the names of all the drugs they are currently taking and receive information of all possible drug interactions. There are sites where patients can answer a series of healthcare profile questions and receive a listing of possible risk factors, or diagnoses associated with some healthcare conditions. There are also online directories where patients find detailed information about individual doctors and hospitals, for example, Joint Commission (JCAHO) hospital ratings, patient evaluations, and reports of malpractice settlements.

Level 7. Interact with volunteer online health professionals: Online patients can send their questions by e-mail to health professionals they have found on the Internet, or they may visit healthcare Web sites (e.g., WebMD), where healthcare clinicians are available to answer health-related questions.

Level 8. Use the paid services of online medical advisors and consultants: Some consumers use online-only services now offered by healthcare practitioners. They may pay for a second opinion or seek answers to their personal healthcare questions. It is becoming popular to seek the advice of an online personal trainer, nutritionist, or weight loss coach. Online consumers might even engage an e-counselor and participate in virtual therapy sessions.

Level 9. Engage in electronic conversations with their local clinicians: There is an increasing number of online consumers who e-mail or communicate via other electronic means with their local brick-and-mortar healthcare provider. The content of these communications often looks like that of a practitioner–patient phone call to solve an immediate problem, but can also provide a means for consumers to prepare questions for a future visit.

Level 10. Receive one-way electronic messages from their clinicians: Some health professionals use information technology tools to send their patients unrequested messages that are not interactive; instead, they may provide targeted behavioral change or patient education materials of the doctor's choosing. Ferguson (2002) noted that the effectiveness of these "pushed messages" may be increased by presenting an "opt-in" approach with feedback or through a more interactive approach, such as described in Level 9.

Today, the trends indicate that electronic tailored information services will continue to become more mainstream as the Information Age evolves. National initiatives such as Healthy People 2020 clearly illustrate this trend. The 2010 release of Healthy People in Health Communities consumer brochure cites new features as "replacing traditional print publication with an interactive Web site ... that allows users to tailor information to their needs and explore evidence-based resources for implementation" (Healthy People 2020, 2010). Because a consumer-centric electronic healthcare record provides a natural base for tailored messages, there will be advances in health education that links personal health information, online information, databases and decision support tools, which in turn will continue to produce consumer-based healthcare products of value.

ISSUES

Your Aunt Mary can't verify the Web site address that describes garlic as a remedy for high blood pressure. She can only show you the post from someone in her online discussion group for the Web site, The Natural Way of Women. Someone in the group suggests an online video to watch, which your Aunt Mary can't play because of her dial-up connection to the Internet. Aunt Mary says that she has received e-mails from other Web sites asking her to provide details of her health history. Your aunt is concerned that her personal information might get into the wrong hands.

Consumers face these types of situations daily in their quest for online healthcare information. They are indicative of several issues associated with CHI. This section discusses the issues of health literacy, disparity in access, and privacy and security.

Health Literacy

Health literacy is becoming increasingly important as consumers directly interact with a complex health system to better manage their own health. Health literacy is defined in *Healthy People 2010* as "the degree to which individuals have the capacity to obtain, process, and understand basic health information and services needed to make appropriate health decisions" (Healthy People 2010). The report goes on to note that consumers trying to make informed decisions are often faced with complex information and treatment choices. In order to ultimately make their decisions, consumers must first carry out a number of tasks, including the ability to locate and evaluate healthcare information.

Locating and evaluating healthcare information have been made more complex due to its rapid growth in volume and availability. Lorence and Abraham (2008) reported that there are over 100,000 indexed health-related Web sites, which health information seekers are likely to visit daily. Consumers have access to a wide range of resources that have the potential for informing their healthcare decisions and thus promoting a greater responsibility for self-care. Although there is agreement that the Internet is a boon for consumers because they have easier access to information, clinicians are also concerned that the poor quality of some information on the Web has the potential to undermine informed decision making. There are growing concerns about the quality, timeliness, and potential misinterpretation of health information available on the Web. These concerns are driving the development of a national and international quality standards agenda to help health professionals and consumers alike access and evaluate high-quality online health information that is accurate, current, valid, appropriate, intelligible, and free of bias (Health on the Net 2008).

Discriminating between what is evidence-based information and commercial rhetoric can be difficult. Many reputable Internet-based healthcare resources and Web sites, including commercial and other privately developed Web sites, meet the Health on the Net (HON) and other quality standards criteria such as those put forth from the American Medical Association (Winkler et al. 2000). However, generally, the most trusted online healthcare resources have been found to be associated with medical schools, medical centers, and federal government Web sites.

Research by Toms and Latter (2007) described how consumers make use of search engines. Their study found that consumers most often initiated their search using a keyword search in a trial and error way, which did not always lead to immediate success. Another study (Lorence & Abraham, 2008) found that the consumers' use of a search engine potentially influenced the types of information they retrieve. Generally, consumers who use healthfinder.gov, a search engine developed by the U.S. Department of Health and Human Services (2011), retrieve more .gov and .org sites than the Google search engine, which returned mostly commercial sites. Eysenbach and Dipegen (2001) described the process of sifting through the volume of information found on Web sites as similar to "drinking through a fire hydrant" (p. 12).

Evaluating the quality of online health information requires literacy skills that are grounded in knowledge about technology and health. Glassman (2008) noted a mounting need for e-health literacy as an indicator of the need to better evaluate the quality of information and services delivered using information technology tools. Further, Healthy People 2010 included a specific goal for improved consumer health literacy. This health goal is related to the need for e-health literacy and the role that it can play in informed decision making. Glassman added that not only must consumers possess basic reading skills in their search for online healthcare resources, they must also have competency in

- Visual literacy (ability to understand graphs, read a label or other visual information),
- Computer literacy (ability to operate a computer),
- Information literacy (ability to obtain and apply relevant information).

In summary, the widespread availability and use of online healthcare resources by consumers have clear benefits and some disadvantages. Quality standards need to be in place to prevent the propagation of inaccurate or outdated online health information. Further, improving e-health literacy among consumers can help them to make decisions based on accurate and timely information.

Disparity in Access

The disparity in access to information technology tools and electronic healthcare resources is commonly referred to as the "digital divide" (U.S. Department of Commerce 1999). The digital divide becomes more critical as the amount and variety of health resources available on the Web increase and as consumers need more sophisticated skills to use electronic resources (Eng et al. 1998). Equitably distributed online healthcare resources, skill in using these resources, and a robust telecommunications infrastructure can contribute to the closing of the digital divide and the overarching goal of Healthy People 2010 to eliminate health disparities.

To understand the importance of closing this divide, consider the impact of widespread access to interactive multimedia healthcare resources. The merging of media (computers, telephones, television, radio, video, print, and audio) and the evolution of the Internet have created a nearly universally networked telecommunication infrastructure. This infrastructure facilitates access to an expanse of health information and health-related services by extending the reach of health communication delivery. The Internet has increased the communication choices available for health practitioners to reach consumers and for consumers to interact with health practitioners and with each other, for example, in online discussion groups.

The Healthy People 2010 Report cites several advantages of using interactive multimedia messages for health communication (Healthy People 2020 2010). For example, (1) accessing personalized health information, (2) getting health information and services 24/7, (3) distributing and updating healthcare content in an efficient and timely manner, (4) contacting real-time expert decision support, and (5) choosing options for treatment.

Despite a rise in the access to these technologies, however, their availability is not ubiquitous. Often individuals who are the most vulnerable continue to have the least access to information, communication technologies, healthcare, and supporting social services. The Healthy People 2010 report cautions of a limited impact of information technologies if underserved communities lack access. While the full health impact of interactive and customized multimedia messages has yet to be determined, interactive communication technologies are increasingly being used to exchange information and support clinical care. Improving access to online healthcare resources and interactive communication has the potential not only to influence the delivery of health services but also to improve health literacy and health status of consumers (Glassman 2008).

Privacy and Security

Another issue in CHI is related to protecting the privacy and security of personal health information. Privacy is defined by the Office of the National Coordinator (ONC) as "an individual's interest in protecting his or her individually identifiable health information and the corresponding obligation of those persons and entities accessing, using or disclosing that information to respect those interests through fair information practices" (ONC 2008). Security is differentiated as "the protection of information and information systems from unauthorized access, use, disclosure, disruption, modification or destruction in order to ensure the integrity, confidentiality and availability of information" (NIST 2002).

The privacy and the security of their personal health information are critical to consumers in any medium; however, individuals can feel particularly vulnerable when their health information is collected and stored electronically and available online. A study conducted by the California Healthcare Foundation found that the privacy policies and practices of many notable consumer health Web sites were deficient in their protection of an individual's healthcare information (Goldman, Hudson, & Smith 2000). This study also found the following: (1) users were not anonymous; (2) privacy policies did not truly protect consumers; (3) privacy policies and practices did not always match, (4) personal health information was not adequately protected, and (5) liability policies were not adequate (Jamison et al., 2006).

Consumer Web sites that adhere to the HON Code of Conduct have been proactive regarding consumers' privacy and security concerns. However, as more interactive healthcare technologies are used, consumer confidence about privacy and security of their information will be challenged (Healthy People 2010). To date, it remains unclear how the privacy and security regulations established by the Health Insurance Portability and Accountability Act of 1996 (HIPAA) will be fully implemented with consumer health Web sites and interactive health communication.

In the future, privacy and security efforts will face even bigger challenges, as personal health information will increasingly be electronically collected and stored during both clinical and nonclinical encounters in a variety of settings, such as schools, mobile clinics, public places, and homes. These data, while de-identified in some instances, will be made available for administrative, financial, clinical, and research purposes. Policies and procedures to protect consumers' information will need to ensure a balance between privacy, confidentiality, and secure access by appropriate parties.

APPLICATIONS

Your Aunt Mary is able to get an appointment with her physician and discuss her concerns. When Aunt Mary returns from her physician's appointment she shows you the new home blood pressure monitor she has been given to check her blood pressure on a daily basis. Because Aunt Mary lives 60 miles from her physician's office you express concern regarding her ability to bring logs in for review. She replies, "Oh, I don't need to bring them anywhere! When I check my blood pressure the results get sent right to them!"

The model of care that your Aunt Mary is using differs from traditional models for chronic disease management. She is using CHI tools. CHI tools include those that the consumer selects and those that are provided by healthcare providers. Consumer-selected tools are further described as free-standing **personal health records** (PHR), smart phone applications, or social networking tools. These technologies differ from those that the healthcare providers might utilize, such as home telehealth monitoring or a PHR associated with the provider's electronic medical record system. Selected CHI applications from categories are described in this section.

Personal Health Records

Today's healthcare consumers are used to having ready access to computerized personal information. Most have utilized automated teller machines (ATM) to access financial information, entered credit card information at online shopping sites, or registered for events using Web portals. However, these same individuals often do not have online access to manage personal health information. This lack of access has been linked to quality and safety issues. In 2001, the Institutes of Medicine described changes needed to enhance safety and quality of healthcare in the United States. Included in those recommendations was patients having "unfettered access to their own medical information" (Committee on Quality of Healthcare in America & Institute of Medicine, 2001).

Despite the growing need for PHRs, there is little agreement on the definition of the PHR. A white paper published by the American Medical Informatics Association utilized a definition developed by the Markle Foundation which defined the PHR as:

> An electronic application through which individuals can access, manage and share their health information, and that of others for whom they are authorized, in a private, secure, and confidential environment. (Markle Foundation 2003)

The Council on Clinical Information Technology of the American Academy of Pediatrics, in its definition of the PHR, specifies that the PHR is a "repository of information from multiple sources" that might include the patient, family, guardians, physicians, and other healthcare providers but is controlled by the individual or designated guardian (Council on Clinical Information Technology 2009).

One key concept to using PHRs is to differentiate them from the electronic medical record (EMR). EMRs are owned, managed, and maintained by the provider while the consumer manages information in the PHR. Consumers typically do not have permission to enter information in the EMR, but might be the major contributor to their PHR. Although PHRs can be paper-based, computer-based and Internet-based, this discussion will center on Internet-based PHRs.

There are two major types of PHRs available, one that is linked to the EMR and the free-standing PHR that is not connected to an EMR. More and more healthcare providers are providing consumers with access to a PHR that is directly connected to the EMR. This provides a situation where the consumer may be able to view information in the EMR along with the ability to utilize online appointment scheduling, secure messaging, and prescription refills. In some cases, consumers can add information to the EMR. Most of EMR vendors now offer some form of PHR that is integrated with their EMR offering.

Consumers who use a free-standing PHR must enter and manage all data themselves. While this provides greater freedom for the consumer, there has been concern voiced that users may not update a free-standing PHR as often as needed or may enter incorrect information (Tang, Ash, Bates, Overhage, & Sands 2006). Widespread use of PHRs cannot be accomplished until these and other fundamental items described below are resolved.

As with EMRs, safety and security of data are of vital importance. In the case of the PHR, where the consumer enters and manages information, additional issues must be addressed. These include rights to access to information entered by adolescents in pediatric practice when sensitive information is entered (Council on Clinical Information Technology 2009), interoperability, data security, and fair access (Kahn, Aulakh, & Bosworth 2009). PHRs that are interoperable with an EMR allow consumers to edit information; standards for notification when data are edited have not yet been widely implemented and must be developed.

Social Networking

Growth of social networking Web sites such as MySpace and Facebook has expanded to include use by individuals seeking information and support for healthcare issues. Social networking groups focusing on particular medical conditions are being accessed by a significant number of health consumers seeking information or support. Following an evaluation of health-related groups on Facebook, four areas of concern were noted: (1) scientific content, (2) anxiety generation, (3) confidentiality issues, and (4) research ethics issues when social networking sites are used to recruit research participants (Farmer, Bruckner Holt, Cook, & Hearing 2009).

Social networking tools specific to health consumers are becoming an important tool for self-management of chronic conditions. Two popular social network sites are inspire.com and patientslikeme.com; both are described here. Inspire.com (Frost & Massagli 2008) is a social networking site designed for individuals and/or caregivers with a variety of health conditions.

Individuals registered at the site can create a profile, join groups focused on different aspects surrounding chronic conditions, and share information.

Patientslikeme.com (http://www.patientslikeme.com) is another social networking site that provides a platform for individuals who have a specific health condition in common to share information about treatments, symptoms, and other issues. Health consumers utilize patientslikeme.com to share information regarding their health condition utilizing discussion boards as well as user access to other users' health profiles. Information is presented to users through graphs and other visual displays allowing for rapid access to information regarding medications, symptoms, and other information. Patientslikeme was initially developed for individuals with amyotrophic lateral sclerosis (ALS) to share information and provide support to families and each other. The site currently provides communities for individuals with ALS as well as a number of other chronic health conditions. Users create a profile that contains:

- Summary representation of current health status
- Diagram that maps functional impairment to areas of the body
- Personal photo
- Autobiographical statement
- Diagnosis history
- Series of charts

Members can then locate others with the same condition with shared medical experiences for discussion of profiles and reports. Data entered by users are aggregated to create graphs and charts to show how one is progressing compared to others wit are similar conditions. Analysis of patient use of the site revealed three categories of comments posted by users: targeted questions, advice and recommendations, and building support relationships. Figure 24–1 shows an example of compiled symptom data from one area of Patientslikeme.com.

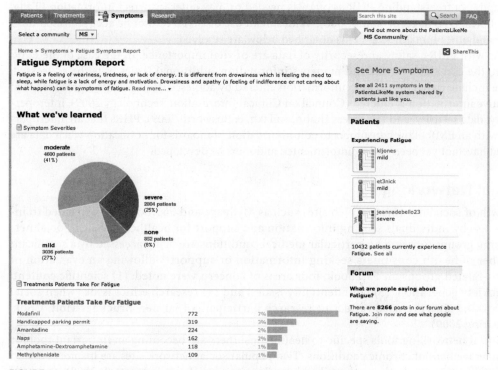

FIGURE 24–1 • Example of Compiled Symptom Data from Patientslikeme.com.
Source: www.patientslikeme.com

Home Telemedicine

The term *home telemedicine* encompasses a number of different tools that can be utilized by consumers to self-monitor and self-manage health conditions. These tools help or enable? home monitoring of vital signs, blood glucose monitoring, Web-based video conferencing, and patient-specific educational sessions. One such tool, the Intel Health Guide is Already implied it is a home tool. (http://www.intel.com/healthcare/ps/healthguide/index.htm) used to provide consumers with a mechanism to better manage chronic health conditions at home (*East Bay Business Times* 2008). Intel Health Guide provides consumers with:

- Real-time interaction with healthcare providers
- Patient education materials that can be accessed as part of a scheduled session or at "teachable moments"
- Two-way video calls
- Integrated vital sign monitoring according to patient needs, including blood pressure monitors, glucometers, pulse oximetry, peak flow meters, and weight scales
- Audio-visual alerts and reminders (http://www.intel.com/healthcare/ps/healthguide/benefits.htm?id=239)

Other home telemedicine projects focus on management of a particular chronic condition but might not be applicable in socioeconomically diverse groups. The IDEATel project had a focus on management of diabetes mellitus (DM) in traditionally underserved communities. Participants in IDEATel were not required to have prior computer experience; home telemedicine equipment was provided by the study. Equipment included a computer with a modem connecting to the Internet through telephone lines, videoconferencing connections, a glucometer, and a blood pressure monitor that could upload results to the participant's EMR, and access to a personal health record that included secure messaging capabilities. Participants also had access to a diabetes-specific educational Web site. Training was provided for participants when the equipment was installed as well as throughout the study as deemed necessary by nurse case managers. Individuals in the intervention group had improvements in hemoglobin A1c, blood pressure, and lipid levels (Shea et al. 2009).

Smart Phone Technology

Use of smart phone service has become nearly universal in the United States. The widespread penetration of smart phones in the consumer market has prompted healthcare providers and business entrepreneurs to investigate how future healthcare services can be delivered using this platform. Like telehealth monitoring, smart phones move healthcare from a provider focus to a patient-centric focus. However, healthcare information and services delivered via smart phones will move one step further. Healthcare, like the patient, will be mobile! This technology holds promise for the future in patient groups who are used to using technology while on the go. For example, mobile healthcare has the potential to be especially useful for adolescents and teens with chronic illness such as asthma. Smart phone technology has the potential to utilize:

- Personalized diary
- Medical regimen information on schedules
- Automated system reminders and tailored messages
- Action plans
- Summary and detailed patient data
- Web portal with provider drill down capability
- Exception reports on noncompliant patients (for the provider)

Boland (2007) pointed out that adolescents tend to have strong smart phone use patterns, have a desire to be more mobile, and were more willing to carry a smaller device for self-management. For example, most adolescents are high-end users of texting. Most current smart phone technology now focuses on short message service (SMS) or text messaging. Use of SMS messaging has been studied in a pulmonary rehabilitation, where participants communicated exercise and symptom logs with clinic staff; preliminary data showed that the program resulted in increased exercise capacity (Nguyen, Gill, Wolpin, Steele, & Benditt 2009). Further, a recent systematic review of use of smart phones, particularly text messaging, showed that there was benefit in improving medication adherence, smoking cessation, and other measures of health outcomes (Krishna, Boren, & Balas 2009). These studies point to the potential for mobile healthcare delivery as a major force in the future.

In summary, many of the consumer health applications in current use focus on disease management. Traditionally, chronic disease management has focused on episodes of care where there is interaction between patients and providers during inpatient stays or visits to an ambulatory care provider. Your Aunt Mary is using health information technology to self-manage her care at home. This shift represents a growing trend in the use of health information technology and CHI tools such as personal health records, telemedicine, telehome health monitoring, social networking, and smart phone applications. There is no doubt that these tools will proliferate and have the potential to significantly impact consumer satisfaction with healthcare as well as health outcomes (Brennan & Starren 2006).

INFORMATICS SPECIALIST ROLES

As you talk to your Aunt Mary about her experience with her new "blood pressure computer," you learn more about how your Aunt Mary has been taught to use her digital monitoring device. You also take a few moments to check out its features and learn first hand how easy it is to use the monitoring device and how it helps your Aunt Mary to feel secure in her ability to communicate with her healthcare provider.

Your Aunt Mary's ability to easily use her blood pressure monitoring device is in part based on its ease of use and her understanding of how and when to use the device. The informatics specialist is in a unique position to promote the integration of consumer informatics into the mainstream of healthcare delivery. Expertise and education in healthcare delivery, human factors, and patient advocacy provides the informatics specialist with the tools to promote the widespread adoption of consumer informatics. This section describes the role of the informatics specialist as an educator about, designer of, and an advocate for the use of consumer informatics in healthcare delivery.

Informatics Specialist as Educator

Healthcare practitioners have a long history of providing health communication and education using a variety of nondigital media such as books and pamphlets (Keselman, Logan, Smith, Leroy, & Zeng-Tritler 2008). More recently, mass media such as newspapers, magazines, and television have been used to deliver health information to the general public. These multiple forms of media have been beneficial as means to effectively and efficiently deliver healthcare education to consumers; however, they have been limited in their one-way communication approach. It is the interactive power of the Internet that has had a major influence on the way that healthcare information is delivered, creating a need for an informatics specialist who can work comfortably in the world of technology and educational literacy.

Technology has provided the infrastructure by which consumers can now have two-way communication with their healthcare provider. However, there are obstacles to interactive technology-driven consumer health communication (Keselman et al. 2008; Zeng & Tse 2006), which revolve around the use of mismatches between consumer and professional healthcare terminology. Specifically, consumers often use common lay-terms such as a "hole in the heart" to describe a complex health condition but that same "hole" may be translated as an atrial septal defect (ASD) diagnosis by a healthcare practitioner. This combination of using vague lay-terms with medical jargon can result in missed or miscommunication. Some experts call this a "vocabulary gap," which forms a barrier for a consumer to using technology to access or send health information (Zeng & Tse 2006). One approach to eliminating this health communication barrier is the development of consumer health vocabularies (CHVs).

Experts (Keselman et al. 2008; Zeng & Tse 2006) note that the use of CHVs has the potential to benefit not only human understanding but also machine processing. Specifically, the use of CHV has the potential to help practitioners use terms that are easily understood and recognizable by the consumer. Conversely, computer systems that may not recognize lay health terms if they are not included in a controlled vocabulary such as the Unified Medical Language System (UMLS) would be able to process searches and retrieve information better if consumers used a standard recognized term.

The informatics specialist as educator can assist in these efforts by contributing to the design of consumer-friendly information retrieval tools, by designing electronic education that is readable at a sixth grade level and by providing consumers with helpful hints about vocabulary translations (hole in the heart *is an* atrial septal defect *or* ASD). Additionally, the informatics specialist as educator can assist in these efforts by including techniques from marketing, entertainment, and news media that will enhance the attractiveness or aesthetics of these healthcare communications.

Informatics Specialist as Designer

The informatics specialist as a designer of health information is in a distinctive position to create and promote the development of effective consumer health digital resources. Evaluation studies (e.g., Keselman, Logan, Smith, Leroy, & Zeng-Treitler 2008) have shown that useful consumer health resources anticipate users' needs and actions and present clear pathways to access information. Other experts (Moen, Gregory, & Brennan 2007) cite the importance of creating consumer health resources that address the assumptions, culture, or context of the consumer.

Evangelista et al. (2006) described a design process that begins with a needs assessment that is grounded in the consumers' needs. Guidelines for Web site development such as Usability. gov (http://www.usability.gov/) also point to the importance of starting with a solid needs assessment. The guidelines also describe the importance of an iterative approach where usability testing is employed throughout the design cycle.

Attention to end-users' needs varies in the design of consumer-health information; however, exemplars do exist. Ritter, Freed, and Haskett (2005) described a process where they performed a task analysis and examined work flow in the design of academic Web sites. The National Cancer Institute (Grama et al. 2005) used a multi-pronged approach to assess consumers' needs and in turn receive user feedback through the CancerNet Web site.

In 2004, iTelehealth completed an NIMH-funded national suicide prevention Web site that focused on designing tools and methodologies to search for authoritative resources that were tailored for the roles of specific intermediaries in the prevention of suicide. The project resulted in an interactive consumer-based Web site that tailored information according to the intermediary type and integrated a resource search feature that was based on combining condition-specific signs and symptoms. The clinical design process for the Preventing Suicide Network is described in Box 24–1.

In summary, the informatics specialist as designer of consumer health information needs to be mindful of end-users' needs and the context in which information is used. Mitchell, Fun, and McCray (2004) outlined three design principles that can serve to guide the informatics specialist in the design of health information: (1) make the site (or information) easy for the public to access with understandable content, (2) interrelate and integrate existing resources extending from consumer health resources to clinical and scientific resources, and (3) create an informatics

BOX 24–1 Case Study: The Preventing Suicide Network

The Preventing Suicide Network (PSN) was developed to provide tailored online resources for individuals in various roles who were intervening or interacting with someone who was suicidal. These role-specific individuals were identified as "intermediaries." The Web site team adopted a design approach linking multiple methods grounded in a traditional Web site performance framework and in an emerging philosophy that emphasized the site's information functionality to end-users. This combined method used participatory design (a strategy characterized by active engagement of the end-user "intermediaries" in various phases of the design) and prototype design (a strategy characterized by responding to scaled-down versions of parts of the product) to get input from actual end-users (see home page of the Web site below).

A multi-phased feedback approach was included in the initial design of the PSN to ensure that potential users would have input into the site's creation. In this multi-phased approach representative users were sought out to test and evaluate the site throughout the process.

Three outcomes were identified:

1. Accurate targeting and comprehensive identification of all intermediaries.
2. Accurate identification of communication relationships between the intermediaries based on mapping strategies.
3. Appropriate use of Web-based technology to provide tailored customized information and resources on suicide prevention to intermediaries.

These outcomes were achieved through pilot evaluation activities carried out by various stake holder groups and end-users such as (1) feedback from the American Association of Suicidology (AAS) Board, where technical approaches and clinical strategies were identified and decided; (2) feasibility interviews with stakeholders who represented the population of suicide prevention intermediaries, and (3) testing of the prototype with other experts and intermediaries who represent different user interests.

Findings from the evaluation activities contributed to specific features that were geared toward meeting the needs of consumers as intermediaries in suicide prevention. These features included:

Main Page Lay-Out
Easy-to-understand navigation links were used for Browse Information; Search Information; and Receive Tailored Information.

A "Lexis/Nexis" type of approach was taken in the organization of content from the main site. Not only was content organized according to the broad categories of Detection, Treatment, Education, and Research but also there was specific content within those pages that was sorted and organized according to intermediary type.

Preference Page
The Preference Page was developed to conduct a tailored search of authoritative resources in the National Library of Medicine. The Preference page reflected not only clinical risks and issues related to suicide, but included search terms most likely to yield information about a suicide-related topic.

Profile Page
The Profile page was developed to gather information about the "registered user" so that tailored resources could be searched for in an ongoing manner and that the results could be pushed via e-mail to the end-user.

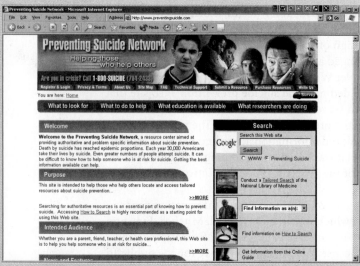

Screen shot reprinted with permission of iTelehealth Inc. Copyright © iTelehealth Inc. January 2010. May not be reproduced or further used without express written permission.

knowledge base to sustain the project. Finally, the ISD must be involved in ongoing evaluation studies to determine how to improve access and use by the public.

Information Specialist as Advocate

The healthcare informatics specialist has the potential to play an important advocacy role through the engagement of consumer use of information technology (IT) tools that support informed healthcare decision making. As the role of CHI has evolved, plans to promote its use have also increased. There is a growing body of scholarly knowledge that is helping to delineate factors for success and proposals such as the e-Health initiative that have been developed to identify best practices. Both efforts support CHI use and adoption.

e-Health Initiative In 2007, the e-Health Initiative (eHI) was developed by a group of stakeholders dedicated to promoting the use of information technology as a means of improving the quality, safety, and efficiency of managing and improving healthcare delivery. The *eHealth Initiative Blueprint: Building Consensus for Common Action* published in 2008 (http://www.ehealthinitiative.org/) represents the consensus of that group on a shared vision and a set of principles (see Figure 24–2).

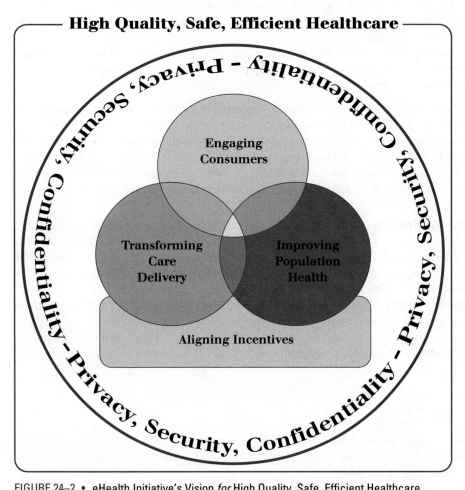

FIGURE 24–2 • eHealth Initiative's Vision *for* High Quality, Safe, Efficient Healthcare
Source: ehealthinitiative.org. (October 17, 2007). eHealth Initiative Blueprint: Building Consensus for Common Action. Available at http://www.ehealthinitiative.org/sites/default/files/file/eHiBlueprint-BuildingConsensusForCommonAction.pdf

Believing that consumers can be engaged in their healthcare by using information and tools that facilitate consumer action and informed decision making, the *eHealth Initiative Blueprint and e-Health Toolkit* were designed to provide helpful information to healthcare leaders in their pursuit of health IT and health information exchange adoption. Successful adoption includes a partnership between healthcare providers and consumers based on the following guiding principles.

- *Consumer engagement in healthcare.* Engaging consumers to use health IT and health information exchange practices to communicate with providers is critical to supporting informed decision making and improving healthcare.
- *Consumer access and control of personal health information.* Controlling access to his or her personal health information is the right of every consumer. Consumers have the right not only to access their personal health information but also to annotate and request corrections.
- *Consumer access to electronic health information tools and services.* Having access to tools that engage consumers through the mobilization of electronic health information should be universal. These tools should also be designed explicitly to meet the needs of diverse consumer groups, including those who are poor, rural, older, physically disabled, or do not speak English.
- *Consumer privacy.* Having the privacy of their personal health information consistent with all applicable federal, state, and local laws is the right of every consumer.
- *Consumer trust.* Making public the policies surrounding the privacy and information use of personal health information is critical. Consumers want assurance that their personal electronic health information is gathered with appropriate consent and stored and used in a secure and auditable way.
- *Consumer participation and transparency.* The functioning of all governing bodies or individuals that oversee, implement, and/or develop policy for the electronic exchange of health information should be made transparent and open.

Recently, the eHealth Initiative took a major step toward consumer-centered health information technology efforts by merging with the Information Therapy Action Alliance. The IxAction Alliance focuses on issues relating to the prescription and use of targeted health information to help consumers make sound health decisions and lead healthy lives. The IxAction Alliance envisions a future healthcare delivery system, where every health decision is made collaboratively by patients and providers. Through its adoption of the IxAction Alliance, eHI is working to make this vision a reality.

Evidence-Based Studies CHI can impact consumers' health only if CHI is accepted and used. As healthcare informatics specialists consider factors that will enhance the successful adoption of CHI, research is beginning to identify attributes that facilitate or hinder CHI acceptance. A recent systematic review (Or & Karsh 2009) investigated variables associated with patient acceptance of CHI (see Table 24–2).

Or and Karsh (2009) further described the need for further research in CHI acceptance. Specifically, they cautioned that many environmental factors have not been studied to date, including lighting, noise, temperature. Additional research will help to further the agenda of CHI acceptance and to ultimately provide consumers with needed resources to make informed healthcare decisions.

THE FUTURE OF CHI

Your Aunt Mary, you, and your children will continue to benefit from advances in CHI tools and information. In the near future healthcare will be tailored to your individual needs in ways that were unheard of just a few years ago.

There is no doubt that consumers will have more frequent opportunities to utilize CHI to find information, communicate with the healthcare team, share health-related data, participate

Factor	Variable Effect on CHI Acceptance
Patient	Age showed no consistent association with acceptance; however, there was some evidence that older adults had less CHI acceptance.
	Gender had no effect.
	Increasing levels of education and prior exposure to computers/health technology increased CHI acceptance.
Human Technology Interface	Perceived usefulness, ease of use, and computer/technology self-efficacy were associated with increased CHI acceptance.
	Perceived anxiety associated with computer use was associated with less CHI acceptance
Organizational	Being a patient in an academic medical center was associated with increased CHI acceptance.
	Satisfaction with medical care services was associated with increased CHI acceptance.
Environmental	Users at home were more accepting of CHI than those in nursing homes.

TABLE 24–2 Variables Associated with Patient Acceptance of CHI

Adapted from Or, C. K. L., & Karsh, B. (2009). A systematic review of patient acceptance of consumer health information technology. *Journal of the American Medical Informatics Association: JAMIA, 16*(4), 550–560. doi:10.1197/jamia.M2888. Used by permission of JAMA.

in virtual communities, and learn more about their health condition. It is difficult to know the impact that CHI will have on the future of healthcare. However, we can consider how the evolution of some specific applications will shape CHI adoption.

Evolution of the Personalized Health Record

There are now several free-standing PHRs available. Microsoft's HealthVault is a well known example. The future of PHRs lies in the ability of the PHR to interface with information contained in the consumers' electronic medical record (EMR) and the reliance on the consumer to enter and maintain information (Lauer 2010). Issues surrounding the shift of data entry from consumer to the provider must be balanced with provisions for data editing by the consumer. A shared responsibility for data entry leads to the need to provide methods to ensure the data are correct and that changes can be monitored (Tang et al. 2006).

As consumers become more familiar with using PHRs and functionality improvements are made, use is predicted to increase. Microsoft's HealthVault is designed utilizing extendable platforms, meaning that future enhancements are possible based on consumer needs and technology development (Sunyaev, Chornyi, Mauro, & Krcmar 2010). Thus, these platforms will be able to mature along with current and future use.

Social Networking

Social networking holds tremendous promise as a consumer health tool; however, disparity in access must be addressed and access to online health information made ubiquitous. In addition, disparities in the future content of patient-focused Web sites must also be addressed. An evaluation (Eddens et al. 2009) of 106 Web sites containing data on nearly 8,000 cancer survivors found that racial/ethnic minority content was present in 9.8% of content. Future social networking tools may be helpful in addressing some of these disparities and may present a novel way for reaching health consumers who may not otherwise have access to or utilize other Internet-based health information (Chou, Hunt, Beckjord, Moser, & Hesse 2009).

Use of virtual world sites such as Second Life continues to grow. Consumer health informatics experts must share their expertise in the design, use, and evaluation of health information provided on virtual reality sites such as Second Life. In 2009 there were 68 health-related areas found on Second Life. Most of these were focused on providing patient education or support. A few were focused on research activities, including recruitment of participants (Beard, Wilson, Morra, & Keelan 2009). These results point to the vast potential for virtual worlds to impact CHI capabilities.

Additionally, condition-specific social networking tools, such as patientslikeme.com and inspire.com, will evolve and provide an expanding forum for individuals to share their experiences and support each other. Enhanced functionality developed through analysis of current use will allow for better matching of individuals with similar conditions, improved health conversations, and inclusion of more health condition communities (Frost & Massagli 2008). As computer and Internet usage becomes more widely available, the use of condition-specific social networking tools will continue to expand. In the future, it may be possible to share information from an individual's PHR to a condition-specific social networking Web site.

Home Monitoring

The future of home telehealth monitoring will depend in part on the integration of telehealth as a healthcare intervention that is recognized and reimbursed. First, telehealth monitoring must be viewed as a viable option to the face-to-face disease management visit, and work flow issues on the provider side need to be addressed (Scherr et al. 2009). The development of standards for data storage and sharing need to be discussed. For example, will telehealth data be stored, viewed, and integrated into the PHR and/or the EMR? Further, the format that the data take, multimedia or text, has implications for how we record all future health encounters. How can text fully capture what multimedia can display so easily in, for example, a wave file?

Additionally, enhancements in usability, interoperability, and consumer access to the tools, needed education, and underlying telecommunication infrastructure also need to be in place (Ackerman, Filart, Burgess, Lee, & Poropatich 2010) for true widespread adoption. Finally, the reimbursement structure for telehealth visits needs to be considered. Currently, telemedicine consults and research-funded demonstration projects are the only telehealth encounters covered by third party payers in the United States.

However, there are home telehealth monitoring tools now in development that may result in radical changes in management of chronic health conditions. Demiris and others reported results of a trial of the "smart home", where integrated sensors transmitted data regarding movement, medication adherence, and sleep patterns in the elderly (Demiris, Oliver, Dickey, Skubic, & Rantz 2008). It appears that there is good acceptance of monitoring as long as the monitors and sensors are unobtrusive and there is sufficient privacy protection.

Smart Phone

Current drivers for future development of smart phone capabilities in consumer informatics include the exponential growth in the number of applications available in the consumer market (Rainie 2010). Healthcare consumers want information that is " . . . tailored to their needs, available when they want it, and delivered how they want it" (Boland 2007). These technologies have the potential to remove the need for patients to remember self-monitoring tasks by using newer technologies that provide automatic prompts and messages via smart phones (Nguyen, Wolpin, Chiang, Cuenco, & Carrieri-Kohlman 2006). Technologies of the future will be focused on providing encouragement and motivation rather than focusing on self-management. One smart phone–based system in development for managing chronic pulmonary diseases includes a pulse oximeter that is connected via Bluetooth to a smart phone (Marshall, Medvedev, & Antonov 2008). Exercise results are then fed to the application, which then provides real time feedback during exercise. A visual display is color coded with a stoplight (normal/borderline/danger) as well as alarms if the danger zone is reached during exercise. Many similar applications are either now available or in development (O'Malley 2011).

Additional research is needed to further cement the position of smart phone technology in consumer informatics. Because management of chronic disease seems to be a key focus for this type of technology and individuals with chronic disease tend to be older, work needs to be done focusing on usability of smart phones in this age group, as screen and font size may be problematic (Scherr et al. 2009).

Personalized Healthcare

Perhaps the most wide-sweeping change in CHI will be that of personalized healthcare. The U.S. Department of Health and Human Services (DHHS) defines personalized healthcare as:

> Medical practices that are targeted to individuals based on their specific genetic code in order to provide a tailored approach. These practices use preventive, diagnostic, and therapeutic interventions that are based on genetic tests and family history information. The goal of personalized healthcare is to improve health outcomes and the healthcare delivery system, as well as the quality of life of patients elsewhere. (U.S. Department of Health and Human Services 2010, paragraph 7)

According to Abrahams and Silver (2009), personalized medicine has the potential to shift the focus of medicine from reaction to prevention, help providers select optimal therapy to make drugs safer, improve clinical trials, rescue drugs that are failing in clinical trials, and reduce the cost of healthcare. Interest in personalized healthcare has grown over the past decade, especially following the discovery that knowledge of individual genetic variation could be used to enhance therapeutic action of some medications with minimized side effects thereby creating a truly tailored pharmaceutical intervention (Jørgensen & Winther 2009).

As more scientific knowledge surrounding genomic-related topics and conditions become known, the need for authoritative, consumer-centric resources will grow. For example, more Web sites like Genetics Home Reference (http://ghr.nlm.nih.gov/), which addresses public health implications of the human genome project (Mitchell, Fun, & McCray 2004), will become more mainstream. This site provides basic information for various genetic conditions and diseases that in turn link to pertinent information available through a variety of resources including Medline Plus and PubMed.

While the ability to identify risk factors and implement targeted interventions based on genetic profiles shows great promise, there is also the need for careful evaluation (Conti, Veenstra, Armstrong, Lesko, & Grosse 2010). Direct-to-consumer genetic testing kits now available make it imperative that both providers and health consumers understand the risks and benefits of such testing (Caulfield, Ries, Ray, Shuman, & Wilson 2010). One of these risks is the potential for employment or insurance discrimination based on one's genetic profile (Hall et al. 2005; Huizenga et al. 2009). As knowledge concerning the human genome expands, consumer informatics applications will need to keep pace with the need to share information on an "as needed" basis while appropriately protecting privacy (Downing, 2009).

Conclusion

It seems clear that as technology continues to evolve, consumers will have even more options for managing their healthcare. More healthcare information will be available online, and opportunities for health-related interactive social networking and communication with providers will become the norm. Technology applications such as the use of sensorized garments that include unobtrusive sensors and monitors that provide real-time feedback regarding vital signs, gait, activity levels, or other information depending on the clinical situation (Bonato 2009) will become more mainstream. And the use of emerging technology in "smart homes," where unobtrusive sensors can allow monitoring of safety issues (falls, poor eating, changes in sleep habits) in the home setting, also has the potential to allow greater independence for older adults (Demiris, Oliver, Dickey, Skubic, & Rantz 2008).

As consumer informatics grows in its popularity, the emerging role of the informatics expert as consumer health e-specialist will also advance. Consumer health informatics truly has the potential to transform healthcare delivery.

CASE STUDY EXERCISE

How would you explain CHI to a class of sophomore nursing students enrolled in a foundations-of-nursing course? Include at least two examples of consumer informatics as well as what the role of the informatics nurse might be with those two examples.

SUMMARY

- The way that consumers access and use health-related information is changing.
- More than one-half of all American adults use online resources to locate personal health information.
- Consumer health informatics (CHI), which studies the use of electronic information and communication from the consumer's perspective to improve medical outcomes and the healthcare decision-making process, has emerged as a subspecialty of medical informatics.
- The move to consumer-driven healthcare decision making creates a greater need for consumer-centered healthcare information.
- The role of health literacy, the degree to which individuals are able to obtain, process, comprehend, and use health information and services, is critical for self-health management.
- e-Health literacy provides consumers with the ability to evaluate the quality of available information and help.
- Recognition of the digital divide and strategies to address are critical in today's healthcare delivery system.
- Protecting the privacy and security of personal health information is critical to consumers.
- Emerging technologies, inclusive of personal health records, social networking (Web 2.0 applications), home telemedicine, and smart phone technology, provide tools that help consumers to manage their own health.
- Informaticists play a role in the design, testing, promotion, acceptance, and use of consumer health applications.

REFERENCES

Abrahams, E., & Silver, M. (2009). The case for personalized medicine. *Journal of Diabetes Science and Technology, 3*(4), 680–684.

Ackerman, M. J., Filart, R., Burgess, L. P., Lee, I., & Poropatich, R. K. (2010). Developing next-generation telehealth tools and technologies: Patients, systems, and data perspectives. *Telemedicine Journal and E-Health: The Official Journal of the American Telemedicine Association, 16*(1), 93–95. doi:10.1089/tmj.2009.0153

American Medical Informatics Association, Consumer Health Informatics Working Group. (2009). *Mission statement.* Retrieved from https://www.amia.org/working-group/consumer-health-informatics

Beard, L., Wilson, K., Morra, D., & Keelan, J. (2009). A survey of health-related activities on second life. *Journal of Medical Internet Research, 11*(2), e17. doi:10.2196/jmir.1192

Boland, P. (2007). The emerging role of cell phone technology in ambulatory care. *The Journal of Ambulatory Care Management, 30*(2), 126–133. doi:10.1097/01.JAC.0000264602.19629.84

Bonato, P. (2009). Advances in wearable technology for rehabilitation. *Studies in Health Technology and Informatics, 145,* 145–159.

Brennan, P., & Starren, J. (2006). Consumer health informatics and telehealth. In E. H. Shortliffe & J. J. Cimino (Eds.), *Biomedical informatics: Computer applications in health care and biomedicine* (pp. 511–536). New York: Springer Science+Business Media.

Caulfield, T., Ries, N. M., Ray, P. N., Shuman, C., & Wilson, B. (2010). Direct-to-consumer genetic testing: Good, bad or benign? *Clinical Genetics, 77*(2), 101–105. doi:10.1111/j.1399-0004.2009.01291.x

Chou, W. S., Hunt, Y. M., Beckjord, E. B., Moser, R. P., & Hesse, B. W. (2009). Social media use in the United States: Implications for health communication. *Journal of Medical Internet Research, 11*(4), e48. doi:10.2196/jmir.1249

Committee on Quality of Healthcare in America & Institute of Medicine. (2001). *Crossing the quality chasm: A new health system for the 21st century.* Washington, DC: National Academies Press.

Conti, R., Veenstra, D. L., Armstrong, K., Lesko, L. J., & Grosse, S. D. (2010). Personalized medicine and genomics: Challenges and opportunities in assessing effectiveness, cost-effectiveness, and future research priorities. *Medical Decision Making: An International Journal of the Society for Medical Decision Making, 30*(3), 328–340. doi:10.1177/0272989X09347014

Council on Clinical Information Technology. (2009). Using personal health records to improve the quality of health care for children. *Pediatrics, 124*(1), 403–409.

Demiris, G., Oliver, D. P., Dickey, G., Skubic, M., & Rantz, M. (2008). Findings from a participatory evaluation of a smart home application for older adults. *Technology and Health Care: Official Journal of the European Society for Engineering and Medicine, 16*(2), 111–118.

Downing, G. J. (2009). Key aspects of health system change on the path to personalized medicine. *Translational Research: The Journal of Laboratory and Clinical Medicine, 154*(6), 272–276. doi:10.1016/j.trsl.2009.09.003

Eakin, B. L., Brady, J. S., & Lusk, S. L. (2001). Creating a tailored, multimedia, computer-based intervention. *Computers in Nursing, 19*(4), 152–160, quiz 161–163.

East Bay Business Times. (2008, July 10). Intel gets FDA clearance on in-home health care device. *San Francisco Business Times.* Retrieved from http://www.bizjournals.com.offcampus.lib.washington.edu/eastbay/stories/2008/07/07/daily64.html?ana=from_rss

Eddens, K. S., Kreuter, M. W., Morgan, J. C., Beatty, K. E., Jasim, S. A., Garibay, L.,...Jupka, K. A. (2009). Disparities by race and ethnicity in cancer survivor stories available on the web. *Journal of Medical Internet Research, 11*(4), e50. doi:10.2196/jmir.1163

Eng. T. R., Maxfield, A., Patrick, K., Deering, M. J., Ratzan, S. C., & Gustafson, D. H. (1998). Access to health information and support: A public highway or private road? *JAMA, 280*(15), 1371–1375.

Evangelista, L. S., Strömberg, A., Westlake, C., Ter-Galstanyan, A., Anderson, N., & Dracup, K. (2006). Developing a web-based education and counseling program for heart failure patients. *Progress in Cardiovascular Nursing, 21*(4), 196–201.

Eysenbach, G. (2000). Consumer health informatics. *British Medical Journal (Clinical Research Ed.), 320*(7251), 1713–1716.

Eysenbach, G., & Dipegen, T. (2001). The role of e-health and consumer health informatics for evidence-based patient choice in the 21st century. *Clinics in Dermatology, 19,* 11–17.

Farmer, A. D., Bruckner Holt, C. E. M., Cook, M. J., & Hearing, S. D. (2009). Social networking sites: A novel portal for communication. *Postgraduate Medical Journal, 85*(1007), 455–459. doi:10.1136/pgmj.2008.074674

Ferguson, T. (2002). What e-patients do online: A tentative taxonomy. Retrieved from http://www.fergusonreport.com/articles/fr00904.htm

Frost, J. H., & Massagli, M. P. (2008). Social uses of personal health information within Patients-LikeMe, an online patient community: What can happen when patients have access to one another's data. *Journal of Medical Internet Research, 10*(3), e15. doi:10.2196/jmir.1053

Glassman, P. (2008). *Health literacy.* National Library of Medicine. Retrieved from http://nnlm.gov/outreach/consumer/hlthlit.html

Goldman, J., Hudson, Z., Smith, R. M. (2000). Report on the privacy policies and practices of health websites. California Healthcare Foundation.

Grama, L. M., Beckwith, M., & Bittinger, W. (2005). The role of user input in shaping online information from the National Cancer Institute. *Journal of Medical Internet Research, 7*(3), e25. doi:10.2196/jmir.7.3.e25

Hall, M. A., McEwen, J. E., Barton, J. C., Walker, A. P., Howe, E. G., Reiss, J. A.,...Thomson, E. J. (2005). Concerns in a primary care population about genetic discrimination by insurers. *Genetics in Medicine: Official Journal of the American College of Medical Genetics, 7*(5), 311–316.

Health on the Net. (2008). *HONCode in brief*. Retrieved from http://www.hon.ch/HONcode/ Conduct.html

Healthy People. (2010). *Goal 11. Health communication*. Retrieved from http://www.healthypeople .gov/document/HTML/Volume1/11HealthCom.htm#_edn28

Healthy People 2020. (2010). *U.S. department of health & human services* [brochure]. Retrieved from http://www.healthypeople.gov/2020/TopicsObjectives2020/pdfs/HP2020_brochure.pdf

Huizenga, C. R., Lowstuter, K., Banks, K. C., Lagos, V. I., Vandergon, V. O., & Weitzel, J. N. (2009). Evolving perspectives on genetic discrimination in health insurance among health care providers. *Familial Cancer, 9*(2), 253–260. doi:10.1007/s10689-009-9308-y

Jamison, D. T., Breman, J. G., Measham, A. R., Alleyne, G., Claeson, M., Evans, D. B., . . . & Musgrove, P. (Eds.). (2006). *Disease control in developing countries* (2nd ed.). New York: A copublication of The World Bank and Oxford University Press.

Jørgensen, J., & Winther, H. (2009). The new era of personalized medicine. *Personalized Medicine, 6*(4), 423–428.

Kahn, J. S., Aulakh, V., & Bosworth, A. (2009). What it takes: Characteristics of the ideal personal health record. *Health Affairs (Project Hope), 28*(2), 369–376. doi:10.1377/hlthaff.28.2.369

Keselman, A., Logan, R., Smith, C. A., Leroy, G., & Zeng-Treitler, Q. (2008). Developing informatics tools and strategies for consumer-centered health communication. *Journal of the American Medical Informatics Association, 15*(4), 473–483. doi:10.1197/jamia.M2744

Krishna, S., Boren, S. A., & Balas, E. A. (2009). Healthcare via cell phones: A systematic review. *Telemedicine Journal and E-Health: The Official Journal of the American Telemedicine Association, 15*(3), 231–240. doi:10.1089/tmj.2008.0099

Lauer, G. (2010). *Consumers not ready for do-it-yourself PHRs experts say*. Retrieved from http://www.ihealthbeat.org/features/2010/consumers-not-ready-for-doityourself-phrs-experts-say.aspx

Lorence, D., & Abraham, J. (2008). A study of undue pain and surfing: Using hierarchical criteria to assess website quality. *Health Informatics Journal, 14*(3), 155–173. doi:10.1177/ 1081180X08092827

Markle Foundation. (2003). *Connecting for health: The personal health working group final report*. Retrieved from http://www.providersedge.com/ehdocs/ehr_articles/The_Personal_Health_ Working_Group_Final_Report.pdf

Marshall, A., Medvedev, O., & Antonov, A. (2008). Use of a smartphone for improved self-management of pulmonary rehabilitation. *International Journal of Telemedicine and Applications, 2008*, 753064. doi: 10.1155/2008/753064

Mayo Clinic Staff. (2011, March 22). *High blood pressure (hypertension)*. Retrieved from http://www.mayoclinic.com/health/high-blood-pressure/DS00100/DSECTION=causes

McDaniel, A. M. (2006). *Consumer health informatics: Using technology to enhance partnerships with our patients*. Retrieved from www.hsrd.research.va.gov/for_researchers/cyber./vci-112106.ppt

Mitchell, J. A., Fun, J., & McCray, A. T. (2004). Design of genetics home reference: A new NLM consumer health resource. *Journal of the American Medical Informatics Association, 11*(6), 439–447. doi:10.1197/jamia.M1549

Moen, A., Gregory, J., & Brennan, P. F. (2007). Cross-cultural factors necessary to enable design of flexible consumer health informatics systems (CHIS). *International Journal of Medical Informatics, 76*(Suppl. 1), S168–S173. doi:10.1016/j.ijmedinf.2006.05.014

Nguyen, H. Q., Gill, D. P., Wolpin, S., Steele, B. G., & Benditt, J. O. (2009). Pilot study of a cell phone-based exercise persistence intervention post-rehabilitation for COPD. *International Journal of Chronic Obstructive Pulmonary Disease, 4*, 301–313.

Nguyen, H. Q., Wolpin, S., Chiang, K., Cuenco, D., & Carrieri-Kohlman, V. (2006). Exercise and symptom monitoring with a mobile device. *AMIA . . . Annual Symposium Proceedings/AMIA Symposium*, 1047.

NIST (2002). *FIPS publication 200: Minimum security requirements for federal information and information systems*. Retrieved from http://csrc.nist.gov/publications/fips/fips200/ FIPS-200-final-march.pdf

O'Malley, K. (2011, November 9). Nancy Finn: Smartphone health care apps storm the market. e.patients.net. Retrieved from http://e-patients.net/archives/2011/11/nancy-finn-smartphone-health-care-apps-storm-the-market.html

ONC (2008). *The ONC—Coordinated federal health IT strategic plan: 2008–2012.* Retrieved from http://healthit.hhs.gov/portal/server.pt/gateway/PTARGS_0_10731_848083_0_0_18/HITStrategicPlan508.pdf

Or, C. K. L., & Karsh, B. (2009). A systematic review of patient acceptance of consumer health information technology. *Journal of the American Medical Informatics Association, 16*(4), 550–560. doi:10.1197/jamia.M2888

Rainie, L. (2010). *Internet, broadband and cell phone statistics.* Pew Internet and American Life Project. Retrieved from http://www.pewinternet.org/Reports/2010/Internet-broadband-and-cell-phone-statistics.aspx

Ritter, F. E., Freed, A. R., & Haskett, O. L. M. (2005). Discovering user information needs: The case of university department web sites. *Interoperations 12L,* 19–27.

Scherr, D., Kastner, P., Kollmann, A., Hallas, A., Auer, J., Krappinger, H.,... MOBITEL Investigators. (2009). Effect of home-based telemonitoring using mobile phone technology on the outcome of heart failure patients after an episode of acute decompensation: Randomized controlled trial. *Journal of Medical Internet Research, 11*(3), e34. doi:10.2196/jmir.1252

Schlachta-Fairchild, L., & Elfrink, V. (2004). Models of health care and the consumer perspective of telehealth in the information age. In R. Nelson & M. J. Ball (Eds.), *Consumer informatics: Applications and strategies in cyber health care* (pp. 95–105). New York: Springer.

Shea, S., Weinstock, R. S., Teresi, J. A., Palmas, W., Starren, J., Cimino, J. J.,... IDEATel Consortium. (2009). A randomized trial comparing telemedicine case management with usual care in older, ethnically diverse, medically underserved patients with diabetes mellitus: 5 year results of the IDEATel study. *Journal of the American Medical Informatics Association, 16*(4), 446–456. doi:10.1197/jamia.M3157

Sunyaev, A., Chornyi, D., Mauro, C., & Krcmar, H. (2010, January 5–8). *Evaluation framework for personal health records: Microsoft Health Vault vs. Google Health.* Paper presented at the 43rd Annual Hawaii International Conference on System Sciences, Honolulu, Hawaii.

Tang, P. C., Ash, J. S., Bates, D. W., Overhage, J. M., & Sands, D. Z. (2006). Personal health records: Definitions, benefits, and strategies for overcoming barriers to adoption. *Journal of the American Medical Informatics Association, 13*(2), 121–126. doi:10.1197/jamia.M2025

Toms, E., & Latter, C. (2007). How consumers search for health information. *Health Informatics Journal, 13*(3), 223–235.

Tu, H. T., & Cohen, G. R. (2008, August). *Striking jump in consumers seeking health care information* (Tracking Report No. 20). Center for Studying Health System Change. Retrieved from http://www.hschange.com/CONTENT/1006/

U.S. Department of Commerce. (1999). Falling through the net: Defining the digital divide. Washington, DC: National Telecommunications and Information Administration. Retrieved from http://www.ntia.doc.gov/ntiahome/fttn99/contents.html

U.S. Department of Health and Human Services. (2010). *Glossary of terms for personalized health care website.* Retrieved from http://www.hhs.gov/myhealthcare/glossary/glossary.html

U.S. Department of Health and Human Services. (2011). Healthfinder.gov. Retrieved from http://www.healthfinder.gov/

Winkler, M. A., Flanagin, A., Chi-Lum, B., White, J., Andrews, K., Kennett, R. L., DeAngelis, C. D., & Musacchio, R. A. (2000). Guidelines for medical and health information sites on the Internet: Principles governing AMA web sites. *Journal of the American Medical Association, 283*(12), 1600–1606.

Zeng, Q. T., & Tse, T. (2006). Exploring and developing consumer health vocabularies. *Journal of the American Medical Informatics Association, 13*(1), 24–29. doi:10.1197/jamia.M1761

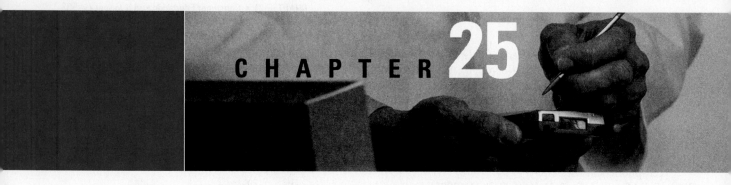

CHAPTER 25

Telehealth

After completing this chapter, you should be able to:

1. Define the term *telehealth*.
2. List the advantages of telehealth.
3. Identify equipment and technology needed to sustain telehealth.
4. Discuss present and proposed telehealth applications.
5. Describe legal and practice issues that affect telehealth.
6. Review the implications of telehealth for nursing and other health professions.
7. Identify several telenursing applications.
8. Discuss some issues pertaining to the practice of telenursing.

Telehealth is the use of telecommunications technologies and electronic information to exchange healthcare information and to provide and support services such as long-distance clinical healthcare to clients. Telehealth is an expansion of telemedicine with preventive, promotive, and curative applications widely used by members of the healthcare community. The American Nurses Association (1996) prefers the term *telehealth* as a more inclusive and accurate description of the services provided. Telehealth services include health promotion, disease prevention, diagnosis, consultation, education, and therapy. Telehealth has the unique capability of achieving health equity by crossing temporal, social, and geographical barriers to healthcare. Computers, interactive video transmissions, teleconferences by telephone or video, and direct links to healthcare instruments are tools used to deliver these services. Electronic, visual, and audio signals sent during these conferences provide information to consultants from remote sites. Many common medical devices have been adapted for use with telemedicine technology. Distant practitioners and clients benefit from the skills and knowledge of the consultants without the need to travel to regional referral centers. Telehealth is a tool that allows healthcare professionals to do the following (Coyle, Duffy, & Martin 2007; Cross 2007; Cunningham & Vande Merwe 2009; Demiris, Edison, & Vijaykumar 2005; Fincher, Ward, Dawkins, Magee, & Willson 2009; Lancaster, Krumm, Ribera, & Klich 2008; Liaw & Humphreys 2006; Lillibridge & Hanna 2008; Lutz, Chumbler, Lyles, Hoffman, & Kobb 2009; Yun & Park 2007):

- Consult with colleagues
- Conduct interviews
- Assess and monitor clients
- View diagnostic images
- Review slides and laboratory reports
- Extend scarce healthcare resources
- Decrease the number of hospital visits for patients with chronic conditions
- Decrease healthcare costs
- Tackle isolation and loneliness
- Provide health education
- Improve case management services
- Improve the equity of access to services
- Improve the quality of client care
- Improve the overall quality of the client's record

Numerous terms have been coined to describe these capabilities (see Box 25–1 for a partial listing).

TERMS RELATED TO TELEHEALTH

Initially *telemedicine* was the predominant term for the delivery of healthcare education and services via the use of telecommunication technologies and computers. It has since largely been replaced by the term *telehealth*. *Telehealth* encompasses telemedicine but is a broader term that emphasizes both the delivery of services and the provision of information and education to healthcare providers and consumers. For example, federal agencies use the Internet to provide healthcare professionals, consumers, and their families with medical information. The Centers for Disease Control and Prevention provides credible online sources for health information. The Agency for Healthcare Research and Quality, formerly known as the Agency for Health Care Policy and Research, places clinical practice guidelines online. The U.S. National Library of Medicine provides information on health, various medical conditions and procedures, clinical trials, and the capability to conduct searches of several databases on its Web site. There also are a number of professional journals and articles available online. Some require subscription; some do not. One example of an online journal is *JNCI Journal*

BOX 25–1   Some Common Telehealth Terms

eCare (E-care). The electronic provision of health information, products, and services online as well as the electronic automation of administrative and clinical aspects of care delivery.

eHealth (E-health). A broad term often used interchangeably with the term *telehealth* to refer to the provision of electronic health information, products, and services using information technologies.

eMedicine (E-medicine). The use of telecommunication and computer technology for the delivery of medical care.

ePrescribing (E-prescribing). Electronic transmission of prescriptions and patient specific clinical information.

Interactive. Describes a technology system that interacts with user input (i.e., interacts with users) and involves information exchange via an online medium.

mHealth (M-Health). The use of mobile devices to collect and provide real-time monitoring of patient health data, and to provide direct provision of care through mobile telemedicine.

Telecardiology. Transmission of cardiac catheterization studies, echocardiograms, and other diagnostic tests in conjunction with electronic stethoscope examinations for second opinions by cardiologists at another site.

Telecare. The remote delivery of healthcare services into the person's home facilitated by communication technologies that include the use of person-centered reactive monitoring devices.

Teleconsultation. Videoconferencing between two healthcare professionals or a healthcare professional and a client. Remote health consultation, whatever the means of transmission.

Tele-diagnosis. The detection of a disease by using data received from monitoring a patient at a distant site.

Tele-education (telelearning). Distance learning via a computer and/or telephone connection.

Telehomecare. The use of telecommunication and computer technologies to monitor and render services and support to home care clients (the use of telecommunication to provide care services to a patient in his or her place or residency).

Telementoring. Real-time advice offered to a practitioner in a remote site via telecommunications technology.

Telenursing. The use of telecommunication and IT for the delivery of nursing services.

Telepathology. Transmission of high-resolution virtual images, often via a robotic microscope, for interpretation by a pathologist at a remote site.

Teleprevention. The use of tele-education technology to provide opportunities to promote health.

Telepsychiatry. Variant of telemedicine that allows observation and interviews of clients at one site by a psychiatrist at another site through videoconferencing.

Telerehabilitation. The use of interactive communication technology to facilitate assessment of patient's functional abilities and provide exercise and rehabilitation therapies.

Teleradiology. Transmission of high-resolution radiological patient images for interpretation or consultation by a radiologist at a distant location.

Telesurgery. Technology that allows surgeons at a remote site to collaborate with experts at a referral center on techniques.

Teletherapy. The use of interactive videoconferencing to provide therapy and counseling.

Teleultrasound. Transmission of ultrasound images for interpretation at a remote site.

of the National Cancer Institute. This publication incorporates a wide range of cancer information from respected sources. It allows readers to browse by topic, and does require a subscription. As a consequence of the information explosion, healthcare professionals and clients gain access to the most current treatment options at essentially the same time. No matter what term is used, the basic premise of telehealth is that it can provide services to underserved communities. Another frequently used term is *eHealth*, which is often used interchangeably with the term *telehealth*. The field of telenursing is part of telehealth. Telenursing is the use of telecommunications and information technology (IT) for the delivery of nursing care.

Teleconferencing

Teleconferencing implies that people at different locations have audio, and possibly video, contact, which is used to carry out telehealth applications. The terms teleconference and videoconference may be used synonymously, because both use telecommunications and computer technology.

Videoconferencing

Videoconferencing implies that people meet face-to-face and view the same images through the use of telecommunications and computer technology even though they are not in the same location. It saves travel time and costs, which actually encourages people to meet more frequently. Videoconferencing is an appealing concept that can be used for many applications, especially distance learning and telehealth (although some applications may require high resolution and audio quality and high-speed transmission). For example, videoconferences provide a means to improve quality and access to care in Alaska, where clinics are connected. Live conferences are used to view critically ill clients, and specially adapted medical equipment is used to collect and send assessment data digitally. Communities benefit by saving travel time and costs for this arrangement, and appropriate care can be initiated in a timely fashion (Smith 2004). For some vulnerable populations, videoconferencing is an effective alternative to traditional psychiatry. For example, cognitive-behavioral therapy was successfully delivered through videoconferencing to children and adolescents with functional abdominal pain (Sato, Clifford, Silverman, & Davies 2009).

Desktop Videoconferencing

Desktop videoconferencing (DTV) is a synchronous, or real-time, encounter that uses a specially equipped personal computer (PC) with telephone line hookup, DSL, or cable connections to allow people to meet face-to-face and/or view papers and images simultaneously. DTV is less expensive than custom-designed videoconference systems, but it may not be acceptable for telehealth applications that require high-resolution or high-speed transmission, such as interpretation of diagnostic images where slower frame rates produce a jerky image or lengthy transmission times.

HISTORICAL BACKGROUND

Telehealth began with the use of telephone consults and has become more sophisticated with each advance in technology. During the past five decades the U.S. government played a major role in the development and promotion of telehealth through various agencies. Interest waned as funding slowed to a trickle in the 1980s, but subsequent technological advancements made telehealth attractive again. Federal monies and the Agriculture Department's 1991 Rural Development Act laid the groundwork to bring the information superhighway to rural areas for education and telehealth purposes.

Historically, the most aggressive development of telehealth in the United States has been by NASA and the military (Brown 2002). NASA provided international telehealth consults for Armenian earthquake victims in 1989. Following the January 12, 2010, Haitian earthquake, telemedicine was part of the coordination efforts for ongoing health services in Haiti. The military has also had several projects to feed medical images from the battlefield to physicians in hospitals and on robotics equipment for telesurgery for improved treatment of casualties.

Another large U.S. telehealth application has been the provision of care to state inmates by the medical branch of the University of Texas at Galveston (Brown 2002). Other states also use telehealth to treat prisoners, avoiding the costs and danger of transporting prisoners. New York piloted a telepsychiatric project that was well received (Manfredi, Shupe, & Batki 2005). The American Psychiatric Association (2010) reports that telepsychiatry is one of the most effective ways to increase access to mental healthcare for rural underserved populations. For example, Walter Reed Army Medical Center (2010) has expanded the availability of mental healthcare to outlying military treatment facilities through use of telepsychiatry for community mental health services.

One major barrier to telehealth was removed with the passage of the Telecommunications Act of 1996, which allowed vendors of cable and telephone services to compete in each others' markets (Schneider 1996). This event helped to open the door to create the information superhighway needed to provide the framework to support telehealth. The Snowe–Rockefeller Amendment required telecommunications carriers to offer services to rural health providers at rates comparable to those charged in urban areas so that affordable healthcare may be available to rural residents.

The American Recovery and Reinvestment Act of 2009 provides for billions of dollars in stimulus funding for research, operations, and grants in the telemedicine, telehealth, and informatics sectors. More than 24 government agencies provide grant monies to fund telehealth, telemedicine, and health information technologies, including the U.S. Departments of Health and Human Services, Homeland Security, Defense, Veterans Affairs, Commerce, Agriculture, Energy, Justice, Interior, Education, Labor, State, and Transportation. There are also private, nonprofit, national, and global groups such as the Center of Excellence for Remote and Medically-Underserved Areas and the Acumen Fund that use entrepreneurial approaches to solve health services problems. The majority of private parties providing funds focus on specific applications, often to promote a particular product. Additional research is needed before there will be widespread acceptance of telehealth applications (Bahaadini, Yogesan, & Wooton 2009; Bonneville & Pare 2006; Gagnon, Lamothe, Hebert, Chanliau, & Fortin 2006). Questions remain about the evidence of the efficacy, cost-benefits, and quality of telehealth applications. These questions arise not so much because of a lack of projects or funding but rather because of a lack of a coordinated approach to the development, research, testing, and evaluation of applications. The Lewin Group (2000) noted that despite an earlier call by the Institute of Medicine (IOM) (1996) to evaluate telemedicine applications in terms of quality of care, outcomes, access to care, healthcare costs, and the perceptions of clients and clinicians, methodology problems remained. These included small sample sizes and a lack of control groups (AHRQ 2001).

Telecommunication technologies are continuing to evolve along with advancements in telehealth. Telehealth will soon become an integral part of healthcare delivery services (AHRQ 2010). The Agency for healthcare Research and Quality is funding organizations across the United States that are investigating telehealth with projects such as improving diagnostic quality and therapeutic decision in ambulatory care settings, using telemedicine to reduce blood pressure in a cost-effective manner, evaluating a automated medication management system for effectiveness in terms of satisfaction and patient medication nonadherence, use of automated telephone self-management support among patients with poorly controlled diabetes, utilizing telemedicine applications for CPAP therapy adherence, and use of an IT-based approach to provide safer pediatric care for children outside the clinical setting. Projects involving chronic conditions that use the bulk of resources or have the greatest barriers to care continue to receive the highest priority for telemedicine research. The National Institute of Nursing Research solicited grant applications to study telehealth technologies that can improve clinical outcomes. The National Cancer Institute's Center to Reduce Cancer Health Disparities has been looking for technology and telehealth applications that can facilitate early detection and screening. Despite the emphasis in this text on U.S. development of telehealth, it is an international phenomenon.

The United States may lead in the development of technologies that enable telehealth, but Australia, Canada, Norway, and Sweden are among the current world leaders in the use of telehealth. Work has been done in Canada on policies and procedures for allied health professionals who provide telehealth services as a means to enhance and expand successes already achieved with telehealth delivery of services and for use by accreditation criteria (Hailey et al. 2005;

Hogenbirk et al. 2006). Topics covered by these policies include the scope and limitations of services, staff responsibilities, training, reporting, professional standards, and cultural considerations. Denmark, Finland, and Sweden are countries leading in deployment of health IT (Castro 2009). According to the World Health Organization (2009), the United States lags behind international best practices in making progress in health IT systems.

DRIVING FORCES

Recent attention to patient safety, cost containment, managed care, disease management, shortages of healthcare providers, uneven access to healthcare services, and an emphasis upon keeping an aging population functional in their own homes makes telehealth an attractive tool to improve the quality of healthcare and save money (Brantley, Laney-Cummings, & Spivack 2004; Introducing: telehealth and telecare 2007; Smith 2004; Stronge, Rogers, & Fisk 2007). Savings may be realized via the following measures:

- Improved access to care, which allows clients to be treated earlier when fewer interventions are required.
- The ability of clients to receive treatment in their own community where services cost less.
- Improved quality of care; expert advice that is more easily available.
- Extending the services of nurse practitioners and physician assistants through ready accessibility to physician services.
- Improved continuity of care through convenient follow-up care.
- Improved quality of client records; the addition of digital information such as monitored vital signs and wound images, which provide better information for treatment decisions and help to decrease errors.
- Time savings; the ability of healthcare professionals to cut down on the amount of time spent in travel and instead spend it in direct client care.

Telehealth is also a marketing tool. Many institutions post health promotion or quality benchmark information on their Web pages with the hope that it will attract new customers. Large institutions offer links with the understanding that additional services will be rendered at their facilities. For example, imagine that a client with symptoms of coronary artery disease is seen at a community hospital that has no facilities for cardiac surgery. The client is more likely to follow up at the larger institution that has established links to the community hospital, because a rapport has been established with the consulting physician. In addition, telehealth services can eliminate the need for visas for international clients. Some facilities provide scheduling and online claim authorization as convenient services. Telehealth services deemed valuable by physicians can also attract new medical staff. As a result of the above factors, many agencies offer telehealth or plan to do so in the near future. Telehealth services need to be addressed in enterprise-wide strategic plans. Box 25–2 lists some additional benefits associated with telehealth.

APPLICATIONS

Telehealth applications vary greatly. Examples include monitoring activities, diagnostic evaluations, decision-support systems, storage and dissemination of records for diagnostic purposes, image compression for efficient storage and retrieval, research, electronic prescriptions, voice recognition for dictation, education of healthcare professionals and consumers, and support of caregivers. Sophisticated equipment is not always necessary. Some applications are "high tech," whereas others are relatively "low tech." Real-time videoconferencing between physicians or healthcare professionals and clients and the transmission of diagnostic images and biometric data are examples of high-tech applications. An example of a low-tech application is a home glucose-monitoring program that uses a touch-tone telephone to report glucose results. Desktop

PCs outfitted with microphones and video cameras can provide telehealth opportunities for applications that do not require high resolution.

Current telehealth technologies can be grouped into at least nine broad categories, although for general discussion purposes, there are two types: store-and-forward and interactive conferencing. Store-and-forward is used to transfer digital images and data from one location to another. It is appropriate for nonemergent situations. It is commonly used for teleradiology and telepathology. Interactive conferencing primarily refers to videoconferencing and is used in place of face-to-face consultation. Interactive conferencing is frequently used for telepsychiatry. Telehealth is not a technology so much as it is a technique for the delivery of services. Increasingly it is perceived as a framework for a comprehensive health system integrating various applications, as well as the management of information, education, and administrative services. Box 25–3 lists some other actual and proposed applications.

BOX 25–3 (*continued*)

- **Mobile unit post-disaster care.** Emergency medical technicians (EMTs) and nurses at the site of a disaster can consult with physicians about the health needs of victims.
- **Education.** Healthcare professionals in geographically remote areas can attend seminars to update their knowledge without extensive travel, expense, or time away from home.
- **Emergency care.** Community hospitals can share information with trauma centers so that the centers can better care for clients and prepare them for transport.
- **Fetal monitoring.** Some high-risk antepartum clients can be monitored from home with greater comfort and decreased expense.
- **Geriatrics.** Videoconference equipment in the home permits home monitoring of medication administration for a client who has memory deficits but who is otherwise able to stay at home.
- **Hypertension management.** Clients receive automated reminders and education feedback regarding hypertension treatment guidelines.
- **Home care.** Once equipment is in the client's home, nurses and physicians may evaluate the client at home without leaving their offices.
- **Hospice.** Palliative and end-of-life services via technology can increase access to services in remote areas or supplement traditional care.
- **Military.** Physicians at remote sites can evaluate injured soldiers in the field via the medic's equipment.
- **Pharmacy.** Data can be accessed at a centralized location.
- **Pathology.** The transmission of slide and tissue samples to other sites makes it easier to obtain a second opinion on biopsy findings.
- **Psychiatry.** Specialists at major medical centers can evaluate clients in outlying emergency departments, hospitals, and clinics via teleconferences.
- **Radiology.** Radiologists can take calls from home and receive images from the hospital on equipment they have in place. Rural hospitals do not need to have a radiologist onsite.
- **School clinics.** School nurses, particularly in remote areas, can quickly consult with other professionals about problems observed.
- **Social work.** Social workers can augment services with telehealth home visits.
- **Speech–language pathology.** More efficient use can be made of scarce speech/language pathologists.
- **Virtual intensive care units.** Remote monitoring capabilities and teleconferencing allow experts at medical centers to monitor patients in distant, rural hospitals, particularly when weather conditions or other factors do not allow transport.
- **Extended emergency services.** Remote monitoring and teleconferencing support allow emergency care physicians to view and monitor ambulance patients, supervise EMTs, and initiate treatments early and redirect patients to the most appropriate facilities, such as burn centers or trauma units, without being seen first in the emergency department.

Online Databases and Tools

Online resources can include the following:

- *Standards of care.* These may include recommended guidelines for care for a particular diagnosis.
- *Evidence-based practice guidelines.* Best practices based upon research findings are increasingly available online for reference and use.

- *Computerized medical diagnosis.* This database assists the physician to match symptoms against suspected diagnoses.
- *Drug information.* One important application is the determination of the most effective, least expensive antibiotic for a particular infection.
- *Electronic prescriptions.* This permits the physician to "write" a prescription that is sent automatically to the pharmacy. It decreases errors associated with poor handwriting and sound-alike drugs. When integration exists among healthcare systems, physicians, and pharmacies, there is no need to enter patient history, allergies, demographic, and insurance information more than once. Electronic prescribing is being adopted in more systems as part of patient safety initiatives.
- *Abstracts and full-text retrieval of literature.* These can be retrieved easily at any time of the day.
- *Research data.* This information is available via literature searches and Web access.
- *Bulletin boards, reference files, and discussion groups on various specialty subjects.*

Ready access to information improves care delivery and decreases related costs. For example, the incorporation of national standards of care and drug information eliminates redundant efforts by individual institutions to prepare their own standards and formularies. It also decreases malpractice claims through adherence to standards of care. Standards of care reflect best practices based on research findings. Online research databases facilitate research through the systematic collection of information on large populations, with potential for data mining at a later time. Further benefits from online resources will be accrued as more projects are implemented to develop common terms to facilitate sharing of data, such as the National Library of Medicine's Unified Medical Language System.

Education

Telehealth affords opportunities to educate healthcare consumers and professionals through increased information accessibility via online resources, including the World Wide Web, distance learning, and clinical instruction. Grand rounds and continuing education are two of the most touted applications for education.

Grand rounds are traditional teaching tools for health professionals in training (Cross, Barnes, & Jawad 2010; Ellis & Mayrose 2003). As the name indicates, a group of practitioners review a client's case history and his or her present condition, at which time they mutually determine the best treatment options. Grand rounds help to maintain clinical knowledge and expertise but are not always available in smaller institutions. Telehealth facilities allow the incorporation of diagnostic images, client interviews, and biometric measurements from outlying hospitals into medical center grand rounds, thereby allowing practitioners from two or more sites to participate.

Videoconferencing allows more practitioners to attend this educational offering than might otherwise be possible. In like fashion, consultations and images from major teaching centers may be made available to remote facilities to enhance the practice of professionals in outlying areas.

Continuing Education

Telehealth offers direct access to traditional continuing education and extemporaneous teaching opportunities with every teleconsultation and distance education offering. Training costs for continuing education may be decreased by bringing people together from many distant sites without travel or lodging expenses or extended time away from their responsibilities.

Home Healthcare

Telecommunication technology can reduce costs and increase choices and the availability of services that can keep people in their own homes longer (Brennan 1996; Garrett & Martini 2007; Hi-tech home help 2007). This is particularly important as the population over age 65 explodes without a concomitant increase in funds for healthcare services (Demiris, Oliver, & Courtney 2006). Telecommunication technology also supports automatic collection of data and allows clinicians to handle more clients than via traditional care models. For example, use of a home monitoring system in Japan provides 24-hour contact and medical response for clients as needed in addition to regularly scheduled visits. Biometric measurements such as heart rate and pattern, blood pressure, respiratory rate, and fetal heart rate can be monitored at another site, with electronic or actual house calls provided as needed. Women with high-risk pregnancies, diabetics, and cardiac and postoperative clients can be monitored at home. Clients who require wound care comprise another population that can be managed well at home through telehealth applications. Nurses can also transmit digital photographs of wounds to certified wound ostomy continence nurses (WCONs). Photographs are stored in the database. The WCON can make recommendations and follow more clients through the use of telehealth than would otherwise be possible. Internet access for home health clients, and their families, provides convenient access to support groups, treatment information, and electronic communication with their healthcare providers, while decreasing feelings of isolation. The REACH (Resources for Enhancing Alzheimer's Caregiver Health) initiative, sponsored by the National Institutes for Health, exemplifies a support program for caregivers that encourages them to engage in relaxation exercises. As the number of the elderly grows, televisits eliminate the discomfort and inconvenience of travel and long waits to be seen by physicians. Equipment needs are dictated by the nature of the monitoring. For example, telemetry requires continuous monitoring, necessitating a dedicated telephone line as well as the monitoring devices supplied by the home healthcare agency. Other clients may require less expensive, low technology monitoring, while another client group requires equipment with videoconference and monitoring capabilities. A Web-based solution for care coordination can integrate information from biometric measures and diagnostic tests and automatically alert the clinician of panic values. The benefits of telehealth technology allow clinicians to cut travel time without decreasing client contact and help to improve the organization of the health record with automatic collection of data and better coordination of care among clinicians. Figure 25–1 depicts a teleconference that connects a home healthcare client, a nurse, and a physician.

The use of sensors can also detect falls and whether the refrigerator has been opened and closed as a means to alert nurses to problems in the homes of elderly and frail individuals.

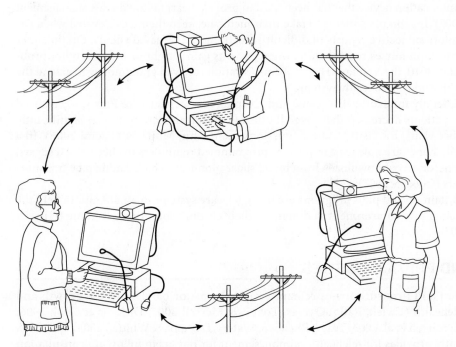

FIGURE 25–1 • Diagram of a teleconference involving client, nurse, and physician at separate sites

Coming trends include the integration of wireless sensors, wearable monitoring technology into telehealth systems, smart homes, and helper robots (Karunanithi 2007; Koch 2006; Lamprinos, Prentza, & Koutsouris 2006).

Some providers of advanced home telemonitoring services have formed partnerships with home care companies that make the technology available to providers. This arrangement eliminates the need for home healthcare companies to invest in the equipment needed to support telehealth.

The American Telemedicine Association developed clinical guidelines for the use of telemedicine for home care that include criteria for patients, care providers, and technology (ATA adopts telehomecare clinical guidelines 2007). These are listed on its Web site (www.atmeda.org/news/guidelines.htm).

Disease Management

The bulk of U.S. healthcare costs results from chronic conditions. For this reason, it is essential to find better ways to manage the health of individuals with chronic medical conditions. Telehealth applications can help. The U.S. Department of Veterans Affairs has several telemedicine initiatives nationally monitoring over 35,000 chronically ill veterans with heart disease, depression, diabetes, post-traumatic stress disorder, pulmonary problems, and other chronic illnesses in their own homes and coordinating regional programs that reduce travel and wait time (Department of Veterans Affairs 2009; Department of Veterans Affairs 2006; Kline & Schofield 2006; Lipowicz 2010; Midwest VA Service 2007; Riverside County 2006; Wertenberger, Yerardi, Drake, & Parlier 2006). Technology ranges from automated reminders to take medications and handheld vital sign monitors to two-way video computers that are equipped with everything from a stethoscope to an electrocardiograph, and a personal health record (PHR) for veterans. Monitoring devices load results into the veteran's PHR. While technology costs maybe substantial, they are significantly less than the cost of an inpatient admission. Links to community health outpatient centers are instantaneous and travel time is significantly reduced. Consequently, telehealth is becoming increasingly popular with veterans.

Similar initiatives have been under way at home care agencies and through private medical centers throughout the country. One example is the use of Health Buddy. Health Buddy is an in-home communication device that has been used to provide heart failure disease management (Rosenberg 2007). It prompts patients to take their medicine, keep their legs elevated when sitting, and monitors subjective reports of difficulty breathing or increased edema. On the other end of the connection nurses receive alerts when patients gain weight or indicate other problems. In February 2010, the Veterans Health Administration received grant money to extend the use of the Health Buddy Telehealth System.

The U.S. federally funded Jewish Home and Hospital Services Lifecare Plus study showed that telehealth patients decreased their overall utilization of healthcare resources significantly with fewer office visits, ER visits, and readmissions (Lehmann, Mintz, & Giacini 2006). In a newer twist cell phones are now used to provide programmed reminders to check blood sugars, take medications, or accept downloads from blood sugar monitors, which can then be transmitted to caregivers (Goedert 2007).

In Great Britain several pilot programs are using telecare systems in an attempt to help the elderly maintain a safe environment and manage their chronic conditions at home (Hi-tech home help 2007).

LEGAL AND PRIVACY ISSUES

Reimbursement and licensure issues remain two of the major barriers to the growth and practice of telehealth (Cwiek, Rafiq, Qamar, Tobey, & Merrell 2007; Dickens & Cook 2006; Kennedy 2005; Starren et al. 2005; Tracy, Rheuban, Waters, DeVany, & Whitten 2008). The CMS (2009a) currently provides for telehealth reimbursement for physician follow-up consultation when communicating with the patient via telehealth (G0425-G0427 reimbursement codes for 2010). The Centers for Medicare & Medicaid Services (CMS) have not formally defined telemedicine for the Medicaid program, and Medicaid does not recognize telemedicine as a distinct service. Medicaid reimbursement for telehealth services is available at the discretion of individual states as a cost-effective alternative to traditional services or as a means to improve access for rural residents (CMS 2009b; Cross 2007; Gray, Stamm, Toevs, Reischl, & Yarrington 2006). Advocates are struggling to increase state Medicaid reimbursement. Several states have passed legislation mandating private insurance coverage of telehealth services (States require reimbursement 2004). Currently 39 states acknowledge at least some reimbursement for telehealth services (Ctel 2011). There are also concerns about the impact of telehealth on record privacy, particularly with the implementation of the Health Insurance Portability and Accountability Act (HIPAA).

Referral and Payment

Brantley et al. (2004) concluded that federal, state, and private sector policies have impeded the advance of telehealth and that an entirely new framework is necessary to determine reimbursement for telehealth services. The Balanced Budget Act of 1997 first authorized Medicare reimbursement for some services that did not traditionally require a face-to-face meeting between client and practitioner, such as radiology or electrocardiogram interpretation. Almost 2 years passed before any reimbursement occurred. There were limitations on who could receive services, what services were covered, who got paid, and how services were reimbursed. Only clients in federally designated rural areas deemed as having a shortage of health professionals were eligible. Store-and-forward technologies were not covered in some cases. And there were issues related to which practitioners were eligible for reimbursement and how they were paid. Reimbursement rules were loosened with the Medicare, Medicaid, and **State Children's Health Insurance Program (SCHIP)** Benefits Improvement and Protection Act of 2000 but not enough to make a significant difference in Medicaid reimbursement or to encourage other third-party payers in the United States to pay for telehealth services. As a result, some physicians and other providers who did teleconsultation did not receive payment for their services. Consequently, increased client volume at referral centers has been regarded as a means to make up for lost revenue.

Support Personnel

While the technology behind telehealth should be easy to use, technical support may be required as new and different skills are required. Support staff should be capable, flexible, and preferably experienced. At the present, questions have not been fully resolved as to who will train healthcare professionals to participate in telehealth and how compensation will be derived for the additional hours associated with installation, training, and use of telehealth technology. There is also an issue of confidentiality. Technical support staff who are present during the exchange of client information need to be aware of institutional policies as well as laws such as HIPAA that are designed to protect client privacy. These individuals should sign the same sort of statement that clinical personnel sign on the receipt of their information system access codes. In the case of home monitoring, support is crucial to help participants feel comfortable with the technology, particularly when using Internet access and Web applications (Cudney, Weinert, & Phillips 2007).

Liability

Telehealth is plagued by a number of liability concerns (ANA 1996; Dickens & Cook 2006). First, there is the possibility that the client may perceive it as inferior because the consulting professional does not perform a hands-on examination. The American Nurses Association (ANA) cautions that telehealth shows great promise as long as it is used to augment, not replace, existing services. Second, professionals who practice across state lines deal with different practice provisions in each state and may be subject to malpractice lawsuits in multiple jurisdictions, raising questions about how that liability might be distributed or which state's practice standards would apply. Theoretically, clients could choose to file suit in the jurisdiction most likely to award damages. The basic question here is, where did the service occur? Third, how might liability be spread among physicians, other healthcare professionals, and technical support persons? And fourth, HIPAA legislation added new concerns to the mix. These issues remain concerns today.

Telehealth has the potential to raise or lower malpractice costs. For example, Pennsylvania's HealthNet recorded teleconferences to provide a complete transcript of the session. Clients were given a videotape for later review and as a means to clarify their comprehension, and the original videotape was kept as part of the client record. The American Nurses Association (1999) called for the development of documentation requirements for telehealth services that addressed treatment recommendations as well as any communication that occurs with other healthcare providers. This strategy should decrease malpractice claims through better documentation and improved client understanding. On the other hand, liability costs may increase if healthcare professionals can be sued in more than one jurisdiction.

Major issues for nurses include questions of liability when information provided over the telephone is misinterpreted, when advice is given across state lines without a license in the state where the client resides, or, particularly, when an unintentional diagnosis comes from the use of an Internet chat room. Liability is unclear in these areas. Regulation of telenursing practice by boards of nursing is difficult when practice crosses state lines. Unless nurses are licensed in every state in which they practice telenursing, respective regulatory boards are unaware of their presence. The majority of states have laws or regulations that require licensure for telehealth practice (Reed 2005).

Authority to practice telenursing across state lines provides the following advantages (National Council of State Boards 1996):

- It establishes the nurse's responsibility and accountability to the board of nursing.
- It establishes legitimacy and availability to practice telenursing.
- It provides jurisdictional authority over the discipline of telenursing in the event that unsafe delivery becomes an issue.

Until this issue has been resolved, nurses must also be cautious when providers from other states give them directions. Several state boards of nursing specifically forbid taking instructions from providers not licensed in the current state.

Box 25–4 summarizes barriers to the practice of telehealth.

BOX 25–4 Barriers to the Use of Telehealth Applications

- **Regulatory barriers.** State laws are either unclear or may forbid practice across state lines.
- **Lack of reimbursement for consultative services.** Most third-party payers do not provide reimbursement unless the client is seen in person.
- **Costs for equipment, network services, and training time.** Equipment capable of transmitting and receiving diagnostic-grade images is still expensive, although costs are declining.
- **Fear of healthcare system changes.** Personnel may fear job loss as more clients can be treated at home and hospital units close.
- **Lack of acceptance by healthcare professionals.** This may stem from liability concerns and discomfort over not seeing a client face-to-face.
- **Lack of acceptance by users.** This may stem from discomfort with technology, the relationship with the provider, and concerns over security of information and confidentiality.

Licensure Issues

Current licensure issues for telemedicine relate to the state in which healthcare professionals are licensed to practice and the jurisdictional boundaries in which services are delivered. Traditionally telemedicine has required multi-state licensure for healthcare professionals, both for their primary state and for the state in which services are rendered. Application for licensure in additional states can be lengthy and expensive, with the ultimate result of restricting access to services. Telehealth advocates want to remove legal barriers to practice through either nationwide or regional licensing or changes in practice acts that permit practitioners from any state to consult with practitioners from another state without the need to be licensed in that second state. The Federation of State Medical Boards drafted legislation to address this issue, calling for the establishment of a registry for telehealth physicians, who would enjoy shorter license application periods and lower fees but have some practice restrictions. Some licensing laws pertaining to telehealth have been enacted or are under consideration, but no resolution has been achieved as yet.

Task forces of the National Council of Nurses suggested multistate licensure as a means to support telenursing. The U.S. Nurse Licensure Compact (NLC) was initiated by the National Council of State Boards of Nursing (NCSBN) in 1997 (NCSBN 2009, 2007). The resulting mutual recognition model allows a nurse in a state that has adopted the compact to practice in other member states but holds the nurse accountable to the practice laws and regulations in the state where telehealth services are provided. As of 2010, 24 states had enacted legislation allowing for nurses to participate in mutual recognition of nurse licensure. No additional compacts have been reported on the NCSBN Web site as of this writing.

The American Nurses Association (1998) did not support this proposed model, however, citing concerns related to discipline, revenue for individual state boards of licensure, and knowledge issues related to allowable practice in other states. Until additional changes are implemented, delivery of services across some state lines via telehealth may be illegal and practitioners must proceed cautiously. The NCSBN was awarded a grant from the Health Resources and Services Administrations Office for the Advancement of telehealth to work on licensure portability (NCSBN 2006). The second licensure issue pertains to what jurisdiction the telehealth practitioner is subject to, the physical space of the practitioner, and the jurisdiction of the recipient (Dickens & Cook 2006).

Confidentiality/Privacy

Although telehealth should not create any greater concerns or risks to medical record privacy than any other form of consultation, records that cross state lines are subject to HIPAA regulations and state privacy laws. Security and confidentiality of telehealth services are crucial to acceptance by consumers and professionals (Hildebrand, Pharow, Engelbrecht, Blobel, Savastano, & Hovsto 2006). For this reason experts have called for the creation of standards for e-health, particularly for security and identity management. Nurses need to be mindful of these issues when technicians, not bound by professional codes of ethics, are present at telehealth sessions. At present, the Office for the Advancement of Telehealth (Department of Health and Human Services) sponsors The Center for Telehealth & E-Health Law Web site; this site provides ongoing information regarding privacy and confidentiality issues in telehealth practice (Ctel 2010a).

OTHER TELEHEALTH ISSUES

There are a number of other important issues related to telehealth. They include the following:

- *Lack of standards.* The lack of plug-and-play interoperability among telehealth devices and point-of-care and other clinical information systems is cited as a major obstacle (Brantley et al. 2004; Charters 2009). There is a need for a standard interface specification that allows telehealth data to be merged easily with information from other clinical information systems. Work is in process on the development of these standards using HL7 messages constructed with Extensible Markup Language.

- *National Health Information Infrastructure (NHII).* In succinct terms, the NHII is all about the secure exchange of healthcare information between a requestor and a provider. While work is in progress the NHII remains a vision at this time. It requires an identity management system, one trusted on a national scale, that will give information providers a means to validate the electronic identity of a requestor. Similar work is presently under way with the U.S. government. Rules are still needed to create electronic IDs for the NHII. The Department of Health and Human Services, the American Telemedicine Association, and the Rand Corporation, among other entities, have been discussing the NHII.

- *Homeland security.* The homeland security community has not given significant consideration to telehealth technology when assessing its needs, strategies, and desired outcomes (Brantley et al. 2004). It can make use of various surveillance systems to analyze symptoms on a large scale for possible biological and chemical attacks.

- *Mainstream acceptance.* Despite its advocates, many healthcare professionals have been slow to accept telehealth applications (Thede 2001; Williams 2007). Their reasons include the perception that telehealth applications are not "real" nursing, that telehealth offers few benefits to them, concerns over privacy and legalities, and fears that telehealth applications will reduce the number of healthcare professionals needed.

- *Accreditation and regulatory requirements.* The Joint Commission on Accreditation of Healthcare Organizations first identified medical staff standards for credentialing and privileging for the practice of telemedicine in 2001 and approved revisions in 2003. Practitioners are required to be credentialed and have privileges at the site where the client is located. Credentialing information from the distant site may be used by the originating site to establish privileges if the distant site is accredited by the Joint Commission. However, this issue for telehealth practitioners remains unresolved as the Joint Commission continues to work on this issue of acceptance of credentialing and privileging decisions by another Joint Commission accredited facility (Ctel 2010b). The Food and Drug Administration has several guidelines for the use of telehealth-related devices.

- *Patient safety.* The majority of discussions that address patient safety emphasize the potential of telehealth to enhance patient safety through applications such as e-prescribing. Some literature makes mention of threats to patient safety when telehealth applications fail to render the same level of care as hands-on care or when problems occur with the use of electrical devices.

- *Limitations.* Despite its many benefits telehealth suffers some limits as well. One is that the quality of transmitted skin tones is dependent upon room lighting. Another is that the distant provider cannot palpate and is dependent upon the skill of the presenter. A third is the lack of smell. Speed and accessibility to information at any time from any place are essential to quality of service (Babulak 2006). Slowdowns or outages in service are not acceptable.

- *Inadequate funding for technology support.* Descriptions of some telehealth applications describe a lack of monies to establish and maintain the technical infrastructure needed (Bond 2006). In some cases, nurses are responsible for the set-up and basic support of telehealth devices. While the wisdom of this approach may be questioned in light of the limited availability of nurses it can be used as an opportunity to establish rapport and comfort with the technology (Starren et al. 2005).

- *Quality of services rendered.* There are two major issues surrounding the quality of telehealth services. One is that services must be at least of the same level of quality as traditional services, particularly for reimbursement services. The second issue is the paradox that geographically isolated populations that stand to derive the largest benefits from telehealth because they have limited access to traditional healthcare services often have the poorest infrastructure, resources, and capability to support telehealth (Liaw and Humphreys 2006).

This situation has been exacerbated by a focus on institutional resources rather than rural poor. Telehealth visits can require extra time for equipment management and transmittal of prescriptions (Boodley 2006). There is also a need for extensive research to establish effectiveness and cost and quality relationships (Miller 2007).

ESTABLISHING A TELEHEALTH LINK

Successful establishment and use of a telehealth link require strategic planning as well as consideration of the following factors: necessary infrastructure, costs and reimbursement, credentialing and privileging by the distant site, human factors, equipment, and technology issues.

Formulating a Telehealth Plan

Any plans for the use of telehealth applications should be in concert with the overall strategic plan of the organization. A telehealth plan minimizes duplicate effort and helps to ensure success. Goals should address the following:

- Current services and deficits
- Telehealth objectives
- Compliance with standards
- Reimbursement policies that favor desired outcomes rather than specific processes
- Periodic review of goals and accomplishments in light of changing technology and needs
- How telecommunication breakdowns will be handled: Will backup be provided? What happens when a power outage in the home severs a link?

The people who will use the system need to be involved in its design from the very beginning. It is wise to start small and expand offerings. Most institutions begin with continuing education and later expand capability. Educational teleconferences require larger rooms that are not suitable for client examinations. Selection of equipment should be based on transmission speed, image resolution, storage capacity, mobility, and ease of use. Higher bandwidth generally improves performance. Equipment should match defined telehealth goals. Box 25–5 lists some strategies to ensure successful teleconferences.

BOX 25–5   Strategies to Ensure Successful Teleconferences

- Select a videoconferencing system to fit your needs, such as a desktop or mobile system or customized room.
- Locate videoconferencing facilities near where they will be used, yet in a quiet, low-traffic area.
- Schedule sessions in advance to avoid time conflicts. Start on time.
- Establish a working knowledge of interactive conferencing features.
- Provide an agenda to keep the conference on track.
- Introduce all participants.
- Set time limits.
- Send materials needed in advance to maintain focus and involve participants.
- Summarize major points at the conclusion.
- Start by asking all participants if they have a good audio and video feed.
- Participate in a conference call as if it were a face-to-face meeting. Enunciate clearly.
- Minimize background noise or use the mute feature.
- Promote interactivity through questions and answers.
- Have technical support available to resolve any problems that might arise.

Building the Supporting Framework Other considerations in telehealth are who will build the infrastructure to support telehealth and what role the federal government should take. Federal and state governments already commit considerable resources to telehealth and related technology. The Department of Commerce, Health Care Financing Administration, Office of Rural Health Policy, and Department of Defense are some of the many federal agencies that have conducted telehealth research and demo programs. Most states have projects in process. The National Information Infrastructure Testbed is a consortium of corporations, universities, and government agencies that views the development of a national information infrastructure as a means to create jobs, promote prosperity, and improve healthcare by reducing redundant procedures and creating an electronic record repository. In their discussion of the infrastructure needed to support telehealth, Nevins and Otley (2002) estimated that a national investment of about $20 to $30 billion was needed. In 2005, Kaushal et al. used estimates from experts to project the cost at $156 billion in capital expenditures over 5 years with another $48 billion in annual operating costs for the creation of a national infrastructure.

Satellite or microwave, telephone lines, or the Internet can support Telehealth transmissions. The cost and speed of the service are interrelated. Satellite and microwave transmission is not feasible for most users. Asynchronous transfer mode (ATM) service is a high-speed data transmission link that can carry large amounts of data quickly. Speeds range from 0.45 megabits per second (Mbps) to 2.48 gigabits per second (Gbps). ATM works well when large sets of data, such as MRIs, need to be exchanged and discussed. Present ATM use is limited for reasons of cost, availability, and lack of standards. Another option for data transmission is switched multi-megabit data service, better known as a T1 line. T1 lines are high-speed telephone lines that may be used to transmit high-quality, full-motion video at speeds up to 1.544 Mbps. T1 services are leased monthly at a fixed charge independent of use. Next in descending order of speed are DSL (digital subscriber lines) and integrated service digital network (ISDN) lines. DSL uses existing copper telephone wires to transfer high bandwidth data. DSL availability has traditionally been limited by distance from the central telephone office. Variants of DSL technology can rival T1 lines for speed of data transmission. ISDN lines carry 128 kilobits per second (kbps), although lines can be bundled for faster speeds. Each ISDN line costs approximately $30 per month plus costs for calls. ISDN lines support medical imaging, database sharing, desktop videoconferencing, and access to the Internet. Telehealth's identification of 384 kbps as its practical minimum bandwidth renders plain old telephone service unsuitable for most applications. Faster access speeds are required for continuing medical education, telemetry, remote consults, and network-based services.

The Internet already carries e-mail for many healthcare professionals and is a powerful tool for obtaining and publishing information. Security and access issues will determine the extent to which client-specific information is interchanged on the Internet. The American Medical Association has published guidelines for e-mail correspondence for clients on its Web site.

Cable also has the potential to bring high-resolution x-ray images to on-call radiologists at home via its broadband capabilities.

Human Factors On-site support and commitment from administrators and healthcare professionals are necessary for successful telehealth practice. Bulik (2008) reported high levels of comfort among practitioners and patients although satisfaction scores were somewhat lower. Palmas, Teresi, Weinstock, and Shea (2008) also found a good level of acceptability among practitioners for telehealth as a tool to manage diabetic patients. Overall, client satisfaction with telehealth services is high, particularly when care is perceived as easier to obtain or otherwise more convenient (Lutz, Chumbler, Llyles, Hoffman, & Kobb 2009; Marcin et al. 2004). Healthcare professionals should provide input about the type of telehealth applications that they would like to see to their professional organizations and healthcare providers. One application, continuing education distance learning programs, has been well received and serves to introduce other applications. As a subspecialty area of practice, telehealth has developed its own set of knowledge and skills that must be incorporated into the orientation process for professionals new to the area (Williams 2007). Specific competencies that must be addressed include training time to develop the technical skills needed to set up and use equipment, professional knowledge, interpersonal skills, documentation, professional development, resource management, and practice and administrative issues. Telehealth and all of its applications are new to most people and time is needed to get accustomed to telehealth practices. An example of this may be seen in teleradiology, where radiologists must learn how to interpret images using a monitor. However, it is possible to enhance images for easier interpretation.

Equipment Equipment must be reliable, accurate, and flexible enough to meet varying needs. One example of this principle may be seen when equipment purchased for continuing education also supports high-resolution images needed for diagnostic images. However, it is not necessary to have all the latest, most expensive technology to start telehealth. Desktop videoconferencing uses specially adapted PCs to operate over telephone lines. These PCs may be merged with existing diagnostic imaging systems and other information systems. While it usually lacks broadcast picture quality, desktop teleconferencing provides an opportunity to practice some telehealth applications at a fairly low cost. Consulting parties may be able to see each other and diagnostic images by splitting the PC screen into segments. Box 25–6 lists components needed to support DTV.

Telehealth Costs Estimates for setting up videoconferencing vary greatly, depending on the type of system and applications chosen. Desktop systems are fairly inexpensive. Better resolution increases costs. Costs include equipment purchase, operation, and maintenance; network services; and time to learn new skills. Time needed to learn how to use telehealth applications is often underestimated.

Technology Issues Many of the early technical problems associated with telehealth have been largely resolved. Present issues include resolution, frame rate, standards, and record storage and location. Resolution is the sharpness or clarity of an image. The resolution needed for interpretation of diagnostic images requires a broad bandwidth that is at least 384 kilobits and 30 frames per second (FPS). Video systems work by rapidly displaying a series of still images referred to as frames. Frames per second, or the frame rate, refers to the number of these images that are captured, transmitted, and displayed in one second. The higher the FPS, the smoother the picture. Broadcast quality transmission is 30 FPS. Lower FPS rates produce marginally acceptable video that may be suitable for purposes other than interpretation of diagnostic images. Many DTV systems do not offer broadcast quality at this time. Bandwidth, the efficiency of compression, and hardware and software limitations all determine videoconference frame

BOX 25–6 Basic DTV Components for Telehealth Applications

- PC
- PC adapter cards
- Camera
- Microphones
- Video overlay cards
- External speakers on existing PCs with broadband switches
- Special adaptive tools, such as an electronic stethoscope

rates. Another issue related to frame rate is the delay that is noted for one videoconferencing party to respond to another. Although this period is only a few seconds long, it must be factored into teleconferences. Another issue related to resolution is the need to digitize x-rays for transmission and storage. For these reasons, teleradiology applications require more costly equipment and telecommunication services.

Healthcare personnel need to shape the development of technological standards by determining the minimal acceptable standards to ensure quality at the lowest possible costs. Acceptance of international standard H.320 for passing audio and video data streams across networks allowed videoconferencing systems from different manufacturers to communicate. H.320 is a standard for the connection and transfer of multimedia data that allows the transmission and reception of image and sound. It supports a wide range of transmission rates. Prior to the adoption of H.320, only systems produced by the same vendor could communicate. Work continues in this area so that continued improvements can be expected. Other important standards for telehealth include the Digital Image Communication in Medicine (DICOM) standard and the Joint Photographic Experts Group (JPEG) compression standard for digital images. DICOM seeks to promote the communication, storage, and integration of digital image information with other hospital information systems, while JPEG is used to compress images as a means to decrease transmission time and storage requirements. Work is under way for the development of plug-and-play standards to integrate and exchange information captured with telehealth technology with that housed in clinical information systems.

Most discussions of telehealth include the electronic health record as a means to make client data readily available and store diagnostic images. Picture archiving communications systems (PACS) are storage systems that permit remote access to diagnostic images at a time convenient to the physician. While PACS technology has been available for a number of years, its early history was troubled. Recent technological improvements make PACS feasible.

TELENURSING

At one time the number of references noted in the literature relative to telenursing was limited even though telenursing has been in existence for decades, using available technology to serve its purposes. For example, the telephone has long been used as a communication tool between nurses and healthcare consumers as well as other professionals. As new technology became available, it was also adapted to educate consumers and peers, maintain professional contacts, and provide care to clients at other sites. As a result, nurses currently use telephones, faxes, computers, smart phones, sophisticated voice and video interactive teleconference systems, and the Internet in the practice of telenursing. Potential applications are varied, but common uses are telephone triage, follow-up calls, and checking biometric measurements. Other examples include education, professional consultations, obtaining test results, and taking physician instructions over the phone. Interactive television or teleconferences enable home health nurses to make electronic house calls to clients in their homes; thus nurses can see more clients per day than would be possible via on-site visits. Some advanced practice nurses maintain a primary practice via telehealth (Boodley 2006). Telenursing currently addresses aging populations and chronic disease problems, community and home-based care needs, geographic health services access problems, and nursing shortage issues.

Globally, there are numerous instances of telenursing (International Council of Nurses 2009a). The International Council of Nurses (ICN) launched the ICN Telenursing Network in Durban South Africa in 2009. Finland's ongoing nationwide project (2008–2012) is focusing on development of unified terms for nursing documentation in electronic health records. England is piloting telehealth services in the case management of patients with chronic obstructive pulmonary disease. Another instance of telenursing is the Telenurse project in Europe, which seeks to standardize the mechanism for describing and communicating nursing care as a means to enable comparisons of nursing practice from one site to another without regard to region or country. In their description of a survey of English-speaking telenurses, Grady and Schlachta-Fairchild (2007) see unlimited opportunities for telenursing, although they note continued issues related to reimbursement, licensure, liability, privacy and confidentiality, quality of care, education, and training for the use of telehealth applications.

The International Telenurses Association was founded in 1995 to promote and support nursing involvement in telehealth and serve as a resource for nurses. The International Council of Nurses published International Competencies for Telenursing in 2007. The ICN (2009b) acknowledges the role of telenurses in addressing health system challenges. The American Nurses Association (1999) published its Core Principles on Telehealth in 1999. These guidelines are intended to help nurses protect client privacy during the delivery of telehealth services. The American Academy of Ambulatory Care Nursing published Telehealth Nursing Practice Essentials in 2009, the Telehealth Nursing Practice Core Course CD-ROM, and its fourth edition of Telehealth Nursing Practice Standards in 2007. Other healthcare providers have also developed policy statements or standards of practice, and special interest groups have formed. Telehealth nursing practice is now considered to be a subspecialty of nursing; although Grady and Schlachta-Fairchild (2007) note that the majority of telenurses are not certified in telemedicine, telenursing, or nursing informatics at present, they believe that basic telehealth principles should be integrated into the basic nursing curriculum, which may lead to certification. A study evaluating the feasibility of telenursing in Korea indicated a need to identify telenursing specialties, create a business model, and develop the infrastructure to support practice (Yun & Park 2007).

Despite all of this work a survey conducted of Australian nursing students just a few years ago found that the majority of the respondents remained largely unaware of what e-health was and how it related to their practice (Edirippulige, Smith, Beattie, Davies, & Wootton 2007; E-health, what health? 2007).

FUTURE DIRECTIONS

Many providers predict that telehealth will change the way that healthcare is delivered and carve out new roles for healthcare providers. Changes have already started. The way that consumer rights and responsibilities are viewed is changing with the increased use of new technology to deliver care (Finch, Mort, May, & Mair 2005). Telehealth offers new means to locate health information and communicate with practitioners through e-mail and interactive chats or videoconferences. It provides new ways to monitor clients. Smart surveillance cameras and analytic software can be used in the home environment to notify caregivers of changes in activity, falls, or lack of movement in the homes of elderly clients. Telehealth cuts down on the need to travel and miss work to seek care. Web-based disease management programs encourage clients to assume greater responsibility for their own care. Applications developed for the military are now available for emergency treatment in some communities. Remote monitoring and use of global positioning systems to direct ambulances to the closest, or best, treatment centers are available now. Mobile technology such as PDAs and point-of-care systems capture data quickly and efficiently facilitate the transmission of data for analysis and use by administrators when they need it, not months or years later. Telehealth services have been slow to take off in the United States primarily due to a lack of reimbursement, but the demand is expected to grow exponentially as Baby Boomers age. Demands for quality, patient safety, and more care options will help change the reimbursement picture, opening the door for more telehealth applications. Brantley et al. (2004) note that better coordination of planning, policy making, and allocation of resources is needed.

Converged devices such as smart phones combine the utility of cell phones and PDAs, allowing users to check e-mail, run applications, and monitor telemetry patients while performing other tasks. These devices provide the potential to increase patient safety, facilitate communication among healthcare professionals, and subsequently reduce liability as orders can be viewed, thus eliminating errors associated with poor handwriting or verbal instructions (Rosenthal 2006).

The Federal Communications Commission (FCC), the National Rural Health Association, the Health Resources and Services Administration Office for the Advancement of Telehealth, and the Healthcare Information and Management Systems Society have been working to demonstrate how telehealth programs and networks can improve the quality of care in underserved populations and to provide grants (Bazzoli 2004; Federal telepractice grants 2006). Until recently, the FCC's telemedicine program has not been well utilized. In 2003, new rules were announced that were designed to improve access for rural healthcare programs. The program enables rural providers to obtain access to modern telecommunication technologies through discounts to telecommunication services charges. These changes are expected to encourage the adoption of more telehealth applications.

Connected health, a new paradigm of care, promises to reduce costs and improve quality by working with clients proactively. People monitor their own health, which results in fewer visits to physicians and inpatient hospital stays (Whitlinger, Ayyagari, McClure, Fisher, & Lopez 2007). Coordinated healthcare is interconnected. Home-based care will continue its exponential growth as a means to help keep older patients in their own homes and better manage their health (Telemedicine's adolescent angst 2007).

There will be additional work on the national and international telehealth research agenda to supplement that started by Grady and Tschirich (2006) and others that will demonstrate the efficacies of the discipline, standard outcomes, and methodologies. This work will occur in conjunction with various stakeholders. Efforts will entail the education and lobbying of groups with research funds such as the National Institute for Nursing Research, the Robert Wood Johnson Foundation, and the Association of Retired Persons.

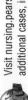

Visit nursing.pearsonhighered.com for additional cases, information, and weblinks.

CASE STUDY EXERCISE

You are the nurse practitioner in St. Theresa's emergency department. A client is brought in with obvious psychiatric problems. You have no psychiatrist available and the nearest psychiatric facility is a 1-hour drive away. St. Theresa is a Tri-State Health Care Alliance Member. Tri-State has telehealth links with the regional hospital, where a psychiatrist is in the emergency department. What steps would you take to initiate a productive teleconference? Justify your response.

SUMMARY

- Telehealth is the use of telecommunication technologies and computers to provide healthcare information and services to clients at another location.
- Telehealth is a broad term that encompasses telemedicine but includes the provision of care and the distribution of information to healthcare providers and consumers.
- Efforts to contain costs, improve the delivery of care to all segments of the population, and meet consumer demands make telehealth an attractive tool. Telehealth can help healthcare providers treat clients earlier when they are not as ill and care costs less, provide services in the local community where it is less expensive, improve follow-up care, improve client access to services, and improve the quality of the client's record.
- Telehealth applications vary greatly and include client monitoring, diagnostic evaluation, decision support and expert systems, storage and dissemination of records, and education of healthcare professionals.

- Teleconferencing and videoconferencing are tools that facilitate the delivery of telehealth services.
- Desktop videoconferencing (DTV) is an important development that enables the expansion of telehealth applications into new areas. DTV uses specially adapted personal computers to link persons at two or more sites.
- Telenursing uses telecommunications and computer technology for the delivery of nursing care and services to clients at other sites.
- Neither telemedicine nor telenursing is new. Applications include education of healthcare consumers and professionals as well as the provision of care. In addition to the use of the telephone for triage and information, clients may be monitored at home via telephone or teleconferences. Telehealth is a tool that helps healthcare providers to work more efficiently.
- Major issues associated with the practice of telehealth and telenursing include a lack of reimbursement, infrastructure, plug-and-play standards, licensure and liability issues, and concerns related to client privacy and confidentiality.
- The successful use of telehealth and telenursing is best ensured through the development and implementation of a plan that addresses current services and deficits, goals, technical requirements, compliance with standards and laws, reimbursement, and strategies to handle telecommunication breakdowns.
- Telehealth and telenursing applications are expected to become more commonplace once reimbursement and licensure barriers are removed and technical standards for the exchange of information between telehealth devices and clinical information systems are established.
- Telehealth has the capacity to revolutionize the delivery of healthcare and has already started to do so.

REFERENCES

Agency for Healthcare Research and Quality (AHRQ). (2001, February). *Telemedicine for the Medicare population: Summary* (Evidence Report/Technology Assessment: Number 24, AHRQ Publication Number 01-E011). Retrieved from http://www.ahrq.gov/clinic/epcsums/telemedsum.htm

Agency for Healthcare Research and Quality (AHRQ). (2010). *Telehealth*. Retrieved from http://www.healthit.ahrq.gov/portal/server.pt

American Nurses Association. (1996, October 9). *Telehealth—Issues for nursing*. Retrieved from http://nursingworld.org/readroom/tele2.htm

American Nurses Association. (1998, June 24). *Multistate regulation of nurses*. Retrieved from http://nursingworld.org/gova/multibg.htm

American Nurses Association. (1999). *Core principles on telehealth*. Washington, DC: American Nurses Publishing.

American Psychiatric Association. (2010). *Topic 4: Telepsychiatry*. Retrieved from http://psych.org/Departments/HSF/UnderservedClearinghouse/Linkeddocuments/telepsychiatry.aspx

ATA adopts telehomecare clinical guidelines. (2007). Retrieved from http://www.atmeda.org/news/guidelines.htm

Babulak, E. (2006). Quality of service provision assessment in the healthcare information and telecommunications infrastructures. *International Journal of Medical Informatics, 75*(3–4), 246–252.

Bahaadini, K., Yogesan, K., & Wooton, R. (2009). Health staff priorities for the future development of telehealth in Western Australia. *Rural and Remote Health, 9*(3), 1164.

Bazzoli, F. (2004, January). Telemedicine gets FCC boost. *Healthcare IT News, 1*(1), 11.

Bond, G. E. (2006). Lessons learned from the implementation of a web-based nursing intervention. *Computers, Informatics, Nursing, 24*(2), 66–74.

Bonneville, L., & Pare, D. J. (2006). Socioeconomic stakes in the development of telemedicine. *Journal of Telemedicine and Telecare, 12*(5), 217–219.

Boodley, C. (2006). Primary care telehealth practice. *Journal of the American Academy of Nurse Practitioners, 18*(8), 343–345.

Brantley, D., Laney-Cummings, K., & Spivack, R. (2004, February). *Innovation, demand and investment in teleheatlh*. A report of the Technology Administration, U.S. Department of Commerce Office of Technology Policy. Retrieved from http://www.technology.gov/reports/TechPolicy/Telehealth/2004Report.pdf

Brennan, P. (1996, October). *Nursing informatics: Technology in the service of patient care*. Paper presented at the meeting of Alpha Rho Chapter of Sigma Theta Tau, Morgantown, WV.

Brown, N. (2002). *Telemedicine coming of age*. Retrieved from http://trc.telemed.org/telemedicine/primer.asp

Bulik, R. (2008). Human factors in primary care telemedicine encounters. *Journal of Telemedicine and Telecare, 14*(4), 169–172. doi:10.1258/jtt.2007.007041

Castro, D. (2009). *Explaining international IT application leadership: Health IT*. Information Technology and Innovation Foundation Report. Retrieved from http://www.itif.org/publications/explaining-international-it-application-leadership-health-it

Center for Telehealth and E-Health Law (Ctel). (2010a). *HIPPA—Privacy & confidentiality*. Retrieved from http://telehealthlawcenter.org/?c=181

Center for Telehealth and E-Health Law (Ctel). (2010b). *Joint Commission telehealth expert to speak at Washington live!* Brown bag telehealth seminar on January 21, 2010. Retrieved from http://telehealthlawcenter.org/?c=125&a=2166

Center for Telehealth and E-Health Law (Ctel). (2011). *Reimbursement main page*. Retrieved from http://www.ctel.org/expertise/reimbursement/

Centers for Medicare & Medicaid Services (CMS). (2009a, September 15). *Telemedicine overview*. Retrieved from http://www.cms.hhs.gov/Telemedicine/

Centers for Medicare & Medicaid Services (CMS). (2009b, December 18). *Pub 100-02 medicare benefit policy*. Retrieved from https://www.cms.gov/transmittals/downloads/R118BP.pdf

Charters, K. (2009). Home telehealth electronic health information lessons learned. *Studies in Health Technology and Informatics, 146*, 719.

Coyle, M., Duffy, J., & Martin, E. (2007). Teaching/learning health promoting behaviors through telehealth. *Nursing Education Perspectives, 28*(1), 18–23.

Cross, F., Barnes, N., & Jawad, A. (2010). Landmark case reports. *Grand Rounds Online Journal*. Retrieved from http://www.grandrounds-e-med.com/index.php

Cross, M. A. (2007). Reaching out to rural residents. *Health Data Management, 15*(6), 62–63.

Cudney, S. A., Weinert, C., & Phillips, L. A. (2007). Telephone technical support: An essential adjunct to computer intervention for rural chronically ill women. *Computers, Informatics, Nursing, 25*(4), 221–227.

Cunningham, B., & Vande Merwe, R. (2009). Virtual grand rounds: A new educational approach in social work that benefits long-term care providers and patients in rural Idaho. *Rural and Remote Health, 9*(1), 1073.

Cwiek, M. A., Rafiq, A., Qamar, A., Tobey, C., & Merrell, R. C. (2007). Telemedicine licensure in the United States: The need for a cooperative regional approach. *Telemedicine Journal and e-Health, 13*(2), 141–147.

Demiris, G., Edison, K., & Vijaykumar, S. (2005). A comparison of communication models of traditional and video-mediated healthcare delivery. *International Journal of Medical Informatics, 74*(10), 851–856.

Demiris, G., Oliver, D. P., & Courtney, K. L. (2006). Ethical considerations for the utilization of telehealth technologies in home and hospice care by the nursing profession. *Nursing Administration Quarterly, 30*(1), 56–66.

Department of Veteran Affairs. (2009, December 17). *VA's innovative telehealth device brings clinical team to veteran's bedside*. Retrieved from http://www.washingtondc.va.gov/news/telehealth-news.aspx

Department of Veteran Affairs—VistA. (2006, July). *Innovations in American government award fact sheet*. Retrieved from http://www.innovations.va.gov/innovations/doc/InnovationFactSheet.pdf

Dickens, B. M., & Cook, R. J. (2006). Legal and ethical issues in telemedicine and robotics. *International Journal of Gynaecology and Obstetrics, 94*(1), 73–78.

Edirippulige, S., Smith, A., Beattie, H., Davies, E., & Wootton, R. (2007). Pre-registration nurses: An investigation of knowledge, experience and comprehension of e-health. *Australian Journal of Advanced Nursing, 25*(2), 78–83.

E-health, what health? (2007, April). *Australian Nursing Journal, 14*(9), 7.

Ellis, D. G., & Mayrose, J. (2003). The success of emergency telemedicine at the State University of New York at Buffalo. *Telemedicine Journal and e-Health, 9*(1), 73–79.

Federal telepractice grants available: Funds will assist underserved rural and urban communities. (2006). *ASHA Leader.* Retrieved from CINAHL with Full Text database.

Finch, T., Mort, M., May, C., & Mair, F. (2005). Telecare: Perspectives on the changing role of patients and citizens. *Journal of Telemedicine and Telecare, 11*(Suppl. 1), 51–53.

Fincher, L., Ward, C., Dawkins, V., Magee, V., & Willson, P. (2009). Using telehealth to educate Parkinson's disease patients about complicated medication regimens. *Journal of Gerontological Nursing, 35*(2), 16–24.

Gagnon, M. P., Lamothe, L., Hebert, M., Chanliau, J., & Fortin, J. P. (2006). Telehomecare for vulnerable populations: The evaluation of new models of care. *Telemedicine Journal and e-Health, 12*(3), 324–331.

Garrett, N., & Martini, E. M. (2007). The boomers are coming: A total cost of care model of the impact of population aging on the cost of chronic conditions in the United States. *Disease Management, 10*(2), 51–60.

Goedert, J. (2007). Bringing I.T. into the home. *Health Data Management, 15*(7), 36, 38, 42.

Grady, J., & Tschirich, P. (2006, October 31). *Creating a national telehealth nursing research agenda.* Retrieved from http://tie.telemed.org/articles/article.asp?path=articles&article=telehealth NursingAgenda_ca_tie06.xml

Grady, J. L., & Schlachta-Fairchild, L. (2007). Report of the 2004–2005 International Telenursing Survey. *Computers, Informatics, Nursing, 25*(5), 266–272.

Gray, G. A., Stamm, B. H., Toevs, S., Reischl, U., & Yarrington, D. (2006). Study of participating and nonparticipating states' telemedicine Medicaid reimbursement status: Its impact on Idaho's policymaking process. *Telemedicine Journal and e-Health, 12*(6), 681–690.

Hailey, D., Foerster, V., Nakagawa, B., Wapshall, T. M., Murtagh, J. A., & Smitten, J., . . . Wong, G. (2005). Achievements and challenges on policies for allied health professionals. *Journal of Telemedicine and Telecare, 11*(Suppl. 2), S39–S41.

Hildebrand, C., Pharow, P., Engelbrecht, R., Blobel, B., Savastano, M., & Hovsto, A. (2006). Bio-health—The need for security and identity management standards in eHealth. *Studies in Health Technology and Informatics, 121,* 327–336.

Hi-tech home help. (2007, July). *Nursing & Residential Care.* Retrieved from CINAHL with Full Text database.

Hogenbirk, J. C., Brockway, P. D., Finley, J., Jennett, P., Yeo, M., & Parker-Taillon, D., . . . Cradduck, T. (2006). Framework for Canadian telehealth guidelines: Summary of the environmental scan. *Journal of Telemedicine and Telecare, 12*(2), 64–70.

Institute of Medicine (IOM). (1996). *Telemedicine: A guide to assess telecommunications in healthcare.* Retrieved from http://books.nap.edu/books/ 0309055318/html/2.html

International Council of Nurses. (2009a, December). *Telenursing network bulletin: No 1.* Retrieved from http://www.icn.ch/telenursing_bulletin.htm

International Council of Nurses. (2009b, April). *Press release: ICN telenursing network launched by the international council of nurses.* Retrieved from http://www.icn.ch/Pro7_09.htm

Introducing: Telehealth and telecare. (2007, July). *British Journal of Community Nursing, 12*(7), 307–307.

Karunanithi, M. (2007). Monitoring technology for the elderly patient. *Expert Review of Medical Devices, 4*(2), 267–277.

Kaushal, R., Blumenthal, B., Poon, E. G., Jha, A. K., Franz, C., & Middleton, B., . . . Cost of National Health Information Network Working Group (2005, August 2). The costs of a national health information network. *Annals of Internal Medicine, 143*(3), 165–173.

Kennedy, C. A. (2005). The challenges of economic evaluations of remote technical health interventions. *Clinical and Investigative Medicine, 28*(2), 71–74.

Kline, S., & Schofield, R. (2006, Spring). Telehealth and care coordination improves outcomes for veterans with heart failure. *Progress in Cardiovascular Nursing, 21*(2), 111–112.

Koch, S. (2006). Meeting the challenges—The role of medical informatics in an ageing society. *Studies in Health Technology and Informatics, 124,* 25–31.

Lamprinos, I. E., Prentza, A., & Koutsouris, D. (2006). Communication protocol requirements of patient personal area networks for telemonitoring. *Technology and Health Care, 14*(3), 171–187.

Lancaster, P., Krumm, M., Ribera, J., & Klich, R. (2008). Remote hearing screenings via telehealth in a rural elementary school. *American Journal of Audiology, 17*(2), 114–122.

Lehmann, C., Mintz, N., & Giacini, J. (2006). Impact of telehealth on healthcare utilization by congestive heart failure patients. *Disease Management and Health Outcomes, 14*(3), 163–169.

The Lewin Group, Inc. (2000, December). *Assessment of approaches to evaluating telemedicine.* Final report prepared for Office of the Assistant Secretary for Planning and Evaluation, Department of Health and Human Services. Retrieved from http://www.aspe.hhs.gov/health/reports/AAET/aaet.htm

Liaw, S., & Humphreys, J. (2006). Rural eHealth paradox: It's not just geography! *Australian Journal of Rural Health, 14*(3), 95–98.

Lillibridge, J., & Hanna, B. (2008). Using telehealth to deliver nursing case management services to HIV/AIDS clients. *The Online Journal of Issues in Nursing, 14*(1). Retrieved from http://www.nursingworld.org/MainMenuCategories/ANAMarketplace/ANAPeriodicals/OJIN/TableofContents/Vol142009/No1Jan09/ArticlePreviousTopic/TelehealthandHIVAIDSClients.aspx

Lipowicz, A. (2010, February 17). VA takes a leap of faith into telehealth: Telehealth has money and support, but does it have a plan? *Federal Computer Week.* Retrieved from http://fcw.com/Articles/2010/02/22/HOME-PAGE-Health-IT-telehealth.aspx

Lutz, B., Chumbler, N., Lyles, T., Hoffman, N., & Kobb, R. (2009). Testing a home-telehealth programme for US veterans recovering from stroke and their family caregivers. *Disability and Rehabilitation, 31*(5), 402–409.

Manfredi, L., Shupe, J., & Batki, S. L. (2005). Rural jail telepsychiatry: A pilot feasibility study. *Telemedicine Journal and e-Health, 11*(5), 574–577.

Marcin, J. P., Ellis, J., Mawis, R., Nagrampa, E., Nesbitt, T. S., & Dimand, R. J. (2004). Using telemedicine to provide pediatric subspecialty care to children with special health care needs in an underserved rural community. *Pediatrics, 113*(1 Pt. 1), 1–6.

Midwest VA service network deploys $2 million telemedicine network. (2007, September 13). *Telemedicine and Telehealth News.* Retrieved from http://tie.telemed.org/news/

Miller, E. A. (2007, July). Solving the disjuncture between research and practice: Telehealth trends in the 21st century. *Health Policy, 82*(2), 133–141.

National Council of State Boards of Nursing (NCSBN). (1996). Telenursing: The regulatory implications for multistate regulation. *Issues, 17*(3), 1, 8–9.

National Council of State Boards of Nursing (NCSBN). (2006, December 14). *NCSBN hosts summit funded by federal grant to promote nurse licensure portability.* Retrieved from https://www.ncsbn.org/1097.htm

National Council of State Boards of Nursing (NCSBN). (2007). *About: Background information about the RN and LPN/VN Nurse Licensure Compact (NLC).* Retrieved from https://www.ncsbn.org/156.htm

National Council of State Boards of Nursing (NCSBN). (2009, July 17). *NCSBN welcomes Missouri as the 24th state to join the Nurse Licensure Compact.* Retrieved from http://www.ncsbn.org/1689.htm

Nevins, R., & Otley, V. C., III. (2002). Demystifying telehealth. *Health Management Technology, 23*(7), 51, 52.

Palmas, W., Teresi, J., Weinstock, R., & Shea, S. (2008). Acceptability to primary care providers of telemedicine in diabetes case management. *Journal of Telemedicine and Telecare, 14*(6), 306–308.

Reed, K. (2005, May). Telemedicine: Benefits to advanced practice nursing and the communities they serve. *Journal of the American Academy of Nurse Practitioners, 17*(5), 176–180.

Riverside County Foundation on Aging for the Riverside County Advisory Council on Aging and Riverside County Office on Aging, in partnership with VNA of the Inland Counties and the Riverside Community Health Foundation. (2006, October). *Using telehealth and other connective technologies to reach and serve older adults and adults with disabilities.* Retrieved from http://www.rcaging.org/opencms/system/galleries/download/ooaging/telehealth_report_oct06.pdf

Rosenberg, H. (2007). Not-for-profit report. Connecting with seniors to reduce hospitalizations. *Nursing Homes: Long Term Care Management, 56*(1), 41–42.

Rosenthal, K. (2006). Enjoy "smarter" patient monitoring. *Nursing Management, 37*(5), 52.

Sato, A. F., Clifford, L. M., Silverman, A. H., & Davies, W. H. (2009). Cognitive-behavioral interventions via telehealth: Applications to pediatric functional abdominal pain. *Children's Health Care, 38*(1), 1–22.

Schneider, P. (1996). Washington word: Telecom reform. *Healthcare Informatics, 12*(3), 93, 691.

Smith, E. (2004). Telehealth in the tundra. *Health Management Technology, 25*(3), 24–26.

Starren, J., Tsai, C., Bakken, S., Aidalay, A., Morin, P. C., Hillman, C., . . . IDEATel Consortium. (2005). The role of nurses in installing telehealth technology in the home. *Computers, Informatics, Nursing, 23*(4), 181–189.

States require reimbursement for telemedicine. (2004, March 19). *Psychiatric News, 39*(6), 14.

Stronge, A. J., Rogers, W. A., & Fisk, A. D. (2007). Human factors considerations in implementing telemedicine systems to accommodate older adults. *Journal of Telemedicine and Telecare, 13*(2), 1–3.

Telemedicine's adolescent angst. (2007). *Hospitals & Health Networks, 81*(6), 66, 68, 70.

Thede, L. Q. (2001). Overview and summary: Telehealth: Promise or peril? *Online Journal of Issues in Nursing, 6*(3). Retrieved from http://nursingworld.org/ojin/topic16/tpc16top.htm

Tracy, J., Rheuban, K., Waters, R. J., DeVany, M., & Whitten, P. (2008). Critical steps to scaling telehealth for national reform. *Telemedicine and e-Health, 14*(9), 990–994.

Walter Reed Army Medical Center. (2010). *Telepsychiatry and community mental health service.* Retrieved from http://www/wramc.army.mil/Patients/healthcare/psychaitry/mentalhealthservice/Pages/default.aspx

Wertenberger, S., Yerardi, R., Drake, A. C., & Parlier, R. (2006). Veterans health administration office of nursing services exploration of positive patient care synergies fueled by consumer demand: Care coordination, advanced clinic access, and patient self-management. *Nursing Administration Quarterly, 30*(2), 137–146.

Whitlinger, D., Ayyagari, D., McClure, D., Fisher, J., & Lopez, F. (2007). Straight talk. Collaboration fosters connected health: A new paradigm of proactive healthcare. *Modern Healthcare, 37*(21), 4–50.

Williams, C. (2007). Telehealth nursing practice. *AAACN Viewpoint, 29*(1), 12.

World Health Organization. (2009, October 6). *eHealth intelligence report: eHealth worldwide.* Retrieved from http://www.who.int/goe/ehir/2009/6_october_2009/en/

Yun, E. K., & Park, H. A. (2007). Strategy development for the implementation of telenursing in Korea. *Computers, Informatics, Nursing, 25*(5), 301–306.

CHAPTER 26

Public Health Informatics

After completing this chapter, you should be able to:

1. Define *public health informatics.*

2. Examine need and support for public health informatics (PHI).

3. Identify resources available to assist in disaster or crisis communication.

4. Examine key issues with respect to information and communication technology (ICT) for populations and healthcare providers.

5. Discuss implications of public health informatics to improve patient and population outcomes.

INTRODUCTION

There is no doubt that technology and healthcare informatics are playing a larger role in the daily lives of healthcare providers in a variety of clinical practice settings, but technology and healthcare informatics are also playing a larger role in society and for individuals as well. For example, there is evidence indicating that more people in the general population are using information technology services, like those from Google, to self-diagnose based on signs and symptoms.

Historically speaking, public health has largely focused on disease surveillance and protection of public health, but recently there has been an increased focus on increased consumer engagement for self-improvement and communication of public health issues and trends to the public (Institute of Medicine 2011). The public health informatics field has expanded significantly over the past 7 years with a clarion call for better national security and integration of information and resources post September 11 (Kukafka 2007). Public health informatics (PHI) will play a major role in these initiatives. The purpose of this chapter is to increase awareness and sensitivity to selected major issues related to PHI and systems to provide public health information to individuals and populations.

PUBLIC HEALTH INFORMATICS

Public health informatics is defined in several ways but one of the most widely accepted definitions of PHI is "the systematic application of information and computer science and technology to public health practice, research and learning" (Yasnoff, O'Carroll, Koo, Linkins, & Kilbourne 2000, p. 67). Public health has always been about disease surveillance and management, particularly the identification of major disease outbreaks. Public health also pinpoints disease causation, distribution of disease, and frequency of disease occurrence or transmission (Macha & McDonough 2012).

PHI is distinguished from other information systems and technology by its emphasis on prevention in populations (Yasnoff, O'Carroll, Koo, Linkins, & Kilbourne 2000, p. 67). The focus on population health is linked to prevention as opposed to diagnosis and treatment. Public health has a governmental context as public health nearly always involves linkages to government agencies at the local, regional, national, or global levels.

Data collection and analysis has always been an essential element for public health, and epidemiologists must gather data from a wide variety of resources to solve and seek out resolution of the epidemiological issue. For example, John Snow was one of the very early epidemiologists who collected and analyzed public health data during the cholera outbreak in England. Through his careful data collection and analysis, Snow was able to track the source of the cholera outbreak to a well from which many citizens obtained their drinking water. It is apparent that in today's global population epidemiologists and healthcare providers are working with larger data sets, making it impossible to do this important work without the assistance of information and computer technology. In fact here is a clear and compelling link between information technology, computer skills, and public health knowledge and practice.

In addition to locating sources of public health information through large data sources, public health informatics assists in tracking and trending health and illness data for surveillance of many actual and potential public health issues. For example, surveillance systems provide accurate, timely, and relevant data about actual or potential health issues, promoting rapid and prompt communication of these issues and threats to a variety of persons and organizations. It is this type of constant public health surveillance and monitoring that saves lives and improves individual and population outcomes as a result of the timely and prompt recognition that an issue exists or is pending. One of the major challenges with PHI is the need to have stronger linkages and interfaces between and among providers and systems to enhance communications particularly related to man-made and natural disasters around the globe.

NEED AND SUPPORT FOR PUBLIC HEALTH INFORMATICS

Effective databases and sources of information for public health systems require application and knowledge from a variety of systems and professions. According to Yasnoff, O'Carroll, Koo, Linkins, and Kilbourne (2000, p. 69), there are four major principles of public health informatics linked to the scope and nature of public health that are distinguishable from other types of informatics; these principles "define, guide, and provide the context for the types of activities and challenges that comprise" the public health informatics field. Box 26–1 identifies the four principles and focus of each.

It is apparent that the ability to communicate between and among many systems is critical from a public health perspective on a continuum from meeting healthcare needs across the life span. This includes being able to communicate on a nationwide level about immunization schedules and medical and health treatment plans for communicable disease and also to know how to serve and meet public health needs in the event of a natural or global disaster like an act of bioterrorism.

With respect to public health communication and tracking of immunizations the Centers for Disease Control and Prevention has begun national initiatives to link public health electronic health records (EHRs) with an immunization tracking system (Centers for Disease Control and Prevention 2011). This tracking system is focused on allowing EHRs of state and local health departments to share data with immunization information systems and integrate these records with the CDC's vaccine tracking system (Centers for Disease Control and Prevention 2011). A major focus of this initiative is to foster communication that facilitates the ability to track, provide reminders, and extend the human and financial resources needed to track immunization records.

There is a wealth of information and data in a variety of sources that can assist the nurse to become more familiar with existing critical infrastructure(s) and particularly with respect to the ability to communicate in the Emergency Services Sector (ESS) of the United States (U.S. Department of Homeland Security 2009). For example, there is discussion of what the critical infrastructure components are for communicating in a crisis, what it means to have critical infrastructure protection, responsibility parties, and the level and type of assistance the Emergency Management and Repose-Information Sharing and Analysis Center can provide in the event of an emergency situation.

Communicating during a crisis presents particular challenges for nurses who may not work in disaster management and public health on a daily basis; however, the United States Homeland Security Web site has a wealth of information for nurses through fact sheets as well as a series of scenario-based workshops that are free of charge and can be completed online. The series of workshops is called "News and Terrorism: Communicating in a Crisis." As part of that series, the National Academies has prepared, in cooperation with the Department, fact sheets on five types of terrorist attacks including chemical, biological, radiological, nuclear, and IED attacks (U.S. Department of Homeland Security, n.d. [a], [b], 2011). These fact sheets offer clear, objective information on these specific types of attacks as well as their impact and dangers, helping nurses focus on specific needs and communication in particular.

Table 26–1 displays Web sites that provide useful information for public health communications in the event of a specific type of crisis or disaster.

BOX 26–1   Four Public Health Informatics Principles

The primary focus of public health informatics should be on applications of science and technology that:

1. Promote the health of populations as opposed to health of individuals;

2. Prevent disease and injury by altering the conditions or the environment putting populations at risk;

3. Explore the potential for prevention of all vulnerable points in the causal chains leading to injury, disease, or disability, and applications should not be restricted to particular social, behavioral, or environmental contexts;

4. Reflect the governmental context in which public health is practiced.

Source: Adapted from Yasnoff, W. A., O'Carroll, P. W., Koo, D., Linkins, R. W., & Kilbourne, E. M. (2000). Public health informatics: Improving and transforming public health in the information age. *Public Health Management Practice, 6*(6), 67–75.

TABLE 26–1	Web Sites to Facilitate Public Health Communications in the Event of a Crisis or Disaster	
Focus	**Information Related to the Site**	**Web Link**
Biological Attack Fact Sheet: Human Pathogens, Biotoxins, and Agricultural Threats	A **biological attack** is the intentional release of a pathogen (disease causing agent) or biotoxin (poisonous substance produced by a living organism) against humans, plants, or animals. An attack against people could be used to cause illness, death, fear, societal disruption, and economic damage. An attack on agricultural plants and animals would primarily cause economic damage, loss of confidence in the food supply, and possible loss of life. It is useful to distinguish between two kinds of biological agents: Transmissible agents that spread from person to person (e.g., smallpox, Ebola) or animal to animal (e.g., foot and mouth disease). Agents that may cause adverse effects in exposed individuals but that do not make those individuals contagious to others (e.g., anthrax, botulinum toxin).	http://www.dhs.gov/xlibrary/assets/prep_biological_fact_sheet.pdf
Chemical Attack	A chemical attack is the spreading of toxic chemicals with the intent to do harm. A wide variety of chemicals could be made, stolen, or otherwise acquired for use in an attack. Industrial chemical plants or the vehicles used to transport chemicals could also be sabotaged. Harmful chemicals that could be used in an attack include: Chemical weapons (warfare agents) developed for military use. Toxic industrial and commercial chemicals that are produced, transported, and stored in the making of petroleum, textiles, plastics, fertilizers, paper, foods, pesticides, household cleaners, and other products. Chemical toxins of biological origin such as ricin. The toxicity of chemicals varies greatly. Some are acutely toxic (cause immediate symptoms); others are not very toxic at all. Chemicals in liquid or vapor form generally lead to greater exposures than chemicals in solid form.	http://www.dhs.gov/xlibrary/assets/prep_chemical_fact_sheet.pdf
Improvised Explosive Attack (IED)	An IED attack is a "homemade" bomb and/or destructive device to destroy, incapacitate, harass, or distract. IEDs are used by criminals, vandals, terrorists, suicide bombers, and insurgents. Because they are improvised, IEDs can come in many forms, ranging from a small pipe bomb to a sophisticated device capable of causing massive damage and loss of life. IEDs can be carried or delivered in a vehicle; carried, placed, or thrown by a person; delivered in a package; or concealed on a roadside. The term *IED* came into common usage during the Iraq War that began in 2003.	http://www.dhs.gov/xlibrary/assets/prep_ied_fact_sheet.pdf
Nuclear Attack	Unlike a "dirty bomb" that disperses radioactive material using conventional explosives, a nuclear attack is the use of a device that produces a nuclear explosion. A nuclear explosion is caused by an uncontrolled chain reaction that splits atomic nuclei (fission) to produce an intense wave of heat, light, air pressure, and radiation, followed by the production and release of radioactive particles. For ground blasts, these radioactive particles are drawn up into a "mushroom cloud" with dust and debris, producing fallout that can expose people at great distances to radiation.	http://www.dhs.gov/xlibrary/assets/prep_nuclear_fact_sheet.pdf

(continued)

Focus	Information Related to the Site	Web Link
TABLE 26–1 *(continued)*		
Radiologic Attack or Radiological Dispersal Device (RDD)	A radiological attack is the spreading of radioactive material with the intent to do harm. Radioactive materials are used every day in laboratories, medical centers, food irradiation plants, and for industrial uses. If stolen or otherwise acquired, many of these materials could be used in a "radiological dispersal device."	http://www.dhs.gov/xlibrary/assets/prep_radiological_fact_sheet.pdf
	Radiological dispersal devices, or dirty bombs: A dirty bomb is one type of RDD that uses a conventional explosion to disperse radioactive material over a targeted area. The terms *dirty bomb* and *RDD* are often used interchangeably in technical literature. However, RDDs could also include other means of dispersal such as placing a container of radioactive material in a public place, or using an airplane to disperse powdered or aerosolized forms of radioactive material.	
	A dirty bomb is not a nuclear bomb. A nuclear bomb creates an explosion that is thousands to millions of times more powerful than any conventional explosive that might be used in a dirty bomb. The resulting mushroom cloud from a nuclear detonation contains fine particles of radioactive dust and other debris that can blanket large areas (tens to hundreds of square miles) with "fallout." By contrast, most of the radioactive particles dispersed by a dirty bomb would likely fall to the ground within a few city blocks or miles of the explosion.	

In addition to providing for communication during a disaster or crisis there is a wealth of information on the use of information technology and efforts to facilitate interoperability and exchange of information through the Healthcare Informatics Technology Standards Panel (HITSP 2009). For example there is extensive discussion on the need for and strategies to enhance partnerships between private and public sectors. HITSP was created for the purpose of "harmonizing and integrating standards that meet clinical and business needs for sharing information among organizations and systems" (HITSP, 2009, para. 1).

A wealth of information exists to facilitate action, decision making, and policy formation related to communications and systems grounded in healthcare technology and informatics.

ISSUES WITH ACCESS AND ADAPTABILITY FOR INFORMATION TECHNOLOGY AND PUBLIC HEALTH

Public health providers have multiple information needs in relationship to healthcare informatics and technology infrastructure. Having the essential components of a health information infrastructure are vital and fundamental underpinnings to increase awareness and sensitivity to the types of data sets needed to provide support and improve outcomes used to make data-driven public health decisions. The ability to improve health outcomes and make data-driven decisions within a new or existing health information infrastructure is critical. For example, there is a clear need for valid and reliable databases. It is essential to consider each of these elements as more systems develop to foster and promote collaboration and communication between new and existing health information systems to promote the public's health. Table 26–2 lists 10 essential elements that need to be considered to have a comprehensive, robust health information system to promote public health informatics.

TABLE 26–2	Ten Essential Elements for Health Information Systems Infrastructure

1. Data definitions
2. Coding classification systems
3. Data transmission capability
4. Health information exchange (HIE)
5. Data storage
6. Data analysis
7. Disease staging
8. Electronic medical records
9. Computerized order entry
10. Decision support systems

IMPLICATIONS OF PUBLIC HEALTH INFORMATICS TO IMPROVE PATIENT AND POPULATION OUTCOMES

Understanding the Information Needs of Consumers

Public health is about protecting health needs of the public, and naturally this requires collaboration and communication between and among healthcare providers on a large scale often at the local, regional, national, and international levels. Information technology provides opportunities to solidify critical linkages between major stakeholders to enhance and facilitate timely and relevant communications between and among all levels of healthcare providers. For example, a local physician may need to know the latest epidemiological data on an outbreak of H1N1 influenza. The ability to access Centers for Disease Control and Prevention updates on outbreaks of H1N1 or to track and trend the epidemiology of the outbreak is critical in management and treatment as well as containment and in some cases eradicating the disease before it rises to epidemic proportions. Therefore, information technology provides a vital tool and a critical link between providers and information sources in a global public health system. As we know one can be in a foreign land in the morning and home in time for dinner with today's global travel, increasing opportunities for the spread of disease.

HEALTHCARE SURVEILLANCE

There is no doubt about the role healthcare informatics and technology play in disease outbreaks and surveillance. "Public health professionals are some of the earliest adopters of computers and other information technologies" particularly with respect to computerized information and databases as well as surveillance systems (Yasnoff, O'Carroll, Koo, Linkins, & Kilbourne 2000, p. 67). Table 26–3 identifies Web sites useful to support surveillance for disease management and services linked to public health informatics to inform decision making and advance management and use of information and public health knowledge to foster and promote population health.

Health and Information Literacy for Diverse Populations and Healthcare Providers

Health literacy is the "degree to which individuals have the capacity to obtain, process, and understand basic health information and services needed to make appropriate health decisions" (U.S. Department of Health and Human Services, 2000, p. iv). This definition remains current

TABLE 26–3 Web Sites Linked to Public Health Surveillance Sites and Resources for Population Health

Source	Web Link	Mission and Focus
Public Health Informatics and Technology Program Office	http://www.cdc.gov/osels/ph_informatics_technology/index.html	Supports health and public health practice by advancing better management and use of information and knowledge.
Public Health Surveillance Program Office	http://www.cdc.gov/osels/ph_surveillance/index.html	The mission of the Public Health Surveillance Program Office (PHSPO) is to advance the science and practice of public health surveillance in support of the CDC mission.
BioSense	http://www.cdc.gov/biosense/	As mandated in the Public Health Security and Bioterrorism Preparedness and Response Act of 2002, the Centers for Disease Control and Prevention's BioSense Program was launched in 2003 to establish an integrated national public health surveillance system for early detection and rapid assessment of potential bioterrorism-related illness.
Biosurveillance Coordination	http://www.cdc.gov/osels/ph_surveillance/bc.html	The U.S. Department of Health and Human Services (DHHS) was charged with the responsibility of enhancing biosurveillance for human health and delegated this responsibility to the CDC. In 2008, the CDC established the Biosurveillance Coordination (BC) unit to oversee the necessary activities to address these mandates.
Behavioral Risk Factor Surveillance	http://www.cdc.gov/brfss/	The Behavioral Risk Factor Surveillance System (BRFSS) is the world's largest, ongoing telephone health survey system, tracking health conditions and risk behaviors in the United States yearly since 1984. Currently, data are collected monthly in all 50 states, the District of Columbia, Puerto Rico, the U.S. Virgin Islands, and Guam.
Distribute	http://isdsdistribute.org/	Tracks and identifies proportion of Emergency Department visits for influenza-like illness (ILI) per week.
Gulf States Population Survey	http://www.cdc.gov/OSELS/ph_surveillance/gsps.html	On April 20, 2010, the BP *Deepwater Horizon* oil rig exploded in the Gulf of Mexico spilling more than 4.9 million barrels of oil into the Gulf. The lives and livelihoods of persons residing in the Gulf coastal communities were affected by this event due to loss of work, disruptions in the fishing and tourism industries, changes in patterns of leisure activities, and the effect on the physical environment in which they live. An ongoing public health concern following the spill is the effect on mental and behavioral health of populations living in and around the Gulf region and the mental health services required to meet that need.
National Electronic Telecommunication System for Surveillance	http://www.cdc.gov/osels/ph_surveillance/nndss/netss.htm	The National Electronic Telecommunications System for Surveillance (NETSS) is a computerized public health surveillance information system that provides the Centers for Disease Control and Prevention with weekly data regarding cases of nationally notifiable diseases.
National Notifiable Diseases Surveillance System	http://www.cdc.gov/osels/ph_surveillance/nndss/index.htm	A notifiable disease is one for which regular, frequent, timely information on individual cases is considered necessary to prevent and control that disease. The list of notifiable diseases varies over time and by state. The list of nationally notifiable diseases is reviewed and modified by the Council of State and Territorial Epidemiologists (CSTE) and CDC once each year.

today and has been used in the Institute of Medicine publication, *Innovations in health literacy research: Workshop summary* (2011).

There is an increased impetus in the United States to ensure that health literacy is considered whenever one is considering revision of an existing healthcare information system or creating and designing a new healthcare information system that can generate health information.

The most generally accepted definition of information literacy is as follows: "In order for a person to be information literate, they must be able to recognize when information is needed and have the ability to locate, evaluate and use effectively the needed information" (American Library Association 1989). There has been quite a bit of conversation on information literacy in academic communities and it is now an important issue in the healthcare community as more consumers access online healthcare information. Of particular concern as we create Information and Communications Technologies (ICT) is the need to consider the literacy levels of the global population and subpopulations in the creation and revision of existing healthcare information systems (Campbell 2004).

There are linkages between an individual's health literacy and health outcomes with positive correlations between poor health literacy and health outcomes, particularly those health outcomes associated with high-risk behaviors and chronic disease. In fact this linkage between health literacy and health outcomes is so strongly correlated that it is reported that "health literacy skills may be the first step in a chain of factors impacting health outcomes" (Paasche-Orlow & Wolf 2007, as cited in Osborn, Paashe-Orlow, Bailey, & Wolf 2011, p. 118). This is certainly an area in which health information technology and informaticians as well as healthcare providers want to continue investigating and researching as well as integrate into health informatics systems and design.

The federal government, healthcare providers, insurers, and other healthcare management teams increasingly use technology to reach out to individual patients and populations to provide information and disseminate reminders regarding healthcare services and products (Goodall, Ward, & Newman 2010). The concern is that not all populations or subpopulations have the resources and capabilities to utilize or benefit from communication using technology and the Internet. Goodall, Ward, and Newman (2010) refer to this concern as the "digital divide" and express concern, and their research examines the use of technology indicating that older people in Australia use information and communication technology less than other age groups. There is a real concern for governments and healthcare agencies relative to the exclusive use of electronic communication for the public as it will exclude select populations from access to important health information.

Not only are there challenges with regard to healthcare information technology for the populations being served but there are also issues to be considered with respect to increasing knowledge and understanding of information needs of healthcare providers and practitioners.

There is a compelling need for healthcare providers and practitioners to have rapid access to databases and critical information in a relevant and timely manner as they make critical healthcare decisions. When developing health information systems infrastructure, one must consider the critical need for public health digital knowledge management systems that reflect the diversity and scope of public health, including support for and integration of digital evidence–based decision support essential to public health work and decision making (Revere et al. 2007).

Another aspect to be considered with respect to patient literacy and healthcare technology is that today some consumers are readily engaged in sorting through Web pages, e-mail, and other instant messaging, including forums, blogs, and wikis, to seek information about health concerns for themselves and others (Abrahamson, Fisher, Turner, Durrance, & Turner 2008). There is a growing body of knowledge to distinguish the needs of those consumer populations who do frequent healthcare Web sites according to the type of user they are. The three types of healthcare users who frequent Web sites to elicit health information for self or others are referred to as lay information mediary (LIM), direct user, and service provider (Abrahamson, Fisher, Turner, Durrance, & Turner 2008). It is interesting to note that one of the major reasons users report for seeking healthcare information on the Internet is that they do not want to bother their healthcare providers with their question.

FUTURE DIRECTIONS

PHI remains a fairly new specialty, but work has been done to identify core informatics competencies needed by all persons working in the public health field, as well as for informaticists working in the field. Basic competencies addressed the use of information for public health practice, the use of IT to support personal effectiveness, and the management of IT projects to improve the effectiveness of the public health system (O'Carroll 2002). This work was significant because it established a baseline for skill sets that must be addressed in the preparation of the workforce. The fact that the public health workforce is drawn from a number of different disciplines makes it difficult to ensure that everyone enters the field with the prerequisite skill sets, however. O'Carroll was also careful to note that these competencies will continue to evolve over time and are not necessarily mutually exclusive of basic competencies identified in other disciplines. The competencies identified for the informaticist in public health (Centers for Disease Control and Prevention and University of Washington's Center for Public Health Informatics 2009) are similar to those identified by the American Nurses Association (2008) in the *Nursing Informatics: Scope & Standards of Practice* and are shown here in Table 26–4.

Support for public health informatics in the general informatics community is present. The American Medical Informatics Association (AMIA) has a workgroup devoted to PHI. There are

---

TABLE 26–4   Core Competencies for Public Health Informaticians

Public Health Informatician	Senior Public Health Informatician
Supports development of strategic direction for public health informatics within the enterprise.	Leads creation of strategic direction for public health informatics.
Participates in development of knowledge management tools for the enterprise.	Leads knowledge management for the enterprise.
Uses informatics standards.	Ensures use of informatics standards.
Ensures that knowledge, information, and data needs of project or program users and stakeholders are met.	Ensures that knowledge, information, and data needs of users and stakeholders are met.
Supports information system development, procurement, and implementation that meet public health program needs.	Ensures that information system development, procurement, and implementation meet public health program needs.
Manages IT operations related to project or program (for public health agencies with internal IT operations).	Ensures IT operations are managed effectively to support public health programs (for public health agencies with internal IT operations).
Monitors IT operations managed by external organizations.	Ensures adequacy of IT operations managed by external organizations.
Communicates with cross-disciplinary leaders and team members.	Communicates with elected officials, policymakers, agency staff, and the public.
Evaluates information systems and applications.	Ensures evaluation of information systems and applications.
Participates in applied public health informatics research for new insights and innovative solutions to health problems.	Conducts applied public health informatics research for new insights and innovative solutions to health problems.
Contributes to development of public health information systems that are interoperable with other relevant information systems.	Ensures that public health information systems are interoperable with other relevant information systems.
Supports use of informatics to integrate clinical health, environmental risk, and population health.	Uses informatics to integrate clinical health, environmental risk, and population health.
Implements solutions that ensure confidentiality, security, and integrity while maximizing availability of information for public health.	Develops solutions that ensure confidentiality, security, and integrity while maximizing availability of information for public health.
Conducts education and training in public health informatics.	Contributes to progress in the field of public health informatics.

Source: Centers for Disease Control and Prevention (CDC) and University of Washington's Center for Public Health Informatics (2009). Competencies for Public Health Informaticians. Atlanta, GA: U.S. Department of Health and Human Services, Centers for Disease Control and Prevention. Retrieved from http://www.cdc.gov/InformaticsCompetencies/downloads/PHI_Competencies.pdf

also two open access journals devoted to the field: the *Online Journal of Public Health Informatics* and *International Journal of Public Health Informatics* (IJPHI).

Safeguarding the public's health clearly requires a workforce prepared in all of the prerequisite skills. In today's world informatics competencies are key to an effective public health system.

CASE STUDY EXERCISE

You are about to present a lecture to your senior nursing students enrolled in their community health class on public health and informatics. What key points would you want to address? Relative to the basic competencies of the workforce? Examples of informatics applications in public health?

SUMMARY

- Public health informatics (PHI) is defined as the systematic application of information and computer science and technology to public health practice, research, and learning.
- Informatics plays a major role in supporting public health functions of disease surveillance, protection of public health, disaster management, and efforts to improve consumer health through improved engagement and education.
- Well-developed informatics competencies among the public health workforce can do much to improve and safeguard the health of the public.
- Initiatives to link EHRs with public health databases will improve tracking for immunization as well as serve as an early alert of threats to public health from disease outbreaks or threats from biological, chemical, or other sources.
- Improved access to information will help to better inform policy decisions.
- Increased use of online resources by the public requires consideration of literacy levels when designing or revising materials for public consumption.
- Additional work is needed to ensure that the current and future public health workforce possess the informatics skills needed to fully support public health.

REFERENCES

Abrahamson, J. A., Fisher, K. E., Turner, A. G., Durrance, J. C., & Turner, T. C. (2008). Lay information mediary behavior uncovered: Exploring how nonprofessionals seek health information for themselves and others online. *Journal of the Medical Library Association, 96*(4), 310–323.

American Nurses Association. (2008). *Nursing informatics: Scope & standards of practice.* Silver Spring, MD: Nursesbooks.org.

Campbell, S. (2004). *Defining information literacy in the 21st century* [Presentation]. Retrieved from http://archive.ifla.org/IV/ifla70/papers/059e-Campbell.pdf

Centers for Disease Control and Prevention. (2011, February). CDC will link public health EHRs with immunization tracking system. Retrieved from http://www.govhealthit.com/news/cdc-will-link-public-health-ehrs-immunization-tracking-system

Centers for Disease Control and Prevention (CDC) and University of Washington's Center for Public Health Informatics. (2009). *Competencies for public health informaticians.* Atlanta, GA: US Department of Health and Human Services, Centers for Disease Control and Prevention. Retrieved from http://www.cdc.gov/InformaticsCompetencies/downloads/PHI_Competencies.pdf

Goodall, K., Ward, P., & Newman, L. (2010). Use of information and communication technology to provide health information: What do older migrants know, and what do they need to know? *Quality in Primary Care, 18*, 27–32.

Healthcare Information Technology Standards Panel (HITSP). (2009). Welcome to http://www.HITSP.org. Retrieved from http://www.hitsp.org/

Institute of Medicine (IOM). (2011). *Innovations in health literacy research: Workshop summary.* Washington, DC: National Academies Press.

Kukafka, R., & Yasnoff, W. A. (2007). Public health informatics. *Journal of Biomedical Informatics, 40*(4), 365–369.

Macha, K., & McDonough, J. P. (2012). *Epidemiology for advanced nursing practice.* Sudbury, MA: Jones & Bartlett Learning LLC.

O'Carroll, P. W. (2002). *Public health informatics competency working group: Informatics competencies for public health professionals.* Seattle, WA: Northwest Center for Public Health Practice.

Osborn, C. Y., Paasche-Orlow, M. K., Bailey, S. C., & Wolf, M. S. (2011). The mechanisms linking health literacy to behavior and health status. *American Journal of Health Behavior, 35*(1), 118–128.

Revere, D., Turner, A. M., Madhavan, A., Rambo, N., Bugni, P. F., Kimball, A. M., & Fuller, S. S. (2007). Understanding the information needs of public health practitioners: A literature review to inform design of an interactive digital knowledge management system. *Journal of Biomedical Informatics, 40*, 410–421.

U.S. Department of Health and Human Services. (2000). *Healthy People 2010.* Washington, DC: U.S. Government Printing Office. Originally developed by Ratzan, S. C., Parker, R. M. (2000). Introduction. In C. R. Selden, M. Zorn, S. C. Ratzan, & R. M. Parker (Eds.), *National Library of Medicine current bibliographies in medicine: Health literacy* (NLM Pub. No. CBM 2000-1). Bethesda, MD: National Institutes of Health, U.S. Department of Health and Human Services.

U.S. Department of Homeland Security. (n.d. [a]). *Communicating in a crisis.* Retrieved from http://www.dhs.gov/files/publications/gc_1262023179771.shtm

U.S. Department of Homeland Security. (n.d. [b]). *Preparedness.* Retrieved from http://www.dhs.gov/files/programs/preparedness.shtm

Yasnoff, W. A., O'Carroll, P. W., Koo, D., Linkins, R. W., & Kilbourne, E. M. (2000). Public health informatics: Improving and transforming public health in the information age. *Public Health Management Practice, 6*(6), 67–75.

CHAPTER 27

Evidence-Based Practice and Research

After completing this chapter, you should be able to:

1. Describe ways that computers and informatics support nurses with the integration of evidence-based practice and the research process.

2. Discuss the necessity of computerized literature searches to translate research into practice.

3. Identify selected software programs for statistical analysis.

4. Discuss impediments to healthcare research related to health information technology.

5. Examine the relevance and impact of technology in translational research.

6. Examine strategies for best practices that engage healthcare professional students to utilize and apply research tools and technology.

7. Discuss implications and the impact of human subject protection and confidentiality on healthcare research.

8. Discuss the role of the healthcare professional in integrating technology into evidence-based practice in a variety of healthcare delivery environments.

There is no doubt about the linkages between informatics and nursing research in contemporary healthcare delivery settings. More healthcare professionals are being called upon to integrate best practice into clinical care to improve patient safety and outcomes. One can hardly pick up a peer-reviewed journal or attend a conference that does not include some discussion about the necessity of integrating evidence into practice. While there is a clear and compelling need for the integration of nursing research into practice, there are challenges and barriers with application of technology and informatics to translate research from the bench to the bedside. The focus of this chapter is to examine some of those challenges and barriers and how to apply technology and informatics to translate research from bench to bedside. There is also emphasis on federal initiatives and policy pushes and impetus for comparative effectiveness research applied to U.S. healthcare delivery. While there are still remaining areas of translation of research from bench to bedside in healthcare, this has been a decade of transformation and reformation in many ways for nurses. Specifically nurses and other healthcare professionals have been able to strengthen their ability and knowledge in translation of original research to improve patient safety and outcomes. It is evident that nurses and health professionals will continue to play a major role in U.S. healthcare system transformation through integration of technology and informatics in the twenty-first century. Nurses and healthcare professionals need to understand how nursing informatics advances one's professional abilities in the quest for new knowledge to advance patient safety and outcomes at all levels of healthcare delivery and to shape health policy well into the future.

THE NEED FOR EVIDENCE-BASED PRACTICE

There is widespread recognition that evidence-based practice (EBP) is essential to transform healthcare by providing proven effective treatments. At present, there is a gap between theory and practice that results in diminished patient care, inefficient practice, and an excessive time lag between the discovery of knowledge and its incorporation into clinical practice (Salmond 2007). The landmark Institute of Medicine (IOM) (2001) report, *Crossing the Quality Chasm*, called for the implementation of EBP as a means to improve the quality of care. Numerous other reports by the IOM, as well as reports from other major healthcare organizations, attest to the need for establishing research priorities. Recently, the IOM (2010) took that step when it identified research priorities for transforming nursing practice, nursing education, and nursing leadership helping to set the stage for increased use of EBP.

There is a growing body of knowledge on computers and informatics support as nurses and other health professionals continue to develop skills and competence in the integration of EBP and the research process. For example, there is increasing scientific evidence of the value of handheld devices like personal digital assistants (PDAs) to improve efforts to bring best practice and evidence-based research to the point of care (Hardwick, Pulido, & Adelson 2007). Another example of the benefits of handheld technology at the point of care is the efficient, effective link that it provides to research evidence-based care, clinical guidelines, and simply calculations, which have the potential to facilitate nurse-to-nurse, provider-to-provider, and provider-to-patient communications and ultimately increase patient safety and improve outcomes (Hardwick, Pulido, & Adelson 2007). There are also health information technology initiatives that use the Internet as a platform for user interaction and collaboration. For example, Web 2.0 provides opportunities for patients to enter, access, update, and monitor their own data and care (Lo & Parham 2010).

Information technology (IT) and systems refer to "technology that has the capacity to accumulate, retrieve, control, convey, or accept information by electronic means" (The Royal Society, 2006 as cited in Bembridge, Levett-Jones, & Jeong 2010, p. 18). Nurses must be engaged in processes to purchase and upgrade IT systems in the twenty-first century and beyond and realize that IT skills and competencies are a necessity in today's healthcare delivery settings. For example, IT and systems have the capacity to increase the speed with which healthcare information can be exchanged, enhance proficiency, as well as foster and promote ability to access large data sets. There is strong and compelling data suggesting that healthcare graduates must be technologically literate and proficient to engage in healthcare technology (Bembridge, Levett-Jones, & Jeong 2010). There is even conversation calling for a new role known as an *informationist* to serve on clinical research teams specifically for subject matter expertise and ability to find clinical evidence-based answers (Grefsheim, Whitmore, Rapp, Rankin, Robison, & Canto 2010).

EBP is applicable to all healthcare disciplines, and it contributes to the evolution of nursing as a profession (Courey, Benson-Soros, Deemer, & Zeller 2006). EBP is only one example of how research can be applied to providing care that integrates nursing experience and intuition with valid and current clinical research to achieve best patient outcomes (Dracup & Bryan-Brown 2006; Drenning 2006; Hanberg & Brown 2006; Salmond 2007). Sigma Theta Tau International (STTI), the Honor Society of Nursing, defines EBP as "an integration of the best evidence available, nursing expertise, and the values and preferences of the individuals, families and communities who are served" (STTI 2005). EBP entails development of best practices based on outcomes and the ability of nurses to access and evaluate current professional literature found in both print and online sources. EBP is a systematic process requiring the following activities (Pipe 2007; Salmond 2007; Zuzelo, McGoldrick, Seminara, & Karbach 2006):

- *Asking a relevant, searchable question.* This determines whether change is needed and helps clarify the problem. An example might include a question asking whether the infection rate associated with central lines is related to the current procedure for central line dressing changes, resulting in policy change based on the findings.
- *Systematically searching for evidence.* This entails a thorough, systematic, exhaustive literature review of studies related to central line dressing change procedures and related infection rates.
- *Critically examining the evidence.* This activity requires practitioners to consider the size and type of studies examined, the quality of research reported, critique of each study examined, results, and recommendations. In the example of the central line dressing change, examining the evidence may lead to recommendations to change the antiseptic agent, the type of dressing material, the frequency at which the dressing is changed, or the dressing change procedure itself; it may also lead to an overall policy review and change.
- *Changing practice as needed.* This requires a redesign of current procedures and work flow as well as timely implementation of needed change. EBP requires sharing results of the examination of evidence and the following up with planned change to educate and acquaint practitioners with the new procedure based on the best evidence.
- *Evaluating the effects of change and maintaining its practice.* This activity involves comparison of pre- and post-change central line infection rates in order to verify the impact or effectiveness of the EBP change. Assuming that problems with the dressing change procedure or wound care material constituted the problem, one would expect infection rates to continue to decline. One of the greatest challenges with EBP change is helping staff break with tradition and integrate the EBP change.

EBP provides a better way to treat patients because it replaces tradition with practices supported by research, improving outcomes (Dracup & Bryan-Brown 2006; Pipe 2007; Shirey 2006). EBP is exciting to research and implement as it removes reliance on the limited knowledge base of individual practitioners, who may or may not be well read and skilled in interpretation and application of research findings into clinical practice settings. There is a tremendous knowledge explosion that presents a unique set of challenges for each care provider, making it virtually impossible for any one individual to remain abreast of all the latest technology and developments in one's specialty area at any given time. EBP provides a shared experience for healthcare professions based on systematic and thorough review of scientific data on a given topic.

EBP also provides an opportunity to standardize best practice, improve adherence to best practices, and reduce the time an individual provider spends gathering and accessing relevant data, as well as making the EBP data available at the bedside at the time it is most needed (Matter 2006). EBP advances patient health and safety, providing quality and excellence through systematic examination of the scientific literature. EBP is reported to contribute to increased job satisfaction and vitality because nurses and professionals in other healthcare disciplines feel better about the quality of care they are delivering (Hockenberry, Wilson, & Barrera 2006). EBP provides a mechanism for hospitals and other healthcare delivery systems to meet research and excellence requirements inherent in the American Association of Colleges of Nursing (AACN), American Nurses Credentialing Center (ANCC), Magnet designation that indicate that a certain level of excellence has been met (Shirey 2006). The ANCC MagnetR Model focuses on "support, conduct, and application of research to clinical and administrative practice" (Ingersoll, Witzel, Berry, & Qualls 2010, p. 226). There are many opportunities for nursing research including EBP and research utilization to solve many issues and provide opportunity for integration of IT to access and evaluate data (Wilson et al. 2004; ANA 2004).

In fact, there are many opportunities for nurses, nurse leaders, and other healthcare professionals to be major stakeholders in planning, designing, implementing, and evaluating of information systems. For example, information systems must have the capability for nurses and other health professionals to create information systems that provide an opportunity for evaluating large bodies of data to inform nursing practice as well as enhance clinical practice (Oroviogoicoechea, Elliot, & Watson 2007). Information systems foster and promote the ability to monitor and evaluate the EBP change, focusing on outcomes and impact particularly related to patient safety and quality of care. This need will be even more compelling with the movement in the United States toward **comparative effectiveness research (CER)**.

CER is the direct comparison of healthcare interventions to determine which work the best as well as those that afford the greatest benefits as well as harm.

THE STATUS OF EVIDENCE-BASED PRACTICE

An extensive body of research knowledge exists now that needs to be incorporated into practice (Drenning 2006). Snyder (2007) reports that nurses view evidence-based research favorably. An increasing number of facilities consider EBP to be part of everyday clinical practice, and a given for ANCC-MagnetR-designated facilities; evidence-based competencies serve to establish the standards of practice and EBP is built into clinical ladders and professional development models (Gardner & Beese-Bjurstrom 2006; Mitchell 2006).

There are still challenges and barriers to the integration of EBP and research utilization in healthcare delivery environments (Brown, Wickline, Ecoff, & Glaser 2008; Carlson & Plonczynski 2008; Walsh 2010). Sigma Theta Tau International (2006) completed a landmark EBP study, finding that nurses need information to provide patient care but that many report lacking the comfort, skills, time, or access to appropriate materials needed to personally engage in EBP. This finding of the Sigma Theta Tau (2006) study is particularly true for nurses who entered practice 5 or more years earlier. There has been continuing work to examine barriers to research utilization over the past 15 years in regard to perceptions of barriers to nurses' use of research and EBP (Carlson & Plonczynski 2008). Increasingly, evidence points to the need for nursing leadership and healthcare administrators to embrace and support organizational cultures to foster and support EBP (Halm 2010). Nurses entering the profession in recent years express familiarity with EBP from their basic education and report feeling more comfortable with the availability of EBP information. Shirey (2006) noted that only 15% of the nursing workforce consistently practiced within an EBP framework. Identified barriers contributing to suboptimal utilization of EBP include the following (Chester 2007; Drenning

2006; Hockenberry, Wilson, & Barrera 2006; Mitchell 2006; Pipe 2007; Pravikoff, Tanner, & Pierce 2005; Salmond 2007; Snyder 2007):

- Failure to link theory to practice
- Limited awareness of EBP
- Lack of literature searching skills
- Lack of confidence with research utilization skills
- Lack of a supportive environment
- Lack of computer access at the bedside
- Lack of effective continuing education to make the transition to EBP

The National League for Nursing completed two similar but separate surveys of nurse administrators and faculty in schools of nursing to determine the level of informatics competencies and related requirements. Survey results indicated that computer literacy was reported as a curricular requirement approximately 60% of the time and information literacy approximately 40% of the time (Skiba & Thompson 2007). These preliminary findings are disturbing because professional leaders and the service sector expect nursing graduates to enter the practice setting with computer and information literacy skills. Even when information literacy programs are well established in nursing education, Courey, Benson-Soros, Deemer, and Zeller (2006) noted that it is imperative for nurse educators to determine whether information literacy actually leads to the promotion of evidence-based nursing practice or if there is a missing link between the two skills. For example, just having exposure to computer and information literacy skills does not guarantee competence in these areas.

STRATEGIES TO PROMOTE EVIDENCE-BASED PRACTICE

EBP requires a shift from the model of clinical practice traditionally grounded in intuition, clinical experience, and pathophysiological rationale to a paradigm where there are linkages between clinical expertise and integration of the best scientific evidence, patient values and preferences, and clinical circumstances (Salmond 2007). At the organizational level, EBP must be incorporated into the philosophy and mission of the organization particularly as it relates to the provision of quality patient care provided by expert clinicians. EBP must be philosophically embraced as an inherent goal of the organization, so there is support for EBP at all levels of the organization. This level of support can only occur when hospital administration and nurse leaders demonstrate a strong commitment through the creation of an environment that infuses and promotes critical thinking, supports autonomous decision making, and values empowerment processes, including shared governance (Zuzelo et al. 2006). Where there is an organizational culture of support as well as incentives linked to engagement in EBP and research utilization, nurses and other health professionals become empowered to promote EBP that truly impacts patient safety and outcomes as well as nurse vitality and professional satisfaction (Tagney & Haines 2009). Nurse managers and leaders are obligated to provide realistic models supporting EBP and ensure the availability of information technology supporting EBP models (Matter 2006; Shirey 2006; Simpson 2006).

Information technology (IT) tools are essential to provide the means to search the literature and apply clinical knowledge, improving practice and safety as well as meeting the standards of excellence required for regulatory and credentialing standards and Magnet status. It is essential that IT tools are accessible at the point of care when needed, providing access to online search engines, journal articles, and databases as well as links through the electronic health record (EHR). Access to essential IT tools requires financial commitment for the technology and subscriptions to database services initially and for upgrades, since there is rapid change in IT. EBP is a shared responsibility among nurses, advanced practice nurses, and nurse researchers (Drenning 2006). The concept of EBP as a basis for nursing practice must be introduced to all nurses during orientation (Dracup & Bryan-Brown 2006; Salmond 2007).

No matter how sophisticated the IT tools and systems are for promoting and facilitating EBP, there is a skill set and competencies nurses and other health professionals must have in order to search for evidence in the literature. The federal government defines *research* as the systematic collection of information in order to increase universal knowledge (Department of Health and Human Services 2009). The use of IT systems to research knowledge and databases for best practice is a different term than carrying out the scientific process. Nurses must have skills and competencies in researching existing data-based research and using systems to inquire about best evidence to inform clinical practice and answer clinical questions (Winsett & Cashion 2007).

The transition to EBP must be supported through ongoing continuing education initiatives to develop and maintain essential skills; this is particularly relevant for staff accustomed to older, more traditional models of practice. One strategy for success in promoting EBP skills is pairing individuals experienced in EBP with novices. This bringing together of novice and expert provides a fertile area for dialogue and partnership to move EBP forward in the organization, and this model often creates excitement and enthusiasm by taking away perceived barriers as well as IT anxiety. Other strategies for infusion of EBP into the organization include journal clubs that provide a forum for nurses to discuss specific articles and scientific research reviews, as well as the opportunity to invite qualified speakers to address EBP topics. Informatics and nursing informatics allow nurses the opportunity to engage in using information technology to examine data-driven research to improve efficiency, safety, and quality of healthcare delivery (Murphy 2010, p. 204).

When scholarly investigations into data-based research are not well planned there are challenges. For example, a thorough review and analysis of existing bodies of scientific knowledge certainly shape and aid in duplication of completed or current research initiatives (Smith 2008). A thorough and comprehensive review of existing data-based literature provides an opportunity to explore the landscape of clinical problems and issues to be investigated for best practice.

Searching existing data and research require skill and precision, and it is relevant to apply search strategies that are thorough. Systematic reviews of literature may already exist as well as meta-analyses of certain clinical issues or topics; there may be no existing systematic review or meta-analysis requiring the nurse or health professional to create that systematic review or meta-analysis. This is a very labor intensive and time-consuming effort, requiring support and resources to conduct a thorough review of the literature. Support and resources may be human and/or financial and require time and concentration for due diligence to this important and essential clinical endeavor. For example, completing a review of the literature on a clinical issue may take weeks to months to realistically plan, implement, and evaluate when done well. This is important to note particularly as nurses and other health professionals must provide the rationale to nurse leaders and managers to garner the needed support for such an undertaking.

Searching databases as part of a systematic review provides an excellent opportunity to engage with other health professionals. For example, one may want to consult with the health system librarian in a large teaching facility or engage with a librarian from a local university or college if the healthcare organization does not have a librarian. Searching databases is a science in and of itself and requires strict discipline to be certain the review of literature is thorough and comprehensive (Golder & Loke 2009). Systematic reviews serve as sources of synthesized knowledge for EBP and the Cochrane Library is one example of a renowned source of systematic reviews. While there are methods for conducting systematic reviews using electronic databases, there is evidence suggesting that even when there are excellent instructions for searching large databases, that search strategies are not being consistently applied by groups producing Cochrane reviews (Yoshi, Plaut, McGraw, Anderson, & Wellik 2009).

Searching large databases like Medline can present real challenges and involves searching literally millions of records. One of the real keys to searching large databases is choosing effective search strategies to delete inefficiencies yet insure accuracy of the search. **Search filters** are collections of hundreds of search terms used to search and retrieve research on particular clinical topics or problems. Search filters are invaluable, allowing the researcher to concentrate on other aspects of a project. It is always important to describe the search filters used in database searches, alerting the reader to those parameters (Glanville 2008). In addition to search filters, there are many stages involved in conducting a thorough and scientific systematic review of databases (Bettany-Saltikov 2010; Flemming & Briggs 2006; Krieger, Richter, & Austin 2008; Lawrence 2007; Whipple, McGowan, Dixon, & Zafar 2009; Younger 2010).

Well-conducted, systematic reviews of literature that have already been completed save nurses and other health professionals substantive amounts of time and energy. Librarians are excellent resources to tap when conducting a review of literature and are often not sought out when in fact they are excellent resources for interprofessional collaboration. There is evidence to suggest that nurses responded very favorably when researchers tested nurses' responses to dissemination of short summaries of systematic reviews to increase nurses' awareness of research results that did not require them to have a research or statistics background (Oermann, Roop, Nordstrom, Galvin, & Floyd 2007). In a systematic review of literature, there are five major activities involved in producing a thorough and comprehensive review of research databases:

1. Knowing how to undertake a comprehensive and systematic search of databases
2. Knowing how to select and appraise studies you want to include in your review of literature
3. Extracting relevant information from the research articles that have been critiqued and found to be scientifically rigorous and meritorious
4. Developing competency and skills in extracting relevant information in accurate and scientifically reliable manner from the research articles; provide a complete and succinct analysis of the findings from the research examined
5. Structuring the results of the systematic review in a clear and succinct manner (Bettany-Saltikov 2010)

Database searches of professional journals and credible EBP Web sites significantly reduce the time and effort one might expend investigating a clinical question. IT provides access to credible and reliable resources, including secondary sources of reviews of the literature by experts as well as EBP guidelines. These secondary sources of reviews and summaries prepared by experts provide clinical practice guidelines and recommendations (AHRQ n.d.). While there has been major impetus in the area of development of clinical guidelines, nurses and healthcare professionals must stay tuned for more in the twenty-first century in this area particularly related to CER. There is a national initiative in the United States examining evidence on effectiveness of treatments rather than on clinical guidelines (Freburger & Carey 2010). For example, the U.S. government is looking more at outcomes and costs of care versus application of specific clinical practice guidelines. CER is really about improving quality and decreasing healthcare costs. CER is focused specifically on determining which clinical guideline or pathway will be most effective both from a clinical perspective and a cost perspective (Cohen 2010, p. 70). This holds significant challenge for patients as well as healthcare providers, and most readers are familiar with the outrage that resulted in November 2009, when the U.S. Preventive Services Task Force (USPSTF) decided that mammograms should be performed routinely only until age 50 and then only every 2 years instead of annually until age 75. This resulted in outrage by many in the general public as well as healthcare professionals. The real issue was the government's attempt to have the USPSTF, an independent panel of nongovernmental medical and scientific experts, evaluate the sensitivity and specificity of mammography screening tests. There was substantial conflict between prior recommendations by many national professional organizations and their clinical guidelines (Cohen 2010). While there is broad utility for the implementation of clinical practice guidelines, it is noteworthy to keep a finger on the pulse of what is happening nationally with CER.

Evidence-based clinical guidelines are often readily available through hospital libraries and the Internet and may be accessed using technology including via mobile handheld devices such as PDAs. PDAs have several attractive features, making them quite portable and allowing the clinician to have access to databases and EBP clinical guidelines at the bedside; there is also increasing evidence that patient safety and nurse satisfaction are increased with PDA use (Cassey 2007; Colevins, Bond, & Clark 2006; Stockwell 2006; Thompson 2005). PDAs are highly regarded by practicing clinicians because they are portable providing current clinical best practice at the bedside. Box 27–1 lists a number of resources that may be accessed via the Internet. In addition to the PDAs that can be taken to the bedside, other strategies for conducting one's own review of the literature and database searches for EBP include:

- *Record the details of the search.* This includes noting the type and names of search strategies and databases used, whether searches were limited by particular languages (and what those were), the search frame (e.g., 1 year ago, 2 years ago), key terms used, and the names of Web sites explored.
- *Maintain notes on each review.* Notes should include the author name(s), title, study question, type of study, findings, and recommendations for clinical applications. The findings and recommendation are evaluated based on the strength of the evidence. Systematic review or meta-analysis of relevant randomized control trials or practice guidelines based on those reviews are the most highly regarded, followed by evidence obtained from a single, well-designed randomized controlled trial. Other studies, expert opinion, and expert committees are accorded less weight (Hockenberry et al. 2006).
- *Prepare a succinct summary of all the studies reviewed.* The summary should include practice recommendations.

In nursing, there is similarity in many of the techniques, processes, and tools used in both research-based practice and EBP. The major difference between the two is that research-based practice does not consider clinical expertise or patient preference while EBP uses expertise to translate

---

BOX 27–1 Selected Resources Supporting Evidence-Based Practice

Centre for Evidence-Based Nursing
http://www.york.ac.uk/healthsciences/centres/evidence/cebn.htm
Site dedicated to furthering evidence-based nursing practice. This site includes systematic reviews and other resources.

The Cochrane Collaboration of the Cochrane Library
www.cochrane.org
Collection of databases that provide reliable systematic reviews of clinical trials and the efficacy of treatments. Full text retrieval access requires subscription. Databases include the Cochrane Database of Systematic Reviews and the Database of Abstracts of Reviews of Effects.

Database of Abstracts of Reviews of Effectiveness
http://www.crd.york.ac.uk/crdweb/
One database in the Cochrane Collaboration. It may also be accessed through the Turning Research Into Practice (TRIP) database.

Evidence-Based Nursing Online
http://ebn.bmjjournals.com/
Provides abstracted, appraised research to subscribers.

Health Information Research Unit
http://hiru.mcmaster.ca
Studies problems of research transfer, develops and tests innovations based on information technology designed to improve the transfer of evidence into practice.

The Joanna Briggs Institute
www.joannabriggs.edu.au/consumer
Australian-based, consumer-focused site with links to other countries. Provides access to evidence-based information, publications, online services, education, and training programs.

BOX 27–1 *(continued)*

National Guideline Clearinghouse
http://www.guideline.gov/
Public resource for evidence-based clinical practice guidelines developed by professional organizations. Available through the U.S. Department of Health and Human Services Agency for Healthcare Research and Quality (AHRQ).

Nursing Best Practice Guidelines
http://www.rnao.org/Page.asp?PageID=861&SiteNodeID=133
Site maintained by the Registered Nurses of Ontario that provides developed guidelines, a toolkit, and guidelines for implementation.

PEDro
http://www.pedro.fhs.usyd.edu.au/
Physiotherapy Evidence Database that offers abstracts of clinical trials, systematic reviews, practice guidelines, and other relevant links.

Sarah Cole Hirsh Institute
http://fpb.case.edu/HirshInstitute/index.shtm
Established by the Frances Payne Bolton School of Nursing, Case Western Reserve University. Provides consulting services, certificates in evidence-based nursing practice, and print and online publications that disseminate EBP information.

SUMSearch
http://SUMSearch.uthscsa.edu
Uses metasearch techniques to simultaneously search the National Library of Medicine, DARE, and the National Guideline Clearinghouse for medical evidence.

Turning Research Into Practice (TRIP) Database
http://www.tripdatabase.com/index.html
Evidence-based medicine site with access to systematic reviews of medical literature, synopses, guidelines, clinical questions, and other relevant links.

Netting the Evidence
http://www.shef.ac.uk/scharr/ir/netting/
Lists multiple Web sites and resources on EBP. It is organized by eight categories: library, searching, appraising, implementing, software, journals, databases, and organizations.

Worldviews on Evidence-Based Nursing
A journal published by Sigma Theta Tau International, the Honor Society of Nursing.

Evidence-Based Practice
http://www.biomed.lib.umn.edu/learn/ebp/
This is a Web site that includes an interprofessional tutorial for students in healthcare fields, medicine, faculty, and anyone interested in EBP.

Medline
http://www.ncbi.nlm.nih.gov/entrez/query.fcgi.
Medline is available through the National Library of Medicine's authoritative and current database of health information for consumers and health professionals and is accessible 24 hours a day.

Agency for Healthcare Quality and Research
http://ahrq.gov/clinic/epc/
Under the Evidence-Based Practice Centers (EPCs) Program of the AHRQ (formerly the Agency for Health Care Policy and Research—AHCPR), 5-year contracts are awarded to institutions in the United States and Canada to serve as EPCs. The EPCs review all relevant scientific literature on clinical, behavioral, and organization and financing topics to produce evidence reports and technology assessments. These reports are used for informing and developing coverage decisions, quality measures, educational materials and tools, guidelines, and research agendas. The EPCs also conduct research on methodology of systematic reviews.

PsychINFO
http://www.ovid.com/site/catalog/DataBase/139.jsp
The American Psychological Association's PsycINFO database is the comprehensive international bibliographic database of psychology. It contains citations and summaries of peer-reviewed journal articles, book chapters, books, dissertations, and technical reports, all in the field of psychology and the psychological aspects of related disciplines, such as medicine, psychiatry, nursing, sociology, education, pharmacology, physiology, linguistics, anthropology, business, and law. Journal coverage, spanning 1806 to present, includes international material selected from more than 1,900 periodicals written in over 35 languages.

evidence into an innovative practice change (Drenning 2006). For example, EBP would involve searching the research to find the best practice based on valid and reliable scientific studies and creating a practice change to implement this best practice—often through developing and implementing a clinical guideline. EBP is also used in policy revision and policy formation. Three of the most frequently cited models for integrating EBP into nursing practice include the Stetler Model, the Iowa Model, and the Rossworm and Larrabee Model (Melnyk & Fineout-Overholt 2005). More and more models for integrating EBP into clinical practice are reported in the literature indicating that others are finding new ways to integrate EBP into clinical practice settings in relevant and meaningful ways.

USING COMPUTERS TO SUPPORT EVIDENCE-BASED PRACTICE AND RESEARCH

Computers are used in infinite ways to support the development of EBP and research, from the earliest stages through the dissemination of findings and the implementation of recommendations and guidelines based on available data and outcomes. While not every student or healthcare professional conducts original research, the current healthcare delivery system calls for nurses and healthcare professionals with skills and competencies in searching literature, who can perform basic statistical analysis enabling a thorough and robust systematic critique of existing research and participate in formation and clinical application of EBP guidelines. More and more nurses and health professionals in both clinical and leadership roles will be called upon to provide data and outcomes evaluation of clinical interventions and shape as well as reform health policy in the United States. Nurses and healthcare professionals are called upon to apply fundamental skills in formal and informal presentations of EBP applications and research. For example, nurses are increasingly expected to share outcomes and impacts of EBP demonstrating outcomes and benefits to patient safety, outcomes, and economics of care at the micro, macro, and meso system levels (Nelson, Batalden, & Godfrey 2007). More and more nurses and healthcare professionals will be part of creating systems of safety and improved patient outcomes at the front line of care which is often described at the micro system level as the "sharp end of care" (Nelson, Batalden, & Godfrey 2007). The micro system level is found at the front line where there are small functional units where staff perform the care or their work. This is opposed to the macro system level, which represents the major divisions of an organization such as the Department of Nursing and the meso system level, the highest level that represents the entire organization led by senior leaders. Nurses and healthcare professionals are being engaged in interprofessional collaboration with colleagues in other disciplines to work together and solve issues at the clinical micro, macro, and meso system levels. Some of the most common computer applications supporting EBP and research for improved patient outcomes are described in the following paragraphs. Box 27–2 summarizes some ways that computers facilitate EBP in the research process.

Identification of Searchable Questions and Research Topics

Constant changes in healthcare and the healthcare delivery system create challenges to keep abreast of the latest findings and recommendations for clinical practice, and there is often a time lag between the discovery of knowledge and its application into the clinical setting. Getting the "bench" research translated into "bedside" care has been estimated by some to be as long as 17 years (AHRQ 2004). It is essential that clinicians narrow the time to get research from the bench to the bedside. More emphasis will be placed on interdisciplinary translation of research in the coming decade.

While translational research is no longer a new concept for many nurse clinicians, there is heightened demand for further exploration and examination of the benefit of scientific contributions including but not limited to the National Institute of Health Roadmap (Woods & Magyary 2010). Some of the major initiatives and funding streams supporting translational research include the National Institutes of Health (NIH) and the AHRQ. Nurses have many opportunities

BOX 27–2 Common Computer Applications Supporting Evidenced-Based Practice and Research

- **Topic identification or searchable questions.** Online literature searches, research reports, e-mail, online communities, and discussion groups can be used to identify areas in need of research.
- **Online literature and database searches.** Electronic searches enable the researcher to identify systematic reviews and prior research in an area, as well as articles pertaining to the theoretical framework for proposed studies.
- **Full text retrieval of articles.** This eliminates the need to physically locate journals and photocopy them.
- **Development of resource files.** Computer files replace handwritten reports and may be searched quickly, allowing researchers to spend valuable time performing research and writing reports instead of performing clerical tasks.
- **Selection or development and revision of a data collection tool.** Online literature searches help researchers locate developed data collection tools. If no suitable tool is found, researchers can develop their own tool using a word processing package and then test it by sending it out via e-mail or the Web.
- **Preparation of the grant/study proposal.** Word processing aids the writing process because revisions can be made quickly.
- **Budget preparation and maintenance.** Spreadsheets and financial planning software assist with this process.
- **Determination of appropriate sample size.** The ability to generalize study findings is related to the size of the sample. Power analysis is the process by which an appropriate sample size may be determined. Software is available for this purpose.
- **Data collection. Computers aid in the collection of data in several ways.** Data may be input into a computer through scanned questionnaires, direct entry of field observations, or the use of an online data collection tool. PDAs and notebook computers aid on-site entry of data, eliminating note and paper tools (Hanberg & Brown 2006).
- **Database utilization.** Databases allow organization and manipulation of collected data.
- **Statistical analysis/qualitative text analysis.** Statistical analysis software performs complex computations, while qualitative text analysis allows searches for particular words and phrases in text, noting frequency of appearance and context.
- **Preparation of the research findings for report.** Word processing and graphics programs enable researchers to present their findings without the need for clerical assistance or graphic artists.
- **Bibliographic database managers.** This type of software aids the preparation of publications through the importation of references from literature databases without the need to rekey and formats citations and reference lists according to the style selected.
- **Electronic dissemination of findings.** Online journals, Web pages, and e-mail permit researchers to share their findings quickly. This contrasts with the traditional publication of study findings in print media that might take a year or more from the time of submission until distribution.

to engage interprofessionally with clinical partners for much needed collaboration through translational research. There are also toolkits to assist clinicians to locate existing evidence-based clinical guidelines or clarify searchable questions with the end goal of developing EBP guidelines. Some of the resources to assist clinicians in translational research are listed in Box 27–3.

As with all things, no one strategy works for everyone and so it is true with nurses and healthcare professionals interested in and passionate about conducting research. A common strategy is the creation of an e-mail list, blog, or wiki, to foster and promote online discussion groups, to provide opportunities for interprofessional mentoring, or to assist others to identify specific areas for EBP or original research. These resources may be specific to a particular subspecialty, including but not limited to critical care nursing, education, and informatics, or to research as an area of concentration. The NURSERES e-mail list group, at listserv.kent.edu/archives/nurseres.html, is a discussion list for nurse researchers. Additional nursing research opportunities are available online at http://www.nursingsociety.org.

Research/ResearchInitatives/Pages/research_finder.aspx provides nurses with names of groups and Web links to various healthcare organizations; it includes a well-defined research section for nurses who have specific research interests and lists upcoming conferences where they may submit their research for peer-reviewed presentation.

Timely and ongoing studies allow healthcare educators, providers, agencies, and alliances to explore and examine information trends and react to market changes proactively. For example,

BOX 27–3   Suggested Healthcare Informatics Research Topics

The development of informatics competencies

- Nursing education and the development of informatics competencies
- Fostering informatics skills among staff nurses
- Data mining and searching for the best evidence
- Use of informatics in knowledge discovery

Clinical data

- Development and efficacy of acuity and classification systems
- Use of point-of-care devices
- The impact of informatics on clients' families and healthcare providers
- EBP guideline development and use, including outcome assessment
- Expert systems, decision trees and support, and artificial intelligence and knowledge engineering
- Client education
- Quality improvement initiatives
- Implementation of ICNP and other standard clinical languages into electronic health records
- Efficacy of telehealth applications
- Tracking resources

Education

- Effectiveness of virtual learning environments
- Models for best practice in unit-based staff development
- Graduate outcome behaviors
- Best pedagogical practice in the nursing classroom
- The impact of mentorship on nurse satisfaction

Device usability and human factors

- Ease of device use
- Device acceptance based upon human factor issues

an exploration of databases might indicate a new trend in nursing practice based on patient outcomes related to best practice in wound care management. This EBP would serve as an opportunity to examine current policy and would create a clinical guideline to change current policy, resulting in improved patient outcomes, fewer inpatient days, and a reduced cost savings to the unit and institution. An example of this was seen when other great opportunity for system change based on EBP was seen when the Centers for Medicare and Medicaid (CMS) shifted from payment to nonpayment for specific events like falls occurring with an inpatient or development of decubitus ulcers during a hospital stay. Many healthcare delivery systems are driving best practice proactively through interprofessional collaboration and translational research in a proactive manner because with shrinking healthcare reimbursement and a tsunami of Baby Boomer's entering the healthcare system there are surely more challenges to come. Box 27–3 lists examples of selected healthcare informatics topics.

Literature Searches

Systematic literature searches provide an effective means of researching primary research in a logical and systematic manner, providing a more efficient and effective means to find credible scientific information than if one were doing a general Web search. This is a relevant concept in the process of locating and examining research because there is opportunity to examine primary data sources in one location (Sigma Theta Tau International 2005). Primary databases for searching nursing literature are the Cumulative Index to Nursing and Allied Health Literature (CINAHL), Medline, and PsychINFO. All three of these primary databases are available for online searches through university and hospital libraries. Students in online educational programs and some of the professional nursing organizations also have free or low-cost access to these online databases to make them readily accessible. For example, Medline is accessed free of charge through the National Library of Medicine's PubMed Web site. CINAHL offers individual subscriptions, although CINAHL does not include medical or basic science journals. Medline incorporates abstracts and references from biomedical journals. PsychINFO is an electronic database produced by the American Psychological Association (APA) that includes the behavioral sciences. It is accessed through the APA Web site. All three of these databases allow users to enter search subjects and then narrow searches by criteria such as language, journal subset, and/or publication year. For example, MEDLINE users can limit a search to nursing journals and/or research reports.

CINAHL provides similar capabilities. These features allow potential researchers to quickly determine whether research has been conducted in their area of interest and to peruse the reported findings. The success of search results is directly related to the choice of the terms selected for search. Search terms or key terms act as filters for records stored in the database. Typically, authors are asked to supply key terms or concepts for their work. Key terms also vary from database to database. PubMed uses key terms known as Mesh headings. Wong, Wilczynski, and Haynes (2006) noted a 70% overlap in terms between Medline and CINAHL, with CINAHL containing terms unique to nursing. In their analytic study, they compared hand searches with CINAHL results to determine the best search strategies to locate research studies and systematic reviews. They used very specific terms such as *exp study design, clinical trial.pt, meta-analysis.mp,* and *meta-analysis.sh.* The use of "meta-analysis," in combination with the letters "mp" to refer to "multiple posting" or "sh" to refer to subject heading, represented the best approach to retrieve systematic reviews in CINAHL. Users may view article abstracts and, in some cases, retrieve the full text for articles online through the use of these and other databases. Box 27–4 summarizes a few advantages and disadvantages associated with online literature searches.

Digital Libraries

A **digital library** extends the missions and techniques of physical libraries through information technology (Barroso, Edlin, Sandelowski, & Lambe 2006). Digital libraries are comprised of a set of electronic resources with the related capabilities to create, store, organize, search, and retrieve information to meet the needs of a community of users. While this sounds very much like online access to databases offered by any public or school library, digital libraries extend the capabilities of information retrieval systems to provide open sharing of information to special users. For example, the SandBar Digital Library (sonweb.unc.edu/sandbar/index.cfm) is funded by a grant from the National Institute of Nursing Research (NINR) and was built by the University of North Carolina. The purpose of digital libraries is to transform large volumes of data into information and knowledge. SandBar integrates findings from qualitative studies of women with HIV infection. The National Electronic Library for Health was a highly publicized digital library in the United Kingdom, but it has since been replaced by the National Library for Health (http://www.library.nhs.uk/Default.aspx); it provides access to evidence-based reviews, guidelines, various databases, news, and updates. Digital libraries are characterized by open access and sharing and frequently increase access to materials that would otherwise be challenging to access. Digital libraries allow users to search or browse a particular research topic. MacCall (2006) noted that clinicians at the bedside need quick access to information with many digital library system searches lasting 1 minute or less. Digital library access will most likely continue to evolve in the coming decade and beyond as clinicians need scientific data literally at their fingertips.

> ### BOX 27–4 Pros and Cons of Online Literature Searches
>
> **Pros**
>
> - Searches may be completed quickly.
>
> - Searches may be done without the aid of a librarian.
>
> - Searches may be limited to specific years, languages, or journal subsets.
>
> - Searches may be general or limited to clinical trials and other research reports.
>
> - Online abstracts allow researchers to quickly determine if a particular article suits their purpose.
>
> - When available, full-text retrieval allows the researcher to obtain articles without searching for volumes on a shelf or waiting for copies to arrive from other sites.
>
> **Cons**
>
> - Searches require a basic level of comfort and skill with online resources and key terms.
>
> - The person conducting the search must be able to narrow the topic area.
>
> - Search results are directly related to the selection of search terms. Poor selection of terms may falsely indicate no or few articles on a given topic or provide a large number of results of limited usefulness.
>
> - The services of a librarian may be needed for improved search results.
>
> - Online searches may not entirely eliminate the need to locate volumes and photocopy articles or wait for copies to arrive from other libraries unless full-text retrieval is available.
>
> - Online retrieval can be expensive for individuals purchasing articles on a per view basis.

Data Collection Tools

Data collection tools may be located via online literature searches and discussion lists. More and more clinical questions are being raised to facilitate quality patient outcomes specifically linked to patient safety and improved outcomes. Increasingly, nurses and healthcare professionals are trying to develop valid and reliable measurement instruments to assess and scientifically measure outcomes as a result of evidence-based interventions. This may appear a daunting task for nurses and healthcare professionals, but it is a necessity to ensure scientific rigor and has many linkages to effectively translating research and evidence-based programs. Researchers commonly focus on having valid and reliable measurement instruments for obvious reasons and so it is equally relevant that nurses and healthcare professionals conducting evaluation of evidence-based outcomes must too have valid and reliable measurement instruments. The more scientific rigor and outcomes measurement of an evidence-based intervention, the more likely the intervention will be adopted by others. Using valid and reliable existing data collection tools and measurement instruments offers benefits of established validity and consistency, and the ability to commence research sooner without spending time to devise and test an instrument. This will likely be an area of continued development and growth in EBP and translational research in the twenty-first century. The purpose of a **data collection tool** is for gathering specific details of an intervention in an organized, systematic, and scientifically robust manner. Credibility and fidelity of data are called into question when data collection tools or measurement instruments are not both valid and reliable. While data collection tools or measurement instruments may vary in purpose in original research and assessment or evaluation of evidence-based outcomes in the clinical setting, the fundamental concepts of scientific rigor are the same.

Data collection can be done in a multiplicity of ways and computers facilitate the data collection process. There are two underlying assumptions inherent in online data collection. The first assumption inherent in online data collection is that subjects are computer literate and the second assumption is that subjects have access to a computer and an Internet provider. Examples of online data-collection tools or measurement instruments include a physical assessment form, a graphics record, or opinion questionnaires. Once a valid and reliable data-collection tool or measurement instrument is determined, permission must be obtained from the author granting permission to use the document. Permission is typically obtained more quickly through e-mail than traditional mail. In the event that a valid and reliable data-collection tool is not available, a valid and reliable data-collection tool or measurement instrument must be created. Construction and validation of a data-collection tool or measurement instrument is time consuming and labor intensive and every effort should be made to use existing tools and measurement instruments already existing. Once the data-collection instrument is constructed, professional e-mail lists, blogs, and wikis, as well as discussion lists and chat rooms may be used to pilot test the instrument, solicit research subjects, and even collect data. E-mail interviews and Web-based surveys offer alternative methods to collect research data electronically. E-mail allows varying degrees of structure in the interview process, as well as ease of transcription via downloading without interpretation error secondary to pauses and inflection. Data collection via the Internet can offer several advantages. These advantages include but are not limited to:

- Interactive forms that can be evaluated for completeness and accuracy of data before submission
- Automated data compilation and exportation to other software
- Fast, cost-effective administration of surveys
- Freedom from geographic boundaries
- Ease associated with sending out reminders to complete survey instruments
- Expanded access to participants.

The Internet user population is not representative of the general population and limits the generalizabilty of the findings. However, because the Internet is not available to everyone, selection bias is a threat to external validity findings because the Internet population is nonrepresentative and because open surveys conducted via the Web net volunteer participants who are most likely self-select subjects. Box 27–5 provides some suggestions for design and administration of Web-based data-collection tools or measurement instruments. As with traditional research methods, ethical issues and issues of fidelity must be considered. The major ethical issues and issues of fidelity in original research and EBP include human subjects protection primarily informed consent, protection of privacy, and avoidance of harm. Computers provide the ability to use cookies to assign a unique identifier to each person viewing a Web-based questionnaire and also afford the researcher the ability to determine response and participation rates and to filter out multiple responses. Researchers using cookies should publish a privacy policy, state that cookies will be sent, explain their purpose, and set an expiration date based on the date that

BOX 27–5   Tips for Design and Administration of Web-Based Data Collection Tools

- Determine the objectives for the tool.
- Write and then edit questions.
- Include title, introduction, purpose of the tool, and an anonymity statement.
- Critique the tool for reading level.
- Ensure that the tool is visually attractive.
- Limit the amount of information on a page.
- Ask evaluators to rate the tool for readability and time required for completion and elicit their suggestions.
- Test the automated data collection process before public posting.
- Pretest the tool before public posting.
- Include a few open-ended questions, and provide a wrap-up.

data collection will end. Researchers must also recognize there will be occasional challenges with online data collection, including programming errors, usability problems, software incompatibilities, and technical problems (Schleyer & Forrest 2000).

Direct Data Input

Data collection is expedited through mobile devices including but not limited to PDAs and notebook computers at the research site. For example, data can be downloaded or transmitted to another computer for compilation and analysis. The ability to download or transmit data to another computer increases accuracy and decreases likelihood of transcription errors and lost or illegible paper notes, facilitating and streamlining data collection and data analysis processes. Interactive data-collection tools offer the advantages of engaging the research subject to validate data. Being able to validate data results in eliminating redundant data entry, and decreasing the time and costs needed for cleaning data to ensure its quality ultimately increasing data accuracy and minimizing cost and time for what might otherwise be a costly and time consuming process.

Data Analysis

Data analysis is the processing of data collected during the course of a study to identify trends and patterns of relationships. This task begins with descriptive statistics in quantitative, and some qualitative, studies. Descriptive statistics permit the researcher to organize the data in meaningful ways that facilitate insight by describing what the data show. Theory development and the generation of hypotheses may emerge from descriptive analysis. In addition to descriptive analysis, there are a number of statistical procedures that a researcher must choose when conducting a study. Until recently, researchers embarking on large studies needed the services of statisticians and large computing centers for data analysis. Many practitioners and students in the healthcare professions thought they were unable to perform meaningful research without these supports. Personal computers now rival larger systems in abilities and can easily link with larger computers, making it easier to conduct research in any setting. There has been a growing recognition that the huge amounts of data collected within business and healthcare systems might be tapped and used for a variety of purposes. The overwhelming volume of data requires computer processing to turn data into useful information.

A variety of terms exist to refer to the use and processing of this data. **Knowledge discovery in databases (KDD)** is a term used in other industries that is now seen in healthcare circles. KDD identifies complex patterns and relationships in collected data. It provides a powerful tool suitable for the analysis of large amounts of data. Commercial packages are available in a range of prices and platforms. KDD may be used to identify risk factors for diseases or efficacy of particular treatment modalities. The confidentiality of individual records may be protected through the use of data perturbation. This is a technique that modifies actual data values to hide confidential information while maintaining the underlying aggregate relationships of the database. Further research is needed on the use of data perturbation and its potential to introduce bias. As healthcare systems continue to expand and explode with large data sets there will be more and more opportunity for KDD to facilitate opportunities to work within these systems and produce population data on a grand scale.

Data mining is another term for the use of database applications to look for previously hidden patterns. Its use is growing; it has been investigated for marketing purposes, tracking the factors underlying medication errors, and improving financial performance. Data mining supports sifting through large volumes of data at rapid speeds in ways that were not previously possible due to size or speed limitations. Data mining allows real-time access to information for a competitive edge. Data mining in conjunction with electronic records can help physicians quickly determine the number of clients in their practice who need examinations and to generate reminders. Application of mined data is contingent on its quality and on maintaining scientific rigor and scientific processes while gathering it.

QUANTITATIVE VERSUS QUALITATIVE RESEARCH

Quantitative research uses objective measurements to study structured questions. Typically large numbers of subjects are used to obtain results to be considered statistically valid. Computers can assist the researcher in determining a power analysis through statistical models to determine the sample size needed for a research project. A major concern with quantitative research is whether research results can be replicated and the findings subsequently applied to larger or other populations. This is in contrast to qualitative research where the researcher is examining a phenomenon of interest through subjective individual interpretation. For example, qualitative research designs provide an opportunity to examine meanings, concepts, definitions, characteristics, metaphors, symbols, and descriptions of things. Qualitative research uses a variety of methods to collect information, including in-depth interviews and focus groups. Both quantitative and qualitative research methods are supported and facilitated through various information technology applications. For example, researchers may use an existing data set through a secondary analysis of data to answer another new research question (Doolan & Froelicher 2009). Researchers may also prefer to use large survey data sets to prepare and manage data that is free access, but one should be aware this process is not a simple one (Aponte 2010). For example, a nurse researcher may perform a secondary analysis of state and territorial healthcare data sets like those provided by the Centers for Disease Control & Prevention focusing on health of Hispanic or Latino populations (Centers for Disease Control & Prevention, ND, http://www.cdc.gov/nchs/fastats/hispanic_health.htm). Another example is using data from the National Health and Nutritional Examination Survey (NHANES) for assessment of epidemiology of populations assessing nutrition status of children (Aponte 2010).

Quantitative Analysis The computational abilities of computers readily lend themselves to statistical analysis of qualitative data and render more accurate results than might be available from hand-calculated statistics. Several software packages are available for quantitative analysis; most evolved during the 1960s and 1970s and permit the importation of data from spreadsheet or database software, and sometimes ASCII files. The majority provide versions of their products for a variety of computer platforms. A partial list follows:

- The System for Statistical Analysis (SAS) comprises several products for the management and analysis of data. It is considered an industry standard.
- MINITAB Statistical Software offers an alternative to SAS. Geared to users at every level, it is widely used by high school and college students and incorporates pull-down menus for ease of use.
- BMDP evolved as a biomedical analysis package. It comes in personal and professional editions and offers an easy-to-use interface for data analysis. BMDP also prompts the user until analysis is complete. It offers a comprehensive library of statistical routines.
- SPSS is another well-known software company. SPSS provides products for most computer platforms; it provides statistics, graphics, and data management and reporting capabilities.
- S-Plus is known for its flexibility in allowing users to define and customize functions. It also offers extensive graphics.
- SYSTAT, unlike some of the other packages discussed, was first developed for PC use.
- DataDesk started as a Macintosh product, but it now is also available for use with Windows.
- JMP started as a Macintosh product and resembles DataDesk. It is available for use with Windows.

Despite the increased use of statistical analysis packages by nurses, some researchers still argue that nurses should work with the traditional users of supercomputers to develop the skills needed to use these resources and to access large data archives held by government and private agencies. Supercomputers offer the ability to quickly peruse huge databases. This belief gave rise to a new branch of nursing science: nurmetrics. **Nurmetrics** uses mathematical forms and statistics to test, estimate, and quantify nursing theories and solutions to problems.

Computer Models Computational nursing, a branch of nurmetrics, uses models and simulation for the application of existing theory and numerical methods to new solutions for nursing problems and for the development of new computational methods. One proposed use of nurmetrics and computational nursing is the formulation and testing of new models for healthcare delivery by using computers. This application is cost effective and can demonstrate how factors such as education may affect health practices and outcomes over time without the need to first implement the program and wait for results. Nursing informatics uses computer science and informatics principles to understand how the structure and function of information may be used to solve problems in nursing administration, nursing education, practice, and research. The College of Nursing at the University of Iowa established the Center for Computational Nursing, which is affiliated with their Institute for Nursing Knowledge.

Qualitative Analysis Computers facilitate organized storage, tabulation, and retrieval of qualitative data. For example, databases like electronic filing cabinets are used to store data; software can locate key words or phrases in a database, sort data in a prescribed fashion, code observations or comments for later retrieval, support researcher notes, and help create and represent conceptual schemes. As notes, coding, sorting, and pasting are automated, researchers have more time to analyze data. Despite these benefits, critics offer the following challenges:

- Qualitative research may be molded to fit the computer program.
- Computers tempt researchers to use large populations, thus sacrificing in-depth study for breadth.

Software is available to support qualitative research by allowing researchers to automate clerical tasks, merge data, code, and link data. QSR International provides several products that facilitate qualitative research, including NUD*IST and Nvivo. Ethnograph is another product that supports importation of text-based qualitative data into word processing packages. HyperRESEARCH and TAMS Analyzer represent other examples of qualitative software. AQUAD is a specialized program for users with an advanced knowledge of qualitative research. Text must first be entered or scanned into a word processor and converted into ASCII. AQUAD permits coding on the screen, and researchers may define linkages they wish to explore. Words or phrases in text and their frequency may be noted. E-mail lists that support qualitative research include QUALRS-L, QUALNET-L, and Qual-software.

Data Presentation: Graphics

Once data analysis is complete, graphics presentation software helps the researcher put study findings into a form that is easy for the reader to follow in written study reports and for the listener to follow when findings are presented at professional meetings and conferences. Graphics presentation software allows the researcher to design and make slides for use at presentations without the services of a media department. Harvard Graphics and PowerPoint are two well-known commercial packages. PDAs can now be used to store slide presentations. Figure 27–1 shows a simple bar graph prepared using a graphics application.

Online Access to Databases

The NIH offers access to several databases useful to nurses interested in research, health policy, and the identification of funded research projects. One of these databases, the Computer Retrieval of Information on Scientific Projects (CRISP), provides information on research grants

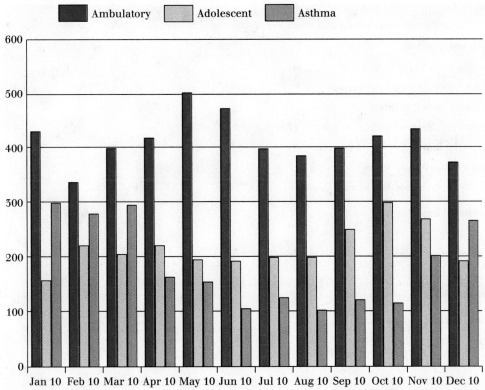

FIGURE 27–1 • Bar graph depicting the number of clinic visits per month for January 2010 through December 2010

supported by the Department of Health and Human Services. CRISP lists the following data for each project: title, grant number, abstract, principal investigator, thesaurus terms, and key words. CRISP is updated weekly and is available at crisp.cit.nih.gov/. Search results may be printed or saved. The Agency for Healthcare Research and Quality sponsors the National Quality Measures Clearinghouse (NQMC). NQMC is a public repository for evidence-based quality measures and measure sets. NQMC may be accessed through the AHRQ Web site at www.ahrq.gov. The intent of this database is to provide detailed information on quality measures and to further their use. Several other agencies provide access to online databases useful to healthcare researchers, educators, clinicians, and administrators. These include the following:

- The National Library of Medicine (NLM) at www.nlm.nih.gov.
- Sigma Theta Tau's Virginia Henderson International Nursing Library (INL) at www.nurs inglibrary.org/portal/main.aspx. The INL provides information on grant opportunities, nurse researchers, meeting proceedings, and access to databases that pertain to nursing research.
- The Cochrane Library at http://www.cochrane.org/reviews/clibintro.htm. The Cochrane Library consists of a regularly updated collection of evidence-based medicine databases, including the Cochrane Database of Systematic Reviews. There are a number of other sites that contain links to databases and research related information. These sites are maintained by government agencies, professional organizations, and publishers, among others. Box 27–6 lists some other sources to consider when seeking research funds. AHRQ is one agency that actively supports research to improve healthcare, particularly studies that can improve patient safety, access to services, and bioterrorism knowledge and preparedness. AHRQ maintains a page for nursing research with links to evidence-based research, funding sources, and news (AHRQ n.d.).

BOX 27-6 Possible Funding Sources for Healthcare Research

Government Agencies

- National Institutes of Health
- National Institute of Nursing Research
- National Library of Medicine
- Substance Abuse and Mental Health Services Administration
- Centers for Disease Control and Prevention
- Food and Drug Administration
- Agency for Healthcare Research and Quality

Professional Organizations

- Sigma Theta Tau
- American Nurses Association
- Oncology Nursing Foundation
- Specialty Groups

Foundations and Organizations

- Robert Wood Johnson Foundation
- Skin Cancer Foundation
- Epilepsy Foundation
- Myasthenia Gravis Foundation
- American Cancer Society
- March of Dimes
- Arthritis Foundation
- Josiah Macy Foundation
- Institute for Healthcare Improvement

Collaborative Research

There are many national initiatives and pushes to translate research from the bench to bedside largely because it takes an average of 17 years to get 14% of all new biomedical discoveries to the bedside and into clinical practice (Westfall, Mold, & Fagnan 2007). Along with these many national initiatives and pushes to translate research from the bench to the bedside, there has been a push also to create and incentivize interprofessional collaboration between and among nurses and healthcare professionals when it comes to translational research. The major impetus behind these national initiatives is to accelerate the translation of scientific research to clinical practice in order to benefit patient outcomes (Chesla 2008; Kon 2008; Morin 2008; Sampselle, Pienta, & Markel 2010; Wilkes & Herbst 2010). One example of a major federal initiative to foster and promote interprofessional collaboration in translation research is development of the Clinical and Translational Science Awards (CTSA). CTSA awards are federal initiatives to engage interprofessional healthcare professional collaboration to address health priorities and inform research agendas. CTSAs are federal initiatives to offer new possibilities to accelerate translation of scientific discoveries to improve and positively impact human health and outcomes (Sampselle, Pienta & Markel 2010).

HISTORY OF TRANSLATIONAL RESEARCH

The term *translation research* appears to have different meanings and definitions depending on the source one examines. Reportedly the term *translational research* first appeared in PubMed in 1993 and was not used much throughout the 1990s (Butler 2008). There did not appear to be a gap in translation of research into practice in the 1950s and 1960s when the majority of basic research and clinical research was performed mainly by physician scientists in academic medical centers and these were the same physician scientists who also cared for patients (Butler 2008). Since the early 2000s, the term translation research is commonly used and there are many national initiatives by the NIH, National Academies of Science as well as private foundations and other key stakeholders to get the results from the bench to the bedside in a more expeditious manner. That said, there is also controversy over the best model with which to make these changes and there are some reporting concerns with the ethics of science with initiatives like the NIH Roadmap (Maienschein, Sunderland, Ankeny, & Robert 2008; Schwab & Satin 2008; Westfall, Mold, & Fagnan 2007; Zerhouni 2007).

The NIH provides billions of support dollars each year on biomedical research and most of that money is allocated to understanding how living organisms work (Westfall, Mold, & Fagnan 2007). The NIH has gone so far as to provide the NIH roadmap, which while there is not unanimous consensus among the entire scientific community on best strategies or the best model for translational research, there is agreement that the gap between research and practice to enhance patient outcomes must be bridged. There are numerous opportunities to be creative and innovative in testing strategies to translate research into practice in all healthcare delivery settings with more and more opportunities surely presenting in the twenty-first century.

Collaborative computing and research foster productivity by allowing individuals at dispersed sites to share ideas and information in real time. Collaborative computing may use e-mail, desktop videoconferencing, other telecommunication tools, digital libraries, or shared databases to join persons of like interests from locations across the globe. Collaborative research fosters and promotes interprofessional collaboration in many ways primarily by facilitating mentorship and support to assist nurses and other healthcare professionals who lack basic competence and comfort with research methods and skills to develop their skills through mentor relationships. The American Academy of Nursing and the AHRQ sponsor the Senior Nurse Scholar in Residence program as a means to encourage a senior nurse researcher to develop areas of investigation that integrate clinical nursing care questions with issues of quality, costs, and access. Information about this program can be found on the AHRQ Web site.

There are initiatives at the NINR to move science forward in more collaborative, synergistic ways than in the past, and the NIH roadmap involves promotion of interdisciplinary teams in addition to clinical and translational research (NINR 2004).

MULTI-INSTITUTIONAL RESEARCH

Automation and uniform languages also aid the simultaneous collection of data from multiple sources. This capability has been limited to healthcare alliances that can, and already do, share data. Predictably there will be even further impetus for the development of national health information networks that can expand linkages to massive databases and solidify those capabilities. The ability to access these large macro databases provides opportunity for multi-institutional research, offering researchers the opportunity to increase the size of their study populations and to eliminate idiosyncrasies associated with a particular place as a contributing factor to the findings. In short, multi-institutional research ensures that findings can be applied to a larger population, increasing the generalizability of one's findings.

COMPARATIVE EFFECTIVENESS RESEARCH

There is no doubt that more and more emphasis is going to be placed on CER. In the last decade there has been major emphasis in nursing and healthcare professions to translate evidence into practice and to assess the effectiveness of those interventions. In February 17, 2009, President Obama signed the American Recovery and Reinvestment Act of 2009 (Steinbrook 2009). The American Recovery and Reinvestment Act of 2009 appropriated $1.1 billion for CER. CER is defined by the IOM (http://www.hrsonline.org/Policy/LegislationTakeAction/iom_report_cer_priorities.cfm) as:

> the generation and synthesis of evidence that compares benefits and harms of alternative methods to prevent, diagnose, treat, and monitor a clinical condition, or to improve delivery of care. The purpose of CER is to assist consumers, clinicians, purchasers, and policy makers to make informed decisions that will improve health care at both the individual and population levels.

The American Recovery and Reinvestment Act of 2009 also directed the IOM to create a priority list of potential areas needed for CER (see Box 27–7). The IOM's list of priorities lists topics by quartile in groups of 25 with the first quartile being considered the highest priority and the fourth quartile the lowest (IOM 2009). It should be noted that topics within the quartiles are not prioritized. The IOM (2010) also issued the report, *Initial national priorities for comparative effectiveness research.*

BOX 27–7   IOM Priority List of CER Areas in the First Quartile

Compare the effectiveness of treatment strategies for atrial fibrillation including surgery, catheter ablation, and pharmacologic treatment.

Compare the effectiveness of the different treatments (e.g., assistive listening devices, cochlear implants, electric-acoustic devices, habilitation and rehabilitation methods [auditory/oral, sign language, and total communication]) for hearing loss in children and adults, especially individuals with diverse cultural, language, medical, and developmental backgrounds.

Compare the effectiveness of primary prevention methods, such as exercise and balance training versus clinical treatments in preventing falls in older adults at varying degrees of risk.

Compare the effectiveness of upper endoscopy utilization and frequency for patients with gastroesophageal reflux disease on morbidity, quality of life, and diagnosis of esophageal adenocarcinoma.

Compare the effectiveness of dissemination and translation techniques to facilitate the use of CER by patients, clinicians, payers, and others.

Compare the effectiveness of comprehensive care coordination programs, such as the medical home, and usual care in managing children and adults with severe chronic disease, especially in populations with known health disparities.

Compare the effectiveness of different strategies of introducing biologics into the treatment algorithm for inflammatory diseases, including Crohn's disease, ulcerative colitis, rheumatoid arthritis, and psoriatic arthritis.

Compare the effectiveness of various screening, prophylaxis, and treatment interventions in eradicating methicillin resistant *Staphylococcus aureus* (MRSA) in communities, institutions, and hospitals.

Compare the effectiveness of strategies (e.g., bio-patches, reducing central line entry, chlorhexidine for all line entries, antibiotic impregnated catheters, treating all line entries via a sterile field) for reducing healthcare associated infections (HAI) including catheter-associated bloodstream infection, ventilator associated pneumonia, and surgical site infections in children and adults.

Compare the effectiveness of management strategies for localized prostate cancer (e.g., active surveillance, radical prostatectomy [conventional, robotic, and laparoscopic], and radiotherapy [conformal, brachytherapy, proton-beam, and intensity-modulated radiotherapy]) on survival, recurrence, side effects, quality of life, and costs.

Establish a prospective registry to compare the effectiveness of treatment strategies for low back pain without neurological deficit or spinal deformity.

Compare the effectiveness and costs of alternative detection and management strategies (e.g., pharmacologic treatment, social/family support, combined pharmacologic and social/family support) for dementia in community-dwelling individuals and their caregivers.

Compare the effectiveness of pharmacologic and nonpharmacologic treatments in managing behavioral disorders in people with Alzheimer's disease and other dementias in home and institutional settings.

Compare the effectiveness of school-based interventions involving meal programs, vending machines, and physical education, at different levels of intensity, in preventing and treating overweight and obesity in children and adolescents.

Compare the effectiveness of various strategies (e.g., clinical interventions, selected social interventions [such as improving the built environment in communities and making healthy foods more available], combined clinical and social interventions) to prevent obesity, hypertension, diabetes, and heart disease in at-risk populations such as the urban poor and American Indians.

Compare the effectiveness of management strategies for ductal carcinoma in situ.

Compare the effectiveness of imaging technologies in diagnosing, staging, and monitoring patients with cancer including positron emission tomography, magnetic resonance imaging, and computed tomography.

Compare the effectiveness of genetic and biomarker testing and usual care in preventing and treating breast, colorectal, prostate, lung, and ovarian cancer, and possibly other clinical conditions for which promising biomarkers exist.

Compare the effectiveness of the various delivery models (e.g., primary care, dental offices, schools, mobile vans) in preventing dental caries in children.

Compare the effectiveness of various primary care treatment strategies (e.g., symptom management, cognitive behavior therapy, biofeedback, social skills, educator/teacher training, parent training, pharmacologic treatment) for attention deficit hyperactivity disorder in children.

Compare the effectiveness of wraparound home and community-based services and residential treatment in managing serious emotional disorders in children and adults.

Compare the effectiveness of interventions (e.g., community-based multi-level interventions, simple health education, usual care) to reduce health disparities in cardiovascular disease, diabetes, cancer, musculoskeletal diseases, and birth outcomes.

Compare the effectiveness of literacy-sensitive disease management programs and usual care in reducing disparities in children and adults with low literacy and chronic disease (e.g., heart disease).

Compare the effectiveness of clinical interventions (e.g., prenatal care, nutritional counseling, smoking cessation, substance abuse treatment, and combinations of these interventions) to reduce incidences of infant mortality, pre-term births, and low birth rates, especially among African American women.

Compare the effectiveness of innovative strategies for preventing unintended pregnancies (e.g., over-the-counter access to oral contraceptives or other hormonal methods, expanding access to long-acting methods for young women, providing free contraceptive methods at public clinics, pharmacies, other locations).

Source: Institute of Medicine. 100 Initial Priority Topics for Comparative Effectiveness Research. Retrieved from http://www.iom.edu/~/media/Files/Report%20 Files/2009/ComparativeEffectivenessResearchPriorities/Stand%20Alone%20List%20of%20100%20CER%20Priorities%20-%20for%20web.pdf

One of the major reasons CER is such a compelling issue presently is that there is a substantial gap between the knowledge needed and the available knowledge for basing medical decisions and with technological advancements that gap is growing larger (IOM 2010). For example, the IOM (2010) reports:

Approaches to clinical research are being substantially outpaced by rapid growth in new health care diagnostic and treatment options and an explosion of new genetics insights that hold real implications for the potential-and the need- to personalize individual interventions. Advances in informatics, large scale data sets, and clinical research methods to assess those data sets hold promise for considerably accelerating the pace, reliability, and applicability of clinical effectiveness research. (http:www.iom.edu/Reports/2010/)

According to the IOM the following are needed to establish a robust, sustainable CER program:

- Continuous evaluation of research priority topics
- Coordination of private and public strategies
- Periodic reports outlining research progress
- Involvement of consumers, patients, caregivers, and healthcare providers in all aspects of CER to ensure its relevance to everyday healthcare delivery
- Large-scale clinical and administrative data networks that enable observational studies of patient care while protecting patient privacy and data security
- Effective strategies to disseminate CER findings and promote their adoption by clinical practices

The bottom line and underlying impetus for CER is that currently clinical research presents healthcare providers with information on the natural history of disease and clinical presentations, as well as diagnostic and treatment options that often have considerable range. It is readily apparent that patients are individuals and in a consumer-driven society, consumers, patients, and caregivers are demanding to decide which course they wish to pursue to evaluate and treat their healthcare conditions. Due to the great diversity in healthcare information needed for informed care one may be astonished to know that in 2011 more than half of the medical treatments delivered lacked clear evidence of proven effectiveness. There is also greater emphasis upon delivering care in a cost-conscious manner to individuals and populations (IOM 2010; Sakala 2009). The American Recovery and Reinvestment Act of 2009 appropriated $300 million of the $1.1 billion in federal appropriations to the AHRQ. Of this $400 million was allocated to the NIH and $400 million to the Secretary of Health and Human Services (American Recovery and Reinvestment Act of 2009, 2009) for the following purpose:

1. Research that compares the clinical outcomes, effectiveness, and appropriateness of items, services, and procedures that are used to prevent, diagnose, treat diseases, disorders, and other health conditions; and
2. The development and use of clinical registries, clinical data networks, and other forms of electronic health data that can be used to generate or obtain outcomes data.

The ultimate goal of CER is to improve healthcare quality for individual patients and populations as well as healthcare providers and other stakeholders with better information regarding risks and benefits of the various treatment options available to them (Freburger & Carey 2010). CER has great potential to be important to many stakeholders including patients, providers, health insurers, employers, governmental agencies, policy makers, and pharmaceutical companies (Schumock & Pickard 2009). It is quite compelling to think that in CER it appears results achieved in clinical effectiveness and from a "cost-benefit" analysis will be more favored than efficacy from original research conducted in artificial environments (Sakala 2009). It is also apparent that CER is quite controversial and nurses and healthcare professionals must stay tuned for the continued dialogue and national agendas on CER in the coming decade. It is abundantly clear that in a national of limited human and financial healthcare resources and disease chronicity costing billions of gross national product each year. The question regarding CER is really about what will be done with CER and how it will be done so there is more data about effective treatment, and while there are interventions that may help some of the population, some subpopulations may be disproportionately affected (Gilbert 2009; Morris & Munro 2009; Traymor 2009).

Projected National Health Expenditures 2009–2019 CMS 2010 (https://www.cms.gov/NationalHealthExpendData/25_NHE_Fact_Sheet.asp):

- Growth in NHE is expected to increase 5.7% in 2009 and average 6.1% per year over the projection period (2009–2019).
- The health share of the Gross Domestic Product is projected to reach 17.3% in 2009 and 19.3% by 2019.
- Medicare spending is projected to grow 8.1% in 2009 and average 6.9% per year over the projection period.
- Medicaid spending is projected to grow 9.9% in 2009 and average 7.9% per year over the projection period.
- Private spending is projected to grow 3.0% in 2009 and average 5.2% per year over the projection period.
- Spending on hospital services is projected to grow 5.9% in 2009 to $761 billion. Average growth of 6.1% per year is expected for the entire projection period.
- Spending on physician and clinical services is projected to grow 6.3% in 2009 to $528 billion. Average growth of 5.4% per year is expected for the entire projection period.
- Spending on prescription drugs is projected to grow 5.2% in 2009.

RESEARCH IN REAL TIME

The potential of hospital information systems to collect large amounts of data almost instantly allows for research in real time, or essentially as events occur. This ability helps institutions react quickly to changes noted in client populations. Some systems can perform routine work while automatically channeling study information into an appropriate database according to particular study protocols. This is a desirable feature that would eliminate redundant data entry; however, at the present, few information systems are flexible enough to do this. This lack of flexibility creates the need to collect, gather, and format data separately each time they are needed for a research study.

The Role of Uniform Languages

The lack of a common language to facilitate data collection and decision making was recognized as a problem in healthcare and nursing several years ago. The Unified Medical Language System project represents an attempt to standardize terms used in healthcare delivery in a way that can be understood, measured, and coded across different settings (NLM 2006). The American Nurses Association had a database steering committee working on the Unified Nursing Language System as a means to develop and use other clinical databases to extend nursing knowledge. A standardized nursing language allows accurate communication among nurses, which aids research and subsequently adds to the body of nursing knowledge. The American Nurses' Association (ANA) (2007) has recognized several standardized languages and terminologies to support nursing practice. These include:

- NANDA for nursing diagnosis
- The Nursing Interventions Classification (NIC)
- The Nursing Outcomes Classification (NOC)
- The Clinical Care Classification (CCC), which is an interface terminology that contains diagnoses, interventions, and outcomes for use in home care
- The Home Health Care Classification (HHCC)
- The Omaha System for capturing community health information
- The Nursing Minimum Data Set (NMDS), which contains clinical data elements
- Nursing Management Minimum Data Set (NMMDS), which contains nursing administrative data elements
- The Patient Care Data Set (PCDS), which has since been retired from use
- The PeriOperative Nursing Data Set (PNDS), a set of diagnoses, interventions, and outcomes for the perioperative area
- ABC codes (Alternative Billing Concept codes) for use in interventions in nursing and other areas
- Logical Observation Identifiers Names and Codes (LOINC) for use of outcome and assessments
- The Systematic Nomenclature of Medicine Clinical Terms (SNOMED CT)
- The International Classification for Nursing Practice (ICNP), which addresses diagnoses, interventions, and outcomes for all of nursing

SNOMED and ICNP are the two most widely accepted standards in nursing. At this time standard languages are fodder for research as well as a tool to enhance research through shared meanings. Research has been done to examine mapping between languages. More research will be needed in this area but ICNP includes all nursing specialties and demonstrates the ability to encompass other standardized nursing languages (ANA 2007; Ryan 2006). In addition to facilitating data collection, uniform languages set the definition of key terms, ensuring that studies can be replicated. Implementation of uniform languages first requires the following:

- Education of staff who are unfamiliar with standardized terms
- Elimination of computer restraints, such as limited characters and lines per field, found with some computer systems

- Database coordination among various clinicians and departments that use terms differently but require access to shared data repositories. This is also known as mapping terms.

IMPEDIMENTS TO HEALTHCARE RESEARCH

From a health information technology perspective, healthcare research has been impeded by slow adoption of data exchange standards and uniform languages, failure to realize a birth-to-death electronic health record, limited interoperability, limited health information exchange, concerns over the confidentiality of private health information, and limited funding. Many technical issues still need to be resolved. From a business perspective, competing organizations have concerns about sharing information within and between healthcare systems. These concerns present barriers to the creation of large databases required to accurately identify trends related to healthcare problems and to develop successful treatment options. The data from large data sets could certainly hold the key to many of the population-focused challenges confronting healthcare delivery systems, including primary, secondary, and tertiary prevention as well as the shift from inpatient to outpatient care delivery settings. Outcomes and impacts from these data could serve as the basis for policy change at local, state, and federal levels as well.

DISSEMINATION OF RESEARCH FINDINGS

Researchers have a professional obligation to share their research findings. This includes dissemination of all types of research and scholarly information, including original research as well as evidence-based research or secondary analysis of data from previously conducted research studies. There are numerous opportunities and venues through which one can share and disseminate research findings, including traditional printed journals, digital libraries, and online publications. The dissemination process for research findings is rather lengthy and may take several weeks from the time a researcher queries a journal to determine if there is interest in the topic from the publishing venue. For example, the query and submission process is shortened with electronic publication. Queries, submissions, reviews, and publication can usually be done electronically via e-mail. The *Journal of Medical Internet Research* is an example of an online publication with a research focus.

Electronic publication makes it possible for more organizations to establish their own journals, and researchers should become familiar with the publication venue that is the best fit for them through conversations with the publisher, mentor, or other colleagues. Preparing research findings for dissemination through peer-reviewed, scholarly publication is facilitated by using a **bibliography database manager (BDM)**. BDM is software that allows the researcher to maintain accurate and current references and properly formats in-text citations as well as the final reference list. BDMs allow importation of references directly from databases. Integration of BDMs requires an Internet connection to the specified database, and in some cases a user ID and password are required to access the database. Selected examples of frequently used BDMs are EndNote, Reference Manager, ProCite, Biblioscape, and the Web-based Zotero.

IMPLICATIONS OF HIPAA AND OTHER LEGISLATION FOR HEALTHCARE RESEARCH

The Health Insurance Portability and Accountability Act (HIPAA) originated in 2003 (Shaughnessy, Beidler, Gibbs, & Michael 2007). The passage of HIPAA brought concerns over its implications for healthcare research, and during the inception of HIPAA, the NIH (2003, 2004) posted explanatory documents online to clarify information for actual and potential researchers. Researchers have experienced barriers due to HIPAA, and it seems that clinical researchers now take what has been described as "extra care" while doing clinical research. As of April 2003, HIPAA, also referred to as the Privacy Rule, requires healthcare providers and insurers to obtain additional documentation from researchers related to assurances of patient safety and confidentiality. The key concern is that human subjects, irrespective of age, are protected with a high degree of confidentiality from the person getting access to their personal information. This means there is increased scrutiny and monitoring of requests for access to health information.

Computers and technology have outpaced the capacity of researchers and persons handling healthcare data related to human subjects to be able to interpret all the data available and to handle these large volumes of data responsibly (Wolf, Paradise, & Caga-anan 2008, p. 361). For example, there may be a need for additional documentation, including written permission from subjects who sign a special authorization form, or a waiver of the authorization requirement from the institutional review board or privacy board. A signed authorization form for research is valid only for a specific research study, not for future projects. Authorization differs from informed consent in that the authorization allows an entity to use or disclose a person's protected health information (PHI) for a specific purpose such as a study, whereas informed consent constitutes permission to participate in the research. The authorization must specify what PHI will be used or disclosed, who can use or disclose it, the purpose of the use or disclosure, and an expiration date. There must also be statements that address the individual's right to revoke the authorization and how that could be accomplished; whether treatment, payment, enrollment, or eligibility of benefits can be based on authorization; and the person's right to know that the Privacy Rule may no longer apply if PHI is re-disclosed by the recipient. The authorization form must be signed and dated. Authorization is not required or may be altered when the covered entity obtains appropriate documentation that an institutional review board or a privacy board has granted a waiver or alteration of authorization requirements. Authorization is not required once information has been de-identified according to Privacy Rule standards. Issues of ethics and integrity related to research information becomes even more challenging and complex with secondary analysis of previously conducted research. Ethics and ethos in all research are important no matter the type of research being conducted.

Researchers are not covered entities unless they are also healthcare providers, employed by a covered entity, or engage in any of the electronic transactions covered under HIPAA. Covered entities include providers that transmit health information electronically for HIPAA transactions, health plans, and clearinghouses. The Privacy Rule allows PHI use or disclosure to researchers to determine if the number and type of study subjects are sufficient to conduct research and if information has been stripped of all or certain identifiers. This second instance is referred to as *limited data*. Covered entities may disclose PHI to researchers to aid in study recruitment. Research started before the enactment of the Privacy Rule may be allowed to continue under a "grandfather" provision. Researchers need to be aware of HIPAA's Privacy Rule because it establishes the conditions under which covered entities can use or disclose PHI. There are implications for the creation and use of databases that contain PHI and that may be used at some future point in time. Researchers may be responsible for drafting the authorization form.

STUDENTS USING COMPUTERS TO SUPPORT EVIDENCE-BASED PRACTICE AND RESEARCH

Students often believe that research has little significance for them, and few actually carry out the entire research process. This is unfortunate because students need to develop information literacy skills, including the ability to locate and understand research reports as a means to engage in EBP. A program outcome essential for healthcare students is that they be skilled in applications facilitating electronic literature searches and in application of fundamentals of statistics to have basic skills and competencies. For example, the American Association of Colleges of Nursing (AACN) MSN Essentials document (AACN 1996) required that a graduate program include:

use of computer hardware and appropriate software, and to understand statistics and research methods, and (use of) information systems for the storage and retrieval of data, consistent with the particular population focus. (p. 7)

For example, one graduate nursing program reported using Microsoft Excel to teach statistics in a graduate advanced nursing program with effectiveness (DiMaria-Ghalili & Ostrow 2009). Since the 1996 MSN Essentials document, the AACN has given considerable attention to the need for informatics competencies for all nursing graduates to enable them to employ EBP, and be savvy consumers of research findings, and when appropriate, conduct research.

Online literature searches provide up-to-date information from peer-reviewed data-based research. It is relevant to keep in mind that a reference book no matter how recently published is already outdated by the publication date as it has references that are 4 or 5 years old by the publication date. Students should also be aware of other resources including digital libraries offering systematic reviews of data-based research findings.

The World Wide Web (WWW) is another popular resource for locating data-based research, and it too offers a wealth of information for both healthcare professionals and consumers. The WWW is widely accessible at educational institutions for students with no access to home Internet access. For example, the WWW has sites of particular interest to healthcare profession students. Healthcare profession students might choose to prepare for a community health teaching project by searching for materials on the WWW as long as they are attentive to the quality of sites selected and dates of publication or revision. It should be noted, however, that the WWW may not provide a comprehensive review of literature needed for a complete and thorough review of literature.

Students enrolled in research courses may have occasion to use software for statistical analysis, presentation of graphics, and proposal and report preparation. Many texts include software with study questions for mastery of research content. Despite the fact that this is considered to be a "digital age" when most students are familiar with a multitude of computer skills, including e-mail, instant messages, Web searches, and file downloads, not all students are equally skilled when it comes to information literacy skills. Reference librarians and faculty are in the ideal position to help foster these skills.

FUTURE DIRECTIONS

Nursing and healthcare both lag behind in the translation of research findings into practice, and it is readily apparent of the implications the role healthcare informatics and technology will play in the twenty-first century and beyond. For example, creation and innovation of new practice models, patient safety outcomes, data driven tests of change, and best practice lie in the ability to work with the resources within our systems. In addition, there will be increasingly more emphasis on evaluations and outcomes of interventions and evaluation of EBP changes as more and more research is translated into practice. For example, the EHR provides the database needed to support research and EBP and has the potential to change and shape care practices. Incorporation of evidence-based guidelines into the EHR and the ability to access data driven information at the bedside puts care and support literally in the hands of clinicians, standardizes evidence-based care, improves quality, and ultimately advances care for patients and satisfaction for providers. The EHR is changing the way in which information is collected and used, ensuring the survival of enterprises with EHR capability. Eventually one imagines an EHR that contains data from birth to death, making tracking and trending of information across one's life span completely possible with remote access from anywhere in the world. It is hard to imagine these "Star Wars" scenarios, but the computers and information technology provides tools and opportunities for system automation unlike ever before. As we move forward in healthcare research and information technology, there will be increased between clinical practice and technology, there are many considerations that can only be provided by a savvy healthcare provider who is knowledgeable in what the challenges and opportunities. Above all else, the outcomes and impacts at the bedside are going to become increasingly more relevant and more important as is the case with comparative evaluation research.

CASE STUDY EXERCISE

You are the staff nurse in a busy medical–surgical department at your community hospital. You and several of your colleagues have an idea that client anxiety is decreased in direct proportion to the amount of teaching that they receive preoperatively. Describe how you might use information technology to look at this issue and prepare a proposal for funding consideration.

SUMMARY

- There is a gap between theory and practice that results in diminished patient care, inefficient practice, and an excessive time lag between the discovery of knowledge and its incorporation into clinical practice. EBP represents the attempt to close this gap.
- EBP is an approach to providing care that integrates nursing experience and intuition with valid and current clinical research to achieve the best patient outcomes.
- EBP asks a relevant question, searches literature for evidence, critically examines the evidence, changes practice as needed, evaluates the effects of change, and maintains the change that was based upon the integration of best practices.
- EBP provides the opportunity to standardize best practices and reduces time that the practitioner spends gathering and assessing data.
- EBP contributes to increased job satisfaction for practitioners secondary to delivery of an improved quality of care.
- Despite the clear need for EBP, barriers remain to its adoption.
- Information technology provides the tools to support EBP and research.
- Research provides the data that allow better allocation of scarce resources and that support the development of knowledge.
- Electronic literature searches, online discussion groups, and digital libraries facilitate both EBP and research through the identification of questions, location of literature, systematic reviews, and resources.
- Data collection instruments may be located, developed, and even administered online.
- Data analysis is facilitated via the use of software for both qualitative and quantitative analyses.
- Nurmetrics is a branch of nursing science that uses mathematical form and statistics to test solutions to problems. One branch of nurmetrics known as computational nursing uses models and simulations to test solutions and proposed models for care.
- Several organizations maintain databases that contain information useful to nurses conducting research, including CRISP, the National Library of Medicine, the *American Journal of Nursing,* and Sigma Theta Tau.
- The implementation of the EHR will provide information required to deliver healthcare more effectively and at lower costs.
- Standardized languages provide a mechanism to ensure common meanings to terms, facilitate data collection, and aid research. The International Classification for Nursing Practice (ICNP) includes all nursing subspecialties and demonstrates the ability to encompass other standardized nursing languages.
- Automation and the implementation of the EHR are expected to increase multi-institutional research efforts as well as research in real time and collaborative research.
- Students in the healthcare professions may reap the benefits of information technology to support EBP.

- Researchers need to be aware of requirements that legislation imposes on them in their conduct of research.
- CER is playing a big part in improving the quality of care while decreasing costs for healthcare.

REFERENCES

Agency for Healthcare Research and Quality (AHRQ). (2004, March). *Closing the quality gap: A critical analysis of quality improvement strategies.* Fact Sheet (AHRQ Publication No. 04-P014), Agency for Healthcare Research and Quality, Rockville, MD. Retrieved from http://www.ahrq.gov/clinic/epc/qgapfact.htm

Agency for Healthcare Research and Quality (AHRQ). (n.d.). *Nursing research.* Retrieved from http://www.ahrq.gov/about/nursing/

American Association of Colleges of Nursing (AACN). (1996). The Essentials of Master's Education for Advanced Nursing Practice. Retrieved from http://www.aacn.nche.edu/education-resources/MasEssentials96.pdf

American Nurses' Association. (2004). Nursing information and data set evaluation center (NIDSECSM). Retrieved from http://www.nursingworld.org/nidsec/

American Nurses' Association. (2007, June 5). *Relationships among ANA recognized data element sets and terminologies.* Retrieved from http://nursingworld.org/npii/relationship.htm

Aponte, J. (2010). Key elements of large survey data sets. *Nursing Economics, 28*(1), 27–36.

Barroso, J., Edlin, A., Sandelowski, M., & Lambe, C. (2006). Bridging the gap between research and practice: The development of a digital library of research syntheses. *Computers, Informatics, Nursing, 24*(2), 85–94.

Bembridge, E., Levett-Jones, T., & Jeong, S. Y. (2010, April/May). The preparation of technologically literate graduates for professional practice. *Contemporary Nurse, 35*(1), 18–25.

Bettany-Saltikov, J. (2010). Learning how to undertake a systematic review: Part 2. *Nursing Standard, 24*(51), 47–56.

Brown, C. W., Wickline, M. A., Ecoff, L., & Glaser, D. (2008). Nursing practice, knowledge, attitudes and perceived barriers to evidence-based practice at an academic medical center. *Journal of Advanced Nursing, 65*(2), 371–381.

Butler, D. (2008). Translational research: Crossing the valley of death. *Nature, 453,* 840–842.

Carlson, C., & Plonczynski, D. J. (2008). Has the BARRIERS scale changed nursing practice? An integrative review. *Journal of Advanced Nursing, 63*(4), 322–333. doi:10.1111/j.1365-2648.2008.04705.x

Cassey, M. Z. (2007, March–April). Keeping up with existing and emerging technologies: An introduction to PDAs. *Nursing Economics, 25*(2), 121–135.

Centers for Disease Control and Prevention. (2010). *Health of Hispanic or Latino population.* Retrieved from http://www.cdc.gov/nchs/faststats/hispanic_health.htm

Chesla, C. (2008). Translational research: Essential contributions from interpretive nursing science. *Research in Nursing & Health, 31,* 381–390.

Chester, L. (2007, March). Many critical care nurses are unaware of evidence-based practice. *American Journal of Critical Care, 16*(2), 106.

Cohen, A. (2010, April). Mammography and comparative effectiveness research: What do you do when you don't like it? *Contemporary OB/GYN,* 70–71.

Colevins, H., Bond, D., & Clark, K. (2006, April). Refresher students hand from handhelds. *Computers in Libraries,* 7–8, 46–48.

Courey, T., Benson-Soros, J., Deemer, K., & Zeller, R. (2006, November). The missing link: Information literacy and evidence-based practice as a new challenge for nurse educators. *Nursing Education Perspectives, 27*(6), 320–323.

DiMaria-Ghalili, R., & Ostrow, C. L. (2009, February). Using Microsoft Excel to teach statistics in a graduate advanced practice nursing program. *Journal of Nursing Education, 48*(2), 106–110.

Doolan, D., & Froelicher, E. S. (2009). Using an existing data set to answer new research questions: A methodological review. *Research and Theory for Nursing Practice: An International Journal, 23*(3), 203–215.

Dracup, K., & Bryan-Brown, C. (2006, July). Evidence-based practice is wonderful... sort of. *American Journal of Critical Care, 15*(4), 356–358.

Drenning, C. (2006, October). Using the best evidence to change practice: Collaboration among nurses, advanced practice nurses, and nurse researchers to achieve evidence-based practice change. *Journal of Nursing Care Quality, 21*(4), 298–301.

Flemming, K., & Briggs, M. (2006). Electronic searching to locate qualitative research: Evaluation of three strategies. *Journal of Advanced Nursing, 57,* 95–100.

Freburger, J., & Carey, T. S. (2010, March). Comparative effectiveness research: Opportunities and challenges for physical therapy. *Physical Therapy, 90*(3), 327–332.

Gardner, C., & Beese-Bjurstrom, S. (2006, June). In our unit: RN-driven, evidence-based practice. *Critical Care Nurse, 26*(3), 80.

Gilbert, S. (2009). The nesting-egg problem: Why comparative effectiveness research is trickier than it looks. *Hastings Center Report, 39(6)* 11–14.

Glanville, J. (2008). Searching shortcuts-finding and appraising search filters. *Health Information on the Internet, 63,* 6–8.

Golder, S., & Loke, Y. K. (2009). Search strategies to identify information on adverse effects: A systematic review. *Journal of the Medical Library Association, 97*(2), 84–92.

Grefsheim, S. W., Whitmore, S. C., Rapp, B. A., Rankin, J. A., Robison, R. R., & Canto, C. C. (2010, April). The informationist: Building evidence for an emerging health profession. *Journal of the Medical Library Association, 98*(2), 147–156.

Halm, M. (2010). "Inside looking in" or "inside looking out"? How leaders shape cultures equipped for evidence-based practice. *American Journal of Critical Care, 19(4),* 375–378.

Hanberg, A., & Brown, S. (2006, November). Bridging the theory—Practice gap with evidence-based practice. *Journal of Continuing Education in Nursing, 37*(6), 248–249.

Hardwick, M. E., Pulido, P. A., & Adelson, W. S. (2007, July/August). The use of handheld technology in nursing research and practice. *Orthopaedic Nursing, 26*(4), 251–255.

Hockenberry, M., Wilson, D., & Barrera, P. (2006, July). Implementing evidence-based nursing practice in a pediatric hospital. *Pediatric Nursing, 32*(4), 371–377.

Ingersoll, G. W., Witzel, P. A., Berry, C., & Qualls, B. (2010, August). Meetings magnet research and evidence-based practice expectations through hospital-based research centers. *Nursing Economics, 28*(4), 226–236.

Institute of Medicine (IOM). (2001). *Crossing the quality chasm: A new health system for the 21st century.* Washington, DC: National Academies Press.

Institute of Medicine (IOM). (2009, June 30). 100 Initial Priority Topics for Comparative Effectiveness Research. Retrieved from http://www.iom.edu/~/media/Files/Report%20Files/2009/ComparativeEffectivenessResearchPriorities/Stand%20Alone%20List%20of%20100%20CER%20Priorities%20-%20for%20web.ashx

Institute of Medicine (IOM). (2010). *Initial national priorities for comparative effectiveness research.* Retrieved from http:www.iom.edu/Reports/2010/

Kon, A. (2008). A clinical and translational science award (CTSA) consortium and the translational research model. *The American Journal of Bioethics, 8*(3), 58–60.

Krieger, M. M., Richter, R. R., & Austin, T. M. (2008). An exploratory analysis of PubMed's free full-text limit on citation retrieval for clinical questions. *Journal of the Medical Library Association, 96*(4), 351–355.

Lawrence, J. (2007). Techniques for searching the CINAHL database using the EBSCO interface. *Association of Operating Room Nurses Journal, 85*(4), 779–791.

Lo, B., & Parham, L. (2010, Spring). The impact of web 2.0 on the doctor-patient relationship. *Journal of Law, Medicine, & Ethics, 38*(1), 17–26.

MacCall, S. L. (2006). Clinical digital libraries project: Design approach and exploratory assessment of timely use in clinical environments. *Journal of the Medical Library Association, 94*(2), 190–197.

Maienschein, J. S., Sunderland, M., Ankeny, R. A., & Robert, J. S. (2008). The ethos and ethics of translational research. *The American Journal of Bioethics, 8*(3), 43–51.

Matter, S. (2006, December). Empower nurses with evidence-based knowledge. *Nursing Management, 37*(12), 34–37.

Melnyk, B. M., & Fineout-Overholt, E. (2005). *Evidence-based practice in nursing & healthcare.* Philadelphia, PA: Lippincott Williams & Wilkins.

Mitchell, P. (2006, June). Research and development in nursing revisited: Nursing science as the basis for evidence-based practice. *Journal of Advanced Nursing, 54*(5), 528–529.

Morin, K. (2008). Translational research: A new social contract that still leaves out public health? *The American Journal of Bioethics, 8*(3), 62–64.

Morris, P. E., & Munro, C. E. (2009). Will comparative effectiveness research increase patient safety in intensive care units? *American Journal of Critical Care, 18*(6), 504–506. doi:10.4037/ajcc200933

Murphy, J. (2010). Nursing informatics: The intersection of nursing, computer, and information sciences. *Nursing Economics, 28*(3), 204–207.

National Institutes of Health. (2003, September). *Privacy boards and the HIPAA privacy rule.* Retrieved from http://privacyruleandresearch.nih.gov/privacy_boards/hipaa_privacy_rule.asp

National Institutes of Health. (2004, February 5). *Clinical research and the HIPAA privacy rule* (NIH Publication Number 04–5495). Retrieved from http://privacyruleandresearch.nih.gov/clin_research.asp

National Library of Medicine (NLM). (2006, May 19). *About the UMLS resources.* Retrieved from http://www.nlm.nih.gov/research/umls/about_umls.html

Nelson, E. C., Batalden, P. B., & Godfrey, M. M. (2007). *Quality by design: A clinical microsystems approach.* San Francisco, CA: Jossey-Bass.

Nijs, N. T., Toppers, A., Defloor, T., Bernaerts, K., Milisen, K., & Van Den Berge, G. (2008). Incidence and risk factors for pressure ulcers in the intensive care unit. *Journal of Clinical Nursing, 18,* 1258–1266.

Oermann, M. R., Roop, J. C., Nordstrom, C. K., Galvin, E. A., & Floyd, J. A. (2007). Effectiveness of an intervention for disseminating Cochrane reviews to nurses. *Medsurg Nursing, 16*(6), 373–377.

Oroviogoicoechea, C. E., Elliott, B., & Watson, R. (2007). Review: Evaluating information systems in nursing. *Journal of Clinical Nursing,* 567–575.

Pipe, T. (2007, July). Optimizing nursing care by integrating theory-driven evidence based practice. *Journal of Nursing Care Quality, 22*(3), 234–238.

Pravikoff, D. S., Tanner, A. B., & Pierce, S. T. (2005). Readiness of U.S. nurses for evidence-based practice. *American Journal of Nursing, 105*(9), 40–51.

Ryan, S. (2006). Interview. Multidisciplinary terminology: The international classification for nursing practice (ICNP), Amy Coenen. *Online Journal of Nursing Informatics, 10*(3), 1–2.

Sakala, C. (2009, December). Letter from North America: The United States government's comparative effectiveness research program. *Birth, 36*(4), 342–344.

Salmond, S. (2007, March). Advancing evidence-based practice: A primer. *Orthopaedic Nursing, 26*(2), 114–125.

Saltikov, B. (2010). Learning how to undertake a systematic review: Part 2. *Nursing Standard, 24*(51), 47–58.

Sampselle, C., Pienta, K., & Markel, D. (2010). The CTSA mandate: Are we there yet? *Research & Theory for Nursing Practice, 24*(1), 64–73. doi:10.1891/1541-6577.24.1.64

Schleyer, T. K. L., & Forrest, J. L. (2000). Methods for the design and administration of web-based surveys. *Journal of the American Medical Informatics Association, 7*(4), 416–425.

Schumock, G., & Pickard, A. (2009). Comparative effectiveness research: Relevance and applications to pharmacy. *American Journal of Health-System Pharmacy: Official Journal of the American Society of Health-System Pharmacists, 66*(14), 1278–1286. doi:10.2146/ajhp090150

Schwab, A., & Satin, D. J. (2008). The realistic costs and benefits of translational research. *The American Journal of Bioethics, 8*(3), 60.

Shaughnessy, M., Beidler, S. M., Gibbs, K., & Michael, K. (2007). Confidentiality challenges and good clinical practices in human subjects research: Striking a balance. *Topics in Stroke Rehabilitation, 14*(2), 1–4.

Shirey, M. (2006, July). Evidence-based practice: How nurse leaders can facilitate innovation. *Nursing Administration Quarterly, 30*(3), 252–265.

Sigma Theta Tau International. (2005, July 6). *Position statement on evidence-based nursing.* Retrieved from http://www.nursingsociety.org/aboutus/PositionPapers/Pages/EBN_positionpaper.aspx

Sigma Theta Tau International. (2006, April). *2006 EBP study summary of findings.* Retrieved from http://www.nursingknowledge.org/Portal/CMSLite/GetFile.aspx?contentID=78260

Simpson, R. (2006, July). Evidence-based practice: How nursing administration makes it happen. *Nursing Administration Quarterly, 30*(3), 291–294.

Skiba, D., & Thompson, B. (2007, September 28). *Report of the NLN survey on informatics compe-tencies in the curriculum.* A paper presented at Evolution or Revolution: Recreating Nursing Education, The National League for Nursing's Annual Education Summit, Phoenix, AZ.

Smith, K. (2008). Building upon existing evidence to shape future research endeavors. *American Journal of Health-System Pharmacy, 65,* 1767–1774.

Snyder, K. (2007, May). Nurses' thoughts on evidence-based practice. *American Journal of Critical Care, 16*(3), 312–312.

Steinbrook, R. (2009). Health care and the American Recovery and Reinvestment Act. *New England Journal of Medicine, 360*(11), 1057–1060. doi:10.1056/NEJMp0900665

Stockwell, D. C. (2006, September). Handheld computing in pediatric practice: Is it for you? *Contemporary Pediatrics, 23*(9), 113–120.

Tagney, J., & Haines, C. (2009). Using evidence-based practice to address gaps in nursing knowledge. *British Journal of Nursing, 18*(8), 484–489.

Thompson, B. W. (2005). HIPAA guidelines for using PDAs. *Nursing, 35*(11), 24.

Traymor, K. (2009). Officials eye comparative effectiveness research. *American Journal of Health-System Pharmacy, 66,* 430–433.

U.S. Department of Health & Human Services. (2009). Code of Federal regulations: Part 46 pro-tection of human subjects. Retrieved from http://www.hhs.gov/ohrp/humansubjects/guidance/45cfr46.html#46.102

Villarruel, A., Gal, T., Eakins, B., Wilkes, A., & Herbst, J. (2010). From research to practice: The importance of community collaboration in the translation process. *Research & Theory for Nursing Practice, 24*(1), 25–34. doi:10.1891/1541-6577.24.1.25

Walsh, N. (2010). Dissemination of evidence into practice: Opportunities and threats. *Primary Health Care, 20*(3), 26–30.

Westfall, J. M., Mold, J., & Fagnan, L. (2007). Practice-based research—"Blue Highways" on the NIH roadmap. *Journal of the American Medical Association, 297*(4), 403–406.

Whipple, E. M., McGowan, J. J., Dixon, B. E., & Zafar, A. (2009). The selection of high-impact health informatics literature: A comparison of results between the content expert and the expert re-searcher. *Journal of the Medical Library Association, 97*(3), 212–218.

Wilson, P. M., Madary, A., Brown, J., Gomez, L., Martin, J., & Molina, T. (2004, September). Using the forces of magnetism to bridge nursing research and practice. *Journal of Nursing Adminis-tration, 34*(9), 393–394.

Winsett, R., & Cashion, A. K. (2007). The nursing research process. *Nephrology Nursing Journal, 34*(6), 635–643.

Wolf, S. P., Paradise, J., & Caga-anan, C. (2008, Summer). The law of incidental findings in hu-man subjects research: Establishing researchers duties. *Journal of Law, Medicine and Ethics,* 361–383.

Wong, S. S., Wilczynski, N. L., & Haynes, R. B. (2006). Optimal CINAHL search strategies for identi-fying therapy studies and review articles. *Journal of Nursing Scholarship, 38*(2), 194–199.

Woods, N. F., & Magyary, D. L. (2010). Translational research: Why nursing's interdisciplinary collaboration is essential. *Research and Theory for Nursing Practice: An International Journal, 24*(1), 9–24. doi:10.1891/1541-6577.24.1.9

Yoshi, A. P., Plaut, D. A., McGraw, K. A., Anderson, M. J., & Wellik, K. E. (2009). Analysis of the reporting of search strategies in Cochrane systematic reviews. *Journal of the Medical Library Association, 97*(1), 21–29.

Younger, P. (2010). Using Google Scholar to conduct a literature search. *Nursing Standard, 24*(45), 40–48.

Zerhouni, E. (2007). Translational research: Moving discovery to practice. *Clinical Pharmacology & Therapeutics, 81*(1), 126–128.

Zuzelo, P., McGoldrick, T., Seminara, P., & Karbach, H. (2006, June). Shared governance and EBP: A logical partnership? *Nursing Management, 37*(6), 45–50.

Glossary

Access code Unique identifier generally provided by a name and password for the specific purpose of restricting computer or information system use to persons who have legitimate authority to view or use information found in the computer or information system.

Accountable care organizations (ACOs) Payment and healthcare delivery reform model that ties provider reimbursement to quality metrics and reductions in the total cost of care for a given patient population.

Administrative information systems Systems that support patient care by managing financial and demographic information and providing reporting capabilities.

Aggregate data Data that are derived from large population groups.

Alphanumeric Numbers and alphabetic characters.

Ambulatory Payment Classification (APC) Describes new reimbursement criteria for ambulatory procedures.

American Recovery and Reinvestment Act of 2009 (ARRA) Legislation that included provisions for health information technology and funding for the Office of the National Coordinator of Health Information Technology (ONCHIT).

Antivirus software Set of computer programs capable of finding and eliminating viruses and other malicious programs from scanned disks, computers, and networks.

Application security Measures designed to protect a set of computer programs and the information that they create or store, such as timed or automatic sign-off, which prevents unauthorized access by others when users forget to sign off the system.

Application service provider (ASP) Third-party entities that manage and distribute software-based services and solutions to customers across a wide area network from a central data center.

Application software Set of programs designed to accomplish a particular task.

Archetypes Re-usable clinical models of content and processes significant for an initiative to develop a life-long electronic record.

Architecture Structure of the central processing unit and its interrelated elements within an information system.

Arden Syntax Standard language used in the healthcare industry for writing rules.

Arithmetic logic unit (ALU) Component of the central processing unit that executes arithmetic instructions.

ARPANET (Advanced Research Projects Agency Network) Precursor of today's Internet which was funded by the U.S. Defense Department.

Asynchronous Transfer Mode (ATM) High-speed data transmission method suitable for voice, data, image, text, and video information that use fiber or twisted pair cable. It is faster than ISDN, but less frequently used for reasons of cost, availability, and a lack of standards.

Attachments Files sent with e-mail messages.

Audit trail Electronic tool that can track system access by individual user, by user class, or by all persons who viewed a specific client record.

Authentication Action that verifies the authority of users to receive specified data.

Authoring tools Software programs that allow persons with little or no programming expertise to create instructional computer programs.

Automatic sign-off Mechanism that logs a user off the computer after a specific period of inactivity.

Backloaded Information that is preloaded into the system before the go-live date.

Backup plan Strategy to ensure availability of key employees and resources to ensure ongoing business and information system processing.

Backup procedure Creation of a second copy of files and information found on a computer, or information system, for the intent of restoring information in the event data are lost or damaged; or an alternative means to accomplish tasks normally done with an information system when that system is not available for some reason.

Backup systems Devices that create copies of system and data files.

Barcode medication administration (BCMA) Process or system used to ensure that the correct patient receives the correct medication in the correct dosage via the correct route and at the correct time. Patients and drugs both have barcode identification codes.

Batch processing Manipulation of large amounts of data into meaningful applications at times when computer demands are lowest as a means to maintain system performance during peak utilization hours. Batch-processed information is not available before processing and is little used today except to run reports.

Benchmarking Continual process of measuring services and practices against the toughest competitors in the industry.

Bennett Bill Although not passed into law, the Medical Records Confidentiality Act of 1995 was a significant piece of legislation because it attempted to establish the role of healthcare providers in the protection of client information; to fix conditions for the inspection, copying, and disclosure of protected information; and to institute legal protection for health-related information.

Bibliography database manager (BDM) Software that allows the importation of references directly from databases. Selected examples include EndNote, Reference Manager, ProCite, Biblioscape, and the Web-based Zotero.

Binary code Series of 1s and 0s.

Binary file transfer (BFT) Set of instructions that represents another standard for file transfer.

Biometrics Unique, measurable characteristic or trait of a human being for automatically recognizing or verifying identity.

BIOS (basic input/output system) Program code start up routine stored in permanent memory.

Bit Smallest unit of data that can be handled by the computer.

Bits per second (bps) Number of bits that can be transferred in 1 second of time.

Bliki A type of Web page that allows collaborative contributions and posts in reverse chronological order.

Blog Abbreviation for Weblog.

Blu-ray High density optical disc format rival to HD-DVD.

Body Main portion of an e-mail message.

Browser Retrieval program that allows the user to search and access hypertext and hypermedia documents on the Web by using HTTP.

Bulletin board systems (BBS) Originally an online service that offered computerized dial-in meeting and announcements, file sharing, and limited discussions. Now it refers to a site used to post announcements.

Business continuity management Process to ensure that organizations can withstand any disruption to normal functioning.

Business continuity planning (BCP) Combines information technology and disaster recovery planning with business functions recovery planning.

Business impact assessment or analysis (BIA) Process of determining the critical functions of the organization and the information vital to maintain operations as well as the applications and databases; hardware; and communications facilities that use, house, or support this information.

Byte Eight bits makes up one byte.

Carpal tunnel syndrome Compression of median nerve as it passes through the wrist along the pathway to the hand resulting in sensory and motor changes to the thumb, index finger, third finger, and radial aspect of the ring finger.

CAPTCHAS Completely automatic public test to tell computers and humans apart.

Central processing unit (CPU) Electronic circuitry that executes computer instructions—reading stored programs one instruction at a time, keeping track of the execution, and directing other computer parts and input and output devices to perform required tasks.

Certificate authority (CA) Trusted third party that issues digital certificates which certify ownership of a public key.

Challenge response software Also known as *CAPTCHAS*, a test to tell computers and humans apart.

Chief information officer (CIO) Person responsible for strategic planning, policy development, budgeting, information security, recruitment and retention of information services staff, and overall management of the enterprise's information systems. computer-related positions.

Chief privacy officer (CPO) Individual responsible for the protection of personal health information of patients as required by federal law.

Classification system Approach that uses mutually exclusive categories for specific purposes such as describing the details of a patient encounter for clinical, administrative, or reimbursement issues.

Client/server Distributed approach to computing where different computers work together to carry out a task. The computer that makes requests is known as the *client*, while the high performance computer that contains requested files is known as the *server*.

Clinical Care Classification System (CCC) Nursing classification designed to document the six steps of the nursing process across the care continuum. Consists of two interconnected terminologies—the CCC of Nursing Diagnosis and Outcomes and the CCC of Nursing Interventions.

Clinical data repository Database where information from many different information systems is stored and managed, allowing retrieval of elements without regard to their point of origin.

Clinical decision support Filtered expert information used to guide decisions for clinical care.

Clinical information analyst Person who synthesizes data and interprets its relationship to clinical interventions.

Clinical information systems (CIS) Large computerized database management systems used to access the patient data that are needed to plan, implement, and evaluate care. May also be known as *patient care information systems*.

Clinical liaisons Clinicians who represent the interests and needs of information system users.

Clinical pathway Suggested blueprint for patient care by diagnosis that includes specific interventions, desired outcomes, and even the projected length of stay of inpatient treatment.

Clinical terminology Concepts that support clinical concepts such as diagnostic studies, history and physical examinations, visit notes, ancillary department information, nursing notes, assessments, flow sheets, vital signs, and outcome measures. Can be mapped to a broader classification system for administrative, regulatory, and fiscal reporting requirements.

Codes Letters, numbers, or a combination thereof, that represents concepts in a computer system.

Codified Concept with an assigned code.

Cognitive walkthrough This usability assessment method is a detailed review of a sequence of real or proposed actions to complete a task in a system.

Cold site Company that maintains electronic records and backup media in secure, climate-controlled storage so that information can be used to restore system capability in the event that information and/or system functionality have been lost.

Comfort zone Situation or place in which the individual is at ease.

Commission on Accreditation of Rehabilitation Facilities (CARF) Healthcare accrediting body with a focus on the improvement of rehabilitative services to people with disabilities and others in need of rehabilitation.

Community Health Information Network (CHIN) Organization that electronically links providers; payers; and purchasers of care for the exchange of financial, clinical, and administrative information via a wide area network in a particular geographic area. Precursor to RHIOs.

Compact discs (CDs) Older form of secondary storage.

Computational nursing Branch of nurmetrics that uses models and simulation to apply existing theory and numerical methods to new solutions for nursing problems.

Computer Electronic device that collects, processes, stores, retrieves, and provides information output under the direction of stored sequences of instructions known as *computer programs*.

Computer-assisted instruction (CAI) Use of a computer to organize and present instruction primarily for use by an individual learner.

Computer-based patient record (CPR) Automated patient record designed to enhance and support patient care through availability of complete and accurate data as well as bodies of knowledge and other aids to care providers.

Computer-based patient record system (CPRS) People, data, rules and procedures, and computer and communications equipment and support facilities that provide the mechanism by which patient records are created, used, stored, and retrieved.

Computer-based training (CBT) Educational format using the computer that is widely used to train persons to use specific computer applications.

Computer forensics Collection of electronic evidence for purposes of litigation and internal investigations.

Computer literacy Familiarity with the use of computers, including software tools such as word processing, spreadsheets, databases, presentation graphics, and e-mail.

Computerized physician (or provider/prescriber) order entry (CPOE) Process by which the physician or provider directly enters orders for patient care into a hospital information system.

Computer viruses Malicious programs spread via computers that can disrupt or destroy data.

Computer vision syndrome (CVS) Eye and vision problems that result from work done in close proximity such as computer work.

Confidentiality Tacit understanding that private information shared in a situation in which a relationship has been established for the purpose of treatment or delivery of services will remain protected.

Concept Expression with a single unambiguous meaning although it may have one or more representations called *synonyms* or *terms*. Used to document ideas and express orders, assessments, and outcomes within an EHR; they are uniquely identified by codes.

Connectivity Process that allows individual users to communicate and share hardware, software, and information using technology such as modems and the Internet.

Consent Process by which an individual authorizes healthcare personnel to process his or her information based on an informed understanding of how this information will be used.

Consumer health informatics Use of electronic information and communication to improve medical outcomes and healthcare decision making from the patient/consumer perspective.

Context sensitive help Additional information available throughout software that provides directions at the screen and field level to help guide end users to complete a particular task.

Contingency planning or continuity planning The process of ensuring the continuation of critical business services regardless of any event that may occur.

Continuity of care document (CCD) Record comprised of contributions from many types of caregivers, with each providing a summary of care provided for the purpose of improved continuity of care when clients move between various points of care.

Continuity planning Essential component of strategic planning designed to maintain business operations.

Control unit Manages instructions to other parts of the computer, including input and output devices.

Critical pathway Approach used in automated nursing information systems for designing screens, generating reminders, and providing guideline interventions and documentation.

Current Procedural Terminology (CPT) Classification system that lists medical services and procedures performed by physicians and is used for physician billing and payer reimbursement.

Cybercrime Commonly refers to the ability to steal personal information stored on computers such as Social Security numbers.

Data Collection of numbers, characters, or facts that are gathered according to some perceived need for analysis and possibly action at a later point in time.

Database File structure that supports the storage of data in an organized fashion and allows data retrieval as meaningful information.

Database administrator (DBA) Person responsible for overseeing all activities related to maintaining a database and optimizing its use.

Data cleansing Use of software to improve the quality of data to ensure that it is accurate enough for use in data mining and warehousing.

Data collection tool Device created for the purpose of accumulating specific details in an organized fashion.

Data dictionary Tool that defines terms used in a system to ensure consistent understanding and application among all users in the institution. This process may also be achieved through the use of an interface engine.

Data exchange standards Set of agreed-on rules that permit the uniform capture and exchange of data between information systems from different vendors and between different healthcare providers.

Data integrity Ability to collect; store; and retrieve correct, complete, and current data so that the data are available to authorized users when needed.

Data management Process of controlling the storage, retrieval, and use of data to optimize accuracy and utility while safeguarding integrity.

Data mining Technique that looks for hidden patterns and relationships in large groups of data using software.

Data privacy Right to choose the conditions and the extent to which information and beliefs are shared with others. Informed consent for the release of medical records represents the application of information privacy.

Data retrieval Process that allows the user to access previously collected and stored data.

Data scrubbing See data cleansing.

Data warehouse Provides a powerful method of managing and analyzing data.

Decision-support software (DSS) Computer programs that organize information to aid choices related to patient care or administrative issues.

Desktop videoconferencing (DTV) Real-time encounter that uses a specially equipped personal computer with an Internet connection to allow face-to-face meetings or simultaneous viewing of the same images.

Digital cameras Means to capture and input still images without film.

Digital Image Communication in Medicine (DICOM) Standard that promotes the communication, storage, and integration of digital images with hospital information systems.

Digital library Set of electronic resources with the related capabilities to create, store, organize, search, and retrieve information to meet the needs of a community of users.

Digital Subscriber Line (DSL) Type of Internet service available over telephone lines that offers greater speed and better connectivity than dial-up service.

Digital signature Mathematical method to demonstrate the authenticity of a digital message or document.

Digital Versatile or Video Discs (DVDs) Secondary storage device.

Disaster Man-made or natural event with the potential to cause considerable damage and possibly loss of life.

Disaster planning Organized approach that anticipates potential problems, maintains security of client information under adverse conditions, and provides an alternative means to support the retrieval and processing of data in the event that the information system fails.

Disaster recovery Processes that help organizations deal with disruptive events.

Disease management Multidisciplinary approach to identify patient populations with, or at risk for, specific medical conditions.

Distance learning Use of print, audio, video, computer, or teleconference capability to connect faculty and students who are located at a minimum of two different sites.

Diskettes Older, largely obsolete form of secondary storage.

Distributed processing Use of a group of independent processors that contain the same information but may be at different sites as a means to maintain information services in the event of a power outage or other disaster.

Document imaging Scanning paper records for conversion to digital files for electronic storage and handling.

Downtime Period of time when an information system is not operational or available for use.

DSL modem Digital Subscriber Line modem.

E-business Refers to services, sales, and business conducted over the Internet.

E-care Broad term used to refer to the automation of all parts of the care delivery process across administrative, clinical, and departmental boundaries.

E-health Wide range of healthcare activities involving the electronic transfer of health-related information on the Internet.

E-learning The delivery of content and stimulation of learning primarily through the use of online telecommunication technologies such as blogs, podcasts, streamed video recorded videos, e-mail, bulletin board systems, electronic whiteboards, inter-relay chat, desktop video conferencing, and the World Wide Web.

E-patient Individual who accesses healthcare information and/or services via the Internet.

Electronic communication Exchange of information through the use of computer equipment and software.

Electronic data interchange (EDI) Communication of data in binary code from one computer to another.

Electronic health record (EHR) Digital version of patient data found in traditional paper records. Increasingly used to refer to a longitudinal record ideally of all healthcare encounters.

Electronic mail (e-mail) Use of computers to transmit messages to one or more persons. Delivery is almost instant, and attachment files may accompany text messages.

Electronic mail (e-mail) software Computer program that assists the user in sending, receiving, and managing e-mail messages.

Electronic medical record (EMR) Legal record created in hospitals and ambulatory settings of a single encounter or visit that is the source of data for the electronic health record.

Electronic patient record (EPR) Electronic client record, but not necessarily a lifetime record, that focuses on relevant information for the current episode of care.

Electronic performance support system (EPSS) An application designed to run at the same time as other applications that may supply information, present job aids, or deliver just-in-time training.

Electronic signature Means to authenticate a computer-generated document through a code or digital signature that is unique to each authorized system user.

Electronic Signatures in Global and National Commerce Act (ESIGN) Legislation that gives electronic signatures the same legal status as hand-written signatures.

Emergency plan Set of actions to deal with disaster situations.

Encryption Process that uses mathematical formulas to code messages when content needs to be kept secure and confidential.

End user Healthcare workers who use an information system to view or document client information.

E-prescribing Electronic transmission of drug prescriptions.

Ergonomics Scientific study of work and space, including details that impact productivity and health.

Error message Computer-generated text that warns the user when entries are missing or improperly constructed for processing. May appear on the monitor screen as data are entered or later via a paper printout.

Evidence-based practice Process by which nurses and other healthcare practitioners use the best available research evidence, clinical expertise, and patient preferences to make clinical decisions.

Expert systems Use of computer artificial intelligence to arrive at a decision that experts in the field would make.

External environment Includes those interested parties and competitors who are outside the healthcare institution.

Extranet Network outside the protected internal network of an organization that uses Internet software and communication protocols for electronic commerce and use by suppliers or customers.

Facebook popular social networking Websites

Fax modem Allows computers to transmit images of letters and drawings over telephone lines.

Feature creep Uncontrolled addition of features or functions without regard to timelines or budget.

File Collection of related data stored and handled as a single entity by the computer.

File deletion software Overwrites files with meaningless information so that sensitive information cannot be accessed.

File Transfer Protocol (FTP) Set of instructions that controls both the physical transfer of data across a network and its appearance on the receiving end.

Firewall Type of gateway designed to protect private network resources from outside hackers, network damage, and theft or misuse of information.

Floppy drives Largely obsolete form of a secondary storage device.

Focused ethnographies Research methods borrowed from anthropology and sociology for conducting investigative fieldwork and analysis of people in cultural–social settings. These can be useful for assessing groups of users and computers.

Frames per second (FPS) Number of still images captured, transmitted, and displayed in one second of time in a video transmission. The higher the FPS, the smoother the picture. Also referred to as *frame rate*.

Freezing Situation in which a computer will not accept further input and does not process what has already been entered.

Frequently asked questions (FAQs) Document or file, used by many World Wide Web sites, that serves to introduce the group or topic, update new users on recent discussions, and eliminate repetition of questions.

Function Task that may be performed manually or automated.

Gateway Combination of hardware and software used to connect local area networks with larger networks.

G-codes or quality data codes (QDC) Special set of nonpayable HCPCS codes for measurement of the quality of care physicians give to their office patients.

Genomics The study of individual's genetic makeup for the purpose of providing treatments that will be effective for that individual.

Gigahertz Represents 1 billion cycles per second in processor speed.

Goal Open-ended statement that describes what is to be accomplished in general terms, often used in the strategic planning process.

Go-live Date when an information system is first used, or the process of starting to use an information system.

Grand rounds Traditional teaching tool for healthcare professionals in training that involves reviewing a client's case history and present condition inclusive of examination findings before a mutual determination of the best treatment options.

Graphical user interface (GUI) A set of menus, windows, and other standard screen devices that are intended to make using a computer as intuitive as possible.

Grid computer Type of computer technology the uses the concept of distributed processing to solve certain classes of computing problems that cannot be solved within reasonable periods of time via other methods.

Hacker Individuals who break into computer systems.

Hard disk drive Provides storage for digital data.

Hardware Physical components of a computer.

Header Section at the top of an electronic mail message that tells who sent the message, when, to whom and at what location, and the address to which a reply should be directed if different from the sender's address.

Healthcare Information Exchange (HIE) Electronic sharing of patient information such as demographic data, allergies, presenting complaint, diagnostic test values, and other relevant data between providers such as primary physicians, specialists, hospitals, and ambulatory care settings according to nationally recognized standards.

Healthcare information system (HIS) Computer hardware and software dedicated to the collection, storage, processing, retrieval, and communication of patient care information in a healthcare organization.

Healthcare information system analyst Person responsible for translating user needs into healthcare information system capability.

Health Insurance Portability and Accountability Act (HIPAA) Also known as the Kennedy–Kassebaum Bill, it is the first federal legislation to protect automatic client records and also mandated that all electronic transactions include only HIPAA compliant codes.

Healthcare terminology standards Strategy to enable and support widespread interoperability among healthcare software applications for the purpose of sharing information.

Health Level 7 (HL7) Standard for the exchange of clinical data between information systems by means of an extensive set of rules that apply to all data sent.

Health literacy Degree to which individuals can obtain, process, and understand basic health information and services needed to make appropriate health decisions.

Help desk First line of user support within an organization. Support service, rather than a specific location, for computer users, often available 24 hours a day by calling a special telephone number. Help desk staff have an information system or computer background and are familiar with all of the software applications and hardware in use.

Helper program Computer application that supports a browser by providing added functionality and performs specific tasks.

Help screens Computer messages displayed on the monitor screen in response to a user's request for assistance by pressing an identified key, or in response to an inappropriate entry by the user. Help screens provide specific directions that the user may follow to reach a desired outcome.

Heuristic evaluations Assessments of a product according to accepted guidelines or published usability principles.

High density optical disc format (HD-DVD) Secondary storage device.

HITECH (Health Information Technology for Economic and Clinical Health Act) Portion of ARRA that amended HIPAA Security and Privacy Rules and provided funds and incentives to increase the use of electronic health records by physicians and hospitals who meet eligibility criteria for Meaningful Use.

Homegrown software Developed by the consumer to meet specific needs usually because no suitable commercial package is available.

Home page First page seen at a particular Web location.

Hospital information system (HIS) Group of information systems used within a hospital or enterprise that support and enhance patient care. The HIS consists of two major types of information systems: clinical and administrative.

Hot site Facility located at a location separate from that of the healthcare provider and which replicates the provider's information systems for the purpose of quickly restoring information system function in the event of a disaster or disruption to services.

Human-computer interaction or HCI The study of how people design, implement, evaluate, and use interactive computer systems.

Human factors The scientific study of the interaction between people, machines, and their work environments.

Hyperlink or link Words, phrases, or images used on Internet pages distinguished from the remainder of the document through the use of highlighting or a different screen color that allow users to skip from point to point within or among documents, escaping conventional linear format.

Hypertext markup language (HTML) Language or set of instructions that is frequently used to write home pages for the Internet and includes text as well as special instructions known as *tags* for the display of text and other media. HTML also includes highlighted references to other documents that the user may choose if additional information about that topic is desired.

Hypertext transfer protocol (HTTP) Transfer protocol used on Internet pages that establishes a TCP/IP connection between the client and server and sends a request in the form of a command when a link or hypertext is clicked with the mouse.

ID management Administrative area that deals with identifying individuals in a system and controlling their access to resources.

Informatics Science and art of turning data into information.

Informatics Nurse A nurse with advanced preparation in information management.

Informatics Nurse Specialist (INS) A nurse who has educational preparation to conduct informatics research and generate informatics theory.

Information Collection of data that have been interpreted and examined for patterns and structure.

Information literacy Ability to recognize when information is needed as well as the skills to find, evaluate, and use needed information effectively.

Information privacy Right to choose the conditions and the extent to which information and beliefs are shared with others. Informed consent for the release of medical records represents the application of information privacy.

Information security Protection of confidential information against threats to its integrity or inadvertent disclosure.

Information system Computer system that uses hardware and software to process data into information in order to solve a problem.

Information system security Protection of information systems and the information housed on them from unauthorized use or threats to integrity.

Information technology General term that refers to the management and processing of information with the assistance of computers.

Input devices Hardware that allows the user to put data into the computer, such as the keyboard, mouse, track ball, touch screen, light pen, microphone, barcode reader, fax/modem card, joystick, and scanner.

Instant messaging (IM) Text-based, real-time communication characterized by abbreviations that occurs via computers, cell phones, or other mobile devices.

Integrated services digital network (ISDN) High-speed data transmission technology that allows simultaneous, digital transfer of voice, video, and data over telephone lines but at higher speeds than available via dial-up or DSL connections.

Integrated video disk (IVD) Outdated technology that combined the interactivity, information management, and decision-making capability of computers with audiovisual capabilities of videodisk or tape to enhance computer learning.

Integration Process by which different information systems are able to exchange data in a fashion that is seamless to the end user.

Interface Computer program that tells two different systems how to exchange data.

Interface engine Software application that allows different computer systems to access and exchange information.

Interface terminology Also known as point-of-care terminology. Consists of terms familiar to clinicians.

Internal environment Includes employees of the institution, as well as physicians and members of the board of directors.

International Classification of Nursing Practice (ICNP) A system that serves to unify various approved nursing languages and classification systems to ensure the acceptance of common meanings across different settings.

International Classification of Disease (ICD–9/ICD–10) System for classification of surgical, diagnostic, and therapeutic procedures.

International standard H.320 Standard for passing audio and video data streams across networks, allowing videoconferencing systems from different manufacturers to communicate.

Internet Worldwide network that connects millions of computers linking governments, university and commercial institutions, and individual users.

Internet relay chat (IRC) Predominantly text-based, interactive form of communication available via the Internet.

Internet service provider (ISP) Company that furnishes Internet access for a fee.

Interoperability The ability of two entities, human or machine, to exchange and predictably use data or information while retaining the original meaning of that data.

Intranet Private computer network that uses Internet protocols and technologies, including Web browsers, servers, and languages, to facilitate collaborative data sharing.

JAVA Programming language that enables the display of moving text, animation, and musical excerpts on Web pages.

Jobs aids Written instructions designed as a reference in training and work settings.

Joint Cognitive Systems Consider the complexity of planned human behavior as opposed to single actions. Joint cognitive systems may imply that information is shared or distributed among humans and technology.

Joint Photographic Experts Group Compression (JPEG) Standard for the compression of digital images for transmission and storage that is also used for diagnostic images.

Joystick Allows the user to control the movement of objects on the screen.

Keyboards Input devices with keys that represent those of a typewriter.

Kilobits (kbps) Data transfer in thousands of bits per second.

Knowledge Synthesis of information derived from several sources to produce a single concept or idea.

Knowledge discovery in databases (KDD) Extraction of implicit, unknown, and potentially useful information from data.

Knowledge management Structured process for the generation, storage, distribution, and application of both tacit knowledge (personal experience) and explicit knowledge (evidence).

Laboratory Information Systems (LIS) Computer system for use by laboratories that provides many benefits as a result of automated order entry.

Laptop computer Streamlined, portable version of the personal computer.

Learning aids Materials intended to supplement or reinforce lecture or computer-based training. Examples may consist of outlines, diagrams, charts, and maps.

Learning object Entity or learning event that can stand alone without losing meaning.

Legacy systems Mainframe vendor-based information systems.

Life cycle Well-defined process that describes the recurring process of developing and maintaining an information system.

Linkedin Popular social networking Websites.

Links Also known as *hypertext,* links are words, phrases, or images used on Internet pages distinguished from the remainder of the document through the use of highlighting or a different screen color that allow users to skip from point to point within or among documents, escaping conventional linear format.

Liquid Crystal Display (LCD) Technology that uses two sheets of polarizing material with a liquid crystal solution between them with each crystal either allowing light to pass through or blocking the light to display text or an image.

Listserv E-mail subscription list program that copies and distributes all e-mail messages to everyone who is a subscriber.

Live data Actual patient and healthcare system.

Local area networks (LANs) Computers, printers, and other devices linked together to share resources and data within a defined area.

Logical Observation Identifiers, Names, and Codes (LOINC) Terminology that includes laboratory and clinical observations.

Macintosh computers (Macs) Computers developed by the Apple, Inc.; considered very user friendly.

Magnet designation Program that recognizes institutions providing quality nursing care.

Magnetic tape drive Secondary storage device used primarily with large mainframe computers.

Mainframes Large computers capable of processing large amounts of data quickly.

Main memory Component of memory that is permanent and remains when power is off. Also known as *read only memory (ROM).*

Malicious software Programs written for the purpose of stealing information, causing annoyance or performing covert actions.

Malware Term used to refer to destructive computer programs including viruses, worms, and Trojan horses.

Mapping Process by which the definition of terms used in one information system are associated with comparable terms in another system, thereby facilitating the exchange of information from one system to another.

Master patient index (MPI) Database that lists all identifiers used in connection with one particular client in a healthcare alliance. Identifiers may include items such as Social Security number, birth date, and name.

Meaningful use Use of health information technology (HIT) legislated by the American Recovery and Reinvestment Act of 2009 to collect specific data with the intent to improve care, engage patients, improve population health, and ensure privacy and security.

Medical informatics Application of informatics to all of the healthcare disciplines as well as the practice of medicine.

Medicare Improvements for Patients and Providers Act (MIPPA) Legislation that called for financial incentives for e-prescribing.

Medicare-severity diagnosis related group (MS-DRG) Classification system that determines the per diem rate for Medicare patients.

Megahertz One megahertz represents 1 million signal voltage cycles per second in processor speed.

Membership fee model Health information exchange model that calls for stakeholders to pay to support shared services for all.

Memory Computer storage device in which programs reside during execution. It comprises main memory and random access memory.

Menu List of related commands that can be selected from a computer screen to accomplish a task.

Metadata Set of data that provides information about how, when, and by whom data are collected, formatted, and stored.

Metasearch engines Tools that search several search engines at one time.

Microcomputer Personal computer that is either a stand-alone machine or is networked to other personal computers.

Microprocessor chip Electronic circuits of the CPU etched onto a silicon chip.

Minicomputer Scaled-down version of a mainframe.

Mission Purpose or reason for an organization's existence, representing the fundamental and unique aspirations that differentiate it from others.

m-learning Popular term that denotes the use of mobile technologies, such as the mobile phone, personal digital assistant (PDA), and iPod for learning purposes.

Mobile computing Devices that can be carried or wheeled from one location to another, often with the capability to transmit and receive information.

Modem Communication device that transmits data over telephone lines from one computer to another.

Monitor Screen that displays text and graphic images.

Monitoring systems Devices that automatically monitor biometrics measurements in critical care and specialty areas.

Motherboard Microprocessor chip that contains the electronic circuits of the CPU etched on a silicon chip, mounted on a board.

Mouse Device that can be moved around on the desktop to direct a pointer on the screen.

Multimedia Presentations that combine text, voice, or sound, and still or video images, as well as hardware and software that support the same.

Multiple function devices Combine functions such as printing, scanning, copying, and Fax.

NANDA International (NANDA-I) Terminology recognized by the American Nurses Association. Represents Nursing Diagnoses as data elements within SNOMED CT.

Nanotechnology Science and technology of engineering devices at the molecular level.

National Health Information Network (NHIN) Office of the National Coordinator (ONC) for Health Information Technology (HIT) initiative to provide the standards, services, and policies that enable secure health information exchange (HIE) over the Internet.

Net An alternate term to refer to the Internet, a worldwide network that connects millions of computers and serves to link government, university, commercial institutions, and individual users.

Netiquette Set of informal rules for polite communication via electronic means.

Network Combination of hardware and software that allows communication and electronic transfer of information between computers.

Network interface card Provides a physical connection between a computer and a network.

News reader software Special browser program needed by individual users to read messages posted on the news group.

Notebook computer Streamlined portable version of the personal computer.

Nurmetrics Branch of nursing science that uses mathematics and statistics to test, estimate, and quantify nursing theories and solutions to problems.

Nursing informatics Use of information and computer technology to support all aspects of nursing practice.

Nursing information system Information system that supports the use and documentation of nursing processes and provides tools for managing the delivery of nursing care.

Nursing Interventions Classification (NIC) Standardized classification of interventions that describes the activities that nurses perform.

Nursing Minimum Data Set (NMDS) Collection of data comprised of nursing diagnoses; interventions; and outcomes that allows comparison of data across different healthcare settings in order to project trends and stimulate research.

Nursing Outcomes Classification (NOC) Classification system that describes patient outcomes sensitive to nursing interventions.

Objective Statement that describes how a goal will be accomplished and the time frame for this activity.

Offline storage Form of data storage that uses secondary storage devices for data that are needed less frequently, or for long-term data storage.

Off-the-shelf software Commercially available software in which someone else bore the cost for its development and testing.

Omaha system American Nurses Association recognized research-based taxonomy that provides a framework for integrating and sharing clinical data. Widely used in settings such as home care, hospice, public health, school health, and prisons.

Online Term indicating a connection to various computer resources, including information systems, the Internet, and the World Wide Web.

Online storage Form of data storage that provides access to current data. An example is a high-speed, hard disk drive.

Online tutorials Detailed instructions available to a user while he or she is using a computer, software application, or information system that show or tell how a particular software application or feature can be implemented.

Ontology System that organizes concepts by meaning describing the definitional structure/relationship and organizes concepts for storage and retrieval of semantically accurate data.

Open architecture Protocols and technology that follow publicly accepted conventions and are employed by multiple vendors, so that various system components can work together.

Open system See open architecture.

Open-source Software available for use and modification by the public at no cost.

Operating system Collection of programs that manage all of the computer's activities.

Optical disk drives They write data to a recording surface media and read it later.

Order entry systems Method by which physician's orders for medications and treatments are entered into the computer and directly transmitted to appropriate areas.

QSEN project Funded project with the aim of preparing future nurses with the knowledge, skills, and attitudes needed to continuously improve the quality and safety of healthcare.

Output devices Hardware that allows the user to see processed data. Terminals or video monitor screens, printers, speakers, and fax/modem boards are types of output devices.

Outsourcing Process in which an organization contracts with outside agencies for services.

Password Alphanumeric code required for access and use of some computers or information systems as a security measure against unauthorized use. Password does not appear on the monitor display when it is keyed in.

Pay for Performance System where providers are rewarded for meeting pre-established targets for the delivery of healthcare services.

PC specialist Person who provides information and training on computers and software.

Peripheral Any piece of hardware attached to a computer.

PeriOperative Nursing Data Set (PNDS) Standardized perioperative nursing vocabulary provides nurses with a clear, precise, and universal language for clinical problems and surgical treatments.

Peripheral device interface cards Provide connection between equipment such as printers to the computer for the exchange of information.

Personal computer (PCs) Known as *desktop computers*. This category provides inexpensive processing power for an individual user.

Personal Computer Memory Card International Association (PCMCIA) card Provides added functionality such as memory to computers.

Personal digital assistants (PDAs) Specialized handheld devices used for calendar and address book functions, access to reference materials, and some input and transmission capabilities.

Personal health information (PHI) Demographic and insurance information, medical history, test and laboratory results, and other data collected by healthcare professionals in order to determine appropriate care. May also be known as *protected health information.*

Personal Health Record (PHR) Lifelong tool for managing health information such as disease conditions, allergies, medications, past surgeries, and other relevant information.

Phishing Ruse to get consumers to divulge personal information through social engineering and technical subterfuge via the use of electronic communication.

Picture archiving communications systems (PACS) Storage systems that permit remote access to diagnostic images at times convenient to the physician.

Plug-in programs Computer applications that have been designed to support browsers by performing specific tasks.

Point-of-care devices Computer access at the actual worksite, which in the delivery of healthcare is at the patient's bedside.

Point-of-care terminology Also known as *interface terminology.* Consists of terms familiar to clinicians.

Point-to-point interface Interface that directly connects two information systems.

Portal Web sites that may require registration, collect information from the user, and offer personalized features for individual users.

Printer Produces a paper copy of computer-generated documents.

Privacy Freedom from intrusion or control over the exposure of self or personal information.

Process interoperability Coordination of business processes at an organization allowing them to work together.

Production environment Point at which a planned information system is actually used to process and retrieve information and support the delivery of services.

Program Set of instructions that tell the computer what to do.

Program and service fee model Health information exchange model that charges stakeholders for participation in services.

Programmers Persons who write the instructions that tell the computer what to do.

Programming languages Set of rules to create the instructions that direct computers to perform specific functions.

Project management Set of practices intended to raise the likelihood that a project will succeed. Includes understanding drivers of change, a feasibility review, defining project scope, determining outcomes, identifying tasks, timelines, responsibilities, and interdependencies and resources needed.

Project scope Defines the size and details of an effort.

Public health informatics Application of information and computer science and technology to public health practice, research, and learning

Public key infrastructure (PKI) Provides a unique code for each user that is embedded into a storage device.

Quality data codes (QDC) or G-codes Special set of nonpayable HCPCS codes for measurement of the quality of care physicians give to their office patients.

Qubit Measurement similar to the bit except that it allows for a superposition of both 1 and 0.

Radio frequency identification (RFID) Technology similar to barcode identification that uses radio waves to transmit data from a tag to a receiver.

Radiology information system (RIS) Provides scheduling of diagnostic tests, communication of patient information, generation of patient instructions and preparation procedures, and file room management.

Random access memory (RAM) Component of memory that can be accessed, used, changed, and rewritten repeatedly while the computer is turned on.

Read-only memory (ROM) Component of memory that contains startup instructions for each time the computer is turned on. ROM is permanent and remains when power is off.

Real-time processing Entry and access to information occurs almost as soon as it is provided.

Recovery plan Organized strategy to restore operations and access to data and information.

Recovery Point Objective (RPO) Point in time to which you must recover data as defined by your organization.

Recovery Time Actual (RTA) Actual amount of time to restore data and functionality based on testing.

Recovery Time Objective (RTO) Acceptable amount of time to restore the function.

Redundant array of independent disks (RAID) Duplicate disks with mirror copies of data.

Reference terminology Set of concepts with definitional relationships that is frequently an ontology and therefore can be used to support data aggregation, disaggregation, retrieval, and analysis.

Refresh rate Term used to refer to the speed with which the screen is repainted from top to bottom.

Regional Health Information Organizations (RHIOs) Regional exchange of health and treatment information of patients among healthcare organizations and providers for the collective good.

Relational database Type of database that relies upon the use of tables to represent data.

Remote access Ability to use the resources contained on a network, or an information system, from a location outside of the facility where it is physically located.

Remote backup service (RBS) Company that provides backup services for customers from an off-site location to an on-site location.

Remote log-on Feature that allows users to access computer resources, such as directories, files, and databases at other locations.

Repetitive motion disorders See *repetitive stress injuries (RSIs)*.

Repetitive stress injuries (RSIs) Results from using the same muscle groups over and over again without rest.

Request for Information (RFI) A document sent to vendors that explains the institution's plans for purchasing and installing an information system with the goal of determining which vendors can meet the organization's basic requirements.

Request for Proposal (RFP) Document sent to vendors detailing the requirements of a potential information system with the purpose of soliciting proposals from vendors that describe their capabilities to meet these requirements.

Request for Quote (RFQ) Statement of need that focuses upon pricing, service levels, and contract terms.

Resolution Term used to refer to the sharpness, or clarity, of an image on a computer monitor. Resolution itself is determined by the number of pixels, or tiny dots or squares, displayed per inch on a monitor screen.

Resource Utilization Groups (RUGs) Per diem system of billing for skilled nursing facility patients.

Response time Amount of time between a user action and the response from the information system.

Return on Investment (RIO) Measure used to determine profits after calculation of all costs.

Roll out Staggered, or rolling, system implementation, sometimes refers to the preceding marketing campaign as well.

RSS (Really Simple Syndication) Markup language that brings users updates from the news and many other Web sites, blogs, and wikis.

Rule Predefined function that generates a clinical alert or reminder.

Sabotage Intentional destruction of computer equipment or records to disrupt services.

Scan The gathering of information from external and internal environments.

Scanner Input device that converts printed pages or graphic images into a file.

Scareware Use of pop-up messages designed to look like legitimate warnings urging users to download software to correct a problem.

Scope Statement in an organization's mission that defines the type of activities and services that it will perform.

Scope creep Unexpected and uncontrolled growth of user expectations as a project progresses.

Search engines Tool to help users find information on the World Wide Web. Each search engine maintains its own index or list of information on the Web and uses its own method of organizing topics.

Search filter Collection of hundreds of search terms used to search and retrieve research on particular clinical topics or problems

Search indexes Automated programs that search the Web when general information is requested.

Secondary storage Form of computer memory that retains data even when the computer is turned off. Examples include hard drives, CDs, DVDs, redundant array of inexpensive disks (RAID), optical disks, and magnetic disks or tape.

Security Officer Person responsible for ensuring that measures exist to protect information privacy.

Semantic interoperability Exchange of data where the meaning remains the same on both ends of the transaction.

Serial Line Internet Protocol (SLIP) Protocol that allows passage of data through communication lines and is used to access the Internet and World Wide Web.

Server Any type of computer that stores files.

Service oriented architecture A set of methods for the design and development of software designed to foster interoperability.

Server-based computing Networking model where all processing occurs on the server.

Service-oriented architecture Modular programming approach that allows re-use of functions.

Short message service (SMS) Means to send short messages to and from mobile phones and handheld devices.

Site license Agreement between the computer lab and the software publisher on the terms of use.

Smart card Storage device for patient information that resembles a plastic credit card. The card is kept by the client and presented to healthcare providers when services are rendered, eliminating redundant data entry and the need to store this information on a network.

Smart technology Integrated technology that saves time, physical burdens, and improves patient outcomes.

Social media Term used to describe Web-based programs and technologies that allow people to interact socially with each other online.

Social networking Web sites that allow users to create a profile within the site and interact with other users of the site.

Software Computer programs or stored sequences of instructions to the computer.

Software shredder Set of computer programs that prevent recovery of deleted, or discarded, computer files by writing meaningless information over them.

Spam Unwanted or "junk" mail.

SPIM Unsolicited messages often containing a link to a Web site that attempts to extract personal information.

Spyware Data collection mechanism that installs itself without the user's permission during Web browsing or downloading software.

Spyware detection software Special software that can detect and eliminate spyware.

Standardized Nursing Languages (SNLs) Common set of terms that have been reviewed and accepted by the American Nurses Association.

Standardized terminologies Structured, controlled languages developed according to terminology development guidelines and approved by an authoritative body.

Strategic planning Development of a comprehensive, long-range plan for guiding the activities and operations of an organization.

Strategic thinking Vision or process that an organization uses to determine what its future should look like.

Strategy Comprehensive plan used by an organization that states how its mission, goals, and objectives will be achieved.

Structured data Data that follow a prescribed format, often presented as discrete data elements.

Supercomputers Largest, most expensive type of computers. They are complex systems that can perform billions of instructions every second.

Superuser Staff person who has become proficient in the use of the system and mentors others.

Survivability Capability of a system as a whole to fulfill its mission, in a timely manner, in the presence of attacks, failures, or accidents.

Switched multimegabit data service (SMDS) High-speed data transmission service that uses telephone lines, also known as a *T1 line*. SMDS is faster than ISDN but slower than ATM.

System check Mechanism provided by a computer system to assist users by prompting them to complete a task, verify information, or prevent entry of inappropriate information.

Systematized Nomenclature of Human and Veterinary Medicine Clinical Terms (SNOMED-CT) Classification system that includes signs and symptoms of disease, diagnoses, and procedures for the integration of all medical information in an electronic medical record.

T1 lines High-speed telephone lines that may be used to transmit high-quality, full-motion video at speeds up to 1.544 Mbps.

Tablet PC Smaller version of a notebook computer but can be carried like a clipboard that accepts text input via a stylet.

Tape drive Copies files from the computer to magnetic tape for storage or transfer to another machine.

Task analysis One of the most well-known collections of usability techniques. Involves systematic methods of determining what users are required to do with systems by accounting for behavioral actions between users and computers. Used to determine the goals of a new system and the role of information technology in user activities.

Technical criteria Hardware and software requirements needed to attain a desired level of overall computer or information system performance.

Technical interoperability Ability to exchange the data from one point to another.

Teleconferencing Use of computers, audio and video equipment, and communication links to provide interaction between two or more persons at two or more sites.

Telehealth Provision of information to healthcare providers and consumers and the delivery of services to clients at remote sites through the use of telecommunication and computer technology.

Telemedicine Use of telecommunication technologies and computers to provide medical information and services to clients at another site.

Telenursing Use of telecommunications and computer technology for the delivery of nursing care to clients at another location.

Terminal Monitor screen and a keyboard once used to input data and receive output from a mainframe computer, now rarely seen.

Test environment Separate software program like that used for the actual application or information system, which permits trial of programming changes prior to their implementation in the actual system, thereby protecting the "real" system from unwanted alterations.

Test plan Refers to strategy to determine viability of plan whether that might be new functions or the restoration of operations after an adverse event.

Thin client technology Computing model that allows PCs to connect to a server using a highly efficient network connection.

Think aloud Usability method where users talk about what they are doing as they interact with an application. Interactions are observed or recorded and analyzed.

Threat source Intent or method that that targets a vulnerability or may trigger a vulnerability.

TIGER Initiative Plan to promote informatics competencies among nurses in order to transform healthcare.

Touchpad Pressure and motion sensitive surface.

Trackball Contains a ball that the user rolls to move the on-screen pointer.

Trainer Person responsible for educating clinical users in one or more applications and may also be required to define and monitor user competencies.

Training Common term used to refer to the introduction of information system skills to workers.

Training environment Separate software application that mirrors the actual information system but permits learners to practice skills without harm to the system or data contained in it. Makes use of fictitious clients and scenarios for instruction and practice.

Training hospital Collection of simulated, or fictitious, client data assembled and stored in a database separate from the actual information system for the purposes of instruction and practice. Incorporates most, if not all, features available on the actual information system.

Training plan Organized approach for the delivery of instruction that should include a philosophy; identification of instructional needs, approaches, and persons responsible for instructional design and delivery; a target date for completion; a budget; and methods for evaluation.

Transaction Fee Model Health information exchange model that charges fees for services or products on the basis of benefit to the participants.

Trusted third party (TTP) or Certificate authority (CA) Term used to refer to an entity that issues digital certificates which certify ownership of a public key.

Twitter Popular social networking Websites

Unified medical language system (UMLS) Attempt to standardize terms used in healthcare delivery. It is a metathesaurus that contains more than a hundred source vocabularies.

Unified nursing language system (UNLS) Attempt to standardize and link nursing databases as a means to extend nursing knowledge.

Uniform Hospital Data Set (UHDS) Most commonly used data set in the United States, even though it does not include data on nursing care and outcomes.

Uniform resource locator (URL) String of characters providing an address that identifies a document's World Wide Web location and the type of server it resides on.

Unique patient identifier Single, universal identifier for client health information that ensures availability of all data associated with a particular client.

Unstructured data Data that do not follow a prescribed format such as that seen in narrative notes.

Usability Specific issues of human performance in achieving specific goals during computer interactions within a particular context.

Usability questionnaires Tools that measure users' perceptions about system usability.

USB flash drives Small portable storage devices that can be plugged into a computer, and then unplugged and transported.

Usenet news groups Popular Internet feature similar to Listservs in content and diversity, with each newsgroup dedicated to a different topic, providing a forum where any user can post messages for discussion and reply.

User class Group of individuals who perform similar functions, and for the purpose of information system training and use, require instruction on how to access and use the same set of system features.

User-generated content (UGC) Any content such as blogs posts, discussion comments, audio, video, digital images, and so forth that have been created by a user of a Web site.

User interface What the user sees when interacting with a computer.

Utility programs Special applications designed to optimize computer operation and control of resident data.

Vendor Company or corporation that designs, develops, sells, and/or supports a product, which in the context of this book is generally a computer, peripheral device, and, more often, an entire information system.

Videoconferencing Face-to-face meeting of persons at separate locations through the use of telecommunications and computer technology.

Virtual Learning Environment (VLE) A system that uses the Internet to assist the educator in developing, managing, and administering educational materials for students.

Virus Malicious program that can disrupt or destroy data.

Vulnerability Flaw or weakness in system procedures, design, implementation, or internal controls that could accidentally or intentionally be used to breach security or violate the system's security policy.

Web Also known as *World Wide Web (WWW)*. Information service for access to Internet resources by content instead of file names via a graphical user interface (GUI) that supports text, images, sound, and links to documents.

Web 2.0 An approach to Web design and development that seeks to foster creativity and collaboration through a variety of services such as blogs, wikis, and social networking sites.

Web-based instruction (WBI) Uses the attributes and resources of the World Wide Web, such as hypertext links and multimedia, for educational purposes.

Web browser or browser Retrieval program that allows the user to search and access hypertext and hypermedia documents on the Web by using HTTP.

Webcam Small camera used by a computer to send images over the Internet.

Webcast Format that allows multiple learners to access a Website.

Webmaster Person responsible for creating and maintaining a World Wide Web site.

Wide area networks (WANs) Large expansive network systems.

Wiki A type of Web page that allows collaborative contributions such as Wikipedia.

Wireless devices Provide the capability to receive and broadcast signals while in transit, sometimes referred to as *mobile computing*.

Wireless modem Communication device that sends and receives information via access points provided with a subscription to wireless service.

Wisdom Application of knowledge to manage and solve problems.

Work breakdown structure (WBS) Plan to develop the project timelines or schedule a hierarchical arrangement of all specific tasks by using project-planning software.

World Wide Web (WWW) Information service for access to Internet resources by content instead of file names via a graphical user interface (GUI) that supports text, images, sound, and links to documents.

Worm Malicious program named for the type of damage left behind. Often uses network communication practices to spread.

Zip drive Now obsolete form of a high-capacity floppy disk drive.

Index